# Essential Malariology
## Fourth Edition

# Essential Malariology

## Fourth Edition

**Edited by**

**David A Warrell**
Director, Nuffield Department of Clinical Medicine, John Radcliffe Hospital,
Oxford, UK

**Herbert M Gilles**
Emeritus Professor of Tropical Medicine, Liverpool School of Tropical
Medicine, Liverpool, UK

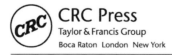

**CRC Press**
Taylor & Francis Group
Boca Raton  London  New York

CRC Press is an imprint of the
Taylor & Francis Group, an **informa** business

CRC Press
Taylor & Francis Group
6000 Broken Sound Parkway NW, Suite 300
Boca Raton, FL 33487-2742

© 2002 by Taylor & Francis Group, LLC
CRC Press is an imprint of Taylor & Francis Group, an Informa business

**Visit the Taylor & Francis Web site at**
**http://www.taylorandfrancis.com**

**and the CRC Press Web site at**
**http://www.crcpress.com**

# Contents

# Preface

A fatal periodic fever associated with marshes and biting insects has been recognized for almost three millennia. Pre-Hippocratic descriptions from Mesopotamia, India and China are recognizable as malaria (Russell, 1955), but it was not until 1880 that Laveran identified the causative organism. The centenary of the science of the study of malaria – malariology – was marked in November 1998 by a memorable celebration at the Accademia Nazionale dei Lincei in Rome, hosted by Professor Mario Coluzzi (Coluzzi and Bradley, 1999) at which the wranglings of the pioneer British and Italian malariologists Ross and Grassi, for recognition as the discoverer of mosquito transmission, were finally laid to rest and our state of knowledge was reassessed in a warm atmosphere of collaboration and colleagueship.

A century of malariology had achieved many important discoveries in the epidemiology, pathogenesis, pathophysiology, treatment and control of malaria. There are now new drugs and proven effective control measures, such as insecticide-treated bed nets, with which to fight the disease.

At the start of the new millennium, the molecular genetics revolution has provided us with an almost complete knowledge of the genomes of *Plasmodium falciparum* (25–30 megabases and 5000–6000 genes on 14 chromosomes; http://www.sanger.ac.uk/Projects/P_falciparum/), *Anopheles gambiae* (http://konops.anodb.gr/AnoDB/) and *Homo sapiens* (http://www.ornl.gov/hgmis/), together with evidence of a dozen or more human genetic polymorphisms that confer some degree of protection against lethal disease (Hill and Weatherall, 1998). Will this information hasten the development of an effective malaria vaccine and a genetically modified mosquito incapable of propagating the parasite?

The twentieth century saw the failure of the World Health Organization's Global Malaria Eradication Campaign (1955–1969) and, as recently as 1980, the late Leonard Bruce-Chwatt included a chapter on 'Malaria eradication' in the first edition of his *Essential Malariology* (Bruce-Chwatt, 1980). That hope has now been abandoned, and from 1954 to 1997 there was no decline in global malarial mortality, currently estimated at about 2 million per year. The incidence of malaria may even have increased during that period, to beyond 500 million cases per year (WHO, 1998). The main burden of malarial morbidity and mortality is borne by pregnant women and young children in sub-Saharan Africa, where the disease is increasingly implicated in social, economic and even intellectual impoverishment (Breman, 2001).

Who could ever forget that limp, cyanosed, comatose 3-year-old brought, too late, to a hospital in Serabu, Sierra Leone; or the similarly moribund 8-year-old discovered in a township hospital in rural Burma (his blood film teeming with malaria parasites unrecognized by local staff because it had been stained at the wrong pH); or the young mother dying in pulmonary oedema after giving birth to a stillborne baby in eastern Thailand? Such personal experiences are humbling reminders of the helplessness and hopelessness of confrontation with advanced disease – a tragedy re-enacted almost daily in many hospitals in tropical countries.

Medical science has not adequately answered the challenge of malaria and there has been a failure of implementation of existing knowledge. However, there have been improvements in political profile and funding. At last, the priority of global malaria control has been recognized; by individual nations, the World Health Organization, the G8 powers, the European Community and charitable sponsors such as the Wellcome Trust and the Gates Foundation. 'Roll Back Malaria' and 'Multilateral Initiative On Malaria' are slogans and rallying points for two of these important initiatives.

Overwhelmed as we are by the terrible human suffering exacted by malaria, we are also amazed and fascinated by the biology, ecology, evasive strategies and adaptive evolution of an extraordinary parasite. This admiration is evident in several of the chapters in this new edition of *Essential Malariology*, a successor to Leonard Bruce-Chwatt's famous monograph. We were delighted to hear that previous editions had proved useful both to laboratory researchers, by providing some idea of the clinical relevance of their work, and to medical staff working at the 'sharp end' of the disease. The aim of the book remains the same: to cover in one volume the basics of most branches of malariology with a strong emphasis on implementing our improved understanding of parasite and vector biology, host immunity and disease pathophysiology in the interests of prevention, treatment and control. With the help of an outstanding team of contributors, we hope to have gone some way towards achieving this aim.

David Warrell and Herbert Gilles
November 2001

## REFERENCES

Breman JG (ed). The intolerable burden of malaria: a new look at the numbers. *Am J Trop Med Hyg* 2001; **64**(Suppl): 1–106.

Bruce-Chwatt LJ. *Essential malariology*. London, William Heinemann, 1980.

Coluzzi M, Bradley D (eds). The malaria challenge after one hundred years of malariology. *Parassitologia* 1999; **41**(1–3): 1–528.

Hill AVS, Weatherall DJ. Host genetic factors in resistance to malaria. In *Malaria: parasite biology, pathogenesis, protection*. Sherman IW, ed. Washington, DC, American Society for Microbiology Press, 1998.

Russell P. *Man's mastery of malaria*. London, Oxford University Press, 1955.

World Health Organization. *The World Health Report 1998*. Geneva, WHO, 1998.

# Contributors

**Peter F Beales MD FFPHM DTM&H FRES MB ChB MRCS LRCP MIScT FFCM**
Visiting Professor of Tropical Hygiene, Faculty of Tropical Medicine, Mahidol University,
Bangkok, Thailand

**Edgar Dorman MA MRCGP MRCOG**
Consultant Obstetrician and Gynaecologist, Homerton University Hospital, London, UK

**Judith E Epstein MD CDR(sel) MC USNR**
Malaria Program, Clinical Trials, Naval Medical Research Center, Silver Springs, MD, USA

**Nick Francis MB BS FRCPath**
Consultant Histopathologist, Hammmersmith Hospitals Trust, and Honorary Senior Lecturer,
Division of Investigative Science, Faculty of Medicine, Imperial College, London, UK

**Herbert M Gilles MD MSc FRCP FFPHM DSc DmedSc**
Professor of Tropical Medicine, Liverpool School of Tropical Medicine, Liverpool, UK

**Stephen L Hoffman MD DTMH**
Senior Vice President, Biologics, Celera Genomics, Rockville, MD, USA

**Marcel Hommel MD PhD**
Alfred Jones and Warrington Yorke, Professor of Tropical Medicine, Liverpool School of Tropical Medicine,
Liverpool, UK

**Kevin Marsh MBChB FRCP DTM&H**
KEMRI-Wellcome Collaborative Programme, Centre for Geographic Medicine Research, Kilifi, Kenya,
and Nuffield Department of Medicine, John Radcliffe Hospital, Oxford, UK

**Malcolm E Molyneux MD FRCP FMedSci**
Director, Malawi-Liverpool-Wellcome Trust Research Programme, College of Medicine,
University of Malawi, Malawi

**Mike W Service BSc PhD DSs CBiol Fibiol**
Emeritus Professor, Liverpool School of Tropical Medicine, Liverpool, UK

**Caroline E Shulman MBBS MRCGP PhD**
Clinical Senior Lecturer, Gates Malaria Programme, London School of Hygiene and Tropical Medicine, London, UK

**Robert E Sinden BSc PhD DSc**
Professor of Parasite Cell Biology, Department of Biological Sciences, Imperial College of Science, Technology and Medicine, London, UK

**Robert W Snow PhD**
Professor of Tropical Public Health at University of Oxford, and Head, Malaria Public Health Group, KEMRI/Wellcome Trust Collaborative Programme, Kenya

**Terrie E Taylor DO**
Professor, Department of Internal Medicine, Michigan State University, E. Lansing, MI, USA, and Director, Blantyre Malaria Project, University of Malawi College of Medicine, Blantyre, Malawi

**Harold Townson BSc(Hons) MSc PhD CIBiol**
Selwyn–Lloyd Professor of Medical Entomology, Liverpool School of Tropical Medicine, Liverpool, UK

**Gareth Turner MA BM BCh DPhil MRCPath**
Clinical Lecturer in Histopathology, Nuffield Department of Clinical Laboratory Sciences and The Oxford-Wellcome Center for Tropical and Infectious Diseases, University of Oxford, The John Radcliffe Hospital, Oxford, UK

**David A Warrell MA DM DSc FRCP FRCPE FMedSci**
Professor of Tropical Medicine and Infectious Diseases and Founding Director of The Centre for Tropical Medicine (Emeritus), University of Oxford, Oxford, UK

**WM Watkins BPharm PhD MRPharmSoc**
Wellcome Resettlement Fellow, Department of Pharmacology & Therapeutics, University of Liverpool, Liverpool, UK

**Peter Winstanley MD FRCP DTM&H**
Professor of Clinical Pharmacology and Consultant Physician, Department of Pharmacology and Therapeutics, University of Liverpool, Liverpool, UK

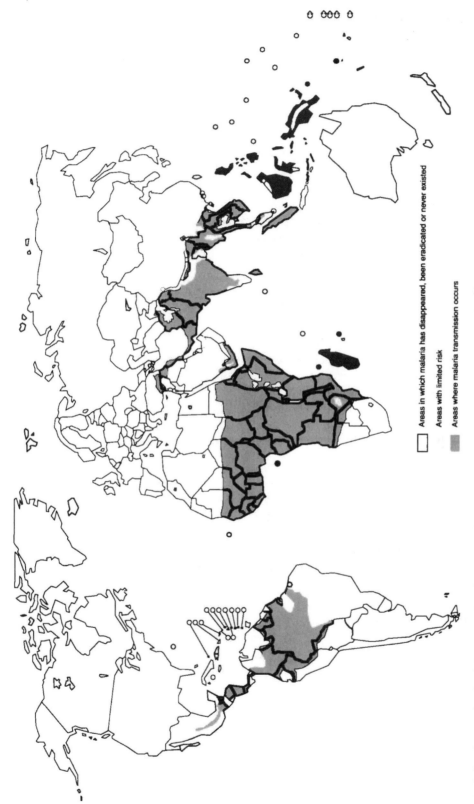

The designations employed and the presentation of material on this map do not imply the expression of any opinion whatsoever on the part of the World Health Organization concerning the legal status of any country, territory, city or area or of its authorities, or concerning the delimitation of its frontiers or boundaries. Dotted lines represent approximate border lines for which there may not yet be full agreement. © World Health Organization 2000.

Areas in which malaria has disappeared, been eradicated or never existed

Areas with limited risk

Areas where malaria transmission occurs

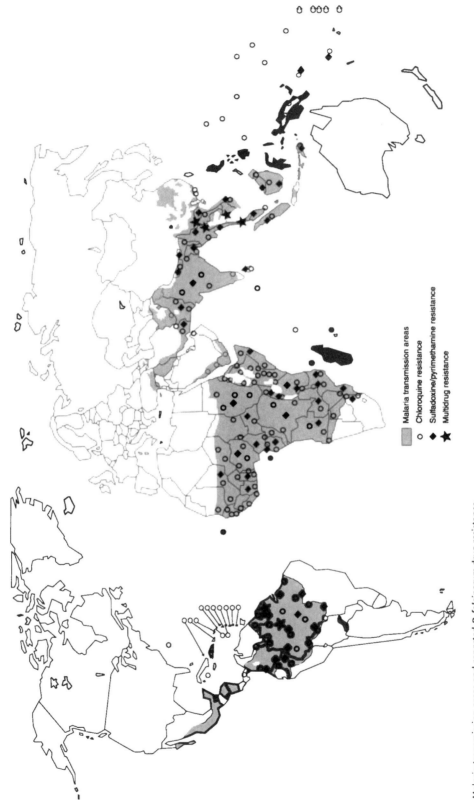

Malaria transmission areas and reported *P. falciparum* drug resistance.
*Source*: International Travel and Health 2001.

Malaria transmission areas

○ Chloroquine resistance

◆ Sulfadoxine/pyrimethamine resistance

★ Multidrug resistance

# Historical outline

HERBERT M GILLES

The great antiquity of malarial infection is confirmed by the fact that well over 100 parasite species similar to those of humans are found in a wide range of vertebrates from reptiles or birds to higher apes. None of these parasites, except for those found in some monkeys, can be transmitted to humans. This high host specificity indicates a long association between the human species and the four particular species of plasmodia that infect humans.

References to seasonal and intermittent fevers exist in the ancient Assyrian, Chinese and Indian religious and medical texts, but their true identity with malaria is uncertain. These afflictions, usually ascribed to the punishment of gods or vengeance by evil spirits, were met by incantations or sacrificial offerings. Hippocrates, who lived in Greece in the fifth century BC, was the earliest physician to discard superstition for logical observation of the relationship between the appearance of the disease and the seasons of the year or the places where his patients lived. He was also the first to describe in detail the clinical picture of malaria and some complications of the disease.

Celsus (25 BC–54 AD) gave a particularly accurate description of the various types of malaria:

> Now quartan fevers have the simpler characteristics. Nearly always they begin with shivering, then heat breaks out and the fever having ended, there are two days free; thus on the fourth day it recurs.
>
> But of tertian fevers, there are two classes. The one, beginning and desisting in the same way as quartan, has merely this distinction, that it affords one day free, and recurs on the third day. The other is far more pernicious; and it does indeed recur on the third day, yet out of forty-eight hours, about thirty-six, sometimes less, sometimes more, are in fact occupied by the paroxysm, nor does the fever entirely cease in the remission, but only becomes less violent.

At the beginning of the seventeenth century came the discovery of the value of 'Peruvian' bark for the treatment of fevers. Morton and Sydenham in England and later Torti in Italy differentiated between the true intermittent fevers and others that failed to respond to the drug, which was then known as 'Jesuit's powder'.

In the eighteenth century, these specific fevers, known in England as 'agues', received the Italian name 'malaria', because it was then widely believed that their cause was related to the foul air common near marshy areas. The French term 'paludisme', indicating a close connection with swamps, was introduced much later. In 1735, the tree producing the Peruvian bark was given its scientific name of *Cinchona* by Linnaeus. But quinine, the active principal of it, was not isolated until 1820, by Pelletier and Caventou in France.

It was in 1880 that Laveran, a French army surgeon in Algeria, first saw and described malaria parasites in the red blood cells of human beings. Soon after that, Romanowsky in Russia developed a new method of staining the malaria parasites in blood films and this, together with the improvement of the microscope, made further studies of plasmodia very much easier.

However, the way in which the disease was transmitted from person to person was still a mystery. The elucidation of the actual mode of transmission was not forthcoming until 1897, when Ronald Ross, working in Secunderabad (India), found a developing form of the malaria parasite in the body of a mosquito that had previously fed on a patient with the plasmodia in his blood. The whole complex picture of the cycle of development of malaria parasites in humans and in the female *Anopheles* mosquito became clear as a result of further studies by the Italians Amico Bignami, Giuseppe Bastianelli and, especially, Battista Grassi in 1898–9.

During the twentieth century, much research was devoted to malaria control. Larvicides in the form of oil of Paris green were introduced to prevent the breeding of mosquitoes in various types of waters. Wider use of these and other methods of mosquito reduction demonstrated the practicability of controlling malaria and yellow fever in Cuba and the Panama Canal Zone, where two American campaigns organized by General William Crawford Gorgas proved to be outstanding successes. Subsequently, Malcolm Watson in Malaya introduced the concept of 'naturalistic control' based on the knowledge of the breeding habits of species of *Anopheles* involved in the local transmission of the disease.

The ravages of malaria experienced during the First World War and the difficulties of securing cheap supplies of quinine stimulated a line of research in Germany aimed at the discovery of synthetic antimalarial drugs. This was brilliantly accomplished in 1924 by Schulemann's discovery of pamaquine. However, a much more valuable drug – Atabrin (mepacrine) – was prepared in 1930 by Kikuth, Mietzsch and Mauss. There can be no doubt that the availability of this compound played a very important role during the Second World War. Other valuable synthetic drugs developed by the Germans, the French, the Americans and the British followed in 1934 (chloroquine), 1944 (proguanil), 1946 (amodiaquine), 1950 (primaquine) and 1952 (pyrimethamine).

In the meantime, another major discovery was to revolutionize the technique of malaria control by spraying insecticides against adult mosquitoes.

At the beginning of the Second World War, Paul Muller discovered in Switzerland the strong insecticidal action of a synthetic compound, dichlorodiphenyl-trichloroethane, which was given the abbreviated name of DDT.

Among other residual insecticides that were introduced soon after DDT, hexachlorocyclohexane (BHC or HCH) and dieldrin should be mentioned.

In 1901, Grassi had formulated the idea that there is a third, cryptic tissue phase following the inoculation of sporozoites by the bite of *Anopheles*. Raffaele in Italy was the first to demonstrate in 1934 the existence of this phase in bird malaria. Then, in 1948, the exo-erythrocytic stages, first of monkey malaria (*Plasmodium cynomolgi*) and then of human malaria (*P. vivax*), were discovered in the UK by Shortt and Garnham. This discovery explained what happens to the parasite during the incubation period and how the relapses of malaria infection occur.

The possibility of global extension of malaria control activities to bring about the final eradication of the disease was contemplated in the 1950s when the results of the application of DDT in Venezuela, Italy, Greece, Guyana, Ceylon and the USA showed great promise.

The concept of malaria eradication was adopted by the World Health Assembly in 1995, and 2 years later the World Health Organization (WHO) launched a global campaign. Its results over the next 15 years were excellent in Europe, North America, some parts of Asia, the former USSR and Australia, and less good in tropical countries. The causes of this lack of progress are many and are fully dealt with in the appropriate section of this book. In 1969, WHO revised the strategy of malaria eradication by stressing the need for greater involvement of general health services and for extension of research on new insecticides, improved surveillance, development of new antimalarial drugs and alternative methods of malaria control.

However, during the past decade there has been a considerable increase of malaria in several tropical areas, where in the past the eradication programmes appeared to advance satisfactorily. This resurgence of the disease was greatest in southern and southeastern Asia, but there was also an increased incidence in Central America and parts of South America; a serious epidemic of malaria occurred in the Asian part of Turkey. In tropical Africa, the malaria situation has also deteriorated. Severe outbreaks have occurred in several countries, with a high mortality and a shift of morbidity to older age groups. Uncontrolled and rapid urbanization has created pockets of transmission in the cities, thus increasing the size of vulnerable groups. Chloroquine resistance of *P. falciparum* has spread throughout the African continent. In Southeast Asia, multidrug resistance is now commonly encountered. Political concern and the will to reduce morbidity and mortality from malaria were mobilized at a Ministerial Conference held in Amsterdam in 1992.

Remarkable progress has been made in scientific activity related to malaria during the past 25 years, since the United Nations Development Programme (UNDP)/World Bank/WHO Tropical Diseases Research and Training Programme extended malaria research over the whole range of the host–parasite relationship, including the mosquito vector, the socio-economic impact of the disease, and the sequencing of the falciparum genome. Progress in drug development – apart from the discovery of mefloquine and artemisinin and its analogues – has been slow and a vaccine remains an elusive, though attainable, target.

In 1997, heads of states of Africa met in Harare, Zimbabwe, and issued a Declaration on Malaria Prevention and Control in the Context of African Economic Recovery and Development. This important African political commitment was endorsed by the leaders of the industrialized G8 nations, with a promise of substantial financial support.

In 1998, WHO announced that malaria was to be one of its top priorities and introduced a new initiative, 'Roll Back Malaria', aimed at developing a sector-wide approach to combat the disease.

Two other major malaria initiatives – the Multilateral Initiatives on Malaria (MIM) aimed at strengthening research capacity in Africa and the African Initiative on Malaria (AIM) – were established.

## MILESTONES IN THE HISTORY OF MALARIA AND ITS CONTROL

The main chronological landmarks in the advance of our knowledge of malaria and the control or eradication of this disease followed three different and yet related roads. This list of major events related to the history of malaria is necessarily arbitrary and incomplete.

## Malaria parasites and their transmission

1847 Dempster in India introduced spleen palpation of children as an index of epidemicity of malaria.

1848 Virchow and Fredrichs in Germany recognized that the presence of pigment in internal organs may be related to deaths from intermittent fevers.

1878 Manson in China showed that a mosquito (*Culex fatigans*) can act as a vector of human filaria.

1880 Laveran in Algeria discovered and described malaria parasites in human blood.

1886 Golgi in Italy described in detail two species of human malaria parasites (*P. vivax* and *P. malariae*).

1889 Danilewski in Russia described the morphology of avian parasites and indicated their wide distribution.

1889–90 Celli and Marchiafava in Italy described *P. falciparum*.

1891 Romanowsky developed his polychrome staining method for demonstrating plasmodia in blood smears.

1894 Manson put forward the theory that malaria is transmitted from person to person by mosquitoes.

1897 Ross discovered pigmented cysts (oocysts) on the stomach wall of an *Anopheles* mosquito (probably *A. stephensi*) in Secunderabad, India.

1897 MacCallum in the USA described the sexual phase of *Haemoproteus* in the blood of a crow, and observed exflagellation of a male gametocyte in *P. falciparum* and the penetration of a female gametocyte by a flagellum.

1898 Ross worked out the complete cycle of bird malaria in naturally infected sparrows in Calcutta.

1898 Grassi, Bignami and Bastianelli in Italy described the cycle of human malaria parasites in *Anopheles* mosquitoes.

1900 Manson, by experiments with human volunteers in the Roman Campagna and in London, confirmed the mosquito–malaria transmission theory.

1901 Grassi forecast the existence of a third phase in the life cycle of the malaria parasite.

1902 Schaudinn announced, incorrectly, the penetration of a red blood cell by a sporozoite, thus apparently refuting Grassi's theory and retarding this line of research for many years.

1922  Stephens identified and described *P. ovale*.

1931  James revived Grassi's theory and suggested that, soon after entering the body, the sporozoite invades reticuloendothelial cells or cells lining the capillary blood vessels.

1934  Raffaele in Italy described tissue forms in *P. elongatum* and concluded that, in avian malaria, there is a schizogonic cycle of development in the reticuloendothelial system as well as in the red blood cells.

1937  James and Tate described schizogonic development of *P. gallinaceum* in fixed tissue cells of the fowl, and showed that the brain is an important place for the localization of the endothelial stages.

1947  Garnham described exo-erythrocytic forms of *P. kochi* (now classed as *Hepatocystis*) in parenchyma cells of the liver of lower monkeys in East Africa.

1948  Shortt, Garnham and Malamos in England described pre-erythrocytic forms of *P. cynomolgi* in parenchyma cells of the liver of *Macaca mulatta* (rhesus) monkeys. Shortt and Garnham also described persistent exo-erythrocytic forms of *P. cynomolgi* in a monkey's liver.

1948  Vincke and Lips in the former Belgian Congo (Zaire) discovered *P. berghei*, the first plasmodium of rodents.

1948  Shortt, Garnham, Covell and Shute described pre-erythrocytic forms of *P. vivax* in the human liver.

1948  Rodhain showed that the chimpanzee is a host of *P. malariae* in Central Africa.

1949  Nikolaev described *P. vivax hibermans*, with a long incubation period.

1949  Shortt, Fairley, Covell, Shute and Garnham described pre-erythrocytic forms of *P. falciparum* in the human liver.

1950  Garnham described pre-erythrocytic forms of *P. inui*, a quartan-like parasite, in a simian liver.

1953  Garnham described pre-erythrocytic forms of *P. ovale* in the human liver.

1965  Cohen and McGregor elucidated the humoral transfer of protective antibodies of *P. falciparum*.

1966  Young discovered the experimental transmissibility of human plasmodia to the Colombian owl monkey (*Aotus trivirgatus*).

1973  A first attempt was made by Clyde to immunize humans with irradiated sporozoites of *P. falciparum* and *P. vivax*.

1976  Continuous *in vitro* culture of *P. falciparum* was developed by Trager and Jensen in the USA.

1977  Carter and Walliker characterized the genetic diversity of strains of *P. falciparum* using enzyme electrophoresis.

1978  Aikawa demonstrated the mechanism of penetration of merozoites into erythrocytes.

1980  Hypnozoites of *P. cynomolgi* were discovered and suggestion made of the role of hypnozoites of *P. vivax* in delayed relapses of human malaria. There was *in vitro* production of mature gametocytes of *P. falciparum* infective to mosquitoes, and production and use of monoclonal antibodies against *P. falciparum* antigens.

1982  There was characterization of polypeptides specific to surface antigens in sporozoites and erythrocytic stages of several animal and human plasmodia.

1983  mRNA was isolated from *P. falciparum* and its DNA was cloned into a bacterium (*Escherichia coli*).

1987  Recombinant DNA *P. falciparum* sporozoite vaccine and synthetic peptide sporozoite vaccine were both tested in volunteers.

1988  Synthetic asexual stage *P. falciparum* peptide vaccine was tested in volunteers.

1992  Field trials began of asexual stage vaccine and of sporozoite vaccine.

1994  Sequencing the falciparum genome began. *P. falciparum* has 14 chromosomes.

1994–96  Vaccine trials of 'SPf66' were unsuccessful in Tanzania, Gambia and Thailand–Myanmar border.

1998  Gardner and colleagues sequenced chromosome 2 of *P. falciparum*.

1999  Bowman and colleagues unveiled chromosome 3 of *P. falciparum*.

## Treatment of malaria

1600  Juan Lopez, a Jesuit missionary, recorded the use of the 'fever tree bark' by Peruvian Indians.

1643  Cardinal Juan de Lugo carried out trials of the Peruvian bark at the Santo Spirito Hospital in Rome.

1649  Cardinal de Lugo supported a wide use of the bark, which became known as Jesuit's powder.

1637–98  Morton and Sydenham in England noted the specific action of the bark in curing certain fevers (agues).

1717 Torti in Italy clearly described the specific action of the bark on intermittent (but no other) fevers.

1735 Condamine, leading the French expedition to Peru, identified the 'Quina-quina' tree.

1747 Linnaeus in Sweden described the tree and gave it the name of *Cinchona*.

1820 Pelletier and Caventou in France isolated the alkaloids quinine and cinchonine from the bark of *Cinchona*.

1854 Hasskarl, a Dutch botanist, brought the seeds of *Cinchona* to Java and began large-scale cultivation in Indonesia.

1872 Markham, an English geographer, started *Cinchona* plantations in the Nilgiri Hills in India.

1914–18 Events during the First World War indicated the shortage of quinine, especially in countries without direct access to *Cinchona* plantations.

1924 Pamaquine (Plasmoquine) was developed in Germany by Schulemann and his colleagues.

1930 Mepacrine (Atabrin) was developed in Germany by Mietzsch and Kikuth.

1934 Chloroquine (Resochin) was developed in Germany.

1944 Proguanil (Paludrine) was developed by Curd, Davey and Rose in England.

1952 Pyrimethamine (Daraprim) was developed by Hitchings in the USA and his co-workers in England.

1956 Primaquine was developed by Elderfield in the USA.

1956 Quinocide was developed by Braude and Stavrovskaya in the former USSR.

1961–65 There were reports from Colombia and Brazil on strains of *P. falciparum* resistant to chloroquine, as well as similar reports from Southeast Asia.

1960–66 The value of sulfones and sulfonamides as antimalarial compounds was rediscovered.

1967–74 The US Army Medical Research and Development Command developed a number of new synthetic antimalarials.

1971–75 Mefloquine was developed and introduced into the treatment of malaria.

1978 Rieckmann introduced a microtest for the detection of chloroquine resistance in *P. falciparum*. Schmidt developed the *Aotus* monkey model for advanced studies of antimalaria compounds.

1974–82 A series of amino-alcohol compounds was developed as possible antimalaria drugs at the US Walter Reed Army Institute for Research.

1979–82 New antimalarials were developed by the Qinghaosu Antimalaria Coordinating Group in China.

1979–82 The appearance of chloroquine resistance in *P. falciparum* was confirmed in several countries in East Africa.

1976–83 A series of derivatives of 8-aminoquinolines with high activity for radical cure of relapsing malaria was developed.

1986 The appearance of chloroquine resistance in *P. falciparum* was confirmed in several countries in West Africa.

1987 *In vitro* chloroquine resistance in *P. falciparum* was reversed by Verapamil and other compounds.

1988 Trioxane derivatives were developed as potential antimalarials. Novel bicyclic peroxide antimalarials related to Yingzhaosu were also developed.

1989 Halofantrine was introduced.

1990 Clinical trials of artesunate and artemether began in countries outside China and Burma.

1990–91 There was global resistance to chloroquine except in Central America. There was also widespread resistance to pyrimethamine-sulfadoxine, and multidrug resistance in South-east Asia.

1991–98 Artemisinin compounds were established as antimalarials. These were effective in multidrug-resistant areas. Artemisinin suppositories were also found to be effective. New combinations were developed: atovaquone–proguanil and chlorproguanil–dapsone.

1997 The Multilateral Initiative on Malaria (MIM) was established.

1999 Combined therapy was strongly advocated by WHO to delay the development of resistance to artemisinin compounds and other new antimalarials.

2000 The Medicines for Malaria Venture (MMV) Foundation was set up and the chloroquine-resistant gene (*PfcR TK767*) was identified.

## Epidemiology and control of malaria

1899 Ross initiated antilarval measures in Sierra Leone.

1899 There was a large-scale demonstration of successful mosquito control by Gorgas and Le Prince in Cuba.

1901–3 Malaria control by antilarval measures in Malaya was initiated by Malcolm Watson. An anti-mosquito campaign was organized by Ross in Ismailia, Egypt.

1904–14  A malaria control campaign was carried out by Gorgas and Le Prince in the Panama Canal Zone.

1908  Ross carried out a survey of malaria in Mauritius and originated the mathematical approach to the transmission of the infection.

1924–26  Roubaud in France, Swellengrebel and Van Thiel in the Netherlands and Falleroni in Italy differentiated the cryptic species of *A. maculipennis* complex and elucidated the importance of mosquito behaviour in the transmission of malaria.

1927  There was the first instance of eradication of an invading vector species (*A. albimanus*) in Barbados.

1935–39  The first large-scale control of rural malaria by imagicidal measures (using pyrethrum spraying) occurred in South Africa, the Netherlands and India.

1936–39  The insecticidal action of DDT (synthesized by Zeidler in Germany in 1874) was discovered by Muller and Wiesman in Switzerland.

1939–40  An invading African mosquito (*A. gambiae*) was eradicated from Brazil.

1942–45  *A. gambiae* was eradicated from northern Egypt.

1942–46  New synthetic insecticides (HCH, dieldrin, chlordane etc.) with residual action were developed.

1946–57  An antimalaria campaign in Cyprus, Sardinia, Guyana, Venezuela and Greece was followed by interruption of transmission.

1947  Beklemishev introduced the concept and practice of landscape epidemiology in the former USSR.

1950–57  Macdonald in the UK and Moshkowski in the former USSR expanded Ronald Ross's mathematical approach to the understanding of the epidemiology of malaria.

1955  The principle of malaria eradication was adopted by the Fourteenth World Health Assembly.

1957  The concept and practice of malaria eradication were defined by the WHO.

1979  The WHO Expert Committee developed the strategy of malaria control and its tactical variants.

1985  The Thirty-eighth World Health Assembly adopted resolution WHA 38.24, which recommended that malaria control should be developed as an integral part of the national primary health care system.

1986  Malaria situations in tropical Africa were stratified for the development of malaria control within primary health care.

1991  A strategy for malaria control was based on major prototypes.

1992  There was a Ministerial Conference on Malaria in Amsterdam. The WHO Global Malaria Strategy was approved.

1997–99  The Harare declaration was  made by heads of states of Africa. There was a Multilateral Initiative on Malaria (MIM), an African Initiative on Malaria (AIM) and the WHO 'Roll Back Malaria' (RBM) initiative.

## Therapeutic malaria

Hippocrates and Galen mentioned that malaria seemed occasionally to have beneficial effects on other diseases. In England, John MacCulloch (1828) described an attempt to 'acquire an ague for removing a previous chronic disorder'. Deliberate infection with malaria for the treatment of general paralysis was proposed by Wagner von Jauregg in Vienna in 1887, although the first trials only started in 1918. The initial method consisted of infecting patients by injecting blood obtained from other individuals suffering from malaria.

In 1922, Warrington Yorke in Liverpool began inducing malaria by the bites of infected mosquitoes, a method that had many advantages over blood inoculation. Therapeutic malaria has been widely used in many countries and with generally satisfactory results. The explanation of the beneficial effects of malaria on late neurosyphilis is not clear. In addition to the possible effect of febrile paroxysms, it is likely that the plasmodial infection stimulates some specific defence mechanism against *Treponema pallidum*. The benefit depends on the degree of fever and on the number of paroxysms.

Many aspects of transfusion malaria were studied in the course of therapeutic malaria. The main difference between the two is that in the former the infection is accidental and presents an added hazard to the recipient of the blood. In therapeutic malaria, the induced infection is deliberate; the species of the parasite is known in advance, the dosage of plasmodia as well as the number of injections are related to the state of health of the patient, and the course of the infection can be easily moderated by the use of appropriate drugs.

It is obvious that the incubation period of therapeutic malaria induced by blood injection depends on the species of the parasite and on the numbers of plasmodia used; it varies between 3 days (0.5–1 million plasmodia) and 10 days (1000–2000 million plasmodia). On the other hand, the true incubation period related to the mosquito transmission of the infection depends primarily on the species of the malaria parasite involved.

Therapeutic malaria was widely practised in many countries between 1920 and 1950. In the past, many thousands of patients have benefited from this treatment. The advent of penicillin for the treatment of syphilis eliminated the use of malaria.

P. vivax has been used in preference to any other species, largely because of the relatively benign infection that it causes. It should be remembered that in malaria induced by injection of infected blood there are no relapses due to the absence of exo-erythrocytic forms in the liver, because the infection takes place without the involvement of sporozoites. Thus, the treatment of induced malaria is relatively simple. However, in some cases, P. malariae, P. falciparum or P. ovale has been employed. A simian malaria parasite, P. knowlesi, has been used occasionally; it causes moderate fever and is easily controlled by drugs.

Various species of Anopheles have been preferred by different specialists for the transmission of induced malaria by mosquitoes. In Europe, A. atroparvus has been most commonly used, although the Indian A. stephensi also proved to be an efficient vector. In the USA, A. quadrimaculatus was generally employed.

Therapeutic malaria provided great opportunities for research in various fields of parasitology, immunology and chemotherapy. In the USA, much of the advance of the chemotherapy of malaria during the past 30 years was due to the existence of human malaria research centres, where the infection could be induced in volunteers. In Brazil, induced malaria was tentatively given for the treatment of non-syphilitic psychiatric disorders.

In the UK over the past 50 years, the scientific contribution of the Malaria Therapy Unit, subsequently known as the Malaria Reference Laboratory, Horton Hospital, has been immense. The characteristics of various strains of the three species of plasmodia were determined; the development of the parasite in different Anopheles species was elucidated; the pattern of relapses in malaria became clearer; considerable knowledge of the immune response to the infection in humans was gained in the course of long-term observations; and the action of various drugs on the course of the disease and its prevention contributed substantially to the development of synthetic antimalarials. In 1948, the discovery of pre-erythrocytic stages of P. vivax was made after the infection of a volunteer with the Madagascar strain of P. vivax and subsequent biopsy of his liver.

A few years later, an international collaborative project studied the parasitological and epidemiological characteristics of P. vivax North Korean strain on patients infected with malaria for therapeutic purposes.

With the discovery in the 1960s that human malaria can be transmitted to the owl monkey (Aotus trivirgatus) and other South American monkeys, and also because of much stricter ethical rules, the importance of deliberately induced malaria to human volunteers declined still further. Nevertheless, for the final testing of some new antimalarial drugs, vaccines or immunological methods, the study of the course of infection in humans is essential.

## SELECTED REFERENCES

Colluzzi M, Bradley D. The malaria challenge after one hundred years of malariology. *Parasitologia* 1999; **41**. Rome, Lombardo Editore.

McGregor IA. Malaria. In *The Wellcome Trust illustrated history of tropical diseases*. Cox FEG, ed. London, The Wellcome Trust, 1996, 230–47.

# 2

# The malaria parasites

ROBERT E SINDEN AND HERBERT M GILLES

The causative organisms of the disease malaria are protozoa of the genus *Plasmodium*, family Plasmodiidae, suborder Haemosporidiidae, order Coccidia. The 120 or so species of *Plasmodium* are found in the blood of mammals, reptiles and birds, and are recognized taxonomically by the presence of two types of asexual division: schizogony, in the vertebrate host; and sporogony, in the insect vector. Within the vertebrate host, schizogony is found both within erythrocytes (erythrocytic schizogony) and in other tissues (exo-erythrocytic schizogony). The great majority of malarial parasites are transmitted by mosquitoes, and the parasites of humans are exclusively transmitted by anophelines. Importantly, the parasites of humans are of two subgenera, *Laverania* and *Plasmodium*. The former subgenus includes *P. falciparum*, the most pathogenic form of malaria, and the closely related *P. reichenowi*, a parasite of the higher primates. The latter subgenus includes the remaining parasites of humans, namely *P. vivax, P. malariae* and *P. ovale*. Parasites of the other mammals also fall into two subgenera: *Plasmodium* and *Vinckeia*; the latter includes the parasites of lemurs and lower mammals. Parasites of birds and reptiles are of the subgenus *Plasmodium* and it is to this ancestral group of parasites that the subgenus *Laverania* may be most closely related (Table 2.1). Three malaria parasites are found exclusively in humans: *P. falciparum* (Welch, 1897), *P. vivax* (Grassi and Feletti, 1890) and *P. ovale* (Stephens, 1922). *P. malariae* (Laveran, 1881) is found in both humans and African apes, and the parasite *P. brazilianum* is probably the same species found in South American monkeys. The diseases caused by the four human parasites have, in the past, been described as follows:

- *P. vivax*: benign tertian, simple tertian, tertian
- *P. malariae*: quartan
- *P. falciparum*: malignant tertian (MT), subtertian, aestivo-autumnal, tropical, pernicious
- *P. ovale*: ovale tertian.

However, it is current practice to use the specific name to describe the disease, i.e. falciparum malaria, vivax malaria etc., though the disease caused by *P. malariae* is still usually referred to as quartan malaria.

Recognizing that human malarial parasites are widely distributed throughout the tropical and subtropical regions of the world, with some 2000 million people in the affected areas and 400–500 million cases annually, it is not unexpected that local differences in parasite biology evolve, leading to the emergence of clearly identifiable geographical variants. These local forms are termed 'isolates', to reflect the fact that they

**Table 2.1** *Plasmodia of primates and other mammals*

| Genus: *Plasmodium* | | |
| --- | --- | --- |
| Sub-genus: *Plasmodium* | | |
| Group: vivax | Species: | *P. vivax,*[a] *P. cynomolgi, P. eylesi, P. gonderi, P. hylobati, P. jefferyi, P. pitheci, P. schwetzi, P. simium, P. sylvaticum, P. youngi* |
| Group: ovale | Species: | *P. ovale,*[a] *P. fieldi, P. simiovale* |
| Group: malariae | Species: | *P. malariae,*[a] *P. brazilianum, P. inui* |
| Group: uncertain | Species | *P. coatneyi, P. fragile* (both with tertian periodicity), *P. knowlesi* (quotidian periodicity) |
| Sub-genus: *Laverania* | Species | *P. falciparum,*[a] *P. reichenowi* |
| Sub-genus: *Vinckeia* | Species | Large number of species (some of them of uncertain taxonomic status) infecting lemurs, rodents, bats and other animals |

[a]Signifies *Plasmodium* spp. of humans.

are samples in time of the parasite population present in any particular locale. Currently, the most important practical facet of parasite variation is the emergence and distribution of metabolic mutants that have been favoured by their resistance to the various antimalarial drugs used in the area. Nowhere is this problem more urgent than in South-east Asia, where multiple drug-resistant parasites have emerged, due in part to the inappropriate use of antimalarials and to the cross-hybridization of separate, uniquely resistant parasites.

When transferred to the laboratory, isolates can be maintained *in vitro*, but these are often polyclonal collections of parasites, which can change rapidly if not managed correctly. Recognizing the genomic plasticity of the parasites, it is advisable to cryopreserve samples of the isolate as soon as possible following their isolation. This is of particular importance if cyclic passage through mosquitoes is considered. Recognizing the polyclonal nature of many isolates, it is also sensible to clone as many of the parasite genotypes present as soon as is practicable.

## LIFE CYCLE AND MORPHOLOGY OF MALARIA PARASITES OF MAMMALS

All malaria parasites require the presence of two hosts to complete their life cycle; by definition, the definitive host (in which sexual development occurs) is the anopheline mosquito and the mammal is the intermediate host. The haploid parasite adopts three very different cellular strategies in the distinct phases of the complex life cycle. Where a strategy is repeated in the life cycle, the stages have largely conserved organelles and cell processes, with stage-specific differences only to complete tasks unique to that stage. The first strategy is the ability to grow replicate extensively (schizogony). This is achieved by the three vegetative stages: the oocyst in the mosquito (where the process is called sporogony); tissue schizogony (also termed exo-erythrocytic schizony or pre-erythrocytic schizogony) in the liver of mammalian hosts or in the reticuloendothelial cells in avian/saurian hosts; and erythrocytic schizogony (Figure 2.1).

The second strategy is parasite dispersal and invasion of the host cells. The parasite stages adopting this strategy are extracellular and are the merozoite, sporozoite and ookinete. The third strategy is sex, which begins with the formation of the gametocytes in the peripheral circulation of the vertebrate host and is completed upon the formation of the ookinete in the mosquito blood meal.

## The parasite in the mosquito

The female anopheline mosquito must take blood meals on a regular basis to support the development of successive batches of eggs. When biting a malaria-infected vertebrate host, she will take up erythrocytes infected with the asexual schizogonic stages and with gametocytes. Gametocytes are the first sexual stages of parasite development and are the gamete-forming cells; they persist as mature forms arrested in $G_0$ of the cell cycle in the peripheral blood of the host. Whereas in most species studied, infectivity of gametocytes is sustained throughout the life of the cell, there are reports that in some mammalian malarial species,

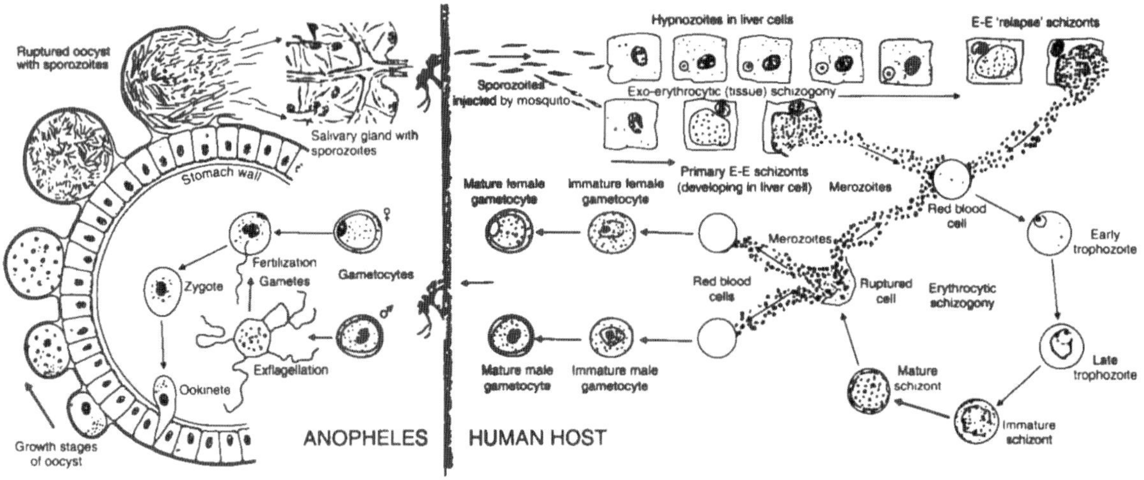

**Figure 2.1** *The life cycle of malaria parasites in the mosquito and in the human host, according to present views on the exo-erythrocytic schizogony.*

e.g. *P. cynomolgi*, infectivity to the mosquito (or gamete-forming ability) follows a circadian pattern that matches the biting behaviour of the mosquito. Evidence for such 'behavioural' strategies is, however, convincing only in the related *Leucocytozoidae*.

Within the gut of the mosquito, the gametocytes are 'immediately' triggered by the fall in temperature ($>5\,^{\circ}$C) and the presence of a mosquito factor recently identified as xanthurenic acid, to begin the formation of gametes. Within 10 minutes, the female gametocytes escape from the erythrocyte by secreting lytic molecules from cytoplasmic 'osmiophilic bodies' into the vacuole containing the parasite and the enveloping red blood cell is broken down. Other changes, e.g. to the plasma membrane of the developing gamete, include the expression of surface antigens, including (in the case of *P. falciparum*) Pfs 230 and 48/45. These are important targets for potential transmission-blocking vaccines, and are known to induce natural transmission-blocking antibodies.

The male gametocyte similarly escapes the enveloping erythrocyte, but simultaneously it undergoes three mitotic divisions inside a single, persistent nucleus. In strict concert with the division of the spindles, the attached cytoplasmic cytoskeletal-organizing centre divides to produce eight kinetosomes, which initiate the formation of eight (22 μm long) axonemes, which are assembled in the cytoplasm. Ultimately, each flagellum becomes motile and drags the attached half-spindle together with its haploid genome into the microgamete, where the DNA condenses in the elongated nucleus. This is the only time in the entire parasite's life cycle when the DNA is condensed, suggesting its packaging proteins may differ from those of most eukaryotic cells. The liberated male gametes move through the viscous blood feed and fuse with the female, forming the zygote. The zygote is uniquely adapted to the environment of the early blood feed, being resistant to complement, but it is nonetheless susceptible to attack by phagocytes in the blood, and to antibodies that recognize the parasite surface. At about 5 hours post-blood feeding, the zygote undergoes a two-step meiosis, during which reassortment and recombination of the 14 chromosomes of the genome can occur. The four individual genotypes, potentially resulting from each recombination event, finally assort when the separate sporozoites emerge from the oocyst some 10–15 days later. By 18–24 hours after blood feeding, the zygote has transformed into an ookinete (Figure 2.2) by a process that is analogous to the formation of a single merozoite or sporozoite (see below). The subcellular organization of the ookinete is directly comparable with the two other motile and invasive stages of the life cycle – the sporozoite and merozoite. The key components that are conserved between the 'zoites' are: a cell surface that is designed to protect the parasite against its environment and which will interact with appropriate host cells, thus inducing invasion; an apical complex comprising the anterior apical rings (the microtubule-organizing centre), subpellicular microtubules, a submembranous skeletal vacuole, and prominent secretory vesicles including rhoptries and

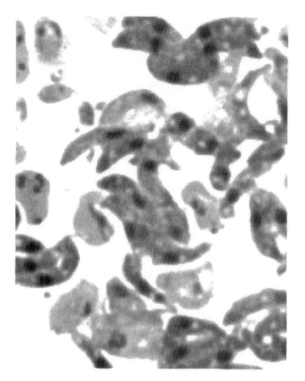

**Figure 2.2** *An ookinete in the stomach of an* Anopheles *mosquito; this stage of the malaria parasite proceeds to the outer epithelium of the mid-gut of the mosquito to form an oocyst. (Wellcome Museum of Medical Science.)*

micronemes – which have been shown to express different stage-specific variants of proteins. These proteins are responsible for the interaction with the host cells, thus mediating invasion. Proteins on the surface of the ookinete have been characterized, of which P25 and P28 are prime candidates for immune attack and are currently being developed as transmission-blocking vaccines.

Stage-specific variation in this conserved structural organization is most notable in the ookinete, and includes *inter alia* the presence of two large, unique organelles – the crystalloids – the function of which remains unknown.

The ookinete traverses the chitinous peritrophic matrix, which it is believed is laid down by the mosquito as a defence against infection. The ookinete does this by secreting a prochitinase enzyme that is subsequently activated in the gut by proteolysis. The ookinete subsequently interacts with the complex microvillar surface of the mid-gut wall, where it appears glycosylated molecules may be important receptors. Invasion of the mid-gut wall requires the

expression of a secretory protein – circumsporozoite, thrombospondin-related protein (CTRP) – but is not dependent upon the expression of major surface proteins P25 and P28. The ookinete reportedly invades only a subset of epithelial cells that express v-ATPase, though evidence for this is not yet conclusive. Within the cytoplasm of the epithelial cell, the ookinete appears to provoke the innate immune response of the mosquito, resulting in the expression of a wide range of immune peptides, e.g. Gram-negative binding protein, defension, and reactive molecules such as nitric oxide. A fraction of the ookinetes emerge through the basal plasma membrane of the mid-gut cell and 'bump into' the collagenous basal lamina. Here, the ookinete comes to rest and initiates its differentiation into an oocyst. It is now some 24–36 hours since the mosquito took its blood feed.

Transformation into an oocyst (Figure 2.3) differs in detail between the different parasites of humans

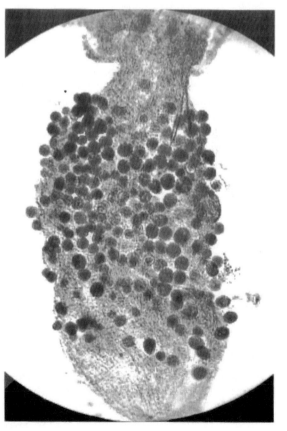

**Figure 2.3** *Mid-gut of an* Anopheles *mosquito heavily infected with oocysts of* P. vivax, ×c. 40. *(Wellcome Museum of Medical Science.)*

**Table 2.2** *Some comparative characteristics of sporogonic and schizogonic stages of the four species of human* Plasmodium

| Species | Duration of sporogony in *Anopheles* (days at 28 °C) | Diameter of mature oocyst | Appearance of pigment in oocyst | Duration of pre-erythrocytic stage (days in humans) | Mean diameter of mature pre-erythrocytic schizont (μm) | Approximate number of merozoites in pre-erythrocytic schizont |
|---|---|---|---|---|---|---|
| *P. vivax* | 8–10 | 50 μm | Feathery | 6–8 | 45 | 10 000 |
| *P. malariae* | 14–16 | 40 μm | Clusters at periphery | 14–16 | 55 | 15 000 |
| *P. ovale* | 12–14 | 45 μm | Crossed lines | 9 | 60 | 15 000 |
| *P. falciparum* | 9–10 | 55 μm | Rows and chains | 5.5–7 | 60 | 30 000 |

*Note.* Previous data on *P. malariae* based on experimental studies on *P. inui* suggested that the number of pre-erythrocytic merozoites was of the order of 2000. The above information derives from the study of *P. malariae* (Bray and Garnham, 1982)

(Table 2.2) and involves the rapid expansion of the cytoplasm as the parasite begins vegetative growth. The nucleus concomitantly undergoes repeated endomitosis, resulting in a large polyploid cell with multiple (and potentially mixed) copies of the haploid genome. All the invasive organelles of the ookinete are resorbed into the cytoplasm and disappear in the following 24 hours. The endoplasmic reticulum, Golgi apparatus and secretory vesicle system denominate the structure of the oocyst during the trophic phase, during which time the oocyst grows almost linearly (in diameter) from about 5 μm to about 50 μm in diameter. As it increases in size, the oocyst distends and eventually ruptures the overlying basal lamina; this may facilitate the escape of the sporozoites when formed.

From about the sixth day onwards, the oocyst begins to undergo segmentation. The first evidence of cell division is when deep invaginations and clefts of the endoplasmic reticulum divide the cytoplasm of the oocyst into sections (sporoblasts). The resulting increase in surface:volume ratio permits the emergence of about 8000 daughter cells (sporozoites) from the sporoblast or oocyst cell surface. Briefly, the nuclei of the oocyst come to lie under the plasma membrane, the microtubule-organizing centre (MTOC) on each pole of the nuclear spindles initiates the formation of the microtubular cytoskeleton, in parallel with the submembranous pellicular vacuole. The secretory organelles of each sporozoite are formed between the MTOC and the nucleus of each developing sporozoite bud. As the nucleus is drawn into the ever-elongating sporozoite, a single mitochondrion and apicoplast are taken in. The rigid sporozoites

become motile and are released into the oocyst. The oocyst wall becomes weakened and the sporozoites emerge through the cyst wall and basal lamina and the majority enter the haemocoele cavity (Figure 2.4).

The ultrastructural/molecular organization of the sporozoite reflects its biology as one of the dispersive and invasive extracellular phases of development. Sporozoites are 10–15 μm long and 1 μm in diameter and have the overall appearance of small nematodes (Figure 2.5). At the anterior end is the apical complex, like that of the ookinete, which is composed of a single subpellicular skeletal vacuole below which lie the subpellicular microtubules (some 12–16 in number,

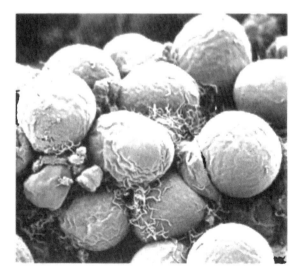

**Figure 2.4** *Scanning electron micrograph of mature oocysts of* P. yoelii *on the mid-gut of* A. stephensi *with numerous emerging sporozoites,* ×2695.

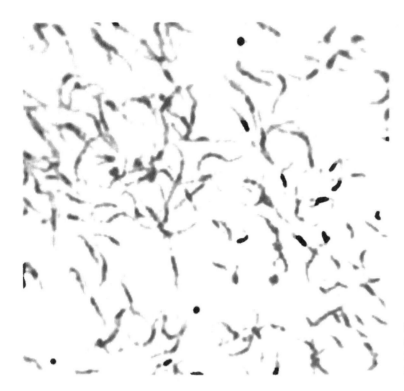

**Figure 2.5** *Sporozoites of* P. falciparum *released from a ruptured mature oocyst, ×1380. (Wellcome Museum of Medical Science.)*

arranged in a typical asymmetric $n + 1$ configuration), which are attached to the apical rings. Within this skeleton, in the anterior third of the cell, lie both the micronemes, which are numerous in the mature sporozoite and contain both circumsporozoite protein (CSP) and thrombospondin-related adhesive protein (TRAP), and the rhoptries, which dominate in the oocyst form of sporozoite. In the middle third of the cell lie the nucleus, mitochondrion and apicoplast, and the posterior third of the cell is occupied by the ribosomes and endoplasmic reticulum (Figure 2.6).

Mosquitoes, and particularly refractory mosquitoes, have an ability to recognize and react to the oocyst and to the ookinete as it emerges from the gut wall. The response is the deposition of melanin formed by the enzyme phenol oxidase from the dopa–dopamine pathway. The melanin deposits are impervious to nutrients and oxygen and the entombed parasites die. In the case of the mature oocyst, these melanized structures are called Ross's black spores.

Sporozoites initially released from the oocyst are morphologically and physiologically distinguishable from those later found in the salivary gland (see Figure 2.5). Oocyst sporozoites are poorly infectious

to the vertebrate host, but will infect mosquito salivary glands. They express the circumsporozoite protein, but express a second surface protein TRAP poorly; by contrast, the salivary gland sporozoites express TRAP at high levels, and will infect the vertebrate host but not salivary glands. These molecular and physiological differences, combined with observations that knock-out parasites that fail to express CSP or TRAP cannot infect the vertebrate host, suggest both CSP and TRAP have important roles in the recognition and/or invasion of host cells (notably the hepatocyte in mammalian malarias). These factors underlie the selection of these two antigens as priority candidates for the formulation of a protective antimalarial vaccine.

The number of sporozoites found in the salivary glands of wild-caught mosquitoes is small (about 1000) compared to the number released from oocysts (normal infections are one to four oocysts producing a total of 8000–32 000 sporozoites). Of these salivary gland sporozoites, normally only about 20 are released in any single mosquito bite – but a single sporozoite has been shown to produce an infection in the vertebrate host.

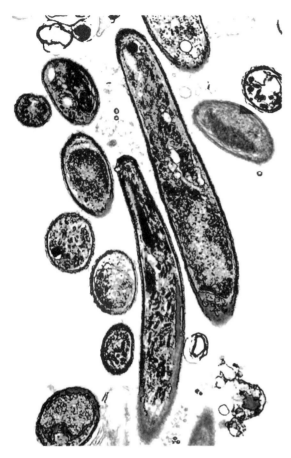

**Figure 2.6** *Sporozoites of* P. cynomolgi. *Electron photomicrograph of longitudinal and cross-sections,* ×21 125. *(Dr M Aikawa, Published in Cochrane et al., 1976.)*

## The parasite in the vertebrate host

### TISSUE PHASE

The tissue phase of avian/saurian parasites differs significantly from that of the mammalian parasites in that it occurs as repeated cycles of growth distributed throughout the mesodermal cells of the reticuloendothelial system. In mammals, the tissue phase is confined to the liver and is a single round of replicative development after which the parasite invades the erythrocytes.

Infectious sporozoites can be recovered from the blood for 30–60 minutes following intravenous inoculation, and can be found invading hepatocytes as quickly as 2 minutes after inoculation. Many sporozoites are ingested by phagocytes, notably Kupffer cells, but may not be destroyed there. Viable sporo- ·

zoites are capable of circumventing the induction of the oxidative burst in the invaded phagocyte and will escape from macrophages *in vitro*.

Interaction of the sporozoite with the hepatocyte *in vitro* has been described in significant detail and clearly involves the interaction of the thrombospondin domains of the CSP and TRAP with the sulphated glycans of the hepatocyte surface. Following this interaction, the sporozoite invades the hepatocyte, where the host cell forms a parasitophorous vacuole that separates the parasite from the cytoplasm of the host cell. Within this vacuole, the sporozoite rounds up (due to the loss of the sporozoite cytoskeleton) into a sphere some 3–5 μm in diameter. Thereafter, development follows one of two routes. Either there is immediate initiation of a vegetative growth leading to primary schizogony, or the rounded cell enters an arrested phase of development termed the hypnozoite, which remains dormant for many days/weeks until an unknown stimulus promotes re-entry into the cell cycle, and schizogony ensues – this delayed primary blood infection is termed a relapse. Relapses are found in relatively few malaria species, including *P. vivax* and *P. ovale* amongst the parasites of humans, and *P. cynomolgi*, a parasite of primates. In *P. vivax* there is a clear variation in the pattern of relapses dependent upon the geographical isolate studied; this subject is extensively reviewed by Garnham (1988).

In the early literature on relapses in mammalian parasites, it was proposed that merozoites from a primary exo-erythrocytic schizont had the ability to re-invade the hepatocyte and thus generate potential relapse populations of parasites, a model not unlike the patterns of tissue development seen in avian parasites. This theory was discounted when the true nature of the hypnozoite was discovered in the 1980s. Recently, however, a novel concept for recrudescence of patent blood infections has been described by Landau *et al.* (1999), who observed, in rodent malaria parasites, novel structures in the lymphatic system that contain merozoites, apparently infectious upon subinoculation to naive hosts. The true role of such structures has yet to be confirmed.

Patterns of primary tissue schizogony differ among the various human malaria parasites (Table 2.2), most notably in the duration of this phase of infection, which can be as short as 5 days (*P. falciparum*) and as long as 16 days (*P. malariae*). The cellular events of tissue schizogony are remarkably reminiscent of the development of the oocyst in the mosquito; indeed, by light microscopy it is difficult to distinguish the internal structures in each. The tissue schizont is inside an hepatocyte and must derive all sustenance from/through it. The cytoplasm of the hepatocyte appears to decrease as the parasite enlarges, but there is as yet no clear evidence that host cell cytoplasm is directly used by the parasite (unlike the erythrocytic schizont). Nonetheless, by the time the schizont is mature it is some 30–70 μm in diameter (Figure 2.7), contains 30 000–50 000 merozoites and greatly distends the infected host cell (see Table 2.2). During the period of trophic growth, it is suggested that a parasite protein (CSP) can interact with the proteasome complexes in the hepatocyte cytoplasm and down-regulate the processing of polypeptides – thereby reducing the probability that parasite peptides will be expressed with major histocompatibility complex (MHC) class 1 antigen on the hepatocyte surface. Irradiated sporozoites, which induce an effective

immune response including CD8+ cytotoxic T cells, invade hepatocytes and develop into degenerate trophozoites. The cytoplasm of hepatocytes infected by such parasites can be shown to contain significant amounts of parasite proteins such as CSP. Mature tissue schizonts in hosts immunized with recombinant liver stage immunogens attract CD8+ cells, and bursting schizonts can be invaded by large numbers of phagocytes. The recognition that the exo-erythrocytic schizont is the target of the human immune response has resulted in a major effort to develop a protective antimalarial vaccine which, contrary to early efforts at anti-sporozoite vaccines, aims to develop a CD8+ response targeted to the hepatocyte, not an antibody response targeted to the sporozoite in the blood. Laboratory studies have shown that cytotoxic T cells recognize the expression of CSP peptides in MHC class 1 antigen on the infected hepatocyte, which, through direct cell contact, results

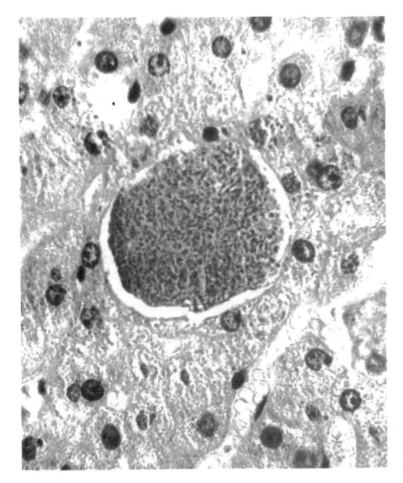

**Figure 2.7** *Pre-erythrocytic schizont of* P. falciparum *in the liver,* ×730.

in the release of interleukin-1 (IL1), IL6 and nitric oxide in the infected cell, thus killing the host cell and the parasite within. Vaccines based on this principle have shown promising effects in the laboratory and are currently under development for human trials.

In the normal developing exo-erythrocytic schizont, the cytoplasm of the parasite becomes subdivided and the ensuing invasive stages (merozoites) develop on the expanded cell surface (analogous to sporozoite formation in the oocyst). The emergent merozoites are small spherical/ovoid cells approximately 1 μm in diameter. Consistent with their small size and brief life span, the merozoites are the 'simplest' of the invasive stages. The microtubule component of the cytoskeleton is reduced to a very few microtubules (typically around two) attached to the apical rings. The secretory organelles are represented by a paired rhoptry, the constituent proteins of which have been extensively characterized and include apical merozoite antigen 1 (AMA-1, a potential vaccine candidate), a few micronemes, and microspheres – which are released post-invasion and are responsible for changes in the structure of the parasitophorous vacuole. Other organelles are similar to those described for the sporozoite. The plasma membrane surface of these merozoites is dominated by the aggregated peptides of merozoite surface 1 protein (MSP-1).

The mass of merozoites released upon rupture of the schizont into the parasitophorous vacuole probably cause the disruption of the parasitophorous vacuole membrane. The merozoites then escape into the residual host cell cytoplasm. Following the subsequent rupture of the hepatocyte plasma membrane, the mixture of cytoplasm and merozoites pours into the sinusoids. Here much of the released material is ingested by Kupffer cells, but some merozoites escape and within a few (about 15) minutes invade the erythrocyte. Invasion of the erythrocyte is very rapid (taking about 30 seconds), and has been defined extensively at the molecular level. Invasion involves a clear cascade of interdependent events. Initial long-range contact is made by means of relatively non-specific mechanisms, including electrostatic interactions. The spacing between host and parasite is at this stage some 150 nm. Thereafter, a tight binding follows. Major ligands in this interaction are: for *P. falciparum* erythrocyte binding antigen 175 (EBA 175) and glycophorin A, amongst others; and for *P. vivax*, EBA 140 and the Duffy antigen (for details see Barnwell and Galinski, 1998). Transition between these two binding states involves re-orientation of the merozoite from random orientation to the direct apposition of the apical end (and thus the secretory pore of the rhoptries and micronemes) against the plasma membrane of the erythrocyte. At this point the tight junction between the parasite and the host cell forms a protein-rich micro-domain in the host membrane in the form of a 'belt' around the tip of the merozoite. This tight junction is then driven by the merozoite actin–myosin network against the cytoskeleton of the parasite towards the posterior of the cell, thus pushing the merozoite into the red blood cell (Figure 2.8). As the merozoite moves into the red blood cell, much of the surface glycocalyx of the parasite is released and shed into the plasma. Following invasion, only a small 19-kDa portion of the carboxy terminus of MSP 1 remains attached, by a glycosyl phosphatidyl inositol (GPI) anchor, to the parasite surface. This fragment, which contains two epidermal growth factor (EGF) domains, is highly conserved between different *P. falciparum* clones, suggesting it is functionally essential to the parasite (unlike the remainder of the molecule, which is highly polymorphic – see below).

Once the merozoite has moved fully inside the red blood cell, it is assumed the red blood cell membranes re-anneal behind the parasite, which now resides inside a parasitophorous vacuole sealed inside the red blood cell. Because the mammalian red blood cell is a non-nucleated cell devoid of MHC class 1 molecules, this represents an immunoprivileged site within the host. Recent controversy has arisen over data suggesting that the point of entry does not seal and thus leaves a permanent duct between parasite and bloodstream through which nutrients and antibodies might travel. The majority opinion, however, is that the evidence for this duct is technically flawed.

Within the parasitophorous vacuole, the merozoite releases the contents of the microspheres through the parasite surface. The contents of these spheres induce proliferation of the parasitophorous vacuole membrane (PVM). It is assumed this expansion allows the more rapid exchange of small molecules between red blood cell cytoplasm and the parasite. The changes induced in the red blood cell by the growing trophozoites become more pronounced as the parasite develops. The species-specific nature of the changes has long been recognized, e.g. Maurer's clefts, Schüffner's dots etc., and is useful in species identification (Figure 2.9). The PVM is clearly a composite structure, derived from both red blood cell and parasite components in

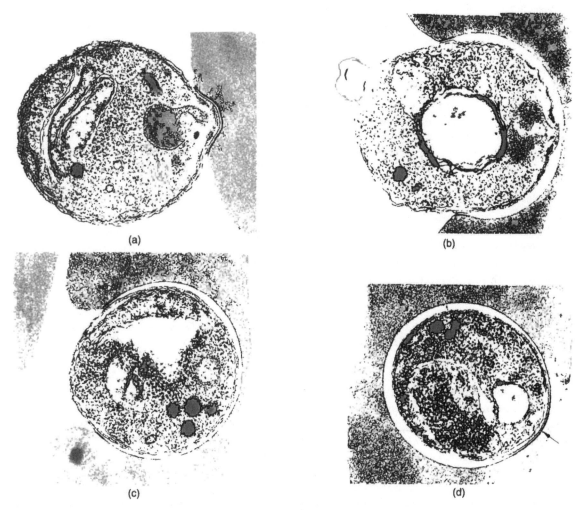

(a)

(b)

(c)

(d)

**Figure 2.8** *(a) Electron micrograph of a longitudinal section of a merozoite of P. knowlesi soon after its contact with the erythrocyte. The erythrocyte membrane is thickened and forms a protein-rich junction with the plasma membrane of the merozoite. The darker, bottle-shaped part of the merozoite near the junction is the rhoptry, which releases its contents on the erythrocyte membrane at the point of attachment, ×48 000. (Dr M Aikawa; published in Aikawa et al., Malaria and the red cell. CIBA Foundation Symposium, 1983.) (b) Electron photomicrograph of a merozoite of P. knowlesi entering an erythrocyte at an advanced stage of the interiorization process. The moving junction formed between the thickened membrane of the erythrocyte and the merozoite brings the latter within the invagination of the erythrocyte. A small projection still connects the apical end of the merozoite and the erythrocyte membrane, ×54 000. (Dr M Aikawa; published in Aikawa et al., 1978.) (c) Electron photomicrograph of a section of a merozoite of P. knowlesi entering an erythrocyte. The merozoite is located within an invagination of the erythrocyte; at the junction points, there is a distinct thickening of the erythrocyte membrane (which is about to seal itself), ×54 000. (Dr M Aikawa; published by Aikawa et al., 1981.) (d) Completion of the entry of the merozoite into the erythrocyte. The membranes of the erythrocyte are sealed, leaving the merozoite within a vacuole lined by the erythrocyte membrane, ×50 000. (Dr M Aikawa; published in Aikawa et al., 1978.)*

that it initially has a markedly reduced number of intramembranous particles (IMPs) compared to either the red blood cell or merozoite plasma membrane.

The pattern of distensions of the PVM differs among parasite species infecting the red blood cell

and is described in the section on parasite diagnosis below. Essentially the distensions fall into two groups: a series of flattened membrane clefts, and specific point modifications at the red blood cell surface. Amongst the latter are the knobs characteristic

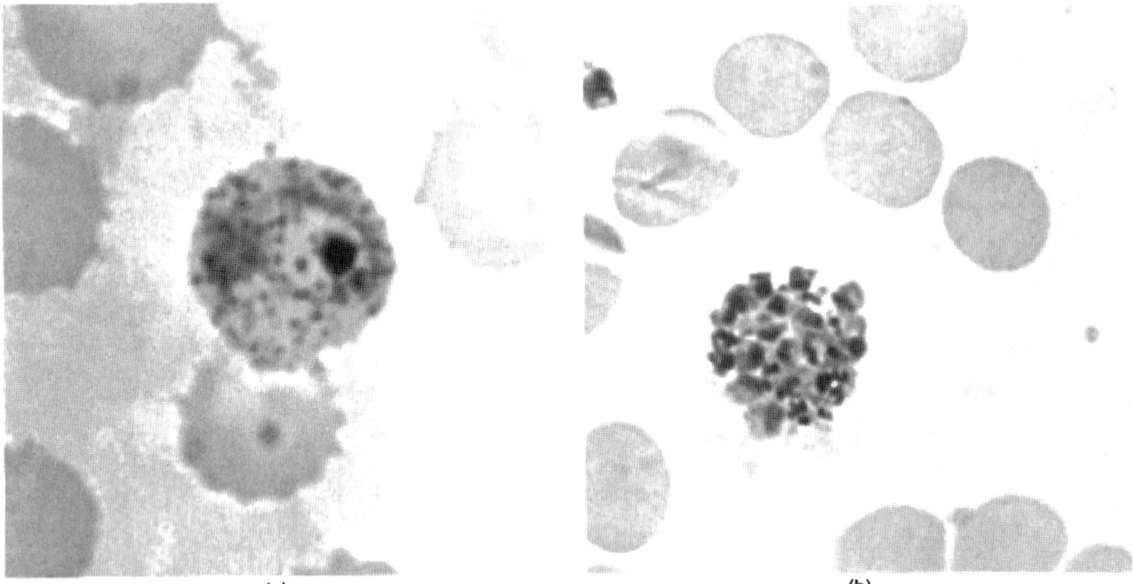

(a)                                                    (b)

**Figure 2.9** Plasmodium vivax. *(a) Trophozoite with pronounced Schüffner's stippling in an enlarged erythrocyte, ×1192. (b) Fully developed schizont with about 20 merozoites ready to burst and to invade new red blood cells, ×833. (Wellcome Museum of Medical Science.)*

of *P. falciparum*, which appear later in the schizogonic cycle. The knobs have been characterized in great detail and the constituent proteins elucidated. Amongst these in *P. falciparum* is PfEMP-1, which was originally recognized as the SICA (surface of the infected cell antigen) antigen. PfEMP-1 is responsible in very large part for the attachment of the schizont-infected red blood cell to the capillary walls of the brain and for the attachment of the immature gametocytes to the deep tissues (notably the bone marrow). There are some 50–60 separate genes encoding PfEMP-1 and the parasite rapidly switches between these. With each new variant there is a transient rise in the parasite density until an immune response controls the rate of re-infection, whereupon the next population is selected. The dynamics as to why it is advantageous to the parasite to 'identify' the infected erythrocyte in this way and to sequester to the brain, thus causing cerebral malaria and death of the host, are fascinating. Clearly, the fact that the parasite has developed such a powerful immune evasion mechanism suggests that there is advantage in retaining this cerebral complication as an effective life strategy.

Redifferentiation of the intra-erythrocytic merozoite into the feeding trophozoite results primarily from the loss of the cytoskeleton and apical complex.

Viewed with the light microscope, trophozoites are irregular parasites of variable (amoeboid) shape and often appearing as flattened discs with the nucleus at one side. When observed in the light microscope *en face*, these parasites have a ring-like appearance and are hence called ring forms. The intra-erythrocytic parasite ingests the cytoplasm of the red blood cell through a unique structure in the cell surface called the cytostome or micropore. The primary phagosome so formed is, in turn, subject to secondary invagination; it is in these small vacuoles that the majority of digestion occurs. As a consequence of the predominant red blood cell protein being haemoglobin, the parasite has a unique problem in successfully disposing of the toxic iron residues of haem. This is achieved by the polymerization of the partial degradation product haematin, which is processed by the enzyme haem polymerase to form crystalline haemozoin. Haem polymerase has been described as a target for the antimalarial drug chloroquine. However, current theories suggest that the primary lethal activity of chloroquine is that it inhibits the maintenance of ionic balance in the cytoplasm and food vacuole. This hypothesis is compatible with the observed reversal of chloroquine resistance by the calcium channel blockers verapamil and its analogue desipramine. Haemozoin is seen with the light microscope as brown crystals of malarial pigment, the distribution of which is another useful criterion to assist in stage and species identification. The pigment remains separated from the parasite cytoplasm by the parasitophorous vacuole membrane. Following the phagocytic activity, the trophozoite increases in size and the protein synthetic machinery, ribosomes, endoplasmic reticulum and dispersed Golgi vesicles expand rapidly and are visible in Giemsa-stained parasites as the blue cytoplasm of the enlarging cell. Thereafter, the nucleus undergoes replication (1/3–2/3 through the cycle) and divides; this is repeated synchronously three to five times, but some daughter nuclei may fail to develop, resulting in variable numbers of parasite nuclei (i.e. other than $2^n$).

Following division, the nuclei of the schizont come to lie under the plasma membrane of the parasite, which by now almost completely occupies the empty shell of the red blood cell. At this time the cytoplasm of the parasite 'retracts' around the nuclei and the daughter merozoites extend out from the surface of the schizont in a manner identical to that in the tissue schizont. In mature schizonts, termed segmenters, the free merozoites lie in the parasitophorous vacuole together with a residual body of schizont cytoplasm that contains all the discarded haemozoin crystals formed from haemoglobin digestion. At the time of rupture of the infected red blood cell, the merozoites and the residual debris are released into the bloodstream. Release of the debris is toxic to the host and, when this occurs in synchronous infections, there is a large toxic stimulus (mediated in part by malaria-specific GPI anchors of parasite surface proteins, and in part by the haemozoin crystals). This in turn results in significant cytokine release by the host, which causes fever. The duration of the asexual schizogonic cycle differs between some of the human malarias (i.e. 48–50 hours in *P. vivax*, *P. ovale* and *P. falciparum*, but 72 hours in *P. malariae*), with the result that the pattern of the fevers observed is species-related. It is these patterns that gave rise to the medical descriptions of the diseases as being of tertian (48-hour) or quartan (72-hour) periodicity. This periodicity is often not apparent early in an infection, because (a) there are fewer parasites present in the blood and (b) different 'broods' of parasites will have arisen from exoerythrocytic schizonts that matured at different rates from sporozoites delivered in the same infected mosquito bite, or (c) multiple infections may have arisen

from repeated bites from different mosquitoes at close intervals. Evidence suggests that fever is itself a positive drive, causing the synchronization of erythrocytic schizogony by temporarily arresting the maturation of the parasite at defined points in the asexual cycle, thus reinforcing the periodicity of fever in older infections.

Whereas the majority of merozoites entering an erythrocyte will develop into asexual schizonts, a small fraction can develop into gametocytes, the first sexual stage of the life cycle. Despite the haploid nature of the parasite genome, gametocytes are sexually dimorphic. Current evidence suggests that commitment to gametocytogenesis varies during the course of an infection. Early data in the rodent malarial parasites showed clearly that the highest rate of commitment was found in the merozoites released from the tissue schizonts, and thereafter fell progressively. This fall was described as being due, at least in part, to the progressive loss of chromosomal integrity, such that, in the artificial situation where parasites were maintained by repeated mechanical blood passage, the ability to form gametocytes was completely lost – such a situation is unlikely to occur in nature. Passage of a poor gametocyte producer through mosquitoes, if successful, reinstates, by selection, the normal ability to produce sexual parasites. Recent work on *P. falciparum* has shown that the induction of gametocytogenesis during the course of an asexual infection is modulated by release of soluble factors which induce gametocytogenesis in a density-dependent manner. Enhanced gametocyte formation has, for more than 40 years, been correlated with a wide range of external causes, all of which, it could be argued, exert 'stress' upon the erythrocytic parasites. These factors include treatment with certain antimalarial drugs (notably chloroquine), with antibody to the asexual parasites, and with parasite lysates. Recognizing that, in a normal infection, each round of asexual schizogony results in a higher number of re-invading merozoites, it is therefore clear why the major peak of gametocyte production follows the major peak of asexual parasitaemia. The spacing between these peaks represents the difference in the maturation time of the asexual parasites and the sexual parasites. Thus, in *P. vivax* and most other malaria parasites, the two peaks tend to be almost co-incident, but in the case of *P. falciparum* and *P. reichenowi*, the gametocyte peak occurs some 9–12 days after the peak asexual infection. This simple biological phenomenon has important implications for the optimal use of antimalarial drugs in the different human parasite species (see below). Current data suggest that the exact time of commitment of the blood-stage parasite to sexual versus asexual development is during the preceding round of schizogony, such that a schizont of generation I will yield merozoites which will all produce *either* asexual or sexual parasites in generation II. Further, if the schizont is sexually committed, it has been shown that all the merozoites produce either male or female cells (i.e. not a mixture). This suggests that commitment occurs at a time point in schizogony at which all progeny cells are affected, i.e. it is produced early when there is only one copy of the genome to be regulated. An alternative is that the regulatory factor is ubiquitous enough to affect all progeny nuclei in the common cytoplasm. Noting this regulation of expression of the sexual phenotype in the blood-stage parasites, it would be intriguing to know whether the same 'rules' exist for the large tissue schizonts.

Gametocytogenesis is best understood in *P. falciparum* – a parasite in which the process is clearly *atypical* for the large majority of malarial parasites, but the protracted 12-day development allows a straightforward temporal analysis of initial sexual differentiation, which is divided into six stages. Stage I gametocytes (days 0–2) are distinguished from the trophozoite because they have begun to lay down a membranous and microtubular subpellicular cytoskeleton. In stage II (days 1–4) the parasite increases in size and the cytoskeleton develops on one side of the cell, forcing it into a typical D shape; in some of these cells, intranuclear microtubules have been described (but mitosis is not seen). Stage III gametocytes (days 2–8) are larger D-shaped cells that now distend the erythrocyte. Stages I–III all appear to show the same sensitivities to antimalarial and antibiotic drugs as do the asexual parasites of the same isolate. Thereafter, the gametocytes become progressively less sensitive to drugs that attack parasite synthetic processes, e.g. chloroquine, but remain sensitive to some drugs that attack energy metabolism, e.g. primaquine, but not to others, e.g. atovaquone/proguanil. Sensitivity of gametocytes to the artemisinine-based drugs is reportedly variable: some workers report that gametocytes are killed, whereas others suggest that the transmission of the parasite to the vector is not blocked. Stage IV gametocytes (days 6–10) become cylindrical, elongated, pointed cells; this is because the microtubular cytoskeleton now surrounds the entire cell. Stage V parasites (days 9–23) are the first to be released into the peripheral bloodstream; these are the typical crescent-shaped cells. The crescentic shape is produced because the parasites, although still invested by a subpellicular membranous 'corsette', have lost the rigid microtubule skeleton; therefore the tubular cell is now flexible and can be bent into the crescentic shape by the enveloping erythrocyte. Male and female cells can be distinguished for the first time in the stage V parasite: the male has a large nucleus, the envelope of which is delimited by haemozoin pigment, the cytoplasm has now lost much of its ribosomal machinery for protein synthesis (and therefore does not stain blue in Giemsa smears), and there are relatively few of the osmiophilic bodies. By contrast, the female gametocyte has a small nucleus which, in Giemsa-stained smears, contains a characteristic magenta dot. The cytoplasm is rich in ribosomes and endoplasmic reticulum (thus blue in Giemsa smears), extensive mitochondria and apicoplast, and numerous osmiophilic bodies. The insensitivity of these cells to most antimalarial drugs reflects the fact that they are arrested in $G_0$ of the cell cycle – which in turn also explains why gametocytes are relatively long-lived compared to the asexual cell. In *P. falciparum*, this life span lies between 2.5 and 22 days, thus maximizing the infectious potential of a gametocyte carrier to the mosquito.

Although the presence of gametocytes is essential for mosquito transmission to occur, it does not guarantee infection, i.e. not all gametocyte carriers are infectious. Reasons for this are dependent on both parasite and host properties. In some malaria species, gametocytes have been described as being 'viable' only at certain times of day, e.g. the evening, which coincides with the biting time of the vector. For this to be mediated solely by parasite physiology would require that (a) the induction of gametocytes was brief and synchronous, (b) the infectiousness (viability) of the gametocytes was very short-lived, and (c) there are no other regulatory factors. This is not consistent with current knowledge, in that gametocytes are relatively long-lived and host factors are critical in the regulation of infectivity. Host factors described to date all relate to the changes induced by the asexual parasitaemia, and include the fall in blood pH induced by lactic acidosis, the concomitant fall in blood bicarbonate levels and, at schizogony, the production of tumour necrosis factor (TNF), interleukins and nitric oxide will transiently suppress infectivity. It is these host-derived factors above all others that result in the poor correlation of gametocytaemia and subsequent mosquito infection in field observations on malaria transmission.

# PARASITE METABOLISM AND THE DESIGN OF ANTIMALARIAL STRATEGIES

Considering the human malarial parasites alone, control strategies have traditionally focused upon two approaches. The clinical approach has the critical objective of management of disease and parasite burden in the infected human host; to date, this has been achieved almost exclusively by the use of chemotherapy. It is to be hoped that vaccines currently under evaluation may lead to new, effective intervention strategies in the future, the objective of this approach being to save the life of the infected person. A second and more indirect approach, here termed 'the biological approach', is to prevent the transmission of the parasite between the mosquito vector and humans. This approach can be multifaceted, involving chemoprophylaxis (to prevent transmission to the mosquito, or from the mosquito to humans), and anti-mosquito strategies, whereby the infectious reservoir is reduced and thus the rate of infectious bites (entomological inoculation rate) is reduced. This can be achieved either by attacking the parasite in the mosquito, the mosquito itself, or by blocking the potential interaction of the mosquito with humans. Current evaluation of the transmission-blocking vaccines that attack the gametes, zygote and ookinete in the mosquito mid-gut suggests that these could be potent components of any future cocktail antimalarial vaccine.

The two basic approaches to attacking the parasite directly are drugs and vaccines. The major problem with the chemotherapeutic approach is that plasmodium, like its human host, is a eukaryotic cell, and therefore successful chemotherapy depends either upon the discovery of the rare, novel targets in the parasite that exist because the parasite has evolved unique solutions to biological problems, or upon the exploitation of differences in the efficiency with which the drug penetrates and interacts with parasite metobolic pathways as opposed to the hosts cells. Such targets for drug intervention may lie in any or all of the parasite's key metabolic pathways.

## Nucleic acid metabolism

The parasite derives its purines from the purine salvage pathway, whereby hypoxanthine in the red blood cell is taken into the parasite, converted to inosine monophosphate and then into guanine and adenosine. The addition of hypoxanthine to media for the culture of the parasite was found to be beneficial for the growth and survival of the parasite, notably the long-lived gametocytes. Pyrimidines are synthesized *de novo*. Two enzymes in this pathway are, unusually, found as a bifunctional protein dihydrofolate reductase–thymidylate synthase. The latter and other enzymes of the folate pathway lead to the formation of dihydropterate and dihydrofolate and can be selectively targeted by potential antimalarial drugs. Prominent examples are sulphanilamide, sulphadimethoxine and dapsone analogues of para-amino-benzoic acid, an essential component of the folate pathway. The presence of the *de-novo* pyrimidine pathway also explains the requirement of the parasite for micro-aerophilic conditions in culture.

## Carbohydrate metabolism

Although glucose metabolism is largely similar to that in the human host, differences described in the enzymes mediating the pathway might lead to the development of new antimalarials. Mitochondrial organization in the malarial parasite is described as differing among species and among life-cycle stages within a species. Specifically, the mitochondria of avian/saurian malarias appear to be cristate throughout the life cycle, whereas those of the mammalian parasites (genus *Plasmodium*) are said to be cristate only in the mosquito stages. In *P. falciparum* there is said to be an intermediate phenotype. Electron transport in the mitochondrion can be targeted by the hydroxynathoquinone group of drugs (e.g. atovaquone). Atovaquone has been shown to be most effective as an inhibitor of schizogony in the tissues and blood of the vertebrate host, and to have a potent transmission-blocking potential in human, but more particularly rodent, parasites. A factor of some significance in the expression of recombinant malarial proteins is that plasmodium 'rarely' glycosylates proteins, 'O'-glycosylation being very rare. The most frequent glycosylation involves the addition of a malaria-specific GPI anchor to some surface proteins. The unusual structure of the glycan core, and additional myristoylation of this structure, may be significant in its potent ability to provoke fever at schizogony.

## Lipid metabolism

Malarial lipid biosynthesis has long been a neglected aspect of parasite biology; however, recent diligent work has described much of the basic pathways of lipid biosynthesis, the composition of parasite and infected red blood cell lipids, and the trafficking of lipids in the parasitized cell. A major development has been the recognition that modification of the infected red blood cell membrane could render this cell susceptible to novel routes of chemotherapy, e.g. the use of ionophores carrying monovalent cations. Although cholesterol and sphingolipid metabolism has not yet been targeted effectively by drugs of adequate therapeutic index, phospholipid metabolism appears to have this potential, notably in the application of inhibitors of choline transport.

## Protein metabolism

Protein synthesis in the malarial parasite appears largely typical of any complex eukaryotic organism with respect to gene structure, transcription regulation, translation control and protein secretion. Facets of biological interest are that the translational regulation of some gamete-stage protein synthesis is achieved by the localization in the gametocyte of pre-synthesized mRNA to discrete areas of the ribosomes/endoplasmic reticulum. The mechanism for molecular regulation of translation control is not yet known, but it emphasizes the extent to which the gametocytes are pre-adapted to the demands of parasite development in the early stages of development in the mosquito mid-gut. A second unusual aspect of the protein synthetic pathway is that plasmodium, unlike most eukaryotic cells and indeed some of its close relatives in the Apicomplexa, does not appear to have a discrete Golgi apparatus; rather, the post-translational mechanisms of protein modification are dispersed to vesicles throughout the cell. Perhaps the most unusual aspect of plasmodium organization relating to protein synthesis is the developmental regulation of the ribosomes. Plasmodium expresses different ribosomal RNA genes in the asexual stages (A-form), and in the mosquito stages (S-form), with perhaps the most detailed study (on *P. vivax*) indicating that a third form is expressed in the ookinete and oocyst (O-form). It will be interesting in the future to determine whether the regulation of parasite differentiation (and thus its viability) via translational control mechanisms (see above) is in any way dependent upon the switching of the ribosome structure which occurs as the parasite moves between host and vector. Should such dependence be demonstrated, the unusual nature of this phenomenon might well render it susceptible to chemotherapeutic attack.

## GENETIC ORGANIZATION OF MALARIAL PARASITES

## Nuclear genome

The malaria parasite is haploid for the majority of the life cycle, being diploid only in the 5–8 hours following fusion of the male and female gamete in the mosquito blood meal. Meiosis, involving a two-step reduction division, chromosomal re-assortment and genetic crossing-over, occurs in the zygote, and is complete before the ookinete invades the mid-gut wall.

Recent international collaboration has resulted in the decision to sequence the entire *P. falciparum* genome. At the time of writing, the full sequences of chromosomes 2 and 3 have been published and the entire nuclear genome will reportedly be completed within 2 years. This detailed knowledge of the genome combined with new 'whole-genome' approaches to the analysis of parasite gene expression can be expected to result in a significant acceleration in drug and vaccine research.

The genetic structure of malaria parasite populations has a significant impact upon the effective management of the disease in endemic areas. The general areas of relevance are: the haploid genome means that mutants, when they arise, are selected for/against immediately; within populations, allelic variation is common; globally, the frequency of individual alleles in endemic populations varies widely (see parasite isolates above) and the majority of people are infected with more than one parasite clone – the degree of polyclonality correlating positively with the local entomological inoculation rate (EIR). Recognizing this within-host and between-host variation, the response to intervention may be expected to be heterogeneous. The presence of many clones in a single patient and in a local population is further justification for the use of drug combinations, which, even for a clonal parasite infection, have the advantage of reducing the probability of selecting parasites resistant to a single antimalarial. Noting the high variation between parasite clones and the polyclonal nature of infections, it is not surprising that there is the potential for rapid genetic recombination in plasmodium and the generation of new genotype combinations. It is this capability for rapid change that is perhaps the greatest long-term challenge for the logical and effective implementation of control strategies, and it points strongly to the use of integrated management strategies where multiple targets are attacked simultaneously.

## Organelle genomes

Malaria parasites have both mitochondria and plastid organelles and are thus phylogenetically related to the Ciliates and Dinoflagellates (the Alveolates). Even though the mitochondrial genome is reduced to a minuscule size (6 kb), with many genes not being represented, it is evident that the mitochondrial genome is functional and that some genes, e.g. *cyt*.b, are differentially up-regulated in the gametocyte stages of the life cycle. At present, this minimal genome is one of scientific fascination as opposed to the focus of potential new intervention strategies, although recognizing that one of the relatively few causal prophylactics/transmission-blocking drugs – primaquine – potentially targets the mitochondrion, this organelle should not be overlooked in future drug development.

The plastid genome is 35 kb in size, which is only 20 per cent size of other plastid DNAs. This small genome encodes an organelle-specific protein synthetic apparatus. The possibility of targeting the activities of this organelle (which is not present in the human host) by novel drugs is clearly attractive. At present it is, however, unclear whether this has been achieved in laboratory studies. Examples of drugs tested to date include members of the dinitroaniline herbicides, which have been shown to affect microtubule assembly; glyphosate, an inhibitor of the Shikimate pathway in plants and algae; and antibiotics that attack the plastid ribosome, such as clindamycin or thiostrepton.

## PARASITE CULTURE

Attempts to grow malarial parasites *in vitro* began very soon after the discovery of the parasite. Significant successes were first recorded in the culture of the tissue stages of avian malarias, followed by the transient maintenance of the sporogonic stages. The breakthrough in the culture of the microaerophilous blood stages was achieved by Trager and Jensen in 1976. Since then, the culture of the blood stages of *P. falciparum* has become an automated process. Other mammalian parasites are now maintained *in vitro*, but at much lower levels of success. Culture of the tissue stages of *P. relictum* and numerous other parasites of primates and mammals and of both the primary and relapse schizonts of *P. vivax* has now been achieved. The sexual stages of *P. falciparum* were initially difficult to culture until the recognition that additional hypoxanthine, and rigorous attention to the maintenance of a constant temperature and pH were essential for these long-lived cells. Culture of the gametes, ookinetes and young oocysts has now been achieved for the rodent malaria parasite *P. berghei*, but not of the mature sporozoite-producing oocyst. In contrast to *P. falciparum* and *P. gallinacium*, oocysts and sporozoites have been generated *in vitro* from the preformed zygote/ookinete, though in this case the presence of both live insect cells and additional extracellular matrix was found to be essential. It is evident in the contrasting successes and failures of culture that there are significant differences in the physiology/molecular organization of the avian and mammalian parasites, and between *P. (Laverania) falciparum* and the other plasmodium parasites of mammals. Recognizing these differences will be the key to the tantalizing possibility that the entire life cycle of malaria parasites will be achieved *in vitro*. The ability to exploit this potential and to contrast development *in vitro* with that *in vivo* will be a powerful tool in the analysis of host–parasite interactions.

## HUMAN PLASMODIA

### *Plasmodium vivax*

This species of malaria parasite of humans occurs throughout most of the temperate zones and also in large areas of the tropics. It is much less common in tropical Africa, especially in West Africa. It causes so-called 'benign tertian' malaria with relapses, the pattern of which varies among the various strains of *P. vivax*.

The existence of the pre-erythrocytic cycle of development of this parasite was proved experimentally in 1948 by Shortt and Garnham, thus confirming the early hypothesis of Grassi and refuting the notoriously erroneous description by Shaudinn (1899) of the penetration of an erythrocyte by a sporozoite. Sporozoites of *P. vivax* differentiate, after invading the liver, either into early, primary tissue schizonts or into hypnozoites, the latter being responsible for late relapses of the infection (see Figure 2.1). Thus, the existence of secondary exo-erythrocytic forms, developing from tissue schizonts and causing relapses of the infection, has now been disproved. The mean duration of the pre-erythrocytic stage of the primary tissue schizonts is 8 days; the number of merozoites in a mature tissue schizont on the eighth day is between 8000 and 20 000.

Some strains of *P. vivax* in the northern hemisphere (such as the Russian one, given the sub-specific name of *P. vivax hibernans* by Nikolaev in 1949) do not produce primary attacks soon after infection, and the first clinical symptoms occur 8–9 months after the infective bite. On the other hand, tropical strains of *P. vivax* tend to cause a number of randomly distributed, short-term relapses following an early primary attack. A delay of primary attack due to *P. vivax* or *P. ovale* infections may also be caused by inadequate chemotherapeutic suppression. There are also so-called intermediate sub-tropical strains with a delayed primary attack or a relapse after 9 months following an infection. It has been suggested that the chronological pattern of the primary attack and subsequent relapses depends on the relative proportion of the early and late sporozoites in a given strain of *P. vivax*. The validity of this attractive hypothesis could be tested by the cloning of haploid parasites from isolates displaying both immediate primary and delayed primary infections. Each clone should exhibit only one of the two phenotypes. Should both be found, it would suggest that it is the environment of individual sporozoites that determines the pattern of development in the liver.

Although the involvement of hypnozoites in the origin of relapses has been supported by much experimental evidence, there are still some unanswered questions. Thus, the stimulus which may activate the latent hypnozoite and provoke the relapse is still unknown. Despite the reported success in culture of both primary tissue schizonts and hypnozoites of *P. vivax*, the experimental possibility of observing the

rare change of a hypnozoite into a growing exo-erythrocytic schizont has yet to be observed.

During the erythrocytic development of *P. vivax*, all blood forms can be found in the circulation and most stages are larger than their counterparts in the other species of human plasmodium. The young trophozoite or ring grows rapidly and soon exhibits the characteristic malaria pigment. The parasite, when alive, has a pronounced amoeboid activity, and the presence of cytoplasmic 'pseudopodia' seen in a stained blood film is typical for this species. A large food vacuole forms a 'hole' in the ring until the division of the nucleus begins. After the nuclei have ceased to divide, the mature schizont, which has, on average, 12–18 merozoites, fills the entire host cell. Segmentation is followed by the rupture of the infected erythrocyte and release into the blood of merozoites and pigment. The merozoites, each measuring about 1.5 μm, invade fresh erythrocytes and the entire asexual erythrocytic cycle is repeated approximately every 48 hours; certain strains show a somewhat shorter periodicity. The degree of infection in vivax malaria rarely exceeds 50 000 per μL of blood as the merozoites can only invade reticulocytes. Infections of one erythrocyte by two or more parasites may be seen, but are not very common.

The periodicity of the asexual cycle of *P. vivax* is typically tertian, with gametocytes developing in the peripheral blood. The course of development of the parasite is well synchronized.

*P. vivax* has a striking effect on the invaded red blood cell, which gradually enlarges and becomes decolorized. A characteristic *stippling* in the form of small, reddish points appears in the infected erythrocyte and is known as Schüffner's dots (Figure 2.9). These are caused by formation of characteristic caveolae in the plasma membrane of the infected red blood cell.

Gametocytes may first be detected in the blood within 3 days after the first appearance of asexual parasites. Both male and female gametocytes are large, round or oval, filling nearly the whole enlarged and 'stippled' host cell (Figure 2.10). The macrogametocyte has a dense cytoplasm, staining dark blue, and a small, compact nucleus; the microgametocyte has a greyish-blue cytoplasm and a large diffuse nucleus. Both contain numerous pigment granules.

The gametocytes develop into gametes in the midgut of the *Anopheles*. After the exflagellation of the male (Figure 2.11) and fertilization of the female

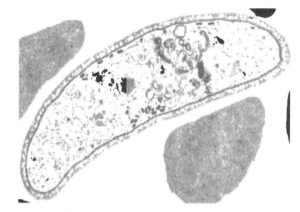

**Figure 2.10** *Electron micrograph of a longitudinal section through a macrogametocyte of* P. falciparum.

gamete, the sporogonic cycle takes 16 days at 20 °C and 8–10 days at 28 °C. Below 15 °C, the completion of the sporogonic cycle is unlikely.

The young oocyst has a light-brown pigment distributed in the form of fine granules without any distinctive pattern. In older oocysts, the granules are often arranged in a single or triple line (see Table 2.2).

## Plasmodium ovale

*Plasmodium ovale* infection produces a tertian pattern of fever similar to that of vivax malaria, but often with prolonged latency, a lesser trend to relapse and generally milder clinical symptoms. It was described in 1922 by Stephens, who saw it in the blood of a soldier who had returned from East Africa. *P. ovale* has been recorded chiefly from tropical Africa, in the west of which it is quite common. It has been reported sporadically from the west Pacific region and from southern China, Burma and South-east Asia. Some of these identifications are not absolutely certain and may relate to simian plasmodium.

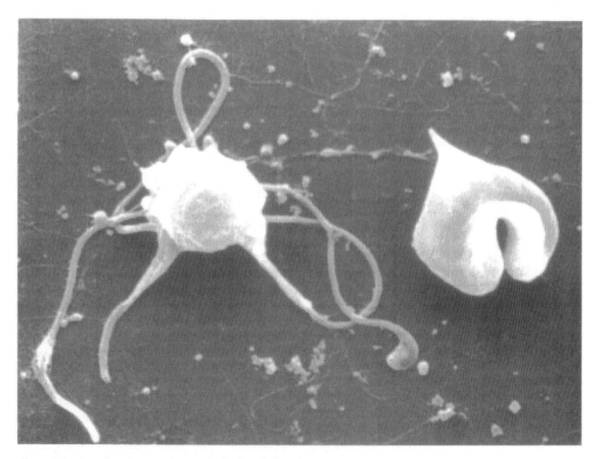

**Figure 2.11** *Scanning electron micrograph of exflagellation of a male gametocyte of* P. yoelii.

The asexual erythrocytic cycle of development of *P. ovale* is similar to that of *P. vivax* and extends over 48 hours. The pre-erythrocytic stage has a general period of 9 days, and the mature liver shizonts, some 60 μm in diameter, contain about 15 000 merozoites; the nucleus of the schizont-containing hepatocyte is often enlarged. The changes produced by the parasite on the infected erythrocytes are similar to those seen in *P. vivax*. The young trophozoites measure about one-third the diameter of the red blood cell. Schüffner's stippling appears quite early and is more pronounced than in the case of *P. vivax*. As the trophozoites grow, they show some resemblance to *P. malariae*; most of them are round and compact, with granules of pigment coarser than in *P. vivax* but not as coarse as in *P. malariae*. At this stage many erythrocytes are slightly enlarged and in thin films many of them assume an oval shape, with ragged or fimbriated margins and heavy stippling.

The schizonts may resemble those of *P. malariae*. They are rounded, compact and when mature contain eight to 10 nuclei, which are arranged peripherally around the central clump of pigment granules. Occasionally, the number of merozoites may be as high as 16.

The gametocytes of *P. ovale* resemble those of *P. malariae*, but the erythrocyte that contains them occasionally assumes an oval shape. The female gametocyte has a small, compact, bluish nucleus; the male's diffuse nucleus stains pale blue with a reddish tinge. The pigment in the oocyst is dark brown and the granules have a tendency to form chains which cross each other in the centre of the cyst. The completion of the sporogonic cycle in the mosquito takes 12–14 days at 28 °C (see Table 2.2).

## *Plasmodium malariae*

*Plasmodium malariae* is the causal organism of quartan malaria, so named because the paroxysms recur on the fourth day, after an interval of 2 days. The parasite differs from the other species affecting humans by its morphological characters and also by its slow development in both the human and the insect host. The course of the disease is not unduly severe, but its persistence is notorious. The geographical range of quartan malaria extends over both tropical and subtropical areas, especially West and East Africa, Guyana and parts of India, but its distribution tends to be patchy.

No direct evidence is available of pre-erythrocytic stages of *P. malariae* after the inoculation of sporozoites into the human host, but the evidence of such a stage has been obtained indirectly by infecting *Anopheles* mosquitoes with human *P. malariae* and inoculating sporozoites into a chimpanzee in whose liver exo-erythrocytic schizonts were demonstrated. *P. malariae* occurs naturally in chimpanzees and these animals may be potential reservoirs of quartan malaria. The old name of *P. rodhaini*, a parasite naturally found in chimpanzees, is synonymous with *P. malariae*. The pre-erythrocytic schizonts in the liver do not reach maturity until the 14th day after inoculation of sporozoites. When the mature schizont discharges the merozoites into the blood circulation, the asexual erythrocytic cycle begins and shows a 72-hour periodicity.

Infection with *P. malariae* has a tendency to persist in the human host for many years, perhaps even for a lifetime; this led to the hypothesis of a succession of several secondary exo-erythrocytic cycles in the liver. However, no late relapse forms of this parasite have been found in livers of chimpanzees infected with quartan plasmodia and the infection is as persistent after the inoculation of infected blood as it is after an injection of sporozoites. This seems to confirm that hypnozoites responsible for late relapses (in *P. vivax*) do not exist in *P. malariae* infections and that re-appearance of parasitaemia with clinical symptoms after periods of latency is presumably due to the recrudescence of the primary attack from erythrocytic forms persisting in very small numbers in internal organs.

The young trophozoites in the blood are not very different from those of *P. vivax*, although their cytoplasm is less attenuated and they stain more deeply. Older trophozoites, when rounded, are about half the size of the host cell. In thin films, the trophozoites may stretch across the entire width of the cell; such band forms are a characteristic feature of *P. malariae*. The pigment granules are numerous, large and dark.

The entire development of the trophozoite takes about 54 hours and, during the succeeding 18 hours, the parasite undergoes the schizogonic development. The nuclei of young schizonts divide repeatedly and finally the mature schizont has an average of eight merozoites (Figure 2.12). The merozoites occupy almost the entire erythrocyte and either form an irregular cluster or are arranged symmetrically

**Figure 2.12** In vitro *culture of* P. falciparum *using the technique of Trager and Jensen (1976). Note a number of fully grown schizonts, some ruptured schizonts and scattered free merozoites in this 48-hour culture, ×870. (Dr AJ Sulzer, Centers for Disease Control, Atlanta.)*

around the centre, in the form of a daisy. The term rosette is often applied to such schizonts.

P. malariae produces no evident changes in the host cells, although they may often appear somewhat smaller than uninfected erythrocytes. A special staining may show the presence of discrete stippling, often called Ziemann's stippling; these may be caused by knob-like protrusions on the red cell surface.

The degree of parasitaemia in quartan malaria is lower than in any other plasmodial infections and in naturally acquired infections the parasite count rarely exceeds 10 000/μL of blood. The 72-hour periodicity of the asexual cycle of development is usually well synchronized with all forms of parasite seen in the blood. The gametocytes probably develop in the internal organs and apparently appear in the peripheral blood only when fully grown. The female gametocyte has a deep-blue cytoplasm and a small, dense nucleus; the male stains pale blue and has a diffuse, larger nucleus. The sporogonic cycle in *Anopheles* takes 30–35 days at 20 °C; it may be as short as 14 days, although the average period is usually longer. The pigment in the oocysts is in the form of large, dark-brown granules

and has a characteristic peripheral distribution. The clumping of the pigment in a small area of the oocyst is of value in identifying the infection in the mosquito (see Table 2.2).

## Plasmodium (Laverania) falciparum

Of all the species of plasmodia that infect humans, P. falciparum is the most highly pathogenic, as indicated by the term *malignant* that is often applied to the type of malaria associated with it. This, in a non-immune subject, usually runs an acute course and, unless promptly treated with specific drugs, frequently terminates fatally.

It is the chief infection in areas of endemic malaria in Africa, and is also responsible for the great regional epidemics that were a feature of malaria in northwest India and Sri Lanka. It is generally confined to tropical or subtropical regions because the development in the mosquito is greatly retarded when the temperature falls below 20 °C. Even at this temperature, about 3 weeks are required for the maturation of sporozoites.

The asexual development of P. falciparum in the liver involves only a single primary schizogonic phase and hypnozoites do not occur. The earliest forms hitherto seen in the liver are schizonts measuring about 30 μm in diameter on the fourth day after infection. The number of merozoites in a mature schizont, which reaches some 60 μm in size, is about 30 000.

The young ring forms of P. falciparum, as usually seen in the peripheral blood, are very small, measuring about one-sixth of the diameter of a red blood cell. In many of the ring forms there may be two chromatin granules, and marginal (accolé) forms are fairly common. There are frequently several ring forms to be seen in a single host cell. This multiple invasion of erythrocytes may result from the tendency of uninfected erythrocytes to clump around a schizont-infected red blood cell in a process termed 'rosetting'.

Although marginal forms, rings with double chromatin dots and multiple infections of red cells may occur in other human plasmodia, they are much more common in P. falciparum and their presence is an important aid to diagnosis.

Later in the attack, the ring forms of P. falciparum may be considerably larger, measuring one-quarter and sometimes nearly one-half the diameter of a red cell, and may be mistaken for parasites of P. malariae.

They may have one or two grains of pigment in their cytoplasm.

In acute infections with numerous parasites, atypical forms are sometimes seen and these have erroneously been described under different specific names. For example, these amoeboid forms have been designated *P. tenue*, but this is not regarded as a valid species.

The succeeding developmental stages of the asexual erythrocytic cycle (trophozoites and schizonts) do not generally occur in the blood, except in severe 'pernicious' cases. The presence of maturing or mature schizonts of *P. falciparum* in a blood film is therefore often an indication for prompt and vigorous treatment. Segmenting forms of *P. falciparum* are easily recognized by having one or at most two solid aggregations of pigment. In other species of human malaria parasites, beyond the half-grown stage there may be 20 or more pigment granules; the form of these pigment granules is affected by antimalarial drugs: chloroquine causes clumping and mefloquine causes them to disappear entirely.

The ring forms and older trophozoites usually disappear from the peripheral circulation after 24 hours and are held (sequestered) in the capillaries of the internal organs, such as the brain, heart, placenta, spleen, intestine or bone marrow, where their further development takes place. This sequestration is caused by an adherence between endothelial lining cells and the knob-like projections on the red blood cell surface; within the knobs, the parasite antigen PfEMP-1 is expressed and it is the interaction of this molecule with molecules on the capillary endothelium such as intracellular adhesion molecule 1 (ICAM-1) that is responsible for sequestration. In the course of 24 hours, the parasites in the capillaries multiply by schizogony. When the schizont is fully grown it occupies about two-thirds of the red cell. Finally, it undergoes segmentation, giving rise to between eight and 24 merozoites, the average number being 16. The mature schizont of *P. falciparum* is smaller than that of any of the other malaria parasites. The parasitaemia reached in falciparum malaria is considerably higher than in the other forms, the density of parasites sometimes exceeding 300 000/μL of blood.

The distribution of the parasites in organs and tissues of the human body varies from case to case, thus accounting for the diversity of clinical manifestations observed in falciparum malaria. Most of the severe and fatal cases show blocking (occlusion) of the capillaries by clumped rosettes of red blood cells harbouring developing parasites, enormous numbers of which can be seen in smears and sections of post-mortem material (see Chapter 10). The presence of high levels of *P. falciparum* antigen and immunoglobulin G (IgG) deposits in the adjacent capillary basement membrane may suggest that the damage to cerebral capillaries could be due to immunopathological mechanisms. Alternatively, the concentration of schizonts in the capillaries could result (at schizogony) in the generation of high local concentrations of TNF. In falciparum malaria, the infected red cells retain their normal size throughout all stages of development of the parasites. Cells harbouring the older trophozoites and schizonts are frequently stippled, with a few coarse reddish dots (Maurer's dots) scattered over about two-thirds of the erythrocyte.

Although erythrocytic schizogony in *P. falciparum* is completed in 48 hours and the periodicity of development is therefore of typically tertian type, there frequently occurs in this species two or more broods of parasites, the segmentation of which is not synchronized, so that the periodicity of symptoms in the patient tends to be irregular.

The development of the gametocytes takes place in the inner organs, but sometimes young forms are seen in the blood. The development of these parasites is described above. Mature crescentic gametocytes usually appear in the peripheral blood for the first time about 10 days after the initial invasion of the blood. In this time the asexual parasites will have undergone four to five rounds of replication in the blood. The female form, or macrogametocyte, is usually a deeper blue colour with Romanowsky stains. The nucleus is small and compact, with a magenta inclusion, and the pigment granules are closely aggregated round it. The male form, or microgametocyte, is either pale blue or tinted with pink, and the nucleus, which can stain dark pink, is large and less compact than in the female. The pigment granules are more widely scattered in the cytoplasm around the nucleus. The number of gametocytes present in falciparum infections is variable, occasionally amounting to 50 000–150 000/μL of blood. Individuals can be infectious to mosquitoes with gametocytaemias as low as 10/μL.

The mosquito phase of *P. falciparum* conforms with that described for mammalian plasmodia in general. Its duration at 20 °C is 22 days; at 23 °C, 15–17 days; and at 28 °C, 9–10 days (see Table 2.2). The pigment in the oocyst is almost black and the granules are relatively large. It usually forms a double circle around the periphery, but it may be arranged as a small circle in the centre, or even as a double straight chain. By the eighth day, much of the pigment becomes obscured, but a few grains can still be seen.

## Mixed infections

Infections due to two or more species of malaria parasites are not uncommon, but they are often overlooked. In endemic malarious areas, mixed infections are particularly frequent; there is a tendency for one species of the parasite to predominate over the other. The most common types of mixed infections are *P. falciparum* and *P. vivax* in subtropical areas; in tropical Africa, *P. falciparum* and *P. malariae* are prevalent, although *P. falciparum* and *P. ovale* are also frequent. On rare occasions all three species can be found in one blood film.

In the past, the best way of diagnosing a mixed infection with more than one species of plasmodia was by a careful and longer than usual microscopical examination of the blood film. Some characteristics of infection with the four species of human plasmodia are given in Table 2.3. More recently, the use of polymerase chain reaction (PCR) techniques to distinguish mixed infections has become reliable, although its ability to distinguish rare parasites in the presence of high parasitaemias of the other species has not yet been fully explored.

## ANIMAL PLASMODIA

## Simian plasmodia

The presence of malaria parasites in the blood of monkeys was observed as early as 1893 and one of these parasites, found in an East African monkey, received the name of *P. kochi* (later renamed *Hepatocystis kochi* by Garnham). In 1907, the discovery of *P. cynomolgi* in *Macaca fascicularis* from Java was of particular interest because of its resemblance to the *P. vivax* of humans; and during the first quarter of the twentieth century a series of other simian plasmodia were found in monkeys in the field or in zoos worldwide. Much of the early work on simian malaria was

done in India, where *P. knowlesi* was isolated in 1932 from *Macaca fascicularis* and subsequently transmitted to humans. The study of plasmodia of higher apes (chimpanzees and gorillas) was given great impetus by Rodhain, who showed in 1940 the identity of *P. malariae* of humans with that of *P. rodhaini* of chimpanzees.

In 1947, Garnham demonstrated the true nature of *H. kochi* in the East African monkey *Cercopithecus aethiops*. He showed that the blood forms of this parasite are composed of gametocytes only, and he discovered the presence in the liver of infected monkeys of the exo-erythrocytic stages of the parasite. The final stage of development in the tissue is a merocyst with a large vacuole; the numerous merozoites present in a simple merocyst invade the bloodstream. This finding was the first step towards the subsequent discovery of exo-erythrocytic stages of the true malaria parasites. The vector of *H. kochi* is a *Culicoides*, as found by Garnham in 1951.

The importance of studies on simian malaria was brilliantly demonstrated by Short and Garnham in 1948. The discovery of exo-erythrocytic stages in the liver of monkeys infected with *P. cynomolgi* pointed the way to finding the tissue stages of *P. vivax* in humans.

Although the relationship between the malaria parasites of monkeys and those of humans had already become obvious in the 1930s, when *P. knowlesi* was used in Romania for malaria therapy by blood infection, the question of simian malaria as a zoonosis only became important in the 1960s. In those years, American workers described the case of an accidental laboratory infection by *P. cynomolgi bastianelli* transmitted from *M. fascicularis* through mosquitoes. The tertian periodicity of the febrile illness and the presence of vivax-like parasites in the blood of the accidentally infected individual drew attention to the possibility of natural transmission of the disease from monkeys to humans.

*P. cynomolgi* infections in the rhesus monkey have occupied an important place in the search for new antimalarials between 1950 and 1960. This model offered a useful biological chemotherapeutic counterpart of *P. vivax* infection of humans. It was due to this model that the identification of primaquine as a radical cure of relapsing malaria became possible. Further work, especially in Malaysia and Brazil, was responsible for a surge of new knowledge of simian malaria. Within 5 years, the number of species of

**Table 2.3** *Some characteristics of infection with four species of human plasmodia*

| Species | Plasmodium vivax | Plasmodium ovale | Plasmodium malariae | Plasmodium falciparum |
|---|---|---|---|---|
| Pre-erythrocytic stage (days) | 6–8 | 9 | 14–16 | 5.5–7 |
| Prepatent period (days) | 11–13 | 10–14 | 15–16 | 9–10 |
| Incubation period (days) | 15 (12–17) or up to 6–12 months | 17 (16–18) or longer | 28 (18–40) or longer | 12 (9–14) |
| Erythrocytic cycle (hours) | 48 (about) | 50 | 72 | 48 |
| Parasitaemia per µL (mm$^3$) | | | | |
| Average | 20 000 | 9 000 | 6 000 | 20 000–500 000 |
| Maximum | 50 000 | 30 000 | 20 000 | 2 000 000 |
| Primary attack[a] | Mild to severe | Mild | Mild | Severe in non-immunes |
| Febrile paroxysm (hours) | 8–12 | 8–12 | 8–10 | 16–36 or longer |
| Relapses | ++ | ++ | – | – |
| Period of recurrence[b] | Variable | Variable | Very long | Short |
| Duration of untreated infection (years) | 1.5–5 | Probably the same as P. vivax | 3–50 | 1–2 |

[a]The severity of infection and the degree of parasitaemia are greatly influenced by the immune responses Chemoprophylaxis may suppress an initial attack for weeks or months.
[b]Patterns of infection and of relapses vary greatly in different strains

plasmodia recognized in lower monkeys increased to about a dozen.

It was soon found that, in addition to the confirmed possibility of transmission to humans of *P. cynomolgi* through mosquitoes, other plasmodia of lower monkeys, such as *P. brazilianum* and *P. inui*, could be transmitted in the same way. Although the possibility of the two-way transmission (monkey–vector–humans) of simian malaria in natural conditions was experimentally established, the proof that it can happen in nature was provided in three cases of human infection with *P. knowlesi* in Malaya and in another case of a similar infection with *P. simium* in Brazil. Recognizing that *P. vivax* does not invade Duffy-negative red blood cells, it is of interest that people of African descent are refractory to infections with *P. cynomolgi*, *P. inui*, *P. knowlesi* and *P. schwetzi*. These exceptional occurrences, while stressing the close relationship between human and some simian *Plasmodium* spp., do not invalidate the fact that in nature the only true reservoir of human malaria parasites is the infected human being.

During the past 20 years, an increasing amount of research has shown not only that some *Plasmodium* spp. of monkeys or apes can be transmitted to humans, but also that human malaria parasites can be successfully transmitted to some lower primates and especially to several species of neotropical monkeys. The latter finding, by Young and his colleagues in Panama in 1960, was of special significance because it opened an entirely new field for experimental chemotherapy of malaria.

*P. vivax*, *P. falciparum* and *P. malariae* can now be transmitted to the Colombian night monkey, *Aotus trivirgatus*. Inoculation with blood forms is the usual procedure. Receptivity is greatly enhanced by splenectomy. Transmission by sporozoites is rarely successful, even in splenectomized *Aotus* monkeys. Other South American monkeys (*Ayeles, Cebus, Saimiri, Saguinus*) are also susceptible to infection with human plasmodia, but the *Aotus* is by far the most useful experimental animal in this respect. A re-transmission of *P. falciparum* from *Aotus* to humans has been achieved. The value of this species is so great that its wide use in various research centres has now led to a great shortage of *Aotus* and to an embargo imposed by some South American governments on the trapping and exportation of these animals.

Some characteristics of the main species of simian malaria parsites are shown in Table 2.4.

## Plasmodia of other mammalian hosts

Mammalian parasites of the genus *Plasmodium* are now classified under the sub-genus *Vinckeia*, which comprises some 20 species found in rodents, lower primates, bats and other mammals. Whereas some of these are of veterinary interest, perhaps the most important roles played by these parasites are as convenient laboratory models of human malarias.

The use of any non-human malarial parasite as a model is fraught with difficulties, for two reasons: (1) none of the hosts is human and the responses of these hosts to infection cannot be taken as definitive for the human condition; (2) (except for *P. reichenowi* and *P. brazilianum*) the parasites are themselves very significantly different from the four species that infect humans. Thus, it is only by the intelligent and objective use of these models that understanding of the human parasites can be advanced.

The rodent malarial parasites have played a central role in malarial research since their discovery in 1948, and now are perhaps the most accessible to molecular and cell research of any species. Particular advantage stems from the fact that the rodent parasite (*P. berghei*), the mouse host, and a convenient vector (*A. stephensi*) can all be genetically manipulated, thus permitting penetrating studies of defined molecular interactions between the parasite and its hosts *in vivo*. The ability to culture the parasite *in vitro* for all stages of the life cycle (with the exception of oocyst-to-sporozoite differentiation) adds further power to this potential. The decision to sequence the entire genome of the most frequently used rodent parasites (*P. berghei*, *P. yoelii* and *P. chabaudi*) and an anopheline vector (*A. gambiae*) will provide significant opportunities for future understanding of host–parasite interactions at the molecular level.

*P. berghei* was discovered in *A. dureni* in the forest gallery in Zaire by Vincke and Lipps in 1948, and subsequently described in the blood of the tree rat, *Thamnomys surdaster*. It is conveniently run in laboratory strains of mice, rats and hamsters, and the natural host can also be colonized, with difficulty. Mosquito transmission proved difficult until it was recognized that mechanical blood passage permitted the development of parasite isolates with poor sexual development, that host responses to high asexual parasitaemias suppressed infectivity and, most importantly, that (being highland forest vectors) mosquito development required temperatures below 24 °C.

**Table 2.4** *Important species of simian plasmodia[a]*

| Species | Natural host | Geographical distribution | Natural vector | Periodicity | Remarks |
|---|---|---|---|---|---|
| P. brazilianum | Alouatta sp. Ateles sp. Cebus sp. Lagotrix sp. and others | Brazil Colombia Panama Peru, Venezuela | A. (Kerteszia) cruzii | Quartan | Several Central and South American monkeys found naturally infected Transmissible to humans |
| P. coatneyi | Macaca fascicularis, | Malaysia | A. hackeri | Tertian | Sub-species |
| P. cynomolgi | Macaca sp. Presbytis sp. | South-east Asia | A. hackeri A. balabacensis and others | Tertian | known as bastianellii Laboratory infections of humans |
| P. fieldi | Macaca nemestrina Macaca follicularis | Malaysia | A. balabacensis A. hackeri | Tertian | |
| P. fragile | Macaca radiata | Sri Lanka, Southern India | A. elegans | Tertian | |
| P. inui | Macaca sp. Presbytis sp. | South-east Asia | A. balabacensis | Quartan | Sub-species known as shortti |
| P. knowlesi | Macaca sp. Presbytis sp. | India South-east Asia | A. hackeri | Quotidian | Transmissible to humans; natural infection reported from Malaysia |
| P. pitheci | Pongo pygmeu (orang-utan) | Borneo | Unknown | Possibly tertian | |
| P. (Laverania) reichenowi | Pan satyrus (chimpanzee) Gorilla sp. | Equatorial Africa Sierra Leone Liberia | Unknown | Tertian | Not transmissible to humans |
| P. rodhaini Synonymous with P. malariae | Pan satyrus Homo sapiens | West and Central Africa | Presumably the same that transmit human malaria | Quartan | |
| P. schwetzi | Pan satyrus Gorilla sp. | West Africa, Cameroon, Lower Congo | Unknown | Tertian | Transmissible to humans |
| P. simium | Alouatta sp. Brachyteles sp. | Brazil | Unknown | Tertian | Natural infection of humans reported |

[a] Partly after Garnham (1966) and Wernsdorfer (1980).
Note. Other species of simian plasmodia not mentioned in this table are: *P. eylesi, P. jefferyi, P. youngi* from Malaysia; *P. gonderi* from West Africa and Cameroon; *P. simiovale* from Sri Lanka and *P. sylvaticum* from Borneo

The *P. berghei* life cycle is as follows: tissue schizogony 43–50 hours; asexual schizogony 22–24 hours; gametocyte development 24–26 hours; ookinete maturation in blood meal and mid-gut invasion 24–30 hours; oocyst maturation (at 21 °C) 18 days; persistence of salivary gland infections up to 39 days at 21 °C. In the asexual phase of blood infections, the parasite preferentially invades reticulocytes, schizogony results in the formation of 6–20 merozoites, and multiple infections are common, particularly at high parasitaemias.

Further studies on the rodents of Africa led to the discovery of *P. vinckei* by Rodhain in 1952, *P. chabaudi* in 1965 and *P. yoelii* in 1966. Six sub-species have been described, many of which were diagnosed by biochemical (isoenzyme) analysis of established (mixed species) laboratory isolates. Mosquito transmission of these species can be achieved using *A. stephensi* as a convenient vector. The differing biology of these parasites requires different management procedures, i.e. *P. chabaudi* is most infectious some 10–14 days after blood infection, whereas *P. yoelii* and *P. berghei* are most infectious prior to the first rise in asexual parasitaemia (i.e. at parasitaemias below 15 per cent). All the above parasites have proved to be most useful to research on basic parasite cell and molecular biology, in the screening and preliminary evaluation of drugs (in the USA some 300 000 compounds have been screened in the past 30 years), and in analysis of the basic immunology of malarial infections. Whereas *P. berghei* is by far the most comprehensively studied and manipulable parasite, *P. chabaudi* is considered by some to be more appropriate for studies on the asexual blood stages because the infections are naturally synchronous. It cannot be overemphasized that caution must be exercised in the direct relevance of such observations to the human situation, because both host and parasite are different.

## Avian plasmodia

Malaria parasites of birds are found in nearly every country in the world. This is largely due to the migratory flights of birds and the widespread occurrence of susceptible mosquito vectors. It was Danilewsky in Russia who, in 1884, first observed malaria parasites in the blood of birds. His major work, published in 1894, indicated the wide distribution of these parasites. Ross in 1897 demonstrated the development of

*P. relictum* in culicine mosquitoes fed on infected sparrows. In 1899–1900, Grassi and other Italian workers described a number of avian malaria parasites and their transmission by mosquitoes.

Over 450 species of birds have now been found infected with malaria parasites. Avian malaria parasites are classified into the sub-genera *Haemamoeba*, *Biovannolaia*, *Novyella* and *Huffia*. They comprise over 40 species, the identification of which is not easy and must be based on observation of various stages of the life cycle and certain biological features.

After the discoveries of Ross and Grassi, it seemed that the knowledge of the life cycle of the malaria parasites was complete, but it soon became obvious that there must be an unknown phase between the introduction of the sporozoite and the appearance of parasites in the blood. Grassi formulated this idea in 1906, but there was no definite proof of the presence of these forms in the body of the host. It was not until 1934–36 that Raffaele described the exo-erythrocytic forms of *P. elongatum* and *P. relictum* in the bone marrow and brain of birds. These findings were soon confirmed in *P. gallinaceum* by James and Tate and were a precursor to the discovery of exo-erythrocytic schizogony in malaria parasites of primates.

The main characteristics that distinguish avian malaria parasites from those of primates are as follows: (1) avian parasites are found in nucleated erythrocytes; (2) they are transmitted mainly by mosquitoes of the genera *Aedes* and *Culex* and very rarely by *Anopheles*; (3) the exo-erythrocytic stages of avian parasites are found in mesodermal tissue, the primary cycle occupies two generations and can arise from blood stages.

Prior to the discovery of the rodent parasites, the avian plasmodia contributed greatly to the early development of antimalarial drugs. One facet of their usefulness was the very early ability to culture the tissue stages *in vitro*; the prolific and repetitive nature of tissue schizogony permitted very high-density cultures to be achieved. Both *in vivo* and *in vitro* studies on *P. cathemerium*, *P. circumflexum*, *P. lophurae*, *P. relictum* and, notably, *P. gallinaceum* have contributed significantly to our current understanding of tissue schizogony and, more recently, to the early phases of the discovery and development of transmission-blocking vaccines. It is perhaps in the discovery of antimalarial drugs where avian malaria made its first major impact. In 1926, Roehl in Germany introduced quantitative methods of assessment of the antimalarial action of new compounds. Roehl's test was based on infecting canaries with *P. relictum*; untreated birds showed parasites in the blood after 4–5 days, whereas birds given quinine by a stomach tube showed no parasitaemia. This method was used as a primary screening test of a number of antimalarial drugs developed in Germany during the 1930s, one product of which was the most effective compound produced to date – chloroquine.

## Plasmodia of other animals

Among other species of animal plasmodium described to date, two were found in Madagascar lemurs, one was discovered in Indian buffalo, three in African and Malaysian deer, and one each in an African squirrel and a fruit bat.

At least 41 species of malaria parasites have been described in reptiles such as lizards, iguanas, skinks and snakes from various, but mainly tropical, parts of the world. The classification of these parasites is difficult because their schizogony takes place in blood cells other than erythrocytes, and their morphology varies according to the host. It is probable that some culicine mosquitoes and phlebotomid flies are the usual vectors. None of these parasites has yet been found to infect common laboratory animals.

## REFERENCES

Aikawa M, Miller LH, Johnson JG, Rabbege J. Erythrocyte entry by malarial parasites. A moving junction between erythrocyte and parasite. *J Cell Biol* 1978; **77**: 72–82.

Aikawa M, Miller LH, Rabbege JR, Epstein N. Freeze fracture study on the erythrocyte membrane during malarial parasite invasion. *J Cell Biol* 1981; **92**: 55–62

Aikawa M, Miller LH. Structural alternation of the erythrocyte membrane during malarial parasite invasion and intraerythrocytic development. In *Malaria and the red cell*. Ciba Foundation Symposium 94. London, Pitman, 1983, 45–63.

Barnwell JW, Galinski MR. Invasion of erythrocytes. In *Malaria: biology, pathogenesis and protection*. Sherman IW, ed. Washington DC, A.S.M. Press, 1998, 93–120.

Bray RS, Garnham PCC. Life-cycle of primate malaria parasites. *Br Med Bull* 1982; **38**: 117–22.

Cochrane AH, Aikawa M, Jeng M, Nussenzweig RS. Antibody-induced ultrastructural changes of malarial sporozoites. *J Immunol* 1976; **116**: 859–67.

Garnham PCC. Exerythrocytic schizogony in *Plasmodium kochi* Laveran. A preliminary note. *Trans R Soc Trop Med Hyg* 1947; **40**: 719–22.

Garnham PCC. An attempt to find the vector of *Hepatocystis (=Plasmodium)* Kochi (Levaditi and Schoen). *Exp Parasitol* 1951; **1**: 94–107.

Garnham PCC. *Malaria parasites and other Haemosporidia*. Oxford, Blackwell Scientific Publications, 1966.

Garnham PCC. Malaria parasites of man: life-cycles and morphology (excluding ultrastructure). In *Principles and practice of malariology*. Wernsdorfer WH, McGregor Sir I, eds. Edinburgh, Churchill Livingstone, 1988, 61–96.

James SP, Tate P. Exo-erythrocytic schizogony in *Plasmodium gallinaceum* Brumpt 1935. *Parasitology* 1938; **30**: 128–39.

Landau I, Chabaud AAG, Mora-Silvera E, Coquelin F, Boulard YR, Snounou G. Survival of rodent malaria merozoites in the lymphatic network: potential role in chronicity of the infection. *Parasite* 1999; **6**: 311–22.

Rodhain J. *Plasmodium vinkei* n. sp. Un deuxième *Plasmodium* parasite de rongeurs sauvage au Katanga. *Annales des Sociétés Belges de Medicine Tropicale* 1952; **32**: 275–9.

Shaudinn F. Untersuchungen über den Generationswechsel bei Coccidien. *Zoologische Jahrbücher* 1899; **13**: 197–292.

Shortt H, Garnham PCC. The pre-erythrocytic development of *Plasmodium cynomolgi* and *Plasmodium vivax*. *Trans R Soc trop Med Hyg* **41**: 785–95.

Tomas AM, Margos G, Dimopoulos G, *et al*. Successful transmission of the malarial parasite through the mosquito requires the expression of P25 or P28: bifunctional, conserved, mutually redundant ookinete surface proteins. *EMBO J 2001*; **20**: 3975–83.

Trager W, Jensen JB. Human malaria parasites in continuous culture. *Science* 1976; **193**: 673–5.

Wernsdorfer WH. The importance of malaria in the world. In *Malaria*, Vol. 1. Kreier JP, ed. New York, London, Academic Press, 1980, 1–93.

Young MD, Porter JA, Johnsen CM. *Plasmodium vivax* transmitted from man to monkey to man. *Science* 1966; **153**: 1006–7.

# 3

# Diagnostic methods in malaria

MARCEL HOMMEL

Malaria may be defined as an illness caused by the development of *Plasmodium* spp. parasites within host red blood cells. It follows that diagnosis might first be suggested by the clinical features presented or described by the patient, then confirmed by evidence of the presence of parasites in the peripheral blood. The correct and timely diagnosis of malaria is critically important because the infection may rapidly develop into a life-threatening form of the disease, requiring urgent medical attention. A history of travel to a malaria-endemic area usually provides a helpful hint.

Microscopy remains the crucial methodology for malaria diagnosis. When performed in optimal conditions, the technique has a remarkable sensitivity (it can detect a parasitaemia as low as 0.0001 per cent), it is specific and enables the identification of the parasite at the species level, and it is quantitative, reasonably easy to perform and cheap (Figure 3.1). A variety of alternatives to microscopy have been described, based on modern technologies, including the quantitative buffy coat technique (QBC®), various antigen detection methods and the polymerase chain reaction (PCR). These may have a place in diagnosis in specific situations, but none has so far out-performed microscopy in all its features.

In situations in which laboratory facilities are not available, a 'presumptive' diagnosis may need to be made on clinical features alone, sometimes with the help of a suitable algorithm developed to suit local conditions. This will enable the physician to start treatment early and confirm the diagnosis later.

A review of diagnostic methods for malaria will, of necessity, have to consider the different situations in which diagnosis is required: in rudimentary field conditions where the only available method is to rely on a basic clinical algorithm; in a district hospital in a tropical environment where microscopy is routinely performed; or in a traveller returning to an industrialized country where sophisticated diagnostic methods may be available alongside microscopy. Finding the parasite is only one of the steps in malaria diagnosis, because infection does not necessarily imply disease and clinical judgement is always required. Thus, the detection of a few parasites in a blood film of a child indigenous to an endemic area demonstrates the presence of infection, but it does not necessarily determine the actual cause for which medical aid was sought – a child may have pneumonia while carrying malaria parasites. The concept of a 'threshold', above which infection generally means disease, is particularly difficult to define, because it is

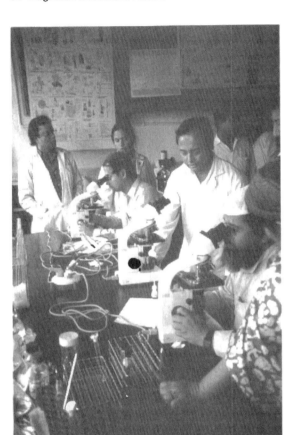

**Figure 3.1** *The microscopical examination of stained blood films is the fundamental technique for finding malaria parasites. This picture shows the training of microscopists in Bangladesh. (M Hommel.)*

variable from one endemic area to another, is age-dependent and needs to be adjusted to the local level of endemicity. Apart from individual diagnosis, methods for detecting malaria parasites or other evidence of malaria infection may be required for epidemiological studies or for the screening blood transfusion units. Finally, in order to evaluate the burden of disease due to malaria in a community, retrospective diagnostic methodologies based on questionnaires ('verbal autopsy') may be of use.

Diagnosis also has a role to play in patient management and in the follow-up of chemotherapy. Apart from the finding of parasites, other laboratory tests may need to be performed to detect signs of poor prognosis (haemoglobin level, blood glucose, lactate, presence of protein or free haemoglobin in the urine)

or to guide chemotherapy (glucose-6-phosphate dehydrogenase, G6PD).

## PRESUMPTIVE DIAGNOSIS AND CLINICAL ALGORITHMS

In many parts of the world, malaria diagnosis and treatment have to be performed without the benefit of laboratory support. Considering the spectacular nature of a typical paroxysm and also the rhythmic pattern of an intermittent fever, it may be thought that malaria is an infection that can be diagnosed with considerable specificity on the basis of the concurrence of these two features. However, this is not the case. The chances of making an accurate diagnosis on clinical grounds alone are probably highest in *P. vivax* infections and lowest in *P. falciparum* infections, in which paroxysms are not well defined and in which the presenting features are often non-specific and may be similar to those of other infections (notably influenza, pneumonia, viral hepatitis or typhoid fever).

In areas of high endemicity, fever is often equated with malaria and treated as such. Such a presumptive diagnosis may be correct in a reasonable percentage of cases during the transmission season, but outside that season (when fever is generally not caused by malaria but is still treated as such), many patients may be inappropriately given antimalarials. In a study performed in Mali in 1991, only 53.9 per cent of cases diagnosed as malaria during the rainy season actually had parasites, but diagnostic efficiency dropped to 4.5 per cent during the dry season (Rougemont *et al.*, 1991). As long as malaria parasites were highly sensitive to chloroquine, a treatment based on such a presumptive diagnosis was a sound and cost-effective approach. A number of studies have shown that a history of intermittent fever, in the absence of otitis, tonsillitis or a respiratory infection, can be a very useful predictor of malaria and, in areas where laboratory facilities are lacking, it can represent the most important tool for reducing malaria-attributable morbidity and mortality. In situations in which chloroquine is no longer the recommended first-line treatment, more toxic and more expensive drugs have to be used and it is necessary either to change policies and ensure that microscopy is widely available or, in situations where this is not feasible, to design basic clinical algorithms that can predict malaria infection with greater precision. Such algorithms are based on the concept that a correct diagnosis can be made by minimally trained health workers and they function best when adapted to local needs (Redd *et al.*, 1996).

A successful algorithm will include the most commonly observed symptoms and signs of the disease (taking local clinical idiosyncrasies into account), as well as the commonest causes for misdiagnosis (for example, the well-known overlap of signs and symptoms between malaria and pneumonia). Fever (or 'hot body'), nail or palmar pallor (a reliable sign of anaemia), together with the finding of splenomegaly, form the basis of the 'malaria score'. The specificity of the score may be improved by a number of negative features, such as the absence of a cough or rash, and a normal chest examination (Trape *et al.*, 1985; Olaleye *et al.*, 1998).

The concept of clinical algorithms can be taken too far. The implementation of algorithms as the routine diagnosis procedure in the context of National Malaria Control Programmes (where the aim of using such an algorithm is, at least in part, to reduce unnecessary treatment and save money) has been criticized by some authors, who feel that presumptive diagnosis can only ever be second best and that laboratory diagnosis should be provided wherever possible. Economic comparisons between presumptive and microscopy-based diagnoses suggest that, contrary to common belief, microscopy may actually be more cost-effective (Jonkman *et al.*, 1995). A more serious criticism is that, if algorithms are considerably more selective than the provision of antimalarial treatment based on fever alone, many African children (whose symptoms and signs do not fit in the algorithm, but who may still have malaria) will be denied treatment for a potentially fatal disease. This would not be justified, even in areas where pyrimethamine-sulphadoxine has replaced chloroquine as the first-line drug (Olivar *et al.*, 1991; Marsh *et al.*, 1996). In areas where endemicity is lower and more seasonal or in areas where quinine has become the first-line drug (as is the case in parts of Southeast Asia), the use of presumptive treatment – even based on a clinical algorithm – is hard to justify. When tested in Thailand, the best clinical algorithm could only predict 49 per cent of true malaria cases (thus leaving half the potentially fatal cases untreated) and was unable to predict whether the infection was falciparum or vivax malaria (Luxemburger *et al.*, 1998).

## BLOOD EXAMINATION FOR MALARIA PARASITES

The only certain means of diagnosing all four of the human malarias is the detection of the *Plasmodium* sp. by microscopic examination of the blood. This examination should be a routine procedure in medical practice, not only in all malarious areas, but also in non-malarious countries, whatever may be the symptoms of primary diagnosis, if the patient has been travelling abroad within a year. The aims of blood examination are to find out:

- if the patient is infected,
- the level of infection,
- which is the infected species.

Each of these findings will have direct implications for patient management.

## Biosafety

It is well established that various pathogens, such as the hepatitis B virus, the human immunodeficiency virus (HIV) and malaria itself, can be transmitted by contact with infected blood during the taking of blood samples. Accordingly, invasive blood sampling techniques such as venepuncture or finger pricking should only be used when the risk is justified by the potential benefit. Health workers who are required to take blood samples for malaria diagnostic purposes should be aware of the potential risks to their patients and themselves and should always follow the recommended biosafety practices to avoid the possibility of cross-infection or autoinfection with these blood pathogens. The risks and recommended precautionary measures are described in detail by Cheesbrough (1998).

## Preparation of blood films

For malaria blood films, use perfectly clean 25 mm × 75 mm glass slides that are free of grease and scratches. Slides that have been previously used should be first soaked in lysol or detergent, then individually rubbed to remove traces of old smears, and finally rinsed and polished. When working in a tropical country, slides should be kept in a dry, dust-free environment.

Blood should be collected as soon as possible if malaria is suspected and before the patient receives antimalarial treatment. (It may be necessary to collect blood on several occasions to detect parasites). Blood may be obtained from the second or third finger (or the heel or big toe in infants). The skin should be cleaned with ether or methylated spirit and allowed to dry. Using a sterile lancet (Microlance), prick the finger or heel, then squeeze gently to obtain a good blood drop (Figure 3.2).

Both a thick film and a thin film should be prepared. The thick film provides the sensitivity (it is about 15 times more sensitive than the thin film and can detect parasitaemia at a level as low as 20 parasites/μL), whereas the thin film provides the specificity by confirming which species of *Plasmodium* is involved. The thick film is not fixed prior to staining, so that red blood cells are lysed, allowing parasites to be seen in a much larger volume of blood.

For a thick film, touch the drop of blood with a glass slide held above it. Then, after reversing the slide, spread the blood evenly with a corner of another slide to make a square or a circular patch of moderate thickness that will just allow one to read

through it. Keep the slide horizontal while drying and protect it from dust and flies (Figures 3.3 and 3.4).

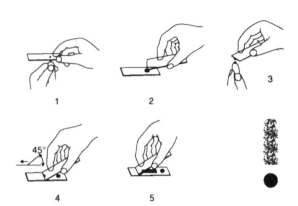

**Figure 3.3** *Preparation of a thin and thick blood film on the same slide. 1. Touch the drop of blood with a clean slide. 2. Spread the drop of blood with the corner of another slide to make a circle or a square about 1 cm². 3. Touch a new drop of blood with the edge of a clean slide. 4. Bring the edge of the slide, carrying the drop of blood, to the surface of the first slide; wait until the blood has spread along the whole edge. 5. Holding the slide at an angle of about 45°, push it forward with a rapid, but not too brisk, movement. Write the slide number with a pencil on the thin film. Wait until the thick film is quite dry. (WHO, 1961.)*

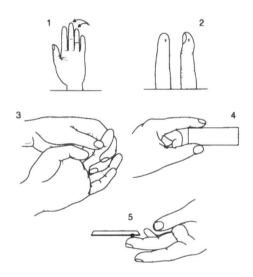

**Figure 3.2** *Details of the correct technique of blood collection for a thin or thick blood film. 1. The second or third finger is generally selected. 2. The site of puncture is the side of the ball of the finger, not too close to the nail bed. 3. If the blood does not flow well, a gentle squeeze will improve it. 4. The slide must always be grasped by its edges. 5. The size of the blood drop is controlled better if the finger touches the slide from below. (WHO, 1961.)*

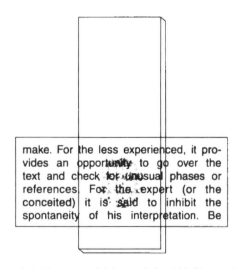

make. For the less experienced, it provides an opportunity to go over the text and check for unusual phases or references. For the expert (or the conceited) it is said to inhibit the spontaneity of his interpretation. Be

**Figure 3.4** *The correct thickness of the thick film can be judged by the legibility of the printed text seen through the slide. The print should be just legible.*

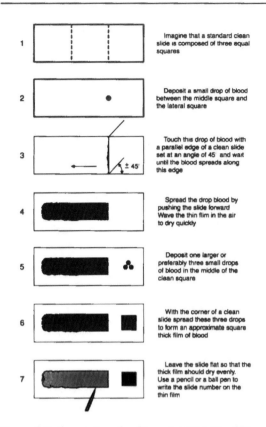

| | |
|---|---|
| 1 | Imagine that a standard clean slide is composed of three equal squares |
| 2 | Deposit a small drop of blood between the middle square and the lateral square |
| 3 | Touch this drop of blood with a parallel edge of a clean slide set at an angle of 45° and wait until the blood spreads along this edge |
| 4 | Spread the drop blood by pushing the slide forward Wave the thin film in the air to dry quickly |
| 5 | Deposit one larger or preferably three small drops of blood in the middle of the clean square |
| 6 | With the corner of a clean slide spread these three drops to form an approximate square thick film of blood |
| 7 | Leave the slide flat so that the thick film should dry evenly. Use a pencil or a ball pen to write the slide number on the thin film |

**Figure 3.5** *Preparation of a thin and a thick blood film on the same slide (alternative method). (WHO, 1961.)*

For a thin film, the drop of blood should be smaller than for the thick film. Apply the smooth edge of another clean glass slide to the drop of blood at an angle of 45°. Touch the drop of blood until it spreads along the edge. Push the spreader forwards, keeping it at the same angle. Dry the thin film by waving it in the air. A properly made thin film should consist of an unbroken layer of single red blood cells with a 'tongue' not touching the edge of the slide (Figures 3.5 and 3.6).

Thin and thick films may be taken on the same slide, and the patient's details can be written with ordinary graphite pencil on the thin film before it dries. Blood films may be stained with Leishman's or with Giemsa stain, the latter being preferred in the tropics. A rapid method of staining thick films is that of Field, using buffered, isotonic Romanowsky stain with eosin as a counterstain (Figures 3.7 and 3.8).

Detailed instructions for the preparation of stains may be found elsewhere (Willcox, 1960; WHO, 1988; Cheesbrough, 1998). Only the most important methods are given here.

## Giemsa stain

Stock solutions of Giemsa may be purchased commercially; some brands are better than others. The stock solution of Giemsa stain is easily prepared from commercially available Giemsa powder:

- Giemsa powder (Azure B type): 3.8 g
- Glycerol, pure: 250 mL
- Methyl alcohol (certified pure): 250 mL.

The stain is prepared best by mixing alcohol and glycerol and then gradually adding small quantities of powder in a porcelain mortar and grinding until most of the powder is dissolved. Some residue may remain and, by leaving the mixture for about a week without filtering, the maximum amount of the stain will be absorbed. The prepared stock solution can then be filtered and should be kept in a glass bottle away from the sunlight.

### DILUTIONS OF GIEMSA STAIN

Stock solutions of Giemsa stain must always be diluted by mixing an appropriate amount of the stain with

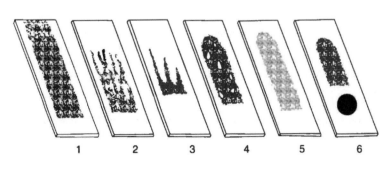

| 1 | 2 | 3 | 4 | 5 | 6 |

**Figure 3.6** *Common faults of the preparation of a thin blood film. 1. Too much blood: the end of the film is lost and the film itself is too thick. 2. An old, devitrified slide or the blood was clotting when the film was made. 3. Uneven contact of the spreader or the edge of the spreader was ragged; the film is too short; there is too little blood. 4. Greasy slide. 5. Good thin film. 6. Thick and thin film on the same slide. (WHO, 1961.)*

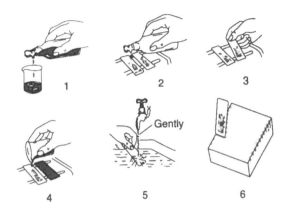

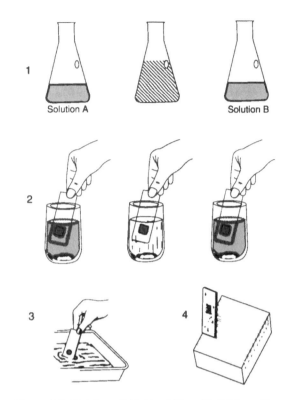

**Figure 3.7** *Staining a thin blood film with Giemsa stain. 1. Prepare the staining solution by diluting the Giemsa stock solution with buffered water in a small beaker. The best solution for reasonably fast staining is two to three drops of Giemsa to each millilitre of water. One slide requires 3–4 mL of diluted stain. 2. Fix the thin film by pouring a few drops of methyl alcohol for a few seconds. 3. Pour off the alcohol and pour on the diluted stain before the film is dry. 4. Stain for 20–30 minutes. 5. Do not pour off the stain but flush off and rinse by holding the slide in a large container with tap water or under a gentle stream of tap water for 10–15 seconds. 6. Place the slide on its end in the slide rack to dry. (WHO, 1961.)*

**Figure 3.8** *Staining a thick blood film with Field's rapid stain. 1. Prepare three containers with solution A, water and solution B. 2. Dip the blood film into solution A and count slowly up to five (about 2–3 seconds). Remove the slide and wash it in a beaker with distilled water or suitable tap water, counting slowly up to 10 (4–6 seconds) or until the stain ceases to run from the slide and film. Dip into solution B and count up to two (1 second). 3. Remove and wash again, waving the slide gently in tap water and counting slowly up to 10. 4. Place on a slide rack to dry. (WHO, 1961.)*

distilled neutral or slightly alkaline water. Buffered saline is preferred because it provides a cleaner background and a better preservation of parasite morphology. A buffer solution that gives a pH of 7.2 is prepared as follows:

- Potassium dihydrogen phosphate $KH_2PO_4$): 0.7 g
- Disodium hydrogen phosphate (Na$_2$HPO$_4$): 1.0 g
- Distilled water: 1 L.

Tablets of phosphate buffer salts can be obtained commercially for 100 mL or 1000 mL of water.

## TECHNIQUE OF STAINING OF FILMS USING GIEMSA STAIN (Figure 3.7)

1. The thin film should be fixed in absolute methyl alcohol for 30 seconds. This can be done simply by immersing the film in methyl alcohol or by putting a few drops on it by means of a pipette. Thick films should be dry, but not by heating the slide. (Important note: thick films are not fixed prior to staining.)

2. The staining solution must be freshly prepared by mixing 5 mL of stock solution with 100 mL of buffered water. For one or two slides, less staining solution is adequate, providing that it will contain 5 per cent of stock stain.
3. Transfer the slide to the staining solution in a Coplin jar or place the slide face downwards in a shallow tray on two glass rods. Stain for 20–30 minutes.
4. Flush the slide with tap water, wipe the back of the slide clean and stand it upright to dry.

*Note*. In emergencies, the staining time can be reduced to 5–10 minutes using a 10 per cent Giemsa solution.

## Technique of staining with Field's stain (Figure 3.8)

The Field's stain is a water-based Romanovsky stain that consists of two solutions (solution A and solution B). This rapid method gives excellent results when the technique is carefully followed.

1. To prepare the Field's stain, either use commercial stain powders or mix the ingredients as follows:

   *Solution A*
   Methylene blue (medicinal) 0.8 g
   Azure I 0.5 g
   Disodium hydrogen phosphate (anhydrous) 5.0 g
   Potassium dihydrogen phosphate 6.25 g
   Distilled water 500 mL
   *Solution B*
   Eosin 1.0 g
   Disodium hydrogen phosphate (anhydrous) 5.0 g
   Potassium dihydrogen phosphate 6.25 g
   Distilled water 500 mL

   First dissolve the phosphate salts in separate containers and add the stain to each container. Leave the appropriate solutions for 24 hours, filter and keep in separate bottles for subsequent use.

2. For the staining of thick films, the Field's method requires the use of three wide-mouth staining jars, about 40 mm in diameter and 100 mm long: one for staining solution A, one for buffered distilled water and one for staining solution B. Neither solution A nor solution B need be diluted prior to staining.
   The technique of staining individual slides is as follows:

   (a) Holding the dried thick film facing downwards, dip the slide for 2 seconds in solution A.
   (b) Drain off the excess stain by touching a corner of the slide on a piece of filter paper or by washing off the stain from the back of the slide with a stream of tap water.
   (c) Dip the slide in the buffer solution until the excess of the blue stain has left the film.
   (d) Dip the slide for 1 second in solution B.
   (e) Wash off the stain with a gentle stream of tap water.
   (f) Stand the slide upright to dry.

3. For the staining of thin films, use solution A at a 1:5 dilution in buffered saline. Place the thin film on a staining rack and first fix it with methanol. Then cover the slide with 0.5 mL of diluted Field's solution B, immediately followed by an equal volume of solution A. Mix the stains on the slide and leave for 1 minute. Wash off the stain with clean water, wipe the back of the slide clean and stand upright to air-dry.

## Examination of blood films

The thick film method, which concentrates by a factor of 20–30 the layers of red blood cells on a small surface, is, in practised hands, by far the best for general clinical use. The parasites are easily detected in the thick film but, because of haemolysis and slow drying used in the preparation of the film, the red blood cells are not visible and only leucocytes and parasites can be recognized. The young trophozoites appear as incomplete rings or spots of blue cytoplasm with a detached red chromatin dot. In the late trophozoites of *P. vivax*, the cytoplasm may be fragmented and Schüffner's stippling may be less obvious; the band forms of *P. malariae* are less characteristic. However, the schizonts and gametocytes of these species retain their usual appearance, as do the crescents of *P. falciparum*.

The interpretation of the parasites seen in a thick film requires some experience, which can be easily acquired, first by studying the morphology of parasites in a thin film and then by searching for corresponding forms in a thick film (Figure 3.9).

Although the thick film is recommended as the routine method for finding parasites, most experienced microscopists supplement it by taking a thin film (often on the same slide). This could be of value when the correct identification of some parasite species is of importance. For staining these double films, Giemsa is the best method.

When looking at a thick film, select areas that are well stained and not too thick. Standard practice requires that the thick film should be examined for at least 5 minutes (corresponding to approximately 100 microscopic fields under oil immersion) (Table 3.1). Some authors advise that the standard duration of examination of the thick film should be extended to 200 oil immersion fields, as this may allow for the detection of very low parasitaemia, which would

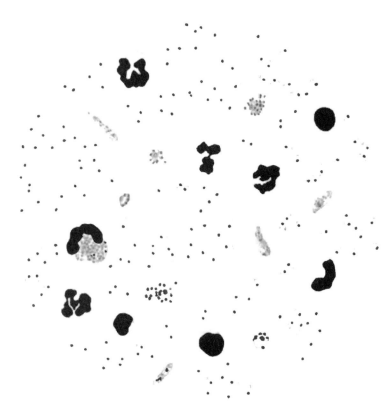

**Figure 3.9** *Heavy infection with P. falciparum in a thick blood film stained by Giemsa. (×440). Note the four 'crescents' of P. falciparum and several developing and fully grown schizonts, as well as one eosinophil, four polymorphonuclear leucocytes, one large and three small leucocytes. The field is studded with hundreds of trophozoites of P. falciparum. (Wellcome Museum of Medical Science.)*

not be seen on the examination of 100 fields. This is a valuable suggestion, achieving some compromise between the need for greater sensitivity of the microscopic examination and the time that is allowable in field practice. An absence of malaria parasites ('negative slide') should not be reported before at least 200 fields of a thick film are examined. In doubtful cases, repeated blood films must be taken every

**Table 3.1** *Quantitative aspects of thick and thin blood films for examination of malaria parasites*

|  | Thin film | Thick film |
|---|---|---|
| Area on slide | 250–450 mm² | 50–90 mm² |
| Blood volume | 1 µL | 3–5 µL |
| Mean thickness | 0.0025 mm | 0.06–0.09 mm |
| Mean difference in concentration | 1 | 20–30 |
| Volume in 100 microscope fields (obj. ×100; ocul. ×6) | 0.005–0.007 µL | 0.1–0.25 µL |
| Time for examination (approximate) | 200–300 fields/20–25 minutes | 100 fields/5 minutes |
| Loss of leucocytes or parasites during staining | None | Leucocytes up to 8% Parasites up to 20% |
| Red blood cells | Fixed | Haemolysed |
| Parasite morphology | Not distorted | Distorted |
| Parasite transfer during mass staining | Impossible | Likely |
| Artefacts | Uncommon | More common |

4 hours and examined; this is particularly important with *P. falciparum* infections, for which the parasites are sequestered in capillaries for 50 per cent of the erythrocytic cycle and therefore not always present in the peripheral blood; thus, the patient may harbour a heavy load of parasites, but no parasites may initially be found if the infection is very synchronous.

Repeated examinations are also necessary to assess the response of the parasite to treatment. It is advisable to have some indication of the density of parasitaemia by counting in a thin blood film the mean number of parasitized erythrocytes in relation to an arbitrary number of red blood cells (e.g. 10 000). Because there are, on average, between 300 and 500 red blood cells in a microscope field under oil immersion, depending on the optical system used and its magnification, a reasonable approximation may be achieved by counting the number of parasites in 20 fields. A more precise method consists of counting the number of parasites and leucocytes in a thick film until several hundred of the latter have been enumerated. If a total white blood cell count of the patient's blood is made, the ratio of parasites to leucocytes will give the number of parasites per microlitre of blood. This is known as the *parasite count*. The estimation of the level of parasitaemia is highly valuable to the clinician and represents an important determinant in choosing the treatment schedule (for example, a parasitaemia above 10 per cent in a non-immune traveller may be an indication for exsanguino-transfusion) and any effective follow-up of treatment efficacy.

For designation of the relative parasite count, a simple code of from one to four crosses is often used by laboratory technicians. For the usual magnification between 500 and 600 times, this is as follows:

- +   1–10 parasites per 100 thick film fields
- ++   11–100 parasites per 100 thick film fields
- +++   1–10 parasites per one thick film field
- ++++   more than 10 parasites per one thick film field

However, such counts are highly susceptible to subjective bias over time and are not recommended for research-related studies.

For all parasite counts, the use of a hand-operated tally counter is necessary. It should always be remembered that examination of 100 thick film fields corresponds to the average volume of only about 0.2 μL of blood. Thus, the part played by chance factors in the microscopic diagnosis of malaria infection

must be recognized. The chance factor rises as the true number of parasites in a unit of blood decreases. Thus, in doubtful cases it is desirable to increase the time devoted to the examination of a single blood slide and, if necessary, to take several blood slides at proper intervals of time.

Based on the examination of 100 microscopic fields under oil immersion, with a magnification of ×500–600, the numerical threshold at which malaria parasites can be detected by an experienced technician in well-stained blood films is about 100 parasites/μL if a thin film technique is used. For a thick film, the threshold is lower – about 10–20 parasites/μL of blood – but here the experience of the microscopist is an important factor.

Technical details for the microscopic examination of blood films are outside the scope of this book and can be found elsewhere. The best-illustrated guides for the staining and identification of human malaria parasites in thick and thin blood films are found in the *Bench Aids for Malaria Diagnosis*, available from the World Health Organization (WHO, 1991) and in papers by Shute (1988), Warhurst and Williams (1996) or Castelli and Carosi (1997).

The diagnostic characteristics of human malaria parasites as seen in a well-stained thick or thin film are given in Tables 3.2, 3.3 and 3.4. The features to look for are:

- The size of the infected red cell (*P. vivax* and *P. ovale* prefer reticulocytes and are therefore found in larger red cells).
- The presence of stippling on the red cell (i.e. Schüffner's dots are characteristic of *P. vivax* and *P. ovale*).
- The morphology of parasites (parasites forming a band across the red cell are a feature of *P. malariae*) and the different parasite stages present (late trophozoites and schizonts of *P. falciparum* are normally absent from the peripheral blood).
- The shape of gametocytes (crescent-shaped gametocytes are characteristic of *P. falciparum*, other species have round gametocytes).
- The quality of pigment (coarse pigment is suggestive of *P. malariae*).
- The level of parasitaemia (a blood film showing only young trophozoites cannot normally be used for the identification of malaria species, but the presence of a large number of parasites and multiple infection of red cells is suggestive of *P. falciparum*).

**Table 3.2** *Appearance of malaria parasites in a thick blood film*

| Stage | Plasmodium vivax (and ovale) | Plasmodium malariae | Plasmodium falciparum |
|---|---|---|---|
| Early trophozoite | Fairly numerous; irregular cytoplasm; fairly large single chromatin bead; often mixed with later stages | Few; more regular cytoplasm; medium-size single chromatin bead; segmenters present occasionally | Often very numerous; delicate cytoplasm; small, sometimes double chromatin bead; no other forms usually present except perhaps crescents |
| Half-grown trophozoite | Great irregularity of cytoplasm which tends to scatter away from single chromatin bead; few small granules of pigment | Regular, compact, deep blue cytoplasm around single chromatin bead; pigment forms early and tends to concentrate | Not common in peripheral blood; regular cytoplasmic ring, broken ring, and comma patterns; single and double chromatin bead |
| Late trophozoite | Considerable cytoplasmic scatter and irregularity; chromatin bead often isolated; fine granular pigment with moderate dispersion and often isolated from cytoplasm; other stages usually present; Schüffner's stippling sometimes seen as a pink halo | Numbers generally few, older stages present; round, compact cytoplasm often obscuring chromatin; scattered pigment relatively abundant | Not in peripheral blood except in very heavy infections; solid, irregularly rounded; chromatin indistinct; pigment concentrated |
| Early schizont or pre-segmenter | Large amount of cytoplasm loosely covering abundant chromatin which is beginning to segment; pigment granules discrete and lightly concentrated in one or two areas; Schüffner's stippling often seen as a pink granular halo, more prominent in *ovale* | Smaller and not so numerous; some scatter of cytoplasm and segmentation of chromatin; pigment in small, separate granules | Seldom in peripheral blood, but if so will be associated with numerous typical ring forms; irregular, fairly compact, dark staining; pigment fused in a single mass |
| Mature schizont (segmenter) | 8–24, usually 12–16 merozoites; relatively large size, early vacuole formation; pigment granular and loose; other stages often present | 6–12, usually 8 merozoites, each with vivid purple, ovoid head of chromatin; early vacuole formation; pigment compact clump of granules | Very rare in peripheral blood; 12–24 or more merozoites, fairly uniform ovoid or round chromatin beads; merozoites grouped or scattered; pigment a single dark mass |
| Gametocyte | Round or oval, relatively large, with fairly uniform cytoplasm, somewhat frayed at edges small rodlet-shaped pigment, irregularly scattered, abundant chromatin, more diffuse in males | Rounded, compact, with abundant peripheral pigment in round granules; single chromatin mass often obscured and more diffuse in males | When mature and normal has distinctive crescentic shape; females longer and more slender with central pigment and chromatin; males fatter and paler, with scattered pigment and diffuse chromatin, coarse grains of pigment |

Mainly after Russell *et al.*, 1963.

*Note.* In properly stained thick films the erythrocytes are lysed and invisible, except for a cloudy, bluish background. Nuclei of white blood cells stain deep mauve; clumps of platelets are pink. The parasites show a dull red or magenta-coloured nucleus and light blue cytoplasm. Species differentiation of very young forms of parasites is often impossible. In *P. vivax* and *P. ovale* infections stippling is usually present. Gametocytes of *P. falciparum* ('crescents') are distinctive but in slowly dried films they are rounded up and can then be confused with schizonts or gametocytes of *P. malariae*.

While in vivax, quartan and ovale malaria all stages of development of malaria parasites can usually be found in the peripheral blood, in falciparum malaria the schizogony takes place in the internal organs and normally only early trophozoites ('rings') appear in the blood. In very severe infections with *P. falciparum*, the appearance of schizonts is a danger signal

**Table 3.3** *Differential characteristics of infected erythrocytes and human plasmodia in stained thin films*

| Characteristics | P. falciparum | P. vivax | P. ovale | P. malariae |
|---|---|---|---|---|
| Infected erythrocyte enlarged | − | + | ± | − |
| Infected erythrocyte not enlarged | + | − | ± | + |
| Infected erythrocyte oval, crenated margin[a] | − | − | + | − |
| Infected erythrocyte decolorized | − | + | + | − |
| Infected erythrocyte, Schüffner's dots[a] (*stippling*) | − | + | + | − |
| Infected erythrocyte, Maurer's dots[a] | + | − | − | − |
| Multiple infections in erythrocytes[a] | + | Rare | − | − |
| Parasite, all forms in peripheral blood | − | + | + | + |
| Parasite, large, coarse rings | − | + | + | + |
| Parasite, double chromatin dots[a] | + | Rare | − | − |
| Parasite, accolé forms[a] | + | Rare | − | − |
| Parasite, band forms[a] | − | − | − | + |
| Parasite, crescentic gametocytes | + | − | − | − |
| Number of merozoites | 8–24 | 12–24 | 8–12 | 6–12 |

[a] Not invariable but suggestive when seen.

Mixed infections, with more than one *Plasmodium* species, are not uncommon and may be a cause for misdiagnosis. For example, if a blood film showing 95 per cent ring-stage parasites and a few late trophozoite 'band forms' characteristic of *P. malariae* is diagnosed as *P. malariae* (not recognizing that it is, in fact, a mixed infection with *P. falciparum*), this may have severe consequences for the patient.

The most common reasons for not finding parasites (when the clinical picture is suggestive of malaria) are that the patient has already taken antimalarial drugs and that the parasites are too few in number to be detected in the peripheral blood. Occasionally, the finding of malaria pigment in monocytes or neutrophils can help to establish the diagnosis.

Care should be taken, when examining the thick film, not to confuse artefacts or blood platelets with malaria parasites. Only a few of the possible errors are mentioned here:

- Ghosts of haemolysed immature erythrocytes (reticulocytes) may be mistaken for Schüffner's stippling of *P. vivax*.
- Clusters of blood platelets may also simulate *P. vivax*; in thin films when several platelets are superimposed and stain differently with Giemsa, they may be mistaken for malaria parasites outside the red blood cell.
- Vegetable spores, yeast, pollen or algae in buffer solution may look like blood parasites.

- Bacteria can contaminate aqueous solutions of Giemsa stain and may interfere with the identification of plasmodia.
- In patients with a degree of anaemia, the nuclear residues of erythrocytes, such as Howell–Jolly bodies, on a background of reticulum of ghosts of immature cells may be easily mistaken for malaria parasites.

In doubtful cases, blood films should be sent to the nearest competent laboratory for confirmation of diagnosis. Human infections with *Babesia* (piroplasmosis or babesiosis) may be easily mistaken for *P. falciparum*. Fortunately, human babesiosis is rare.

Despite its shortcomings, microscopy has qualitative and quantitative features that most other techniques do not possess. When carefully examined by an experienced microscopist, a thin film with *P. falciparum* can provide clues regarding the degree of disease severity, which include not only the high level of parasitaemia but also the presence of more 'mature' ring-stage parasites (linked to the existence of a greater sequestered biomass of parasites) (White *et al.*, 1992), the presence of an unusually high number of circulating schizonts, or the presence of visible malarial pigment in neutrophils or monocytes. All three features have been suggested as predictors of poor prognosis. In a study in Thailand, the presence of pigment in more than 5 per cent of neutrophils was a predictor of fatal outcome, with 77 per cent

**Table 3.4** *Changes in the red blood cells infected with human malaria parasites as seen in the thin blood film*

| P. vivax | P. malariae | P. falciparum | P. ovale |
|---|---|---|---|
| Larger than normal, paler, often slightly distorted. Schüffner's dots present in nearly all infected cells except for very young rings. Multiple infection by several parasites not uncommon. Pigment brownish in short, scattered rods | About normal size or slightly smaller. Stippling not seen by normal staining. No multiple infection of erythrocyte, as a rule. Pigment seen even in early stages, dark granules rather than rods, often seen at the periphery of the cell | Normal in size. Multiple infections of erythrocyte very frequent. Some cells yellowish, seem to have a thicker rim (brassy cells). No Schüffner's stippling but irregular clefts (Maurer's dots) may be seen in overstained films. Pigment granular with tendency to coalesce. In gametocytes (crescents), the outline of erythrocyte barely seen | Many infected erythrocytes enlarged and definitely oval in shape while the parasite is round or elongated. The outline of infected cells often ragged (fimbriated). Schüffner's dots prominent at all stages of the parasite. Pigment brownish, similar to that of P. vivax |

accuracy (Nguyen Hoan Phu *et al.*, 1995), whereas one report from Nigeria showed that the average percentage of neutrophils with pigments was 6.5 per cent in mild malaria, compared to 27 per cent in cerebral malaria (Amodu *et al.*, 1998).

## Quality control

Satisfactory diagnosis of malaria by light microscopy requires the availability of a functioning, wellmaintained microscope, an adequate source of illumination and an operator experienced and competent in the preparation and staining of blood films, as well as in the recognition and identification of the characteristic stages of malaria parasites.

Whenever possible, a binocular microscope with a substage illumination should be used in preference to a monocular instrument. The use of a wide-angle eyepiece to obtain a better coverage of the microscopic field of an oil immersion is of great value and thoroughly recommended, providing adequate illumination is available. The optimum definition/magnification for malaria diagnosis with most standard microscopes is ×600–700, i.e. ×6 or ×7 eyepieces and ×100 oil immersion lens (spring loaded for protection).

Substandard equipment, which is irregularly maintained, can seriously affect the effectiveness of microscopy.

In many countries, even at the level of fairly well-equipped laboratories and major hospitals, the competence of microscopists often leaves much to be desired. To retain competence, it is necessary that good supervision and regular re-training take place. Operating fatigue is also a limiting factor and it has been suggested that the examination of 50 thick films daily is the absolute maximum for any microscopists, and that no more than 20 films should be examined without a break of at least 30 minutes of non-microscope activity (Milne *et al.*, 1994).

Inappropriate technology, use of the wrong stain concentration and method of preparation, or the wrong pH buffer can seriously affect the quality of microscopy. The detection of malaria parasites uses differential stains, where nuclear material is red and cytoplasm is blue, with clearly visible blood stippling; this appearance will only occur if the pH of the buffer is 7.2. Inappropriate staining is often a problem when automated staining procedures are used in haematological laboratories: parasites are often hardly visible and the low pH used (pH 6.8 or less) does not show Schüffner dots in *P. vivax* films.

## Special methods for sampling infected blood

Various procedures have been suggested to improve and facilitate the conventional ways of obtaining infected red cells and examining stained blood slides under the microscope. The examination of smears from the bone marrow, obtained by sternal puncture as a supplementary diagnostic method, has no advantage over the usual blood examination. The formerly advocated method of 'provocation' by the injection of 0.5 mL of 1:1000 solution of adrenaline (which was supposed to produce a contraction of the spleen and the appearance of parasites in the blood) is of no value for the diagnosis of malaria and may be dangerous when used in patients with high blood pressure. It has been stated, particularly by Chinese researchers, that sequestered forms of *P. falciparum* could be found in bloodless exudate from scarified skin and that intradermal smears may therefore be of value in assessing the degree of severity of falciparum malaria. In reality, the sensitivity of the procedure is only marginally better than the examination of peripheral blood, and the relative difference in parasite stages is so difficult to interpret as to be of no practical benefit for patient management (Silamut and White, 1993; White, 1998).

Amongst methods for concentrating parasites before examination, the centrifugation of heparinized blood may be of value. Late trophozoites, schizonts and gametocytes are concentrated in the buffy coat after centrifugation (the procedure is particularly useful to detect *P. vivax*, *P. malariae* or *P. ovale* when parasitaemia is very low, but is not useful for the detection of *P. falciparum*).

Centrifugation can be done in capillary tubes, which are then broken to make a blood film of the buffy coat. When using this technique, it should be remembered that breaking capillary tubes containing human blood is a safety hazard.

For post-mortem examinations, if death from malaria is suspected and no full autopsy can be carried out, a specimen can be obtained from a puncture of the spleen or brain. For the latter specimen, a large-bore needle can be pushed through the supra-orbital plate into the brain and a smear, obtained by suction, should be spread on the slide, fixed, and stained in the usual way.

## Fluorescence microscopy techniques

The main problem with microscopical diagnosis is that it is time-consuming and needs to be performed by skilled microscopists. Various methods have been designed to improve upon the examination of blood films in order to reduce the time spent reading the slides or to enable less well-trained personnel to achieve equally reliable results. The staining of films with acridine orange or with benzothiocarboxy-purine, which can be read either on a fluorescence microscope or on a microscope equipped with an interference filter system, allows a quicker screening of films, because parasites are more readily recognized and a lower power lens may be used (Kawamoto, 1991; Makler *et al.*, 1991).

The QBC® method is also based on acridine-orange staining, but in this case the blood is centrifuged in a specially designed and patented microhaematocrit tube fitted with a plastic float that spreads the buffy coat against the edge of the tube. Parasites and leucocytes take up the dye, which is fluorescent when examined under ultraviolet light, using a Paralens objective (Figure 3.10; Spielman *et al.*, 1988).

This elegant method is easy to perform, fast and easy to read, but requires specialized equipment (a microcentrifuge and a fluorescence attachment for the microscope) and the purchase of expensive QBC capillary tubes. The sensitivity of QBC, when used in field conditions, is comparable to that of thick film examination (Wongsrichalanai *et al.*, 1991). The major advantage of QBC is that the technique is normally available in haematology laboratories for leucocyte counting and, in many industrialized countries, it is in haematology laboratories that initial tests for malaria are performed (the speed and ease of performance of QBC are particularly appreciated when the test is performed by 'on call' staff). The high costs of QBC tubes and the need for additional equipment rule out its use in rural clinics in the tropics.

Both acridine-orange staining techniques are inferior to Romanovsky for the precise identification of malaria species or their accurate enumeration.

## DETECTION OF MALARIAL ANTIGEN

A positive antigen detection assay would be expected to detect a current infection. The ideal target antigen

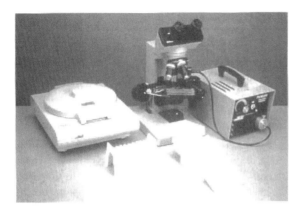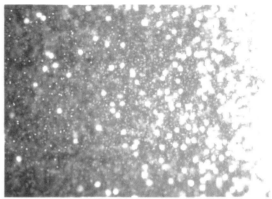

**Figure 3.10** *Quantitative buffy coat (QBC). (a) Equipment required for the QBC test. (b) Blood infected with P.* falciparum *as seen in QBC capillary tubes. The large fluorescent cells are white blood cells; the small fluorescent dots in the dark area are ring-stage parasites within non-fluorescing erythrocytes. (Reproduced with permission of Becton–Dickinson Tropical Disease Diagnostics, USA.)*

should be abundant in the blood (or other bodily fluids, such as the urine) to maximize sensitivity, be malaria-specific without cross-reactions with other micro-organisms, and should not persist after parasitaemia disappears. If the assay is to be designed to be useful in field conditions (e.g. to replace microscopy at the primary care level), it should also be robust, cheap, easy to perform and to interpret. In addition, it would be useful if the assay was to some extent quantitative, though bearing in mind that a quantitative assay is always more difficult to interpret. Such an assay does not yet exist, but a number of assays have been described that possess at least some of these features.

Experimental tests for detecting malarial antigens were originally based on either an antigen-capture or an **antigen-competition** format, and used the enzyme-linked immunosorbent assay (ELISA) methodology. Once optimal reagents have been identified (i.e. monoclonal or polyclonal antibodies to specific malarial antigens), the assay may be simplified for field use. Only methods based on the detection of histidine-rich protein-2 (HRP-2) and the parasite lactate dehydrogenase (pLDH) have so far been commercialized, in both cases using an immunochromatographic ('dipstick') test format. This new generation of easy-to-perform tests has been developed to diagnose falciparum malaria rapidly and reliably without the need for a microscope. The most recently developed tests can also detect other malaria species.

## The HRP-2 detection methods

*Pf*HRP-2 is a molecule present in the parasite throughout the erythrocytic cycle. A monoclonal antibody to HRP-2 is bound to the nitrocellulose/glass-fibre dipstick (forming a line across the strip) and, when in contact with lysed infected blood, the antibody captures the specific antigen of *P. falciparum*. The positivity of the test is visualized by a polyclonal anti-HRP-2 antibody labelled with a coloured marker, which produces a visible line on the dipstick. Two versions of the test are commercially available: ParaSight™-F, manufactured by Becton Dickinson (Cockeysville, USA) and ICT Malaria Pf™, manufactured by ICT Diagnostics (Sydney, Australia).

ParaSight™-F was the first rapid malaria antigen detection test to be developed. It has been extensively evaluated in tropical and developing countries, in stable and unstable areas of malaria transmission and in both laboratory and non-laboratory situations (Shiff *et al.*, 1993).

### TEST METHOD AND PRINCIPLE

1. Capillary blood is collected and dispensed into a small tube containing a red cell lysing agent.
2. A test strip is placed in the tube. As the lysed blood travels up the strip by chromatography, HRP-2 antigen in the specimen binds to the antibody.
3. The reaction is visualized by adding a pink-red-coloured detector reagent containing sulpho-

rhodamine B dye and polyclonal antibody raised against *P. falciparum* HRP-2. As the reagent travels up the strip, it attaches to the captured HRP-2 antigen, producing a pink-coloured line.

4. After adding a wash solution to clear the lysed blood, the pink line is seen against a white background, indicating a positive test for *P. falciparum*.

5. A positive control is contained on the strip. It is seen as a broken pink line above the test line, proving that the test has been performed correctly and the detector reagent is working satisfactorily.

The whole test only takes 10 minutes and evaluations of the test have shown ParaSight™-F to be both sensitive and specific, performing as well as, and often better than, microscopy in field situations. Although an experienced microscopist working under optimal conditions is able to detect as few as 10–20 parasites/μL in a thick blood film, this level of sensitivity is rarely achieved in most district laboratories. Craig and Sharp (1997) found a sensitivity of 84 parasites/μL for Giemsa thick films and a sensitivity of 30 parasites/μL for ParaSight™-F. Most evaluations have estimated sensitivity to be between 81 per cent and 99.5 per cent, with variations being found in different areas of malaria transmission. In most cases, antigenaemia following successful treatment persists for at least 1 week (in 70 per cent of patients) and sometimes for as long as 28 days.

The ICT test is exceptionally easy to perform and most field workers prefer it to ParaSight™-F because it has fewer test stages and the test strip is mounted on a cleverly designed card; it takes about 5 minutes to perform. In terms of sensitivity and specificity, ICT and ParaSight™-F are indistinguishable (Pieroni *et al.*, 1998). ICT Diagnostics also manufactures test kits for travellers visiting falciparum-malaria endemic areas. These kits, called Malapac Travel Tests, also contain materials for collecting blood.

Evaluations so far carried out have shown ICT Malaria Pf™ to be sensitive and specific (Figure 3.11).

## pLDH detection methods

The metabolic malaria parasite enzyme pLDH is actively produced by all human malaria parasite species during their growth in red cells. The detection of pLDH, originally developed as a way to monitor

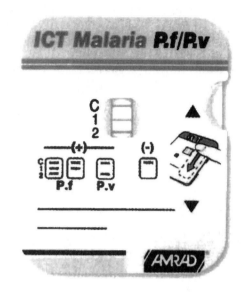

**Figure 3.11** *Commercial ICT presentation of immunochromatographic kit for the detection of* P. falciparum *and* P. vivax.

*in vitro* drug susceptibility assays, has the potential of being useful for the detection of *Plasmodium* parasitaemia. The principle of the assay is that pLDH has different biochemical characteristics from human LDH and may therefore be differentially measured using a simple colorimetric assay. Such assays are not species-specific, can detect a parasitaemia as low as 0.1 per cent (a level of parasitaemia just below the threshold of 10 000 parasites/mL and thus potentially useful as a marker for clinical malaria in endemic areas), and can be used as quantitative assays above that threshold (Knobloch and Henk, 1995). An immuno-capture version of the pLDH activity assay (ICpLDH) improves the sensitivity and ease of performance of the test.

The principle of OptiMAL, manufactured by Flow Inc. (Portland, USA), is based on the detection of pLDH enzyme using a series of monoclonal and polyclonal antibodies. It is the most recently developed immunochromatographic rapid malaria strip test (Piper *et al.*, 1999). Differentiation of malaria species in the OptiMAL test is based on antigenic differences between pLDH isoforms. Unlike HRP-2, pLDH does not persist in the blood, but clears at about the same time as the parasites following successful treatment. The test is therefore of use for monitoring responses to drug therapy and for detecting drug-resistant malaria because pLDH reflects the presence of viable malaria parasites in the blood. If less sensitive than HPR-2 tests (with a threshold of 100–200 parasites/µL), the test produces fewer false positives in patients with rheumatoid factor.

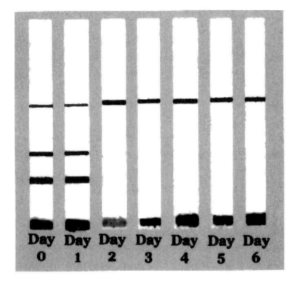

**Figure 3.12** *Results of OptiMAL test on subsequent daily samples from the same patient from initial diagnosis until 6 days after treatment showing the positive reaction and the rapid negativation of the test after treatment. (Courtesy of Dr M Makler.)*

The test is rapid and easy to perform (Figure 3.12). Evaluations published so far indicate that the test is sensitive and able to speciate *P. vivax* and *P. falciparum* (but cannot identify *P. vivax* in mixed infections). A study performed in Honduras showed that OptiMal had sensitivities of 94 per cent and 88 per cent and specificities of 100 per cent and 99 per cent, respectively, when compared to the examination of Giemsa-stained thick blood films for the detection of *P. vivax* and *P. falciparum*. In this study, OptiMal correctly identified *P. falciparum* more often than the two HRP-2 tests (Palmer *et al.*, 1998).

Table 3.5 compares the characteristics of Giemsa-stained and acridine-orange-stained blood films, QBC and ParaSight-F, based on data collected in a survey in KwaZulu, South Africa (Craig and Sharp, 1997). Such a comparison confirms that neither QBC nor antigen detection tests can as yet replace microscopy. Thick blood film examination is as sensitive and more specific, it allows estimation of parasitaemia and distinction between parasite stages, it covers all species and becomes rapidly negative after treatment. This does not mean that QBC and antigen detection have no role to play in malaria diagnosis. In industrialized countries, the tests are paradoxically used more and more as a first-line method in sophisticated laboratories that have not maintained competency in malaria microscopy; confirmatory diagnosis is then performed in a specialized centre. In tropical countries and situations in which microscopy is not yet available, antigen tests are increasingly used

**Table 3.5** *Comparison between diagnostic tests*

| | Giemsa | AO | QBC | ParaSight-F |
|---|---|---|---|---|
| Sensitivity[a] | 84/µL | 30/µL | 143/µL | 84/µL |
| | 91% | 93% | 89% | 96% |
| Specificity | 100% | >95% | >95% | >95% |
| Species identification | Clear | Unreliable | Unreliable | Pf specific |
| Parasite count | Accurate | Accurate | Good | Not quantitative |
| Speed | Slow | Moderate | Moderate | Fast |
| Cost[b] | US$0.03 | US$0.03 | US$1.70 | >US$2.25 |
| Equipment required | Microscope | Microscope | Microscope | None |
| | Laboratory | Laboratory | Laboratory | |
| | Electricity | Electricity | Electricity | |
| | | AO filters | Microcentrifuge | |
| | | Halogen lamp | Florescence attachment | |

[a] Sensitivity compared to a gold standard of 800 Giemsa-stained thin film field examined by microscopy.
[b] These are minimal costs because the price of tests varies from country to country (for example, in the UK, the cost of ParaSight-F is >US$5.00) and does not include the salary costs of trained microscopists (high in industrialized countries, low in tropical countries).
AO = acridine-orange; QBC = quantitative buffy coat.

as a means to reduce inappropriate antimalarial chemotherapy. The tests have been used with success in remote tribal groups in forested areas of central India, in refugee camps on the Thai-Myanmar border, in mining communities in Cambodia and Venezuela, and at primary health care level in Sri Lanka. The use of antigen detection tests in hyperendemic or holoendemic zones in Africa is more questionable, because the tests are not quantitative and the finding of parasites alone is not sufficient for a diagnosis of clinical malaria. However, one study in Zimbabwe indicated that mistreatment was reduced by 81 per cent when ParaSight-F was used compared to presumptive clinical diagnosis.

## SEROLOGY

Serological methods have been in use since the early 1960s, when indirect fluorescent antibody tests (IFAT) and indirect haemagglutination assays (IHA) were described (Voller, 1988). Because such tests detect antimalarial antibodies, they cannot distinguish between current or past infection and are therefore of limited value as a guide to the treatment or management of the disease (Gillespie and Chiodini, 1988). At best, a negative serological assay may help to eliminate the possibility of malaria, because it has been shown that antibody levels become detectable a few days after the blood is invaded. The main uses of serological tests are for retrospective studies, particularly for epidemiological purposes, and for tracing asymptomatic infections in blood donors.

### Indirect fluorescent antibody test

The indirect fluorescent antibody test (IFAT) is the main method for routine serodiagnosis, because it is relatively easy to make antigen slides for all human malarial parasites, and commercial IFAT slides for malaria are available from various sources (Voller and O'Neill, 1971). Homologous antigens used in the IFAT consist of human malaria parasites of a given plasmodial species and preferably erythrocytic schizonts obtained from humans, from experimentally infected animals (owl or squirrel monkeys, or chimpanzees) or from an in vitro culture. Cultured P. falciparum is a most convenient and stable source of antigen.

In the IFAT procedure, the antigen consists of infected blood bound to a 12-spot Teflon-coated microscope slide. A drop of 1:100 dilution of washed infected red cells is placed on each spot and allowed to dry. The slide is then stored at −20 °C (or, preferably, −70 °C). Just before use, the slide is thawed in a wet chamber to allow red cells to lyse, dried and (optionally) fixed in cold acetone. The slide is covered first with one of the serial dilutions of the test serum (collected after finger prick in a capillary tube, for subsequent separation of serum, or collected on filter paper and dried before an eventual elution using physiological saline). It then receives a solution of antihuman immunoglobulin labelled with fluorescein isothiocyanate containing 1:10 000 Evans' blue as a counterstain. After washing and drying, the slides are examined by fluorescence microscopy. Antibody in the test serum reacts with antigen of the malaria parasites and the antiglobulin reaction with the antibody is indicated by the fluorescence of the parasites. Fluorescence of the last serial dilution is given as a 'titre' of the antibody present. Generally, fluorescence at a dilution of over 1:20 is regarded as a positive test. This method has the advantage of giving a visual picture of parasites used as an antigen. Moreover, the slides with the antigen film can be easily prepared and stored at −20 °C for long periods.

Although different species of Plasmodium have some antigens in common, it is recommended to use species-specific antigen for maximum test sensitivity. This is possible in the case of IFAT, for which the blood from infected humans with P. vivax or P. malariae can be used as antigen, but is generally not possible for tests using a soluble antigen. (However, the simian P. cynomolgi or P. simiae may be used for P. vivax, and P. brazilianum for P. malariae.)

The disadvantages of IFAT are the requirement for a fluorescence microscope, the subjectivity of the reading and the fact that the method is relatively labour intensive, which limits its application to specialized centres with a relatively small throughput of samples.

### Enzyme-linked immunosorbent assay

ELISA uses a soluble malarial antigen (generally prepared from asexual stages of P. falciparum), coated on the wells of a microtitre plate (Voller et al., 1974). This enables a large number of samples to be processed at the same time and produces quantitative results when the assay is read on a spectrophotometer (portable, battery-operated ELISA readers are available for field use).

For the preparation of crude extracts of malaria parasites to be used as antigen for ELISA, an *in vitro* culture rich in schizonts (at a parasitaemia of 10 per cent or more) is sedimented by centrifugation and the washed red cells are then lysed in cold hypotonic buffer to release the haemoglobin, leaving the parasites intact. The parasites are disrupted by sonication or repeated freeze–thawing, then sedimented by high-speed centrifugation and the supernatant used as the stock soluble antigen, which is stored in aliquots at $-70\,°C$ until use. The optimal antigen concentration is determined by chequer-board titration against positive and negative control sera. Each well of a 96-well polystyrene plate is coated overnight at $4\,°C$ with 200 $\mu$L of the optimal dilution of soluble antigen in carbonate buffer at pH 9.6. After washing, the plates can be used immediately or stored dry at $4\,°C$ for several years. Test serum dilutions (at 1:100 or 1:200 dilution in phosphate-buffered saline plus 0.05 per cent Tween 20) are added to the wells, incubated for 2 hours at room temperature and washed. A dilution of enzyme-labelled antihuman immunoglubulin (diluted following the manufacturer's instructions) is added to each well for 2 hours and washed as before. Finally, a freshly prepared substrate solution is added to each well until the expected colour intensity has been reached by standard positive control serum. The colour intensity of the content of each well may be measured visually (when the test is performed in field conditions and when looking for approximate positive/negative tests), but normally the absorbance is measured on a spectrophotometer at the suitable wavelength. The most commonly used conjugate/substrate combinations are:

(i) alkaline phosphatase-labelled antihuman immunoglobulin with para-nitrophenyl phosphate substrate;
(ii) horseradish peroxidase-labelled antihuman immunoglobulin with ortho-phenylene diamine substrate.

Substrates are available commercially in easy-to-use presentations.

In addition to crude extracts of malarial antigens, ELISA has been applied to a variety of defined, synthetic or recombinant malarial antigens (e.g. MSP-1,

RESA or CSP) (Del Giudice *et al.*, 1987). Such studies have been useful to elucidate the role of target malarial antigen in immunity and protection.

A variety of other serological test formats have been explored, including radio-immunoassays, latex agglutination, indirect haemagglutination, solid-phase dipstick and membrane dot-blot, which may have specific advantages in given situations. (For details on these techniques, see Voller, 1988.)

## Collection of capillary blood on paper for serology

The simple protocol for the collection of blood on filter paper for serology as described by Dr C.C. Draper of the Ross Institute, London School of Hygiene and Tropical Medicine, is as follows.

1. Whatman No. 3 chromatography paper cut into strips of about 14 × 9 cm should be stored in self-sealing polythene bags, each containing up to 10 pieces. For use in humid climates, it is preferable, before cutting them into strips, to soak the sheets of paper in 1/10 000 thiomersal (Merthiolate), to act as a fungicide, and to allow them to dry thoroughly.
2. A finger or ear lobe is cleaned. If cleaning fluid is used, this should be dried. A deep prick is made and drops of blood are allowed to fall onto the paper, so that the skin does not touch the paper. A minimum of two to three spots of not less than 50 $\mu$L each are collected from every subject. If necessary, several drops of blood may be allowed to fall on top of each other on the same spot of the paper and to soak in until this is about 1 cm in diameter. Each of the drops should be allowed to spread out on its own. Up to five sets of blood samples from different subjects can be put on one piece of paper. Each set must be clearly marked, with a reference number.
3. Papers should be protected from dirt and flies, e.g. by standing them on their sides inside a covered bowl. These should be allowed to dry thoroughly at room temperature or by holding them in gentle heat (not more than 37 °C). Under field conditions, this is often not practicable. The partially dried papers are then taken back to the laboratory, preferably within a few hours, where they are thoroughly dried and then sealed in the polythene bags. The

bags are stored as soon as possible in a refrigerator (4 °C) or, preferably, deep freeze (−20 °C or less). Under these conditions, specific immunoglobulins are probably stable for at least several months. As long as the papers are well dried, the bags can probably be kept at ambient temperature for several weeks without serious degradation of the immunoglobulins.

4. At the serological laboratory, a calibrated paper punch is used to cut out circles of paper containing the equivalent of 50 μL of blood. When eluted in 0.4 μL of diluent, this will given an approximate 1/16 dilution of serum.

5. Slightly greater precision (of doubtful value for most survey work and taking more time) may be obtained by taking up measured amounts of 50 mL of blood in a pipette or capillary tube and expelling these on to a paper. (This obviates the need for a calibrated punch when the processing of the blood samples takes place in the laboratory.)

## MOLECULAR METHODS

The application of DNA or RNA hybridization to malaria diagnosis has several advantages over traditional methods and, whereas the methodology is unlikely ever to be useful at the peripheral level of health care in its present form, it may have a place as a research tool to monitor malaria control programmes, to perform quality control checks on microscopical diagnosis or to determine the distribution of important genes (e.g. genes associated with drug resistance).

The presence of parasites in the blood means that there is parasite DNA and RNA present, and various methods based on the principle of nucleic acid hybridization have been developed to detect this. In these methods, a known sequence of nucleic acid (oligonucleotide) is synthesized and labelled with either radioactive $^{32}P$ or a non-radioactive colorimetric reagent, and this 'probe' is used to detect parasite nucleic acid, taking advantage of the fact that complementary sequences will hybridize (Franzen et al., 1984). The simplest version of this technique is the use of DNA probes to detect parasites directly in a drop of patient's blood immobilized on a filter paper. In this test format, the sensitivity and speci-

ficity of the technique depend largely upon the choice of nucleic acid sequence. In order to achieve a higher degree of sensitivity, most of the first-generation DNA probes were directed towards repetitive sequences of parasite genes (e.g. the rep20 subtelomeric repeat of P. falciparum). Since the availability of amplification methods, such as the PCR, for which the number of copies of any target sequence may be increased many times, the sensitivity of nucleic acid probes has exponentially increased. This has made it possible to use probes against non-repetitive sequences, which are useful, for example, to examine the association of Pfmdr genes with chloroquine resistance or to use species-specific small subunit ribosomal RNA sequences to differentiate between P. falciparum, P. vivax, P. ovale or P. malariae (Figure 3.13; Snounou et al., 1993).

The gain in sensitivity of PCR over the original dot DNA probes has meant an increased technical complexity, including the need for PCR equipment to automatically perform the thermal recycling used for amplification and the need to separate the amplified material by agarose electrophoresis. In addition, the risk of sample contamination is an intrinsic problem with any form of amplification, and scrupulous care is necessary in the handling of samples to avoid this. Many technical refinements of the PCR method have been described, some of which have been applied to malaria diagnosis (e.g. the use of methods

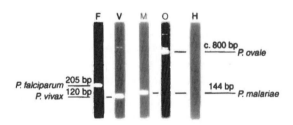

**Figure 3.13** *Polymerase chain reaction (PCR) detection of human* Plasmodium *species. (Courtesy of Dr G. Snounou, Imperial College School of Medicine, London.) Genomic DNA purified from the four human malaria parasites was separately subjected to nested PCR analysis and PCR products were resolved by electrophoresis on a 2% agarose gel and visualized under ultraviolet light after ethidium bromide staining. A characteristic DNA band is observed for each of the malaria species; no species PCR products are observed when oligonucleotide primers specific to one parasite species are used with DNA templates from any of the other three malaria species, or from uninfected human blood.*

for the detection of immobilized amplified nucleic acid or liquid-phase hybridization, which provide a test format akin to ELISA methods) (Oliveira *et al.*, 1995). Various ways have also been described to make the PCR technique more user-friendly for use in field conditions by reducing the manipulation of the samples and the likely contamination of specimens (e.g. by the collection of blood on filter paper) (Long *et al.*, 1995; Singh *et al.*, 1996).

The PCR technique has been reported to be capable of detecting parasitaemia of less than 0.00002 per cent when used in the best possible conditions. It is theoretically capable of detecting the presence of a single parasite in the sample, although this is rarely achieved, partly because the blood contains poorly defined products that may inhibit the PCR reaction. The detection of a parasitaemia of 0.00002 per cent, which corresponds to one parasite per mm$^3$ or five parasites per 5-$\mu$L sample of blood, is a detection threshold at least five times lower than the detection threshold achieved by means of a thick film performed in optimal conditions (i.e. 0.0001 per cent), assuming that a competent microscopist has spent at least 10 minutes examining 100 fields of an adequately stained thick film, i.e. a 0.2 mL fraction of a 5–10 mL drop of blood. A sensitivity of one parasite per 20 mL of blood (as reported by Tirasophon *et al.*, 1991) would, therefore, correspond to a sensitivity 100 times better than that of a thick film. In reality, the sensitivity of PCR is rarely as good, particularly when performed in field conditions, and may be considered comparable or only marginally better than that of the microscopical examination of a thick film. In contrast, the specificity of PCR is generally considered to be better than that of microscopy, and this feature is particularly helpful for studies of mixed malarial infections. The use of nested PCR in field surveys has shown that mixed infections were far more common than reports based on microscopy alone would have suggested, and that the global prevalence of *P. ovale* and *P. malariae* (two parasites commonly found as the minority population of mixed infection with *P. falciparum* or *P. vivax*) was much wider than generally believed (Kawamoto *et al.*, 1999).

## VERBAL AUTOPSY

Retrospective diagnosis of malaria as a cause of death is particularly difficult in countries where malaria is not a reportable disease and where hospital records are non-existent or unreliable. The technique of verbal autopsy is widely used to determine the predominant causes of mortality in a given community and to assess the impact of an intervention against a specific disease (Snow *et al.*, 1992). This approach has been used to estimate the role of malaria as a cause of death in African children, with variable results and a specificity of only 50–80 per cent. This lack of specificity is not surprising because the same algorithms used by medical staff to establish a presumptive diagnosis are used in this case by bereaved relatives to answer a questionnaire. The verbal autopsy algorithms used for cerebral malaria (fever, loss of consciousness or convulsions) are among the more reliable ones. Despite the shortcomings of the verbal autopsy approach, such data are used to estimate the overall impact of malaria on mortality.

## APPRAISAL OF THE RELATIVE VALUE OF DIAGNOSTIC METHODS

Whatever the method used, a diagnostic test should be able to correctly differentiate between individuals who are infected and those who are not. Consequently, the validity of a test is usually determined by its sensitivity (i.e. the test with the highest sensitivity has the lowest number of false negatives) and its specificity (i.e. the test with the highest specificity has the lowest number of false positives). In reality, it is generally more important to know the ability of a positive assay to predict the probability of infection, i.e. its positive predictive value.

### Individual diagnosis

In most situations, the 'gold standard' for individual diagnosis is the microscopical examination of thick and thin films. There are, however, situations where this may not apply (Payne, 1988).

In areas of high endemicity, clinical diagnosis alone is usually the only feasible and cost-effective method for recommending the first line of treatment. In a country where the annual budget for health per individual is US$2, it is difficult to justify diagnostic assays costing US$1 or more if the full treatment dose of Fansidar is only US$0.04. Even if this first-line treatment was given inappropriately in 75 per cent of cases, this would still mean that six patients were treated appropriately for the cost of one diagnostic test (Foster, 1991). Unfortunately, modern diagnostic assays are all likely to cost more than US$1 and the use of less costly microscopy requires a health care infrastructure and expertise that often do not exist. When microscopy is not available, the use of dipstick antigen detection tests may be of value, particularly in areas of low endemicity, where infection usually coincides with disease.

Semi-immune individuals may harbour malaria parasites without symptoms of disease and in many hyperendemic and holoendemic areas of sub-Saharan Africa, 60 or 70 per cent of the population may have a positive parasitaemia at any given time. When microscopy is used in areas of high endemicity, it is therefore necessary to define the *clinical threshold* for each situation, i.e. a level above which parasitaemia may have a clinical significance. A parasitaemia above 5000–10 000 parasites/$\mu$L is usually suggested as a guideline, but precise counting may not always be feasible. Coosemans and colleagues (1994) have proposed the sensible 'rule of thumb' that a 100 per cent field positivity on a thick film may be used as a good morbidity indicator. Because antigen detection tests are not quantitative in their present format, their use is of limited value in high-endemicity areas (where over 50 per cent of the population may carry parasites), except when used in conjunction with a well-tried clinical algorithm.

There is a correlation between density of parasitaemia and severity of malaria. It is considered that any *P. falciparum* parasitaemia above 250 000/$\mu$L (approximatively 5 per cent of red blood cells) should be taken as a sign of severity requiring emergency treatment. The presence of schizonts in the peripheral blood is also considered a sign of severity. Because *P. falciparum* matures in internal organs ('sequestration'), a severe form of malaria may occur at a time when the parasites in the peripheral blood are scanty or even absent (Silamut and White, 1993). It is therefore necessary to examine serial blood films at intervals of 6–12 hours to confirm the diagnosis. The finding of pigment in monocytes may help the diagnosis (WHO, 2000). There are suggestions that antigen detection tests may be useful in helping to make a positive diagnosis during the window when parasites are sequestered, but this requires further data.

Non-immune travellers to malaria-endemic countries who have chosen, against medical advice, not to take preventive antimalarials (and instead carry curative doses of quinine, halofantrine or artemisinine as 'back pocket treatment') may also be tempted to use individual test kits (such as the ICT Malapac) as an indicator of when to take their treatment dose. This practice may be justified when travelling in areas where the risk of infection is low, but where antimalarial resistance is high, the traveller must be aware of the serious potential hazards of such a practice.

## Epidemiological surveillance

Active or passive surveillance of malaria prevalence is an important tool for malaria control, particularly when the efficacy of control measures is being evaluated. Microscopy and, by extension, antigen detection or PCR have serious limitations for such an evaluation, because these techniques only measure a 'point prevalence' of the infection at the time of the survey (which is particularly unhelpful in a situation in which malaria transmission is seasonal). In contrast, sero-epidemiology may help to delineate those areas where there is malaria transmission, provide information on species prevalence or age-related prevalence, and chart the changes that are taking place as a result of the control intervention. Malaria serology is particularly valuable when a control intervention has been in operation for some time. By estimating the seroprevalence in new entrants to the population, it is possible to detect residual, low levels of transmission when other methods of study such as parasite rate and spleen rate become relatively insensitive.

In countries where malaria incidence is very low, but where the risk of resurgence or epidemic outbreaks still exists, malaria diagnosis may still be recommended routinely for every case of fever as part of the national control programme (as is the case in China). Microscopy used in such situations is disheartening for the microscopists (with only 1:10 000 positive slides or less) and eventually becomes counter-productive when microscopists become unable to recognize a positive blood film. This is a situation in which non-microscopic methods of diagnosis (including serology and antigen detection) are of particular value.

Another issue in diagnosis for epidemiological purposes is the follow-up of the distribution in a community of isolates with specific features (e.g. antigens of interest, in the context of a vaccination programme or drug-resistance markers, for the definition of treatment policies). PCR (whose specificity can be changed at will by changing the primer sequences used) is ideally suited for this purpose and molecular epidemiology employing such tools is increasingly being used for isolate-specific surveys.

## Transfusion malaria

The transmission of malaria by blood transfusion is a serious risk, because the diagnosis of malaria in the recipient, being unexpected, is often missed. Microscopic examination of donor blood is highly unsatisfactory, because most donor infections are at a sub-microscopic level. Outside endemic areas, the policy of screening the donor's history for known episodes of clinical malaria or for tropical travel in the past 5 years is generally sufficient. In view of the increasing frequency of tropical travel, the policy in some countries is to reject only donors whose malaria serology is positive (generally using IFAT with homologous antigens for *P. falciparum*, *P. vivax* and *P. malariae* for maximum assay sensitivity). This screening method is not perfect, but a negative serology gives a high probability of freedom from infection. The use of PCR (recently explored by the Blood Transfusion Centre of Ho Chi Minh City in Vietnam: Vu thi Ty Hang *et al.*, 1995) is not, despite its much increased sensitivity, a complete guarantee of safe blood, because the absence of parasites in a 20-$\mu$L sample does not exclude the possibility of infection in the remaining 450 mL of the blood unit. In endemic areas, the only safe prevention of transfusion malaria is appropriate preventive antimalarial therapy of the recipient.

## REFERENCES

Amodu OK, Adeyemo AA, Olumese PE, Gbadegesin G. Intraleucocytic malaria pigment and clinical severity. *Trans R Soc Trop Med Hyg* 1998; **92**: 54–6.

Castelli F, Carosi G. Diagnosis of malaria infection. In *Handbook of malaria infection in the tropics*. Carosi G, Castelli F, eds. Health Cooperation Papers No. 15. Bologna, Associazione Italiana, 1997, 53–71.

Cheesbrough M. District laboratory practice in tropical countries. Part 1. Tropical Health Technology, 1998.

Coosemans M, Van der Stuyft P, Delacollette C. A hundred per cent of fields positive in a thick film: a useful indicator of relative changes in morbidity in areas with seasonal malaria. *Ann Trop Med Parasitol* 1994; **88**: 581–6.

Craig MR, Sharp BL. Comparative evaluation of four techniques for the diagnosis of *Plasmodium falciparum* infections. *Trans R Soc Trop Med Hyg* 1997; **91**: 279–82.

Foster SO. Pricing, distribution and use of antimalarial drugs. *Bull World Health Organ* 1991; **69**: 349–63.

Franzen L, Shabo B, Perlmann H, *et al.* Analysis of clinical specimens by hybridization with a probe containing repetitive DNA for *Plasmodium falciparum* malaria. *Lancet* 1984; **i**: 525–7.

Gillespie SH, Chiodini P. Is serology helpful in the diagnosis of malaria. *Serodiagnosis and Immunotherapy in Infectious Disease* 1988; **2**: 157–160.

Hang VTT, Be TV, Tran PN, *et al.* Screening donor blood for malaria by polymerase chain reaction. *Trans R Soc Trop Med Hyg* 1995; **89**: 44–7.

Jonkman A, Chibwe RA, Khoromana CO, *et al.* Cost-saving through microscopy-based versus presumptive diagnosis of malaria in adult outpatients in Malawi. *Bull World Health Org* 1995; **73**: 223–7.

Kawamoto F. Rapid detection of *Plasmodium* by a new thick smear method using transmission fluorescence microscopy: direct staining with acridine orange. *J Protozool Res* 1991; **1**: 27–34.

Kawamoto F, Liu Q, Ferreira MU, Tantular IS. How prevalent are *Plasmodium ovale* and P. *malariae* in East Asia? *Parasitol Today* 1999; **15**: 422–6.

Knobloch J, Henk M. Screening for malaria by determination of parasite-specific lactate dehydrogenase. *Trans R Soc Trop Med Hyg* 1995; **89**: 269–70.

Long GW, Fries L, Watt GH, Hoffmal SL. Polymerase chain reaction amplification from *Plasmodium falciparum* on dried blood spots. *Am J Trop Med Hyg* 1995; **52**: 344–6.

Luxemburger C, Nosten F, Kyle DE, Kiricharoen L, Chongsuphajaisiddhi T, White NJ. Clinical features cannot predict a diagnosis of malaria or differentiate the infecting species in children living in an area of low transmission. *Trans R Soc Trop Med Hyg* 1998; **92**: 45–9.

Makler MT, Ries LK, Ries J, Horton RJ, Hinrichs DJ. Detection of *Plasmodium falciparum* infection with the fluorescent dye benzothiocarboxypurine. *Am J Trop Med Hyg* 1991; **44**: 11–16.

Marsh K, English M, Peshu N, Crawley J, Snow R. Algorithm for malaria in Africa. *Lancet* 1996; **347**: 1327–8.

Milne IM, Kyi MS, Chiodini P, Warhurst DC. Accuracy of routine laboratory diagnosis of malaria in the United Kingdom. *J Clin Pathol* 1994; **47**: 740–2.

Olaleye BO, Williams LA, D'Alessandro U, *et al.* Clinical predictors of malaria in Gambian children with fever or a history of fever. *Trans R Soc Trop Med Hyg* 1998; **92**: 300–4.

Olivar M, Develoux M, Abari AC, Loutan L. Presumptive diagnosis of malaria results in a significant risk of mistreatment in urban Sahel. *Trans R Soc Trop Med Hyg* 1991; **85**: 729–30.

Oliveira DA, Holloway BP, Durigon EL, Collins WE, Lal AA. Polymerase chain reaction and a liquid-phase, non-isotopic hybridization for species-specific and sensitive detection of malaria infection. *Am J Trop Med Hyg* 1995; **52**: 139–44.

Palmer CJ, Lindo JF, Klaskala WL, Evaluation of the OptiMal test for rapid diagnosis of *Plasmodium vivax* and *Plasmodium falciparum* malaria. *J Clin Microbiol* 1998; **36**: 203–6.

Payne D. Use and limitations of light microscopy for diagnosing malaria at the primary health care level. *Bull World Health Organ* 1988; **66**: 621–6.

Phu NH, Day N, Diep PT, Ferguson DJ, White NJ. Intraleucocytic malaria pigment and prognosis in severe malaria. *Trans R Soc Trop Med Hyg* 1995; **89**: 200–4.

Pieroni P, Mills CD, Ohrt C, Harrington A, Kain KC. Comparison of the Parasight™-F test and the ICT Malaria Pf™ test with the polymerase chain reaction for the diagnosis of *Plasmodium falciparum* malaria in travellers. *Trans R Soc Trop Med Hyg* 1998; **92**: 166–9.

Piper R, Lebras J, Wentworth L, Hunt-Cooke A, Chiodini P, Makler M. Immunocapture diagnostic assays for malaria using *Plasmodium* lactate dehydrogenase (pLDH). *Am J Trop Med Hyg* 1999; **60**: 109–18.

Redd SC, Kazembe PN, Luby SP, *et al.* Clinical algorithm for treatment of *Plasmodium falciparum* malaria in children. *Lancet* 1996; **347**: 223–7.

Rougemont A, Breslow N, Brenner E, *et al.* Epidemiological basis for clinical diagnosis of childhood malaria in endemic zone in West Africa. *Lancet* 1991; **338**: 1292–5.

Russell PF, West LS, Manxwell RD, Macdonald G. *Practical malariology*, 2nd edn. London, Oxford University Press.

Shiff CI, Premij Z, Minjas JN. The rapid ParaSight™-F test. A new diagnostic tool for *Plasmodium falciparum* infection. *Trans R Soc Trop Med Hyg* 1993; **87**: 29–31.

Shute GT. The microscopic diagnosis of malaria. In *Malaria. Principles and practice of malariology*, Vol. 1.

Wernsdorfer WH, McGregor I, eds. Edinburgh, Churchill Livingstone, 1988, 781–814.

Silamut K, White NJ. Relation of the stage of parasite development in the peripheral blood to prognosis in severe falciparum malaria. *Trans R Soc Trop Med Hyg* 1993; **87**: 436–43.

Singh B, Cox-Singh J, Miller AO, Abdullah MS, Snounou G, Rahman HA. Detection of malaria in Malaysia by nested polymerase chain reaction amplification of dried blood spots on filter papers. *Trans R Soc Trop Med Hyg* 1996; **90**: 519–21.

Snounou G, Viriyakosol S, Jarra W, Thaithong S, Brown KN. Identification of the four human malaria parasite species in field samples by the polymerase chain reaction and detection of a high prevalence of mixed infections. *Mol Biochem Parasitol* 1993; **58**: 283–92.

Snow, RW, Armstrong, JR, Forster, D, Childhood deaths in Africa: uses and limitations of verbal autopsies. *Lancet* 1992; **340**: 351–5.

Spielman A, Perrone JB, Teklehaimanot A, Balcha F, Wardlaw F, Levine RA. Malaria diagnosis by direct observation of centrifuged samples. *Am J Trop Med Hyg* 1988; **39**: 337–42.

Tirasophon W, Ponglikitmongkol M, Wilairat P, Boosaeng V, Panyim S. A novel detection of a single *Plasmodium falciparum* in infected blood. *Biochem Biophys Res Commun* 1991; **175**: 179–84.

Trape J-F, Peelman O, Morault-Peelman B. Criteria for diagnosing clinical malaria among a semi-immune population exposed to intense and perennial transmission. *Trans R Soc Trop Med Hyg* 1985; **79**: 435–42.

Voller A. The immunodiagnosis of malaria. In *Malaria. Principles* and *practice of malariology,* Vol. 1. Wernsdorfer WH, McGregor I, eds. Edinburgh, Churchill Livingstone, 1988, 815–25.

Voller A, O'Neill P. Immunofluorescence method suitable for large scale application to malaria. *Bull World Health Organ* 1971; **45**: 524–9.

Voller A, Bidwell DE, Huldt G, Engvall, EA. A microplate method of enzyme linked immunosorbent assay and its application to malaria. *Bull World Health Org* 1974; **51**: 209–10.

Warhurst DC, Williams JE. Laboratory diagnosis of malaria. *J Clin Pathol* 1996; **49**: 533–8.

White NJ. Malaria. In *Manson's tropical diseases*, 20th edition. Cook G, ed. London, WB Saunders, 1998, 1087–164.

White NJ, Chapman D, Watt G. The effects of multiplication and synchronicity on the vascular distribution of parasites in falciparum malaria. *Trans R Soc Trop Med Hyg* 1992; **86**: 590–7.

WHO. Severe and complicated malaria. *Trans R Soc Trop Med Hyg* 2000; **94**(Suppl. 1): 1–90.

WHO. *Bench aids for the diagnosis of malaria.* Geneva, World Health Organization, 1988.

WHO. *Basic malaria microscopy.* Part 1. Learner's guide. Geneva, World Health Organization, 1991.

Willcox A. *Manual for the microscopical diagnosis of malaria* in man, 2nd edition. Washington, DC, US Department of Health, Education and Welfare, Public Health Services, 1960.

Wongsrichalanai C, Namsiripongpun V, Webster KH, *et al.* Acridine orange fluorescent microscopy and the detection of malaria in populations with low density parasitaemia. *Am J Trop Med Hyg* 1991; **44**: 17–20.

# 4

# The *Anopheles* vector

MIKE W SERVICE AND HAROLD TOWNSON

Since it was first shown, 100 years ago, that the malaria parasite is transmitted through the bite of a mosquito, it has been recognized that knowledge of the mosquito is of major importance in malaria control. Simple techniques of reducing mosquito survival, such as spraying interior wall surfaces with residual insecticides, have in some countries led to the total eradication of malaria or greatly reduced its public health importance. However, successful programmes have always been based on a sound knowledge of the mosquito species concerned and the details of their biology and behaviour. This chapter considers the biology of the malaria vectors, emphasizing features important to an understanding of malaria epidemiology and control, and describes the more important methods used by entomologists to collect and study them.

Although there are some 3200 species of mosquitoes belonging to 42 genera, only one genus, *Anopheles*, is able to transmit human malaria. *Anopheles* mosquitoes can also transmit filariasis and some arboviruses, but these other infections are more often carried by culicine mosquitoes. All mosquitoes are placed in the family Culicidae of the order Diptera, with the genus *Anopheles* in a subfamily Anophelinae (anophelines), which includes two other genera, *Chagasia*, found in South and Central America, and *Bironella*, from the Australasian region, neither of which is of medical importance. The genus *Anopheles* contains around 430 known species, of which perhaps 70 are malaria vectors, but only 40 of these are thought to be of any major importance. Though most common in tropical and subtropical regions, *Anopheles* mosquitoes have an almost worldwide distribution, but are notably absent from the Pacific east of Vanuatu (170°E), including Polynesia. Typically, *Anopheles* are not found at altitudes above 2500 m. The genus is divided into six subgenera, four of which include disease vectors.

Natural susceptibility to malaria infection in a particular mosquito species depends on a range of intrinsic physiological and biochemical processes, many of which are poorly understood. However, ecological factors such as frequency of feeding on people, longevity of adult female mosquitoes, and vector population density in relation to humans are important determinants of the transmission potential of a species.

## MORPHOLOGY OF *ANOPHELES*

The external morphology of adults and larvae provides the means for recognizing both the genus *Anopheles* and its constituent species. During its growth and metamorphosis, the mosquito passes through the four distinct stages: egg, larva, pupa and adult (Figure 4.1). The immature stages are aquatic, depending on free water for their survival and development.

### Eggs

The eggs are about 0.5 mm long and typically boat-shaped. In nearly all species, the egg is provided with a pair of air-filled, lateral floats that allow it to float on the water surface (Figure 4.2). The egg is covered with a grey-black exochorion, the patterning of which is sometimes useful for identification of species. The collections of water in which adult females lay their eggs, and which provide the larval and pupal habitat, are commonly known as breeding sites.

### Larvae

Eggs hatch within 48 hours in tropical conditions. The emerging larvae feed on bacteria, yeasts, protozoa and other micro-organisms as well as on particulate organic matter in the water, all of which they filter out with their mouth brushes. Larvae move actively with a wriggling motion. Growth takes place through a series of moults, during which the larvae pass through four larval instars.

The main body of the larva is white to pale brown in colour, contrasting with the dark brown head capsule, which bears a pair of eyes and the conspicuous mouth brushes used to sweep food particles into the mouth (Figure 4.3). The thorax has several groups of long hairs that are useful in species identification. The abdomen is composed of 10 segments, but only nine are visible. The first six to seven segments usually have a pair of palmate hairs or float-hairs on the dorsal surface; segments one to eight may also carry a dark, oval tergal plate and, in some species, small accessory tergal plates. The presence of palmate hairs or tergal plates suffices to identify mosquito larvae as those of *Anopheles*. Most abdominal segments have groups of conspicuous lateral hairs that are often feather-like. The penultimate visible segment has a pair of round spiracular openings to the respiratory system, allowing air to be breathed when the larva is at the water surface (Figure 4.4). This is the most obvious diagnostic characteristic, distinguishing anophelines from other mosquitoes, which carry their spiracular openings at the tip of a prominent respiratory tube, the siphon. During feeding and breathing at the water surface, the anopheline larva, assisted by the palmate hairs, lies parallel to the water surface, a characteristic that distinguishes it from culicine mosquitoes (see Figure 4.1). Most methods of identification of larvae to species are based on the fourth instar, earlier instars being difficult or impossible to identify. Prior to pupation, the fourth-instar larva ceases to feed, becomes quiescent and then moults to become the pupa.

### Pupae

The pupa is comma-shaped and differs in appearance from the larva. The anterior part consists of a fused head and thorax, the cephalothorax, on the dorsal surface of which is a pair of short, apically flared respiratory trumpets (see Figure 4.1). The abdomen has eight freely moveable, visible segments, which terminate in a pair of oval, flattened paddles. Anopheline pupae differ from those of other mosquitoes by having, in addition to various fine hairs, a short peg-like hair at the posterior corners of most abdominal segments, but their identification to species is usually impossible. Pupae do not feed during their brief life of some 2–4 days (in the tropics). They remain at the water surface, taking in air through their trumpets, unless disturbed, when they swim down to the bottom with characteristic jerky movements. Just prior to adult emergence, the pupa becomes quiescent at the water surface, the upper part of the integument then splits open and the adult emerges to rest briefly at the water surface before taking to flight.

### Adults

The adults (Figure 4.5) are the stages most frequently encountered and carry a number of morphological features useful in diagnosis (Figure 4.6). The head bears a pair of prominent compound eyes and a pair

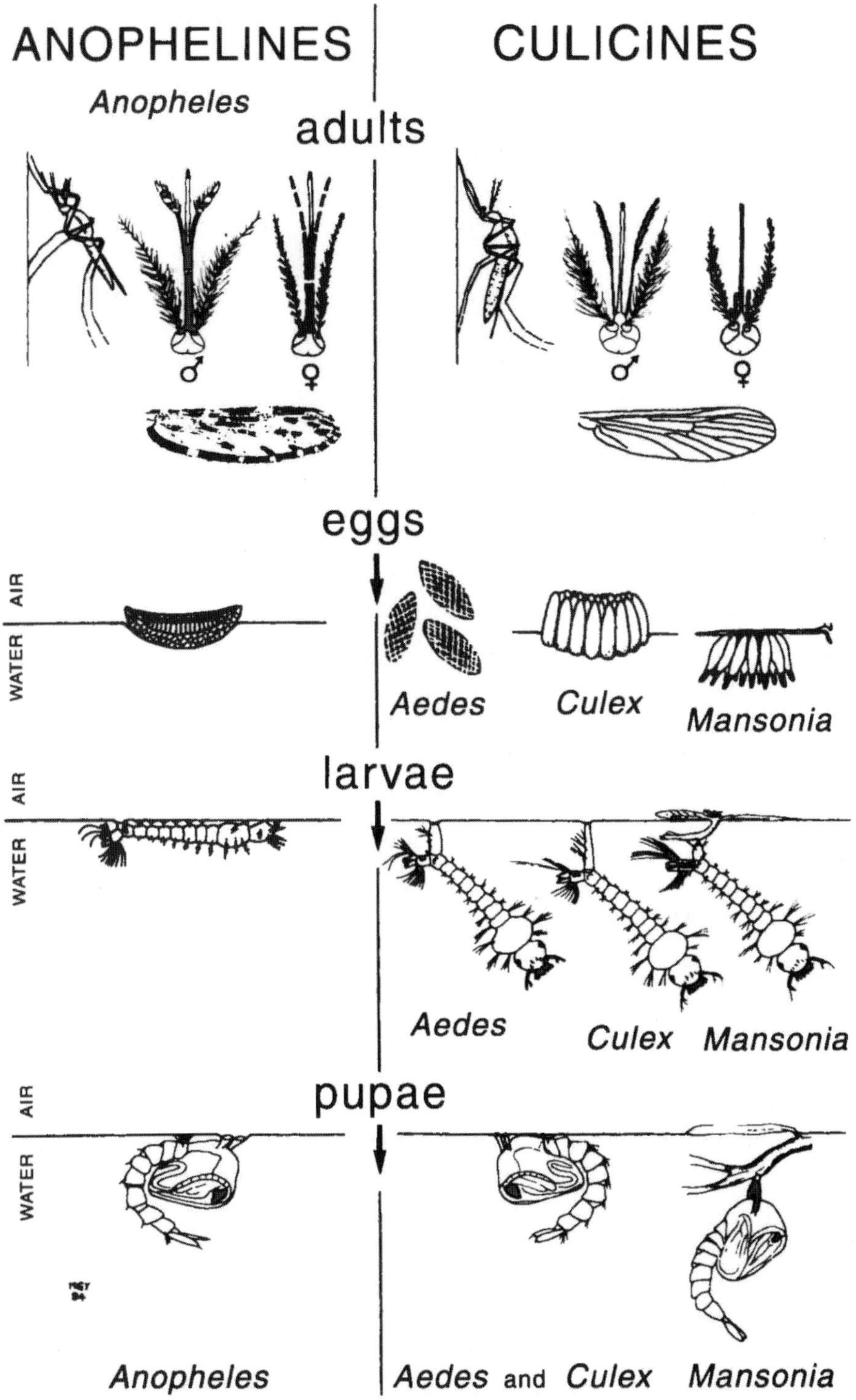
ANOPHELINES
CULICINES
Anopheles
adults
♂
♀
♂
♀
eggs
AIR
WATER
Aedes
Culex
Mansonia
larvae
AIR
WATER
Aedes
Culex
Mansonia
pupae
AIR
WATER
Anopheles
Aedes and Culex
Mansonia

**Figure 4.1**
*Differentiation of anopheline and culicine mosquitoes at various stages in their life cycle.*

of filamentous, segmented antennae that are plumose in the males but sparsely feathered in the females. The antennae carry numerous sense organs, including receptors in females that are involved in host location. Antennae are also involved in sound detection and probably assist males in locating

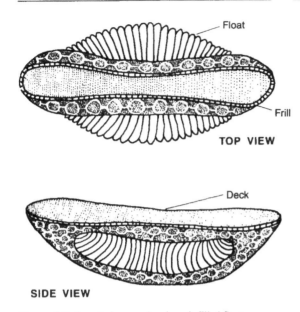

TOP VIEW

SIDE VIEW

**Figure 4.2** Anopheles *egg showing air-filled floats.*

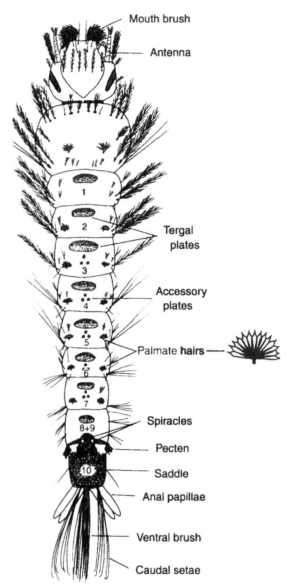

**Figure 4.3** *Dorsal view of an* Anopheles *larva: note the palmate hairs and tergal plates, which are diagnostic of the genus.*

females. Situated one on each side of the forward-projecting proboscis is a pair of sensory structures, the palps, which are about as long as the proboscis in both sexes (see Figures 4.1 and 4.6). The palps are covered with appressed scales that give them a dark or black hue. In the female they are more or less of equal thickness throughout their length, whereas in the males they are distinctly swollen or clubbed apically (see Figure 4.1). The palps often have narrow to broad rings of pale and dark scales, giving an ornamentation characteristic of a particular species or group of species. In culicine mosquitoes, the palps of females are usually short or very short and in males, although about as long as the proboscis, they are not swollen apically. The palps also carry important sense organs used in host location in females. The mouthparts collectively form the proboscis, the largest component of which is the gutter-shaped labium, which bears a small pair of apical labella (Figure 4.7). The labium sheathes the other structures of the mouthparts (stylets). These comprise the paired and toothed mandibles, the paired and toothed maxillae and the single hollow hypopharynx (Figure 4.7), which conducts saliva from the salivary glands to the wound made in the skin when the female is feeding. The dorsal labrum closes the open side of the labium and forms an open-sided cylinder that carries the blood into the digestive system. When the mosquito bites in order to feed, all com-

ponents of the proboscis, except the labium, penetrate the skin. The ingestion of blood up the labrum is achieved by contraction of a pair of muscular organs, the cibarial and pharyngeal pumps.

The thorax has three pairs of legs, the parts of which are shown in Figure 4.6. There is a single pair of wings, the hind wings being represented by a small pair of drumstick-shaped halteres. The wings of all mosquitoes have a characteristic arrangement of veins

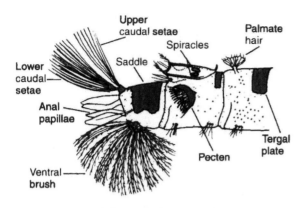

**Figure 4.4** *Lateral view of the last abdominal segments of an* Anopheles *larva, showing spiracular openings to the respiratory system.*

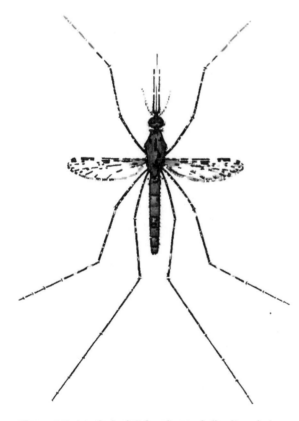

**Figure 4.5** *A typical adult female anopheline* (Anopheles gambiae). *(Source: JD Gillett, Common African mosquitos. London, W Heinemann Medical Books, 1972, p. 27.)*

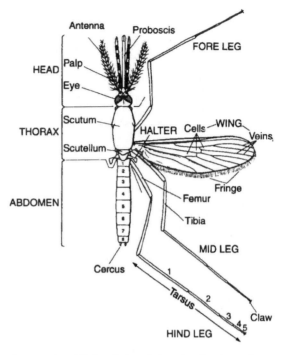

**Figure 4.6** *Adult female* Anopheles, *showing the main morphological features.*

*maculipennis* complex, have spotted wings, that is dark and pale scales arranged in blocks or areas on the veins (Figure 4.8). When present, this characteristic is diagnostic of anopheline mosquitoes. Behind the main part of the thorax is a small, trilobed scutellum that usually carries scales on each lobe.

The abdomen has eight visible segments, which, unlike those of culicine mosquitoes, are mostly devoid of scales. The last segment terminates in a pair of small, finger-like cerci in females, and in males a pair of prominent claspers that are used to seize females during mating.

Most anopheline adults rest and feed with the body making an inclined angle to the surface on which they stand, whereas culicine mosquitoes stand with the abdomen more or less parallel to the surface (see Figure 4.1).

## INTERNAL ANATOMY OF *ANOPHELES*

Certain internal structures of adult anophelines are relevant to the study of malaria transmission (Figure 4.9).

covered with small pale and dark scales. The patterns of these scales, as with those on the palps and legs, are often useful in species identification. Most *Anopheles* species, but with notable exceptions such as *Anopheles*

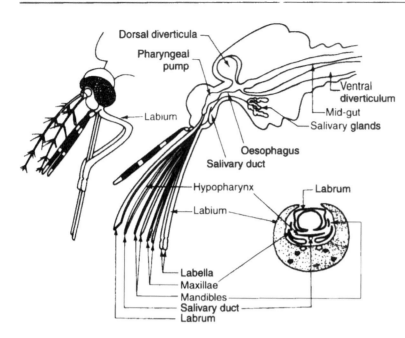

**Figure 4.7** *The mouthparts of an adult female* Anopheles, *including a cross-section through the proboscis.*

A pair of three-lobed salivary glands is situated in the anterior thorax. The three lobes differ in internal structure and it is known that the secretory products of the glands are differentially synthesized in the median and lateral lobes and between the distal and proximal regions of the lobes. The secretions of the glands also vary depending on whether the mosquito is feeding on blood or sugar. During feeding, these glands secrete a number of enzymes as well as anti-haemastatic and vasodilatory components to assist feeding. Ducts from each lobe unite to form a single duct from each gland, which then combine to form the common salivary duct through which the saliva is carried during feeding. The sporozoite stage of the malaria parasite migrates through the haemocoele (body cavity) of the mosquito after the rupture of the oocyst stage on the gut wall and enters the glands in the distal

region. When saliva is induced to flow during a feed, the sporozoites are stimulated to enter the salivary duct, to be swept along with the saliva into a new human host. It is believed that very few sporozoites enter the human skin during feeding of an infective mosquito, perhaps as few as 5–50.

The alimentary canal consists of three main parts: the fore-gut, mid-gut and hind-gut. Liquids imbibed during feeding are sucked up through the labrum and pass through the cibarium and pharynx into the oesophagus. Sugary liquids are passed to a ventral diverticulum, or crop, where they are stored, being passed to the stomach (mid-gut) for digestion as and when required. However, when the female feeds on blood, this passes through the oesophagus directly to the mid-gut, where the meal is digested. If the blood meal contains the sexual stages (gametocytes) of the malaria parasite, fusion of gametes

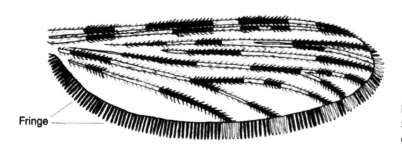

**Figure 4.8** *The wing of* Anopheles, *showing the black and white scales arranged in blocks.*

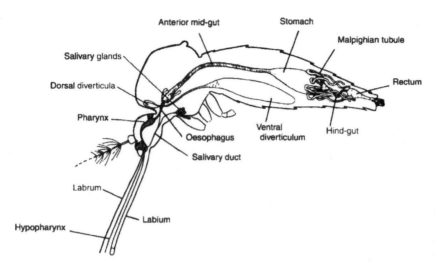

**Figure 4.9** *A schematic diagram showing the the alimentary canal and other internal structures of an adult female* Anopheles.

occurs within the mid-gut to form a wandering zygote, the ookinete. This then leaves the blood meal, migrates through the gut wall and comes to lie just beneath the basement lamina adjacent to the haemocoele. It then transforms to the oocyst stage, within which, by a process of schizogony, sporozoites are produced.

In the mosquito, the initial phase of diuresis and nitrogen excretion occurs in the five malpighian tubules. The resultant fluid is discharged into the hind-gut, being modified in the rectum before being discharged from the anus as urine. The dog heartworm, *Dirofilaria*, which occasionally infects humans, undergoes part of its development in the malpighian tubules of mosquitoes.

In the male, a pair of testes occupies the posterior part of the abdomen. Adjacent accessory glands secrete substances that can induce a short-term monogamy when they are introduced into females during insemination. The common genital duct leads into an ejaculatory duct and thence to the complex structure of the external genitalia with a central phallosome and two prominent claspers.

In the female, a pair of ovaries is situated in the posterior part of the abdomen, each ovary comprising some 50–200 ovarioles. At every blood meal, each ovariole has the potential to produce a new egg, but, in practice, only half do so. In newly emerged females, the ovaries are small, but after a blood meal, nutrients from the digested blood are transported to the developing follicle and are incorporated into the developing oocyte. As a result, the ovaries swell until they come to occupy much of the posterior third of the

abdominal cavity. An oviduct leads from each ovary to unite in the common oviduct, into the distal part of which the sperm duct opens (Figure 4.10). This duct comes from a single, spherical, sclerotized spermatheca in which the spermatozoa that are introduced during mating are stored for the duration of the life of the female.

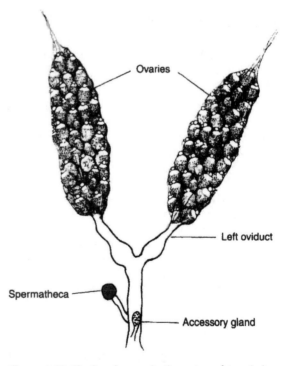

**Figure 4.10** *The female reproductive system of* Anopheles.

## BIOLOGY OF *ANOPHELES*

### Blood feeding and the gonotrophic cycle

Because egg production and blood feeding are intimately linked and blood feeding is also essential to the acquisition and transfer of malaria infection, malaria entomologists have paid special attention to this physiological phenomenon termed the gonotrophic cycle. If the duration of this cycle is known, the number of gonotrophic cycles can serve as a proxy for the physiological age of the mosquito, an important determinant in malaria epidemiology.

Adults usually mate within 1–2 days after their emergence. Mating normally occurs in the evenings and in many species is preceded by the formation of swarms of males. Females entering the swarm are apparently recognized by their lower wing-beat frequency. During copulation, a male passes spermatozoa into the female, which in turn passes them to her spermatheca. Usually, these spermatozoa are sufficient for the fertilization of all egg batches laid during the life of the female, although females sometimes mate more than once.

Most female anophelines are anautogenous, i.e. a female must obtain a blood meal to provide the pro-

teins and amino acids required for the maturation of the eggs. However, females of a few species are autogenous, i.e. they can mature and lay their first batch of eggs without a blood meal, although blood is essential for all subsequent ovipositions. After feeding, the swollen abdomen appears bright red and the mosquito is referred to as *blood-fed*. As digestion occurs, the abdomen darkens and the ovaries enlarge and appear whitish through the abdomen. At the halfway stage, when much of the blood has been digested and ovarian development is half completed, the mosquito is termed *half-gravid* or *semi-gravid* (Figure 4.11). When all blood has been digested and the eggs in the ovaries have matured, much of the dilated abdomen appears whitish and the mosquito is now *gravid*. After the female lays her eggs, the abdomen is again thin and appears empty and the female is classified as *unfed*. It is this cycle from unfed to blood-fed to half-gravid to gravid to unfed again that is called the gonotrophic cycle and it is repeated several times (often four to five times) until the female dies. The duration of the gonotrophic cycle is dependent on temperature and, in the tropics, at temperatures above 23 °C, it usually lasts 2–3 days, but in the colder temperate climates it may take many days or even weeks. Females of some species, including the important African malaria vector *A. gambiae*, may require two blood meals before the first batch

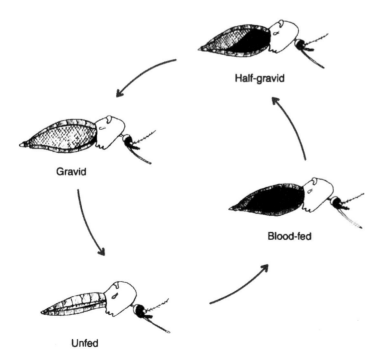

**Figure 4.11** *Stages in the gonotrophic cycle of a female mosquito.*

of eggs can develop. Rarely, a species may require three to four blood meals. After her first blood meal, if ovarian development is not complete, the female is referred to as *pre-gravid*. In subsequent gonotrophic cycles, a batch of eggs is produced after each blood meal. It is possible to estimate the number of gonotrophic cycles from dissection of the ovaries and this technique provides a comparative measure of the survival of mosquito populations.

Plant sugars are a major energy resource for mosquitoes and both males and females will feed on nectar, sugary exudates from fruit, honeydew and even damaged or intact plant tissues. Although male mosquitoes have a conspicuous proboscis, the mandibles are reduced or absent in many species and the stylets are unable to pierce the skin of vertebrates. Thus, plant juices are the only food resource for males.

## Blood feeding behaviour

The females of most species of *Anopheles* feed on warm-blooded animals, predominantly mammals. Some species prefer to feed on humans and are termed anthropophagic or anthropophilic, whereas others favour animals, such as cattle, and are termed zoophagic or zoophilic. However, these traits are not absolute, for whereas most species may be predominantly anthropophagic or zoophagic, they are not usually exclusively so. *Anopheles* are attracted to their hosts by a range of stimuli, including exhaled carbon dioxide, lactic acid, other host odours, warmth and moisture. The distance over which a mosquito is attracted varies with species, meteorological conditions and topography, but is usually between 7 m and 20 m. Some people are more attractive to mosquitoes than others, but the reasons remain largely unknown, although odour substances from the skin of different humans differ in their attractiveness to *Anopheles*. Adults are bitten more often than infants and children, perhaps because of their larger size. Having located a suitable host, the female mosquito alights and makes a minute incision in the skin with her mandibles and maxillae, before inserting her labrum. Once this has located and penetrated a capillary vessel, blood feeding commences and is usually completed within 1 minute.

Throughout the penetration and feeding process, the mosquito pumps saliva down the hypopharynx into the wound. This saliva contains a complex mixture of anti-haemostatic and vasodilatory compounds to aid feeding. These salivary constituents also help produce the characteristic skin reactions to mosquito bites.

In anophelines, feeding takes place, almost without exception, between dusk and dawn, but some species may feed during the day in densely shaded woods and forests. Some have early peaks of biting, as with *A. albimanus* in Central America (1900–2100 hours), whereas others, such as *A. gambiae* in Africa, are late feeders (2400–0300 hours). The readiness of mosquitoes to feed at a particular time of night depends to some extent on environmental conditions, such as temperature, wind speed and moonlight, but the times of biting (biting cycles) are determined mainly by in-built circadian rhythms.

Some malaria vectors feed mainly outside and are termed exophagic; other species may feed readily, or even predominantly, inside houses and are called endophagic. After engorging on blood, the female mosquito usually seeks shelter in which to rest and digest her blood meal, and to develop her eggs. Some anophelines rest inside houses, both before and after feeding, and are termed endophilic. Others rest in various outdoor sites, in vegetation, in rodent holes, on earthen banks, between buttress roots of trees, in cracks in the ground, in excavation pits, in granaries or cow sheds, on fencing around cattle enclosures or in culverts, and are termed exophilic. Few *Anopheles* exhibit exclusively one set of behaviour patterns. For example, although in Africa *A. gambiae* may be predominantly anthropophagic, endophagic and endophilic, in some areas cattle may be much more numerous than humans and so the mosquitoes will become zoophagic, exophagic and, perhaps, exophilic.

The time and place of biting can be of epidemiological importance and influence control measures. A vector that feeds early in the evenings, outside, can transmit malaria to young children as well as to adults, but one that bites outside later at night when young children are predominantly indoors will be less important in this respect. It is therefore important to study the customs of the people and their sleeping habits as well as the behaviour of the vectors. For example, in the hot, dry seasons, substantial numbers of people may sleep outside and, as a consequence, be more frequently bitten by exophagic vectors. Furthermore, the use of insecticide-impregnated bed-nets indoors will be of little value if the vector bites predominantly outdoors. The resting behaviour of adults is also an important consideration in planning control measures. In many malaria control operations, the interior surfaces of houses, such as walls and ceilings, are sprayed with a residual insecticide to kill mosquitoes resting on them. However, this strategy would not be effective in killing the vectors if they were predominantly exophilic.

The quantity of blood ingested at a single feed depends largely on the mosquito's size, but ranges from about 1 mg to 2.5 mg, which approximates to the weight of the unfed female. However, anophelines are able to increase the volume of blood they take in through diuresis. Thus, the blood ingested is concentrated by the discharge of a few drops of clear liquid from the anus. In nature, the volumes of blood ingested may be markedly limited by the defensive behaviour of the host.

The blood ingested by female mosquitoes is primarily used for egg production, but it may also be used as an energy resource. Nectar meals are less frequently sought when a mosquito is digesting its blood meal. Typically, each blood meal leads to the development of a batch of eggs. The process of blood feeding followed by full development of the ovaries is termed gonotrophic concordance, to distinguish it from gonotrophic dissociation. This latter term is applied when the ovaries fail to mature after a blood meal, such as in *A. atroparvus* of Europe, which hibernate during the cooler months, a strategy found mainly in temperate species. Another condition, known as gonotrophic discordance, describes the situation in which blood feeding leads to the maturation of eggs but the gravid female delays oviposition, with or without subsequent re-feeding. This condition is seen in those tropical species that undergo a process of aestivation during periods of drought, such as *A. arabiensis* in the northern Sudan, or *A. culicifacies* and *A. stephensi* in the Indian subcontinent.

## OVIPOSITION

Depending on the species, and on the quality and size of the blood meal, a female *Anopheles* lays 50–200 eggs during a single oviposition, usually at night. Successive egg batches tend to decrease in size and there may be seasonal variations in the numbers of eggs laid. *Anopheles* eggs cannot withstand desiccation and usually hatch in 2–3 days, but in some species eggs remain alive for 16 days or longer on wet mud, and then hatch within seconds when flooded.

## ADULT LONGEVITY

The survival and longevity of an adult female depend to some extent on environmental factors such as temperature and relative humidity, but also vary among species. Although innate mortality rises with age, predators and disease are probably the most important causes of death. When the mean temperature exceeds 35 °C, or the humidity is less than 50 per cent, the longevity of *Anopheles* is drastically reduced, unless the adults can find a more favourable microclimate within their resting sites. The average duration of life of a female *Anopheles* in the tropics is about 10–14 days. Occasionally, the average life will be nearer 3 weeks and, in temperate regions, anopheline adults may live many weeks, or even months in species that hibernate during the winter. Males live for a shorter time than females.

Adult longevity is of paramount importance in malaria epidemiology. For example, if the mean daily survival fraction of a vector population is 0.65, then $0.65^{10}$ (only around 1 per cent) will survive the 10 days needed for the development of *P. falciparum* to the infective sporozoites in the salivary glands. The importance of this concept is explained more fully in the next chapter.

## FLIGHT RANGE

*Anopheles* adults are not usually found more than 2–3 km from their breeding sites, at least in large numbers. Distances flown are largely determined by the environment: if suitable larval habitats and hosts are nearby, females have little need to fly far. However, strong winds may carry *Anopheles* up to 30 km or more. In Egypt, *A. pharoensis* has been found 72 km from the nearest breeding place, and swarms of *A. pulcherrimus* have invaded a ship 25 km off the Arabian coast. Adults may also be transported long distances by hitching rides on aeroplanes, ships, trains or vehicles. The carriage of exotic, malaria-infected *Anopheles* by aircraft to temperate areas has been responsible for so-called airport malaria in several European countries. Generally, the control of anophelines within a radius of 2 km from airports, docks and other transportation systems where immigrant mosquitoes may be resting or breeding should provide adequate protection against their further dispersal.

For the study of anopheline dispersal or flight range, adult mosquitoes may be marked with different-coloured paints or fluorescent powders, or made radioactive by dosing larval rearing waters with radionuclides of phosphorus or strontium, and then released. Recaptured marked adults can be visibly recognized by their coloured marks, and radioactive ones detected by Geiger–Müller or scintillation counters, or by their 'fogging' of photographic film.

Service (1997) reviews mosquito dispersal, and further details of marking and recapture methods can be found in Service (1993).

## SEASONAL FLUCTUATIONS IN POPULATION SIZE

Seasonal fluctuations in environmental factors such as rainfall, temperature and humidity affect the survival rate of anophelines and their population size. In most tropical countries, breeding continues throughout the year, albeit at a greatly reduced rate in the dry season due to the paucity of larval habitats. The onset of the rains or monsoon season usually creates a proliferation of potential breeding places and the numbers of adult *Anopheles* can increase explosively. Large populations are usually maintained throughout the rains and for some weeks afterwards, then anopheline numbers gradually decrease. In contrast, for species breeding in the margins of streams, population sizes may decrease with the onset of the main rains. Atypical weather can have dire consequences. For example, excessive rainfall and high temperatures in Ethiopia in 1958 resulted in exceptionally large numbers of *A. arabiensis*, followed by a disastrous malaria epidemic involving an estimated 3 million cases and 150 000 deaths. In contrast, a severe drought in south-western Sri Lanka in 1934–5 created numerous pools in partially dried streams that were colonized by *A. culicifacies*. Their excessive numbers resulted in a severe malaria epidemic, causing about

80 000 deaths among 2–3 million cases. The El Niño southern oscillation has recently been shown to be associated with epidemic malaria in Africa.

In hot regions, during the dry season when larval habitats are scarce, females of some species may seek shelter in cool, damp places, such as on the walls of wells. Although continuing to blood feed, they do not lay eggs until the beginning of the rains, although fully developed eggs may be present in their ovaries. Such seasonal behaviour is termed aestivation. *Anopheles arabiensis* is thought to survive the dry season in Khartoum and Omdurman in the Sudan by aestivating. In temperate areas, but also in some hot countries that experience seasonal cool periods, females may seek shelter from the cold in hibernation sites, such as caves, buildings or rodent burrows. Before hibernation, females of some species may undertake a pre-hibernation flight, which is longer than their normal ones. In Israel, 14-km pre-hibernation flights have been recorded in *A. sacharovi* and, in California, *A. freeborni* may fly up to 42 km to seek out hibernation sites. Before hibernation, a last blood meal is taken from which abdominal fat reserves, not eggs, are formed. If there is complete hibernation, females remain inactive in their sheltered sites until warmer weather returns. However, in some species there is only partial hibernation and females need to emerge periodically from their shelters to take blood meals to renew their fat reserves. Such incomplete hibernation occurs in *A. sacharovi* at the beginning of hibernation in Israel, and in *A. atroparvus*, feeding of which in the winter has resulted in cases of malaria in the Netherlands, Germany and England. Only fertilized females successfully hibernate. In some species, such as the European *A. claviger* and *A. plumbeus*, adults die with the onset of the cold season and the population over-winters as larvae.

## LARVAL AND PUPAL BIOLOGY

The duration of the larval period depends mainly on temperature and, in the hot tropics, may last some 7–11 days. In colder seasons and in the temperate regions, the larval period may extend to several weeks or months. The pupal stage typically lasts 2–4 days, although in colder climates this may extend to a week or more. The total duration of the aquatic cycle from egg to adult emergence varies from 7 days at 31 °C to 20 days at 20 °C.

## LARVAL HABITATS

There is a great diversity in the types of water utilized by different anopheline species. Some larval habitats may be temporary, such as small ponds, pools and puddles, others may be more permanent, such as marshes and borrow pits (depressions created by excavating soil). Although most aquatic habitats are freshwater, some *Anopheles* species breed in saline waters. Most anophelines avoid organically polluted waters, such as those contaminated with human or animal faeces or rotting vegetation. Many species have a relatively narrow range of habitats, with some species preferring those fully exposed to the sun, whereas others are more or less restricted to shade.

Many anophelines are found in freshwater ponds and small collections of water such as pools and puddles that lack vegetation (e.g. *A. gambiae* in Africa and *A. stephensi* in India; Figure 4.12). Others are found in marshes or large ponds with floating or emergent vegetation (e.g. *A. nili* and *A. funestus* of Africa and *A. albimanus* in Central America). Mosquitoes are not found in fast-flowing streams, but a few anophelines, such as *A. pseudopunctipennis* in South America, *A. superpictus* in Europe, *A. minimus* in Asia and *A. maculatus* in Malaysia, breed in the shallow, relatively still waters at the edges of streams or in springs and seepages. A few species (e.g. *A. plumbeus* in Europe) prefer rain-filled tree holes. Certain species of the subgenus *Kerteszia* (e.g. *A. bellator* and *A. cruzii* in Central

and South America) select water-containing leaf axils of bromeliad plants growing on trees (Figure 4.13). Several species are found mainly in saline waters, including *A. atroparvus* in Europe, *A. aquasalis* in Latin America, *A. sundaicus* and *A. litoralis* in Southeast Asia, and *A. melas* and *A. merus* in West and East Africa. Artificial containers, such as water pots, are generally unsuitable for most anopheline species, although *A. stephensi* in India is often found in water tanks and cisterns sited on roofs of buildings, as well as in tin cans, pots and wells. For some species, larvae occur in a great diversity of habitats. In Africa, the larvae of *A. gambiae* can be found in roadside pools, small puddles and hoof prints as well as in borrow pits and rice fields and, very occasionally, in water-filled village pots.

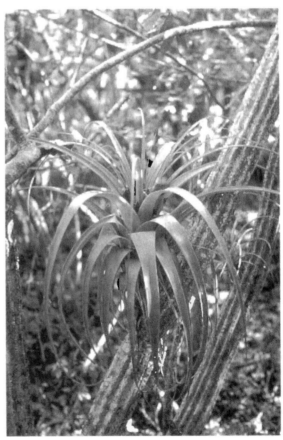

**Figure 4.13** *A South American bromeliad (shown growing on a cactus, although more usually they grow on trees). A few anopheline species, such as* Anopheles bellator *and* Anopheles cruzii, *breed in water collected in their leaf axils. (Photograph by MW Service.)*

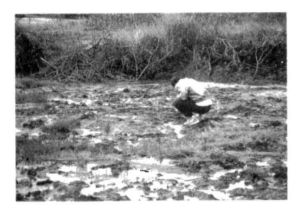

**Figure 4.12** *Small, temporary, ground pools, a typical larval habitat of several anopheline species, including* Anopheles gambiae. *(Photograph by MW Service.)*

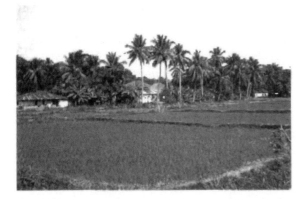

**Figure 4.14** *Rice fields, a common larval habitat of several anopheline species, such as* Anopheles culicifacies, Anopheles gambiae *and* Anopheles aconitus. *(Photograph by MW Service.)*

Man-made malaria is a term applied to many human activities that provide habitats suitable for malaria vectors, so favouring increased incidence of disease. Road building and track laying for trains, for example, create puddles and ditches, and gem mining results in pits that fill with rainwater. Land under agricultural irrigation, such as flooded rice fields (Figure 4.14), is colonized by several important malaria vectors, including *A. gambiae* and *A. arabiensis* in Africa, *A. culicifacies* and *A. subpictus* in the Indian subcontinent, *A. sinensis* in China, *A. aconitus* in much of South-east Asia, *A. darlingi* in Central America and *A. freeborni* in the USA. Breeding in rice fields can result in increased intensity of malaria transmission and extend transmission into the dry season.

## SPECIES COMPLEXES

Many species of anopheline mosquito can be reliably identified by their morphology, but an increasing number of species defined on morphological criteria are found on closer inspection to consist of several, reproductively isolated entities that constitute good biological species. Such sibling species, despite their apparent similarity, may differ in important biological characteristics that influence their role in the transmission of malaria. A group of several such species, with a common line of descent, comprise a species complex. The discovery over

50 years ago that the European malaria vector *A. maculipennis* consisted of several biologically distinct species helped explain the puzzle of anophelism without malaria, and was a landmark in the study of malaria vectors.

The recognition of sibling species complexes is important because the constituent members may differ in their host preference, breeding sites, preferred sites for resting or feeding and even their capacity to transmit malaria. The *A. gambiae* complex, which includes the most important malaria vectors in Africa, has been studied more than any other vector species complex and well illustrates the practical importance of distinguishing sibling species. The complex consists of seven described species, six of them formally named, although it is believed that additional cryptic species occur in the savannah regions of West Africa. The two most important species in the complex are *A. gambiae* and *A. arabiensis*. The former predominates in humid areas, prefers feeding on humans and resting indoors and is a highly efficient malaria vector. In contrast, *A. arabiensis*, although found in the humid zones, is more tolerant of the drier savannah regions. Whereas it readily bites humans and may rest indoors, it often feeds on cattle and rests outdoors, particularly in man-made structures. It, too, is an efficient vector, second only in importance to *A. gambiae*. Both these species are widespread over much of Africa, whereas *A. quadriannulatus* (now recognized as comprising two species, A and B) is restricted to north-eastern and southern Africa. In southern Africa, it is considered to be both exophilic and wholly zoophagic, and consequently not a vector. The two brackish-water, and mainly coastal, species *A. melas* of West Africa and *A. merus* of East and southern Africa are more zoophagic and exophilic than *A. gambiae* and malaria vectors of lesser importance. The remaining species, *A. bwambae*, is known only from the Semliki forest on the Rift Valley escarpment in western Uganda, where it breeds in seepage water from geothermal springs. It is therefore a very localized and minor vector. In many parts of Africa, mosquitoes of the complex occur in mixed, sympatric populations, comprising two or even three species. Although the reproductive barriers between the species are strong, occasionally hybridization does occur where species occur in sympatry, and this leads to introgression, a limited exchange of genes.

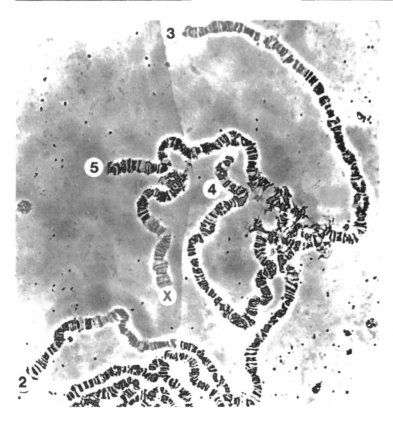

**Figure 4.15** *Polytene chromosomes from adult ovarian nurse cells of* Anopheles gambiae, *showing the species-diagnostic X arm and the four autosomal arms (2–5). (With permission from Richard Hunt and Maureen Coetzee.)*

The techniques used to recognize the existence of sibling species are diverse. The cross-mating of forms suspected to be separate species was the first method employed with malaria vectors and provides a sound basis for recognizing good biological species. Studies of the giant polytene chromosomes found in the larval salivary glands and ovarian nurse cells of the adult female often reveal species-specific karyotypes (Figure 4.15) and this method has been widely used. A limitation is that adult females must be half-gravid for their chromosomes to be useful. Increasingly, molecular techniques are being applied and, in some cases, these have led to polymerase chain reaction (PCR)-based methods for identification (Figure 4.16). These can be readily used with dry specimens, even quite old museum specimens, as well as specimens preserved by other means (Townson *et al.*, 1999). Because this is a rapidly advancing field of study, any attempt at a comprehensive summary of anopheline sibling species is likely to be quickly out of date. Table 4.1 illustrates selected examples from major regions of endemic malaria. The estimated number of species within a

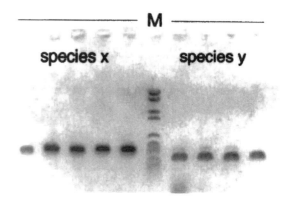

**Figure 4.16** *The identification of nine female mosquitoes drawn from two species (here arbitrarily labelled x and y) within the* Anopheles fluviatilis *complex, using a PCR reaction based on species differences in ribosomal DNA sequence. DNA extracted from individual dry mosquitoes is amplified with a cocktail of two species-specific primers and one primer homologous to both species. The PCR products are then run in agarose gels along with molecular weight markers (lane M), to reveal a DNA product with a species-characteristic number of base-pairs. (Copyright H. Townson.)*

**Table 4.1** *Examples of anopheline sibling species from major regions of endemic malaria*

| Species complexes | No. of species | Zoogeographical region |
|---|---|---|
| gambiae | 7+ | Afrotropical |
| maculipennis | 8 | Palaearctic |
| | 5 | Nearctic |
| albitarsis | 4 | Neotropical and Nearctic |
| nuneztovari | 3 | Neotropical |
| culicifacies | 5 | Oriental |
| dirus | 7 | Oriental |
| fluviatilis | 4 | Oriental |
| minimus | 4 | Oriental |
| sinensis | 2 | Oriental |
| subpictus | 4 | Oriental |
| punctulatus | 11 | Australasian |

complex is provisional and likely to be an underestimate. Furthermore, not all authorities define the boundaries to the complexes in the same manner.

## DISTRIBUTION OF *ANOPHELES* VECTORS

*Anopheles* mosquitoes are sometimes classified as primary and secondary vectors, but a species regarded as a primary vector in some areas may be only a secondary vector in others. Identification of *Anopheles* to species is an important task for the epidemiologist, and the major publications containing taxonomic keys for the identification of anopheline mosquitoes in different geographical regions are listed in an annex to the references for this chapter.

## Survey methods

Larval surveys are undertaken usually to identify where vectors are breeding; insecticidal or non-insecticidal control methods may then be directed at the larvae. Adult anophelines are collected for a variety of reasons, including the estimation of biting rates on humans, proportions feeding on humans or animals, location of their resting places indoors or outdoors, changes in their relative population size caused by season or control measures, estimation of dispersal distances, age-structure and adult longevity, calculation of sporo-zoite rates, and *Anopheles* susceptibility to insecticides. Numerous methods have been devised for collecting the immature stages and adults of anophelines (WHO, 1992; Service, 1993).

*Anopheles* eggs are very rarely seen in larval habitats and their collection is not described. Pupae are difficult to identify to species so it is best to rear out adults.

## Larval collections

### GROUND COLLECTIONS OF WATER

Mosquito larvae are disturbed by shadows and movement of the water, which cause them to swim downwards; therefore, the collector should wait for them to resurface before attempting to collect them. For mosquito larvae and pupae in ground collections of water, the most commonly used tool is a dipper, often a soup ladle. Mosquito larvae usually have a very patchy distribution and most aggregate along the edges of water collections or around clumps of emergent or floating vegetation. The dipper should be gently lowered into the breeding place and water and the larvae allowed to flow into it. The number of dips taken depends on the size and diversity of the habitat and on whether simple detection of breeding places or some measure of larval density is required. Probably about 10 dips are appropriate for small ponds up to 4 m in diameter. Aquatic nets are useful in detecting anopheline breeding when larval density is low.

For very small collections of water such as in cattle hoof prints and puddles, visual inspection should reveal whether larvae are present. The larvae can then be collected by direct pipetting.

### WELLS

Because the water level is usually far below ground level, long-handled dippers, but more usually nets or buckets attached to a cord, are used. After submerging them, and allowing 3–4 minutes for any anopheline larvae to resurface, the net or bucket is gently pulled up along the sides of the well.

### TREE-HOLES AND BROMELIADS

Only a very few anophelines, such as *A. plumbeus* in Europe, *A. barberi* in North America and *A. barianensis* in India and Pakistan, breed in tree-holes, and just a few, such as *A. bellator* and *A. cruzii*, breed in water-filled leaf axils of bromeliads growing on trees, or sometimes cacti in tropical America (see Figure 4.13). The water is removed from such sites with pipettes or siphoned out to allow larval sampling.

## Transportation of larvae

The number of larvae in each dip should be recorded separately to allow calculation of the standard error of the mean number of larvae collected per dip from the different habitats. The collected larvae can be pipetted into plastic vials or into small, snap-sealing, plastic envelopes. To minimize mortality, containers of larvae should be kept out of direct sunlight by placing them in an insulated coolbox. Relevant collection data, such as locality, type of breeding place and date, should be written in pencil on a slip of paper included in each container.

## Adult collections

### HUMAN BAIT CATCHES

To determine the species and numbers of *Anopheles* biting people in an area, collections on human bait, sometimes euphemistically called landing counts, have traditionally been performed. However, there are increasingly strong ethical objections to such an approach. Although collectors are expected to catch

mosquitoes before they bite, it is almost inevitable that they are sometimes bitten, and this exposes them to the risk of acquiring malaria or other vector-borne infections. Antimalarial drugs can reduce the risk of malaria, but not of other diseases. Unfortunately, no other sampling technique gives such reliable estimates of mosquito–human contact, although light-traps hung alongside occupied bed-nets have proven a useful alternative in some countries, for example for *A. gambiae* in Tanzania (Lines *et al.*, 1991).

Because of the nocturnal biting behaviour of malaria vectors, human bait collections are undertaken from 1800 hours to 0600 hours, or for shorter periods in the night. They can be performed inside houses to measure endophagic biting or outdoors to monitor exophagic behaviour. A more realistic measure of the degree of biting experienced by a population is often obtained if bait catches are performed outside houses until most people go indoors, and then indoors. The procedure consists of sitting down and exposing the legs to host-seeking anophelines. When these land on any area of the body, and before they start biting, they are captured with an oral aspirator (sucking tube), then carefully blown into cardboard cartons covered with mosquito netting. Alternatively, a test-tube can be placed carefully over a mosquito that has alighted, which results in it flying up into the tube, which is then plugged with cotton wool. A hurricane lamp is useful in giving background illumination and a torch used intermittently helps locate mosquitoes on the body. It helps if two people sit together, catching from themselves and their companion. Collectors tire after 3–4 hours, and are best rotated with a fresh team after such an interval. The total numbers of mosquitoes caught each hour should be recorded separately so that the hours of maximum biting are obtained for the different species. Human bait catches performed in different months can monitor seasonal fluctuations in biting density.

### BED-NET COLLECTIONS

All-night collections from human bait not only pose a possible risk to collectors, but are also labour intensive and expensive. For these reasons, other methods have been sought. An animal bait that is attractive to malaria vectors, such as a cow, can be placed under a mosquito net that is either raised 10–15 cm from the ground or has a door-like opening on one side to let in host-seeking mosquitoes. After feeding on the enclosed bait, the engorged mosquitoes tend to rest within the net and can be collected in the early morning or at intervals throughout the night. A similar method can be used with human bait, the person being completely enclosed within an inner net to protect against biting, but such arrangements usually reduce the numbers caught and retained within the outer net.

## HOUSE-RESTING (ENDOPHILIC) MOSQUITOES

Malaria vectors that rest in houses before and/or after blood feeding can be collected in the early morning by two procedures. The first entails collectors searching, with the aid of torches, for mosquitoes resting indoors on walls, roofs, ceilings and furniture, particularly in bedrooms, and transferring them by aspirator to cardboard cartons. If house-resting densities are low, very few will be caught, but an advantage is that the mosquitoes are caught alive, making them available for insecticide-resistance testing or experiments.

The other method is the pyrethrum spray-sheet collection, which is often the most effective method for collecting endophilic mosquitoes, although it is less useful where houses have a very open structure, as when constructed of bamboo. Collections are usually started early in the mornings (e.g. 0700 hours). First, all occupants, animals, food, stored water and small items of furniture are removed from the house. Then white sheets are spread over the floor and over any furniture that has not been removed, and windows and doors are closed. One person space-sprays the room, or house, with 0.1–0.2 per cent pyrethrum in kerosene (paraffin), usually synergized with piperonyl butoxide, using a small hand sprayer. Certain formulations of pyrethrum concentrate contain emulsifiers and can be diluted for spraying with water instead of kerosene. At the same time, another person walks round the outside of the house spraying the eaves and other escape routes to deter mosquitoes from flying out. After 10 minutes or more, the house is re-entered and mosquitoes are collected from the floor sheets.

The mean number of unfed, blood-fed, half-gravid and gravid females per house can be calculated. If the number of blood-engorged anophelines is divided by the number of occupants, this gives an estimation of the number biting per person per night, but excludes mosquitoes that have bitten and then flown out of the house. The presence of male anophelines indicates that larval habitats are nearby.

## LIGHT-TRAPS

Some, but not all, malaria vectors can be caught in simple light-traps placed inside houses, animal sheds or even outside in cattle enclosures. Center for Disease Control (CDC) light-traps (Figure 4.17) are a useful alternative to human bait collections in Africa when positioned alongside a person sleeping under an unimpregnated bed-net. The light-trap can be suspended by string from the ceilings or roofs of bedrooms near the head of a bed, or from a post or tree branch in a cattle enclosure. If occupants sleep under nets, this usually increases the catch. It may be necessary to grease the string to prevent ants entering the trap and devouring the catch. In addition to collecting endophilic species, light-traps are useful in catching species that leave houses after feeding, and which consequently would not be caught in pyrethrum spray-sheet or other indoor collections.

## EXIT TRAPS

Various types of traps can be fitted to houses to catch a sample of the mosquitoes leaving them. The simplest exit trap consists of a 30-cm cube metal or wooden frame covered with mosquito netting, but incorporating an inverted netting funnel in one side, narrowing to a 2-cm diameter opening. Such traps can be placed in doors or windows of bedrooms (Figure 4.18) at dusk to catch samples of the

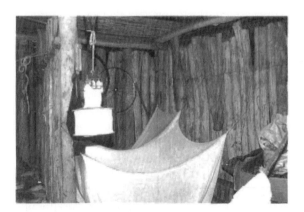

**Figure 4.17** *A battery-operated light-trap placed near a mosquito net in a bedroom of a village hut in Guatemala to sample indoor biting and resting anophelines. (Photograph by MW Service.)*

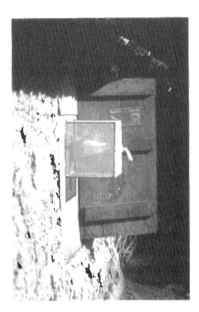

**Figure 4.18** *An exit trap fitted to the window opening of a house in Sierra Leone to catch anopheline mosquitoes leaving the house. (Photograph by MW Service.)*

mosquitoes leaving the house during the night. Traps are removed or emptied early the following morning. The size of the catch will depend in part on the number of other openings through which indoor-resting mosquitoes may escape. Exit traps are inefficient in houses with an open type of construction. The presence of blood-fed anophelines in exit traps indicates deliberate exophily.

### OUTDOOR-RESTING COLLECTIONS

Using aspirators and torches, searches can be made for exophilic *Anopheles* in a variety of natural and man-made outdoor resting sites. These include animal burrows, hollow trees, cracks and crevices in the ground, amongst rock fissures, from earth banks, buttress roots, fences and culverts. A net with a strong bag that is not easily torn can be used to sweep-net low vegetation. After several sweeps, the net is folded over to prevent insects escaping and lightly sprayed with a knock-down spray, such as an aqueous preparation of natural pyrethrum, then placed in a large plastic bag. After a few minutes, the net is opened and the catch shaken into a white tray to allow the collection of dead and dying mosquitoes.

Several types of artificial resting sites can be constructed to attract exophilic *Anopheles*; the best is the pit-shelter. A hole, 1.75–2 m deep, is dug beneath trees or bushes so that its opening (1.5 × 1.5 m) is shaded from the sun. A series of 20-cm deep cavities are dug horizontally in all four sides of the pit. Outdoor-resting mosquitoes are collected from these small excavations and from the sides of the pit. Fencing or thorn enclosures surrounding the pits prevent animals and young children falling into them. Clearly, if the water table is high, the pits become flooded and useless.

## Transportation of adults

Live anopheline adults collected from the field can be carried in cardboard or plastic cartons such as cups or beakers, the openings of which are covered with mosquito netting, on top of which is taped a moist piece of cotton wool. Cartons need to be protected from the sun and transported to the laboratory in a coolbox. Relevant collection data should be written on the outside of the cartons.

Dead mosquitoes, such as those collected from pyrethrum space-spray collections or by sweep-netting vegetation, should be placed on filter paper covering wet cotton wool in plastic Petri dishes and these placed in a coolbox. On arrival at the laboratory, if the mosquitoes cannot be processed immediately (e.g. for detection of sporozoites or identification of blood meals), the Petri dishes should be transferred to a refrigerator.

## Blood meal identification

The abdomens of wild-caught, blood-engorged mosquitoes or half-gravid females with some remaining undigested blood can be squashed onto filter paper, which is stored in a desiccator or refrigerator until tested. The dried blood is extracted subsequently in buffer and tested by an enzyme-linked immunosorbent assay (ELISA) method (Service *et al.*, 1986) to determine whether the blood is of human origin. Further tests can be undertaken to determine whether the blood is from bovids, equids, goats, dogs, birds etc., but this considerably increases the costs. The proportion of *Anopheles* giving a positive reaction for human blood is the Human Blood Index, which is a valuable guide to the potential importance of an *Anopheles* species as a malaria vector. Sampling bias must be taken into consideration in interpreting the results. For example, it is to be expected that a high proportion of adults caught from houses will have fed on humans and most of those caught from cattle sheds will have fed on cattle. The collection of blood-engorged mosquitoes from outdoor resting sites may give a sample that is more representative of the feeding behaviour of a species.

## Sporozoite detection

The presence of sporozoites in mosquitoes can be determined either microscopically, following dissection of the salivary glands (see Figure 2.5), or by immunological methods performed on the crushed thorax.

Dissection of the mosquito is not difficult, but the removal of the salivary glands is more difficult than that of the gut and requires some practice (Figure 4.19).

The sequence of operations is as follows:

1. Transfer the mosquito to a narrow test-tube and stun it by rapping the end of the tube several times sharply on the palm of the hand. Identify the species of the *Anopheles* (for unfamiliar species, this may require the mosquito to be killed) and record relevant collection details.
2. Holding the mosquito by one wing, remove the legs one at a time and then pull off one wing.

With the insect on a microscope slide, remove the remaining wing with a dissecting needle.
3. Place the insect in the centre of a dry microscope slide and cleanly cut off the head. Place a small drop of normal saline (0.85 per cent), just touching the neck end of the thorax.
4. Under a low-power binocular microscope, hold the thorax firm with a needle and, with a blunt needle in the other hand, gently press the thorax close to the neck to express the glands into the saline.
5. Remove the remainder of the mosquito to a drop of saline on a fresh slide for dissection of the midgut. Lower one corner of a small (about 18 mm) square cover glass on the glands. This restricts the saline to a small area and makes it easier to locate the glands in subsequent steps.
6. Rupture the cells of the glands by gently pressing on the cover glass with a dissecting needle and examine under the high-power objective ($\times$40) of a compound microscope for sporozoites, which are about 12 $\mu$m long. Sporozoites are feebly motile, often showing slow bending movement.

Although gland dissections are routine in many laboratories, microscopical detection of sporozoites does not indicate which species of human malarial parasite is involved. Furthermore, in regions such as South-east Asia, many anophelines transmit rodent

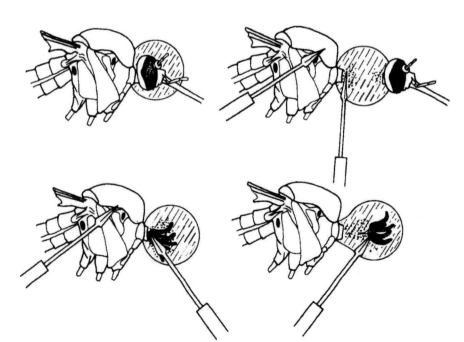

**Figure 4.19** *Procedures in the dissection of the salivary glands from an adult female* Anopheles *and their examination for malaria sporozoites. (Source: MW Service. A guide to medical entomology. London, Macmillan, 1980, p. 186.)*

or simian malarias, and it is not possible to differentiate their sporozoites morphologically from those of human malaria. However, immunological tests can differentiate between the sporozoites of human and non-human malarias. Furthermore, ELISA tests, using monoclonal antibodies to the circumsporozoite protein, can differentiate between infections of *P. falciparum* and *P. vivax* and, in some cases, different strains of these parasites. As yet, tests for the other two human malaria species have not been adequately tested under field conditions. Another advantage of ELISA tests is that they can be performed on dry specimens. However, to minimize misleading positive results due to sporozoites that have not reached the salivary glands, the abdomen should be excluded from the test. Only the thorax, or head and thorax, should be ground up and tested. Monoclonal antibodies to circumsporozoite protein are not yet widely available and testing may be expensive if reagents have to be bought. Dissection of the salivary glands and microscopic identification of sporozoites may be somewhat slower, but is inexpensive. New PCR-based methods of detecting malaria parasites in mosquitoes are becoming available, but are not yet in routine use (Snounou *et al.*, 1993).

## Oocyst dissections

The presence of oocysts on the stomach wall (see Figure 2.3) shows that the mosquito has fed on someone with gametocytes in his or her blood and that the parasites are beginning to undergo cyclical development in the mosquito (see Figure 2.1). Finding oocysts does not incriminate the mosquito as a vector, because further development to the sporozoite stage may be unable to proceed, or the mosquito may die before this is achieved. The presence of oocysts shows the mosquito is infected, indicating a potential vector, but not that it is infective.

Dissection of the mosquito mid-gut is not difficult, but requires some practice (Figure 4.20). If the glands have been dissected with sufficient care, the mid-gut can easily be dissected from the remaining parts of the mosquito.

The sequence of operations is as follows:

1. Place the remaining thorax and abdomen of the mosquito on a drop of normal (0.85 per cent) saline on a microscope slide.

2. Hold the thorax steady with one needle and nick the integument above and below on either segment six or seven.

3. Still holding the thorax with one needle, place the other across the tip of the abdomen and, with steady, gentle traction, draw out the abdominal contents into the saline until the mid-gut and malpighian tubules come into view. Cut across the anterior portion of the gut so as to leave a little of the oesophagus attached.

4. Steady the anterior part of the gut with a needle and, with the other, cut through the gut just at the junction with the malpighian tubules so that they and the hindgut can be discarded. Also discard the ovaries and any remaining integument.

5. Gently place one edge of a cover glass on the slide so that the glass covers the isolated mid-gut and, with the opposite edge resting on the point of the needle, gently lower the cover glass until the mid-gut has flattened and expanded.

6. Examine the mid-gut under a compound microscope for the presence of oocysts, first using a low-power objective ($\times$10), before changing to high power ($\times$40) to confirm the presence and appearance of the oocysts.

Oocysts lie on the outer surface of the gut, just beneath the basement membrane, and appear as clear, round or oval bodies, containing distinct granules. In the early oocysts some 3–4 days after infection, the granules of malaria pigment are concentrated in the centre, but subsequently the pigment granules become more dispersed. In larger oocysts (30–60 $\mu$m in diameter), the developing sporozoites are easily visible. The sporozoites of mature oocysts are readily released by gentle pressure on the cover glass.

Occasionally, during dissections, clusters of dark, round, oval or often banana-shaped bodies are seen on the gut walls. These are the famous 'Ross's black spores', and represent dead parasites, probably early oocysts but sometimes sporozoites, that have been encapsulated and melanized by the mosquito's immune system.

When sporozoites are found in the salivary glands, the mosquito is assumed to be infective, i.e. capable of transmitting malaria. The percentage of females with sporozoites is termed the sporozoite rate. The percentage showing oocysts on dissection (i.e. infected mosquitoes) is the oocyst rate. There may be considerable seasonal variations in sporozoite rates, reflecting, in part, changes in adult survival rates of the mosquitoes.

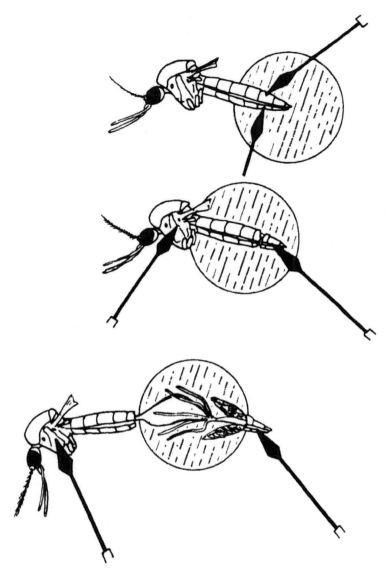

**Figure 4.20** *Procedures in the dissection of an adult female* Anopheles *for removal of the mid-gut, which is then examined for the presence of malaria oocysts. (Source: MW Service.* A guide to medical entomology. *London, Macmillan, 1980, p. 185.)*

An important parameter is the entomological inoculation rate (EIR), which is the sporozoite rate multiplied by the average number of mosquitoes of that species biting a person per unit of time. This allows a better comparison of the importance of different mosquito species in transmitting malaria than does comparison of just sporozoite rates. In sub-Saharan Africa, sporozoite rates of about 3–5 per cent are common in an efficient vector such as *A. gambiae*, but much lower rates (0.01–0.1 per cent) are usually encountered in Neotropical and Asian species. In the latter case, thousands of mosquitoes may have to be examined before a positive is found. Doing this

by dissection and gland examination is extremely tedious, and ELISA tests are better in such circumstances.

## Age-grading methods

Determination of the age of female mosquitoes is important for understanding malaria epidemiology and assessing the efficacy of vector control programmes. Most anti-mosquito measures aim at reducing the average longevity of adult female mosquitoes, because reductions in longevity reduce transmission exponentially. Physiological age is easier to determine than calendar age, but often age in days of a female adult can be estimated from her physiological age, which can be determined from inspecting the ovaries. The simplest method involves an examination of the tracheoles covering the ovaries of unfed females to determine whether a mosquito has or has not laid eggs. Those that have not laid are classified as nulliparous and retain tightly coiled tracheoles (skeins), whereas those that have laid at least one batch of eggs are referred to as parous and have their tracheoles unwound (Figure 4.21).

The technique is as follows:

1. A freshly killed mosquito is placed on a microscope slide and the posterior part of the abdomen surrounded by a drop of tap or distilled water (not saline).
2. Nicks are made on either side of segments six or seven and the contents of the abdomen pulled out, as described in step 3 for oocyst dissection (p. 78).
3. The two ovaries are isolated and transferred to a small drop of water (not saline), where they are allowed to dry out. In drying, air is drawn into the tracheae and the whole tracheal system becomes visible, including the finest tracheoles supplying the ovaries.
4. Paired ovaries from about 10 females can be neatly arranged side by side in a line on a single slide. Specimens prepared in this way can withstand long storage, allowing results to be re-checked where necessary.

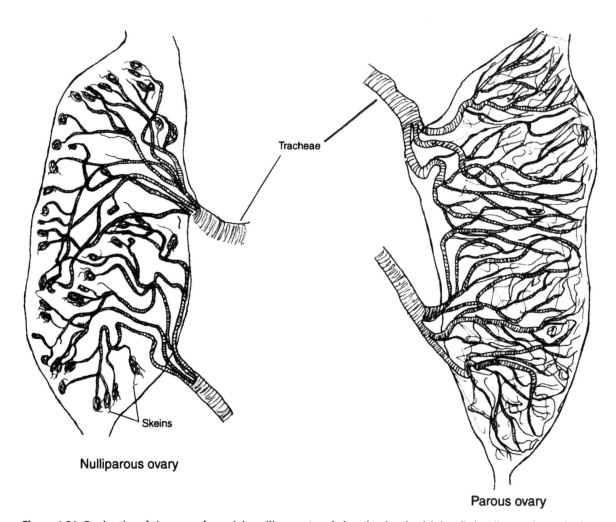

Tracheae

Skeins

Nulliparous ovary

Parous ovary

**Figure 4.21** *Tracheation of the ovary of an adult, nulliparous* Anopheles, *showing the tightly coiled endings to the tracheoles (skeins) and the ovary of a parous female with uncoiled endings. (Drawn by MW Service.)*

Once the ovaries have completely dried out, they can be examined under the low power of a compound microscope. If the ends of the tracheoles that cover the ovary are tightly wound or coiled into round or elongate skeins (Figure 4.21), this shows the female has never laid eggs. If the tracheoles are uncoiled (Figure 4.21), they come from a female that has laid one or more batches of eggs. The unwinding of the skeins is caused by the stretching that results from maturation of the eggs. This unwinding is irreversible and so serves to distinguish the ovaries of parous mosquitoes.

The proportion of parous individuals usually changes seasonally. Absence or scarcity of nullipars indicates that no, or very few, new mosquitoes are emerging from breeding places, as might be expected in the dry season. Vector control measures such as residual house spraying reduce the proportion of parous females by shortening adult longevity. Various methods, based on the proportion parous in a population, have been proposed to estimate the probability of daily survival of females (see Service, 1993), an important entomological parameter in malaria epidemiology (see p. 87).

A potentially more precise age-grading technique involves counting the number of dilatations in the part of the ovariole most distal to the follicle in unfed females. Their number is considered to correspond to the number of ovipositions a female has completed (Detinova, 1962). However, this method is technically difficult and time-consuming, and the results need to be interpreted with care. Therefore, it is rarely used in routine entomological surveys.

# BIBLIOGRAPHY

Beier JC, Perkins PV, Koros JK, *et al.* Malaria sporozoite detection by dissection and ELISA to assess infectivity of Afrotropical *Anopheles* (Diptera: Culicidae). *J Med Entomol* 1990; **27**: 377–84.

Bock GR, Cardew G. *Olfaction in mosquito–host interactions.* Chichester, Ciba Foundation Symposium 200, John Wiley, 1996.

Burkot TR. Non-random host selection by anopheline mosquitoes. *Parasitol Today* 1988; **4**: 156–62.

Burkot TR, Dye C, Graves PM. An analysis of some factors determining the sporozoite rates, human blood indexes, and biting rates of members of the *Anopheles punctulatus* complex in Papua New Guinea. *Am J Trop Med Hyg* 1989; **40**: 229–34.

Clements AN. *The biology of mosquitoes.* Vol. 1. *Development, nutrition and reproduction.* London, Chapman & Hall, 1992.

Clements AN. *The biology of mosquitoes.* Vol. 2. *Sensory reception and behaviour.* Wallingford, CABI Publishing, 1999.

Coluzzi M. Malaria vector analysis and control. *Parasitol Today* 1992; **8**: 113–18.

Coluzzi, M, Petrarca V, Di Deco M. Chromosomal inversion intergradation and incipient speciation in *Anopheles gambiae. Boll Zool* 1985; **52**: 45–63.

Delforme DR, Wirtz RA, Loong KP, Lewis GE. Identification of sporozoites in *Anopheles maculatus* from Malaysia by enzyme-linked immunosorbent assays. *Trop Biomed* 1989; **6**: 21–6.

Detinova TS. *Age-grouping methods in Diptera of medical importance. With special reference to some vectors of malaria.* Monograph Series No. 47. Geneva, World Health Organization, 1962.

Dye C. The analysis of parasite transmission by blood-sucking insects. *Annu Rev Entomol* 1992; **37**: 1–19.

Laird M. *The natural history of larval mosquito habitats.* London, Academic Press, 1988.

Lines JD, Curtis CF, Wilkes TJ, Njunwa KJ. Monitoring human-bait mosquitoes (Diptera: Culicidae) in Tanzania with light-traps hung beside mosquito nets. *Bull Entomol Res* 1991; **81**: 77–84.

Pant, CP, Houba V, Engers, HD. Bloodmeal identification in vectors. *Parasitol Today* 1987; **3**: 324–6.

Robert V, Petrarca V, Carnevale P, Ovazza L, Coluzzi M. Analyse cytogénétique du complexe *Anopheles gambiae* dans la région de Bobo-Dioulasso (Burkina Faso). *Ann Parasitol Humaine Comparée* 1989; **64**: 290–311.

Robert V, Verhav JP, Ponnudurai T, Louwe L, Scholtens P, Carnevale P. Study of the distribution of circumsporozoite antigen in *Anopheles gambiae* infected with *Plasmodium falciparum* using enzyme-linked immunosorbent assay. *Trans R Soc Trop Med Hyg* 1988; **82**: 389–91.

Scott JA, Brogdon WG, Collins FH. Identification of single specimens in the *Anopheles gambiae* complex by the polymerase chain reaction. *Am J Trop Med Hyg* 1993; **49**: 520–9.

Service MW. *Mosquito ecology. Field sampling methods,* 2nd edition. London, Chapman & Hall, 1993.

Service MW. Mosquito (Diptera: Culicidae) dispersal – the long and short of it. *J Med Entomol* 1997; **34**: 579–88.

Service MW, Voller A, Bidwell DE. The enzyme-linked immunosorbent assay (ELISA) test for the identification of blood-meals of haematophagous insects. *Bull Entomol Res* 1986; **76**: 321–30.

Snounou G, Viriyakosol S, Jarra W. Identification of the four human malaria species in field samples by the polymerase chain reaction and detection of high prevalence of mixed infections. *Mol Biochem Parasitol* 1993; **61**: 315–20.

Townson H, Harbach RE, Callan TA. DNA identification of museum specimens of the *Anopheles gambiae* complex: an evaluation of PCR as a tool for resolving the formal taxonomy of sibling species complexes. *System Entomol* 1999; **24**: 95–100.

White GB. Malaria vector ecology and genetics. In *Malaria*. Cohen S, ed. London, British Medical Bulletin, 1982; **38**: 115–218.

World Health Organization. *Entomological field techniques for malaria control. Part 1. Learner's guide.* Geneva, World Health Organization, 1992.

Zahar AR. *Vector bionomics in the epidemiology and control of malaria. Part I. The WHO African region and the southern WHO eastern Mediterranean region. Section I: Malaria vectors of the Afrotropical region – general information. Section II: An overview of malaria control problems and the recent malaria situation.* Mimeographed document VBC/84.6 and MAP/84.3. Geneva, World Health Organization, 1984.

Zahar AR. *Vector bionomics in the epidemiology and control of malaria. Part I. The WHO African region and the southern WHO eastern Mediterranean region. Section III: Vector bionomics, malaria epidemiology and control by geographical areas. (A) West Africa.* Mimeographed document VBC/85.1 and MAP/85.1. Geneva, World Health Organization, 1985.

Zahar AR. *Vector bionomics in the epidemiology and control of malaria. Part I. The WHO African region and the southern WHO eastern Mediterranean region. Section III: Vector bionomics, malaria epidemiology and control by geographical areas. (B) Equatorial Africa. (C) Southern Africa.* Mimeographed document VBC/85.2 and MAP/85.2. Geneva, World Health Organization, 1985.

Zahar AR. *Vector bionomics in the epidemiology and control of malaria. Part I. The WHO African region and the southern WHO eastern Mediterranean region. Section III: Vector bionomics, malaria epidemiology and control by geographic areas. (D) East Africa. (E) Eastern Outer Islands. (F) Southwestern Arabia.* Mimeographed document VBC/85.3 and MAP/85.3 Geneva, World Health Organization, 1985.

Zahar AR. *Vector bionomics in the epidemiology and control of malaria. Part II. The WHO European region and the WHO eastern Mediterranean region. Volume I. Vector laboratory studies.* Mimeographed document VBC/88.5 and MAP/88.2. Geneva, World Health Organization, 1988.

Zahar AR. *Vector bionomics in the epidemiology and control of malaria. Part II. The WHO European region and the WHO eastern Mediterranean region. Volume II. Applied field studies. Section I: An overview of the recent malaria situation and current problems. Section II: Vector distribution.* Mimeographed document VBC/90.1 and MAP/90.1. Geneva, World Health Organization, 1990.

Zahar AR. *Vector bionomics in the epidemiology and control of malaria. Part II. The WHO European and the WHO eastern Mediterranean region. Volume II. Applied field studies. Section III: Vector bionomics, malaria epidemiology and control by geographical areas. (A) The Mediterranean Basin.* Mimeographed document VBC/90.2 and MAP/90.2. Geneva, World Health Organization, 1990.

Zahar AR. *Vector bionomics in the epidemiology and control of malaria. Part II. The WHO European region and the WHO eastern Mediterranean region. Volume II. Applied field studies. Section III. Vector bionomics, malaria epidemiology and control by geographical areas. (B) Asia west of India.* Mimeographed document VBC/90.3 and MAP/90.3. Geneva, World Health Organization, 1991.

Zahar AR. *Vector bionomics in the epidemiology and control of malaria. Part III. The WHO South-east Asia region and the western Pacific region. Volume I. Classified bibliography 1970–1991.* Mimeographed document CTD/MAL/94.1. Geneva, World Health Organization, 1994.

Zahar AR. *Vector bionomics in the epidemiology and control of malaria. Part III. The WHO South-east Asia region and the western Pacific region. Volume II. (i) Leading literature – General review 1970–1994.* Mimeographed document CTD/MAL/96.1. Geneva, World Health Organization, 1996.

## Taxonomic references for identification of *Anopheles* species

### AFROTROPICAL REGION

Anon. *Les anophèles de la région afro-tropicale.* CD-Rom. [In English, French and Portuguese]. Paris, ORSTOM, 1998.

Gillies MT, Coetzee M. *A supplement to the Anophelinae of Africa south of the Sahara (Afrotropical region)*, No. 55. Johannesburg, South African Institute for Medical Research, 1987.

Gillies MT, de Meillon B. *The Anophelinae of Africa south of the Sahara (Ethiopian Zoogeographical Region)*, No. 54. Johannesburg, South African Institute for Medical Research, 1968.

Grjebine A. Insectes Diptères Culicidae Anophelinae. *Faune de Madagascar* 1966; **22**: 1–487.

## AUSTRALASIAN REGION

Belkin JN. *The mosquitoes of the South Pacific (Diptera, Culicidae)*, Vols 1 and 2. Berkeley and Los Angeles, University of California Press, 1962.

Lee DJ, Hicks MM, Griffiths M, *et al. The Culicidae of the Australasian region*. Vol. 5, *Nomenclature, synonymy, literature, distribution, biology and relation to disease. Genus Anopheles. subgenera Anopheles, Cellia.* Monograph Series, Entomology Monograph No. 2. Canberra, Commonwealth Department of Health, School of Public Health and Tropical Medicine, Australian Government Publishing Service, 1987.

## NEOTROPICAL REGION

Cagampang-Ramos A, Darsie RF. Illustrated keys to the *Anopheles* mosquitoes of the Philippine islands. San Francisco: *USAF Fifth Epidemiological Flight, PACAF, Technical Report* 1970; **70–1**: 1–49.

Clark-Gil S, Darsie RF. The mosquitoes of Guatemala. Their identification, distribution and bionomics, with keys to adult females and larvae in English and Spanish. *Mosquito Systematics* 1983; **15**: 151–284.

Cova-Garcia P. *Notas sobre los anofelinos de Venezuela y su identifación*, segunda edicion. Caracas, Editoria Grafos, 1961.

Darsie PF. Mosquitoes of Argentina. Part I. Keys for identification of adult females and fourth stage larvae in English and Spanish (Diptera, Culicidae). *Mosquito Systematics* 1985; **17**: 153–253. [References cited in this paper are in Mitchell and Darsie, 1985.]

Faran ME, Linthicum KJ. A handbook of the Amazonian species of *Anopheles (Nysorrynchus)* (Diptera: Culicidae). *Mosquito Systematics* 1981; **13**: 1–91.

Forattini OP. *Entomologia médica*: Vol. 1, *Parte geral, Diptera, Anophelini.* São Paulo, Faculdade de Higiene e Saúde Pública, 1962.

García Avila I, Gutsevich AV, Gonzalez Broche R. Determinación de las especies de mosquitos (Culicidae) de Cuba, según preparados microscópicos de la cabeza de las hembras (excetuades las especies del género *Culex*). *Poeyana* 1981; **231**: 1–12.

Goreham JR, Stojanovich CJ. Clave illustrada para los mosquitos anofelinos de sudamerica occidental. Illustrated keys to the anopheline mosquitoes of western South America. *Mosquito Systematics* 1973; **5**: 97–156.

Mitchell CJ, Darsie RF. Mosquitoes of Argentina. Part II: Geographic distribution and bibliography (Diptera, Culicidae). *Mosquito Systematics* 1985; **17**: 279–360.

Vargas L, Martínez Palacios A. *Anofelinos Mexicanos taxonomia y distribución.* Mexico, DF, Secretaria de Salubridad y Asistencia, 1956.

Wilkerson RC, Strickman D. Illustrated key to the female anopheline mosquitoes of Central America and Mexico. *J Am Mosquito Control Assoc* 1990; **6**: 7–34.

Xavier SH, Mattos SS. Distribuição geográfica dos culicineos no Brasil (Diptera, Culicidae). I. Estado de Goias. *Rev Brasileira Malariol Doenças Trop* 1965; **17**: 269–91.

Xavier SH, Mattos SS. Geographical distribution of the Culicinae in Brazil. III. State of Pará (Diptera, Culicidae). *Mosquito Systematics* 1975; **7**: 234–68.

## ORIENTAL REGION

Borel E. Les moustiques de la Cochinchine et du Sud-Annam. *Collect Soc Pathol Exotique, Monographie* 1930; **3**.

Darsie RF, Pradhan SP. The mosquitoes of Nepal; their identification, distribution and biology. *Mosquito Systematics* 1990; **22**: 69–130.

Das BP, Rajagopal R, Akiyama J. Pictorial key to the species of Indian anopheline mosquitoes. *J Pure Appl Zool* 1989; **2**: 131–62.

Harrison BA, Scanlon JE. Medical entomological studies – II. The subgenus *Anopheles* in Thailand (Diptera: Culicidae). *Contributions Am Entomol Soc* 1975; **12**(1): 1–307.

Rao TR. *The anophelines of India*, revised edition. Delhi, Malaria Research Council, 1984.

Rattanarithikul R, Panthusiri P. Illustrated keys to the medically important mosquitos of Thailand. *Southeast Asian J Trop Med Public Health* 1994; **25** (Suppl.): 1–66.

Reid JA. *Anopheline mosquitoes of Malaya and Borneo.* Studies from the Institute for Medical Research, No. 31. Kuala Lumpur, Government of Malaysia, 1968.

## PALAEARCTIC REGION

Danilov VN. Mosquitoes (Diptera, Culicidae) of Afghanistan. Communication I. Identification tables of females. *Meditsinkaya Parazitologiya i Parazitarnÿe Bolezni* 1985; **2**: 67–72. [In Russian, English summary.]

Danilov VN. Mosquitoes of Afghanistan. 2. A key to fourth-stage larvae. *Meditsinkaya Parazitologiya Parazitarnÿe Bolezni* 1985; **4**: 51–5. [In Russian, English summary.]

Glick JJ. Illustrated key to the female *Anopheles* of south-western Asia and Egypt (Diptera: Culicidae). *Mosquito Systematics* 1992; **24**: 125–53.

Guy Y. Les *Anophèles* du Maroc. *Mémoires Soc Sci Naturelles et Physiques du Maroc (n.s.) (Zoologie)* 1959; **7**: 1–235.

Lu BL, Li BS. Identification of Chinese mosquitoes. In *Identification handbook for medically important animals in China*. Lu BS, ed. Beijing, People's Health Publication Company, 1982. [In Chinese.]

Mattingly PF, Knight KL. The mosquitoes of Arabia I. *Bull Br Museum (Natural History) (B)* 1956; **21**: 89–141.

Postiglione M, Tabanli B, Ramsdale CD. The *Anopheles* of Turkey. *Riv Parassitol* 1973; **34**: 127–57.

# 5

# The epidemiology of malaria

ROBERT W SNOW AND HERBERT M GILLES

## GEOGRAPHICAL DISTRIBUTION AND PUBLIC HEALTH SIGNIFICANCE

Indigenous malaria has been recorded as far north as 64°N latitude (Archangel in the former USSR) and as far south as 32°S latitude (Cordoba in Argentina). It has occurred in the Dead Sea area at 400 m below and at 2800 m above sea level in Cocha-Mbamba (Bolivia). Within these limits of latitude and altitude there are large areas free of malaria, which is essentially a focal disease, because its transmission depends greatly on local environmental and other conditions.

*Plasmodium vivax* has the widest geographical range; it is prevalent in many temperate zones, but also in the subtropics and tropics. *Plasmodium falciparum* is the commonest species throughout the tropics and subtropics. *P. malariae* is patchily present over the same range as *P. falciparum*, but much less common. *P. ovale* is found chiefly in tropical Africa, but also occasionally in the West Pacific.

Natural transmission of malaria infection occurs through exposure to the bites of infective female *Anopheles* mosquitoes. The source of human malaria infection is nearly always a human subject, whether a sick person or a symptomless carrier of the parasite. With the possible exception of chimpanzees in tropical Africa, which may harbour *P. malariae* infection, no other animal reservoir of human plasmodia is known to exist. However, there have been a few cases of natural or accidental infection of humans with some plasmodia of simian origin.

The alternation between the human and the mosquito host represents the biological cycle of transmission of the malaria parasite. The transmission of the infection by the mosquito from the human carrier (donor) to the human victim (recipient) represents the chain of transmission. The infection, however, may also be transmitted accidentally; this occurs not infrequently as a result of blood transfusion when the donor harbours malaria parasites. Drug addicts using the same hypodermic needle have also been known to infect one another.

It has recently been estimated that approximately 1 million people may have died from the direct consequences of *P. falciparum* in Africa during 1995 (Snow *et al.*, 1999). Malaria not only poses a risk to survival, but the repeated clinical consequences of infection during early life place a burden on households, the health service and ultimately the economic development of communities and nations. Gallup and Sachs (1998) have argued that the persistence of endemic malaria in the tropics and subtropics significantly contributes to a perpetual state of depressed economic growth. These macro-estimates and associations provide clear support for a renewed effort launched by the World Health Organization (WHO), aimed at halving malaria mortality by the year 2010, referred to as the Roll Back Malaria (RBM) Initiative. This goal has been conceived at a time when existing, affordable therapeutics are rapidly failing, health service provision is breaking down, there are few immediate prospects of widespread vaccination and poverty continues to afflict most endemic countries.

Prior to the recent RBM Initiative, the most significant period in the history of malaria control was the outcome of a series of conferences held by WHO during the late 1940s and early 1950s. Supporters of global eradication were adamant that all endemic countries could achieve the successes afforded by co-ordinated mass action, particularly with the use of dichlorodiphenyl- trichloroethane (DDT) in South America, India and isolated areas of Africa (such as Freetown, Sierra Leone). During this period, there was a rapid expansion in our knowledge of the bio-mathematical relationships between malaria vectors and infection risks in humans. The 20 years following eradication efforts witnessed great achievements in South America, North America, the Mediterranean, Indian sub-continent, Pacific and South-east Asia. Only limited successes were achieved in Africa. For whatever reason, the guiding principle that the parasite's cycle between human and vector could be forever broken everywhere in the world was recognized as impracticable. The WHO redefined the agenda from parasite eradication to disease control (see Chapter 6). At this juncture, despite our detailed understanding of the bionomics of infection between primary and secondary hosts, it was not possible to provide a quantifiable framework of the relative risks of the morbid, developmental or fatal risks among the human population. This has posed a barrier to

constructing an epidemiological framework to empower public health decision-making for the effective targeting of cost-effective stratagems.

This chapter considers both the traditional 'infection' epidemiology and more recent approaches to defining the epidemiological basis of malaria as a disease. Ninety per cent of the world's malaria deaths probably occur in Africa due to *P. falciparum*. There is therefore a discernible emphasis in this chapter on the epidemiology of malaria as it affects Africa. This does not belie the significance of *P. vivax*, whose geographical distribution is much wider than that of *P. falciparum*, and special attention is given to this parasite's health impact following new research in South-east Asia and the Pacific.

## DEFINING MALARIA INFECTION RISKS AMONG HUMAN POPULATIONS

The term endemicity refers to a general statement indicating the amount or severity of malaria in an area or community. Epidemic malaria is a term that indicates a periodic or sharp increase in the amount of malaria in a given indigenous community. Any precise information about the degree of endemicity must be based on quantitative and statistical concepts.

Malaria is often classified according to whether transmission is stable or unstable. These two concepts form a continuum of differing epidemiological scenarios. The term stable implies equilibrium and, on the whole, the prevalence of infection is persistently high and endemicity is relatively insensitive to environmental changes. Under stable endemic conditions, variation in transmission is minimal over many years, although seasonal fluctuations do occur and transmission can continue even with very few vectors. High levels of immunity develop within the population due to regular and often continuous transmission.

Unstable malaria, on the other hand, is characterized by great variability in space and time. Collective immunity is low and there is a propensity for epidemics to occur. The disease is also characterized by recession and recurrence, and by periods when disease incidence is low alternating irregularly with times of high incidence. Unstable malaria is a particular feature of *P. vivax*; however, sharp outbreaks of severe *P. falciparum* do occur.

## The stability index

Davidson proposed an index of stability based on the malaria vector's human biting habit and its expectancy of life:

$$\frac{a}{-\log_e p}$$

where *a* is the average number of human blood meals taken by the female *Anopheles* in a day (the human biting habit) and $1/\log_e p$ the life expectancy of the mosquito (*p* being the probability of the vector surviving 1 day). Values of over 2.5 indicate stability and values of less than 0.5 indicate instability.

## The basic reproductive rate

Transmission potential may be quantified based upon the basic reproduction rate ($R_o$) of the disease. $R_o$ is defined as the average number of successful offspring that the parasite is intrinsically capable of producing. It is expressed as the average number of secondary infections produced from one infected individual introduced into a non-immune host population. The average basic reproduction rate determines endemicity. For the parasite to survive successfully, $R_o$ must be greater than 1; $R_o$ values of less than 1 indicate diminishing disease risks and a tendency toward unstable conditions. $R_o$ combines measures of mosquito infectivity and survival and is calculated using the formula:

$$\frac{ma^2 b p^n}{-r(\log_e p)}$$

where *ma* represents the man-biting rate, *p* is the probability of the mosquito surviving through 1 day, *n* is the incubation period to infectivity in the mosquito, and *r* is the proportion of cases recovering in 1 day.

## The vectorial capacity

The vectorial capacity (*C*) is a transmission probability index that reflects the mean number of probable inoculations transmitted from one case of malaria in a unit of time. It is based on $R_o$, but incorporates the duration of sporogony, vector density and duration of infectivity in humans and is therefore a better indicator of stability. To sustain malaria, there needs to be a sizeable population of vectors, and their longevity is therefore a key factor. In general, vectors tend to die as a result of external factors before completing their full life span, and only a small proportion of mosquitoes survive long enough to transmit disease. The female *Anopheles* takes a blood meal once every 2–4 days. The length between blood meals is dependent on temperature and also on the preference of the vector for biting humans. Sporogony lasts 8–25 days for the most efficient human malaria parasites. This duration is genetically determined and temperature dependent. The average life expectancy of vectors of human malaria is 20–25 days and the average daily death rate is 4–5 per cent. These estimations have been made by direct observation of different anopheline species and are taken into consideration in the determination of the vectorial capacity, which is defined mathematically as:

$$C = \frac{ma^2 p^n}{-\log_e p}$$

where *m* is the relative density of female anophelines, *a* the probability that the mosquito will take a human blood meal during a particular day, and $p^n$ the proportion of vectors surviving the parasite's incubation period (i.e. *p*, the probability of vector survival, and *n*, the number of days the vector lives). The probability of daily survival is key in determining endemicity levels. For *A. gambiae* and *A. funestus*, an average daily survival rate of >60 per cent has been shown to be associated with stable endemicity.

## MEASURES OF STABLE *P. FALCIPARUM* TRANSMISSION

### Parasite rate

One useful, and widely used, measure of malaria endemicity is the prevalence of peripheral blood-stage

**Table 5.1** *Confidence intervals at 95 per cent probability level corresponding to varying sample percentages from 5 per cent to 95 per cent.*

| Sample size | Percentage observed in sample | | | | | |
| --- | --- | --- | --- | --- | --- | --- |
| | **5%** | **10%** | **20%** | **30%** | **40%** | **50%** |
| 50 | | 3–22 | 10–34 | 18–45 | 26–55 | 36–64 |
| 60 | 1–14 | 3–20 | 11–32 | 19–43 | 28–54 | 37–63 |
| 80 | 1–12 | 4–19 | 12–30 | 20–41 | 29–51 | 39–61 |
| 100 | 2–11 | 5–18 | 13–29 | 21–40 | 30–50 | 40–60 |
| 200 | 2–9 | 6–14 | 16–26 | 24–38 | 33–47 | 43–57 |
| 300 | 3–8 | 7–14 | 16–25 | 25–36 | 35–46 | 44–56 |
| 400 | 3–8 | 7–13 | 16–24 | 26–35 | 35–45 | 45–55 |
| 500 | 3–7 | 8–13 | 17–24 | 26–34 | 36–44 | 46–54 |
| 1000 | 4–7 | 8–12 | 18–23 | 27–33 | 37–43 | 47–53 |
| | **60%** | **70%** | **80%** | **90%** | **95%** | |
| 50 | 45–74 | 55–82 | 66–90 | 78–97 | | |
| 60 | 46–72 | 57–81 | 68–89 | 80–97 | 86–90 | |
| 80 | 49–71 | 59–80 | 70–88 | 81–96 | 88–99 | |
| 100 | 50–70 | 60–79 | 71–87 | 82–95 | 89–98 | |
| 200 | 53–67 | 62–76 | 74–84 | 86–94 | 91–98 | |
| 300 | 54–65 | 64–75 | 75–84 | 86–93 | 92–97 | |
| 400 | 55–65 | 65–74 | 76–84 | 87–93 | 92–97 | |
| 500 | 56–64 | 66–74 | 76–83 | 87–92 | 93–97 | |
| 1000 | 57–63 | 67–73 | 77–82 | 88–92 | 93–96 | |

infections among a community. This is strictly a ratio and not a rate and provides only a crude indication of transmission intensity as it is categorical rather than a continuous variable. Saturation of infection combined with the longevity of infection does not allow for an estimate of the incidence of infection, with the exception of the study of infants (see below). Information is best collected through random, community-based samples. The use of clinic attendees, school children or non-random samples biases estimates of community infection rates. The techniques of blood examination are discussed in Chapter 3. Parasite counts should be made for each *Plasmodium* and their sexual versus asexual forms separately. The average microscopist can examine 100 thick-film, high-magnification fields in 5 minutes. This represents about 0.1–0.25 μL of blood, and some scanty infections may escape detection. To improve parasite detection, polymerase chain reaction (PCR) techniques or dipsticks can be used (Chapter 3). However, such approaches make comparisons with previous microscopic methods difficult during comparative studies. A rubric for sample-size estimation is provided in Table 5.1. The use of serological tests for epidemiological purposes is discussed in Chapter 3.

In some surveys, particularly morbidity surveys (see below), it may be useful to know the degree of malarial infection. The term parasite count is the number of parasites seen on an average in a number (such as 100) of high-power magnification fields, or in relation to the number of red blood cells. Usually, the parasite count is given in relation to 1 μL of blood after a suitable conversion. The parasite count may also be calculated in relation to the number (400–500) of white blood cells seen in 100 fields, when the number of these cells per microlitre is known.

During the 1950s, the WHO derived a classification of endemicity based upon the spleen rate (another proxy marker of malaria endemicity). This classification was later revised by Metselaar and Van Thiel in relation to the parasite rate. These defini-

**Table 5.2** *Classifications of endemicity*

| Type | Spleen rates | Parasite rates | Description |
|---|---|---|---|
| Hypoendemicity | Not exceeding 10% in children aged 2–9 years | Not exceeding 10% in children aged 2–9 years but may be higher for part of the year | Areas where there is little transmission and the effects, during an average year, upon the general population are unimportant |
| Mesoendemicity | Between 11% and 50% in children aged 2–9 years | Between 11% and 50% in children aged 2–9 years | Typically found among rural communities in subtropical zones where wide geographical variations in transmission risk exist |
| Hyperendemicity | Constantly over 50% in children aged 2–9 years; also high in adults (over 25%) | Constantly over 50% among children aged 2–9 years | Areas where transmission is intense but seasonal where the immunity is insufficient in all age groups |
| Holoendemicity | Constantly over 75% in children aged 2–9 years, but low in adults | Constantly over 75% among infants aged 0–11 months | Perennial, intense transmission resulting in a considerable degree of immunity outside early childhood |

tions of hypoendemic, mesoendemic, hyperendemic and holoendemic malaria are described in Table 5.2. The cut-offs of either spleen or parasite rates are arbitrary and do not capture the seasonal nature in transmission, and thus the annual changes in spleen or parasite rates. More importantly, they do not distinguish between areas that may experience 20 new infections per person per annum compared to those where over 200 new infections are received by the population each year, both potentially classified as holoendemic on the basis of a cross-sectional parasitological survey. Some common terms used in malaria epidemiology are given in Table 5.3.

**Table 5.3** *Some terms used in malaria epidemiology*

| | |
|---|---|
| Anophelism without malaria | This term applies to a situation in which there are *Anopheles* mosquitoes but no evidence of human malaria. This can occur when the mosquito is zoophilic; the climatic conditions do not allow the development of the parasite, the vector population is too low; the vectorial capacity does not support the parasite or control measures are effective |
| Indigenous malaria | Malaria is natural to an area or country |
| Autochthonous malaria[a] | Malaria contracted locally |
| Imported malaria[b] | Malaria acquired outside the specified area in which it is found |
| Introduced malaria | Secondary cases contracted locally but derived from an imported case |
| Induced malaria | Accidental or deliberate infection by blood transfusion, needles, organ transplantation |

[a] 62 000 cases of autochthonous malaria in Europe were reported to WHO in 1998.
[b] *P. vivax* malaria has re-emerged in some of the states of the former USSR (Armenia, Tajikistan, Azerbaijan) and near the demilitarized zone of the Republic of Korea.

## The entomological inoculation rate

The activity of the anopheline vector of malaria provides the basis for calculating the entomological inoculation rate (EIR):

$$h' = mas$$

where $h'$ is the number of infective mosquito bites received per person per unit time; $m$ is the anopheline density in relation to humans; $a$ is the average number of persons bitten by one mosquito in a day; and $s$ is the proportion of mosquitoes with sporozoites in their salivary glands. Usually, EIR values are expressed per year to capture the seasonal nature of vector activity. To provide reliable estimates of vector infection risk, field surveys must derive estimates of the biting rate and the sporozoite index at a monthly (or higher) frequency, for at least a year, or for known months of transmission.

The most direct way to measure the human biting rate (the product of $ma$) is the human bait catch (see Chapter 4). This involves a team waiting in a given location, usually throughout the night, collecting all the mosquitoes that attempt to feed on exposed individuals. Despite being expensive and technically difficult to replicate, it is unique in that it directly samples human-biting mosquitoes. Other sampling methods, such as pyrethrum spray collections, light and exit traps, depend on mosquito behaviours that are less directly associated with feeding on humans.

Measurements of the sporozoite index ($s$) require the number of infective mosquitoes (those with sporozoites in their salivary glands) in the local population to be determined. Ideally, but not always, the index is derived from the biting rate sample. The traditional method was to dissect all sampled mosquitoes for their salivary glands and subject them to procedures designed to help reveal potential sporozoites under the microscope. More recently, the enzyme-linked immunosorbent assay (ELISA) techniques, which detect *Plasmodium*-specific circumsporozoite antigens from mosquito head and/or thorax samples, is used due to its greater sensitivity and species specificity.

The annualized EIR is a favoured measure for assessing malaria endemicity as it reflects the *incidence* of new infections received by the human popu-

lation from the local vector population. The EIR is subject to climatic and ecological constraints, described below. By way of example of the diversity of EIRs recorded across stable endemic areas of Africa, studies have recorded from one infective bite every 3 years to several infective bites every night (Hay *et al.*, 2000).

## Force of infection

Entomological studies have for many years provided the mainstay of transmission intensity measurement. However, in areas of low transmission, sampling techniques become insensitive and errors in calculation transmission indices become large. The logistic requirements for intensive entomological surveillance, reflecting seasonal patterns and marked geographic over-dispersion of vectors, are considerable.

Unlike other infectious diseases, the prevalence of infection in a population reaches saturation very quickly, making any estimate of the incidence of infection difficult from cross-sectional surveys. However, MacDonald first proposed an estimate of the force of infection using infant parasite conversion rates for malaria.

The force of infection ($h$) among infants can be estimated by using a simple, constant-risk, catalytic conversion model:

$$X(a) = 1 - e^{-ha}$$

where $X(a)$ denotes the proportion of individuals of age $a$ that have been exposed (infected at least once) to the parasite. Randomly selected infants aged from birth through to the first birthday can be examined for the presence of blood-stage infection using microscopy. Structuring the proportion of infected infants by month of life can be used to define the cumulative exposure to infection and convert prevalence into incidence of infection using the catalytic conversion model.

Strictly, the proportion positive for a given marker is determined by the balance between the force of infection and the rate of reversion to the negative state. Therefore, a constant-risk catalytic conversion model can be used to estimate the force of infection only by assuming that recovery rates from infection within this period are negligible. Draper and others working in Tanzania during the 1970s estimated the force of infection from serologic surveys simply by assuming that conversion from seropositive to seronegative is uncommon. More recently, combinations of parasite prevalence and malaria-specific immunoglobulin M (IgM) sero-prevalence have been used to assess changes in the force of infection due to the introduction of insecticide-treated bed-nets.

Studies by Walton in Freetown in Sierra Leone during the 1930s confirmed a crude correlation between entomologic challenge and infant parasite conversion rates, but data from the Garki project in Nigeria suggest that the relationships may be non-linear.

## MATHEMATICAL MODELS USED FOR UNDERSTANDING CONTROL

Early mathematical models were conceived during the eradication era essentially to understand how $R_0$ could be reduced below unity, thus interrupting transmission. An expanded model which included a number of endemic levels in relation to the whole range of vectorial capacity involved in transmitting *P. falciparum* was developed as a result of the Garki project in northern Nigeria, carried out in 1973–80 with the support of WHO (Molineaux and Grammicia, 1980).

The model's main output variable was the prevalence of *P. falciparum* parasitaemia as a function of season and age group of the population. It was fitted to data obtained after 1 year of baseline observation and 2 years of insecticidal spraying with proxopur (Arprocarb). The model can be used to indicate the relationship between the prevalence of *P. falciparum* and vectorial capacity, when the latter undergoes natural or man-made changes (e.g. control).

It was hoped that these models would be useful for planning and evaluating malaria control operations. There has been little evidence, however, of their subsequent practical use, primarily as the outputs of the models do not relate to any public health measure.

## DETERMINANTS OF TRANSMISSION

Epidemiological features of malaria in a community depend on the amount and duration of trans-mission and on the diversity of the parasite species involved. Climate, local ecology and active control affect the ability of parasites and vectors to co-exist long enough to enable transmission to occur. The frequency of transmission, or endemicity, depends upon the density and infectivity of anopheline vectors and also on the fluctuations of the sources of infection, namely gametocyte carriers. These features are also dependent upon a range of climatic, physical and population characteristics of a given community. The following sections review some of these factors.

## Temperature

The development of both the vector and parasite is temperature dependent. The female *Anopheles* is not immediately infective after taking a blood meal and the parasite requires a period of time within the mosquito for its development to an infective stage. This period is termed the extrinsic incubation period and its duration under favourable conditions of the vector is dependent on ambient temperature and humidity. Optimum conditions for sporogony are between 25 °C and 30 °C and it ceases below 16 °C (Figure 5.1). Above 35 °C, sporogony slows down considerably and it is also delayed by intermittent low temperatures, with the period immediately after the infective bite being

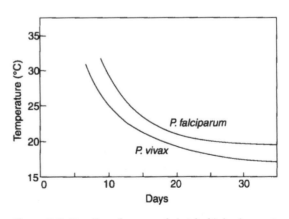

**Figure 5.1** *Duration of sporogonic (extrinsic) development of malaria parasites in* Anopheles *in relation to environmental temperature (MacDonald, 1957). At 25 °C:* P. vivax *10 days;* P. falciparum *12 days;* P. ovale *16 days;* P. malariae *28 days.*

the most sensitive to drops in temperature. High temperatures are associated with more rapid development of vectors and also with increased frequency of feeding by female anophelines. Extreme high temperatures are associated with the development of smaller and less fecund adult mosquitoes, and thermal death of mosquitoes occurs at 40–42 °C.

## Altitude and frost

Altitude and temperature are strongly correlated and for every 100-m increase in altitude, temperature drops by 0.5 °C. Altitude-limiting levels for transmission have been described at approximately 1700–1800 m in the Congo. Lindsay and Martens (1998) consider malaria to be absent above 1500 m, which is contrary to early descriptions of malaria in Kenya, where transmission and epidemics at 1680 m and 1950 m have been described. Overall, the use of altitude as a marker of endemicity or disease risk is complex. Nevertheless, there is a tendency within the literature to refer to 'highland malaria' in East Africa and the Horn of Africa. The parasite is very sensitive to drops in temperature during sporogony and a period of frost during the development cycle may prevent sporogony altogether, as seen in studies in southern Africa, where *A. gambiae s.l.* disappeared completely when winter temperatures dropped below 5 °C.

## Rainfall and humidity

The relationship between mosquito abundance and rainfall is complex and best studied when temperature is not limiting. Studies have demonstrated the association between *A. gambiae s.l.* abundance and rainfall. The female *Anopheles* requires surface water in which to lay her eggs and in which the larvae hatch after 2–3 days. *A. gambiae s.l.* are observed to breed more prolifically in temporary and turbid water bodies, such as those formed by rain, whereas in permanent water bodies predation becomes important. *A. funestus*, in contrast, prefer more permanent water bodies. Both temporary and permanent water bodies are dependent on rain. Rain is also related to humidity and saturation deficit, both of

which affect mosquito survival (adult vector longevity increases with humidities over 60 per cent). By contrast, excessive rainfall may transform small streams into rapid torrents and thus strand many larvae and pupae on the edges of the water channel.

Rainfall effects are most noticeable during epidemic outbreaks in which the rise in cases of malaria is in proportion to the amount of precipitation. In arid areas, though optimum temperatures are found, malaria transmission occurs only when seasonal periods of rainfall provide temporary breeding sites for vectors, as is experienced in the arid areas of the East Africa, the Horn of Africa and Sahel of Africa.

There is good reason for using rainfall to indicate the probable presence of vectors, their survival and the potential for malaria transmission, but a direct, predictable relationship does not exist.

## Malaria seasons

The interaction between temperature and rainfall is responsible for the seasonal features of malaria transmission in many parts of the world. In general, where periods of maximum precipitation coincide with those of maximum temperature, transmission will be highest. Almost every malaria setting shows some seasonal variation in infection risk from local mosquito vectors. These seasonal changes in risks can last for a few weeks or several months. The duration of these malaria seasons also has a direct influence on the annualized risks of parasite exposure a given community is likely to experience.

## Man-made environmental changes and agricultural patterns

The construction of dams, formation of reservoirs and irrigation systems and agricultural practices provide important influences on human settlement, land use and disease risk. The relationship between the amount of rainfall and the development of breeding sites is dependent on several factors, such as the slope of the land, run-off and soil type, and the suitability of these breeding sites will be further affected by the availability of shade, vegetation, salinity and predators.

Deforestation and the development of new breeding sites led to at least a doubling of malaria risk during the construction of the Trans-Amazonian Highway during the early 1970s. The recent development of micro-dams in the Tigray highlands of Ethiopia led to a seven-fold increase in the risk of malaria for villages located closest to these dams.

Certain crops, notably rice, provide suitable environments for vector breeding. Such activities, particularly if widespread, could have an effect on the distribution of malaria, although evidence for this is mixed. In Madhya Pradesh, India, the density of *A. culicifacies* was inversely related to the increasing distance from the rice agro-ecosystem. Similar observations have been made for rice systems near Bobo-Dioulasso in Burkina Faso. The density of *A. gambiae* was 10 times higher near the rice fields compared to the surrounding savannah, yet the sporozoite rate among these vectors was 10 times lower and the expected increase in malaria incidence was not observed.

## Population displacement, urbanization and mobility

One hundred thousand people were displaced from the Bandama valley in Cote d'Ivoire when Lake Kossou was created. Estimates of the numbers of displaced people in India as a result of the Narmada valley project range from 300 000 to 1 million. Such displacement of people along newly created breeding sites exposes communities to new transmission conditions that may result in increased infection risks.

Regional conflicts result in large-scale population movements to avoid the ravages of war. The recent exodus from the hills and mountains of Burundi of people traditionally unexposed to malaria into endemic conditions in Tanzania resulted in an epidemic of severe malaria among these refugees. Similar conditions prevailed among the Karen refugees as they left Burma for Thailand.

Urbanization is a rapidly proliferating demographic feature of most parts of the developing world. There are several examples of the effects of urbanization on vector populations, most notably in Kinshasa, Democratic Republic of Congo and Brazzaville, Congo. Whereas the risks of infection may be much reduced for urban dwellers, they need only travel to the periphery of these urban settlements to experience a considerable increase in risk. Mobility among non-immune urban residents in traditionally endemic countries poses a special risk.

## Socio-economic and housing factors

Several household factors have been identified as increasing human–vector contact within a given ecological environment. These have included the presence of open eaves or the lack of ceilings, population density and the presence of animals close to the house. In Sri Lanka, the risk of infection with either *P. vivax* or *P. falciparum* was halved among residents of houses with complete walls and ceilings compared to that among residents of 'poor' housing.

## Zoophily

Some mosquito species are predominantly zoophilic. The choice of animal, bird or human blood is probably genetically, developmentally and opportunistically determined. Thus, there are examples of populations of zoophilic species building up to such an extent that they 'spill over' to the human population and become secondary vectors of malaria. Conversely, there are also situations in which the animal population has been depleted and a normally zoophilic species has become a human malaria vector. In China, animals are traditionally kept at the periphery of the village between the rice fields or other breeding places and human dwellings, and therefore the mosquitoes bite the animals instead of the humans – zooprophylaxis.

## Personal protection

Both education and available income in households are likely to determine the use of bed-nets, bed-net insecticide treatment services, insect repellents and mosquito coils. These personal protection methods have all been shown to significantly reduce the risks of infection and clinical disease.

## Effect of vector control and drugs

A good example of the effect of active vector control on the risk of infection was demonstrated in the Pare-Taveta settlement scheme in Tanzania. During the 1950s, this area was the focus of a residual house-spraying project using Dieldrin. Adequate rainfall coupled with irrigation of rice fields provided suitable conditions for the breeding of *A. funestus* and *A. gambiae*, and pre-intervention parasite rates among children aged 2–9 years was 64 per cent. After 3 years of spraying, parasite rates declined to 16 per cent.

For refugees located along the Thai-Burmese border, first-line recommendations for malaria therapy were changed in 1994 from mefloquine to a combination of mefloquine and artesunate. The introduction of this combination therapy was associated with an 18.5-fold reduction in gametocyte carriage rates, halving the *P. falciparum* transmission rates in the area (Nosten *et al.*, 2000).

A pragmatic approach to the epidemiological stratification of malaria has been developed and is given in Table 5.4 (WHO, 1993).

## MODELS OF MALARIA RISK USING GEOGRAPHIC INFORMATION SYSTEMS AND REMOTE SENSING

Geographic information systems (GIS) are new computer software tools that are being used increas-

**Table 5.4** *Epidemiological prototypes related to ecological and socio-economic conditions*

African savannah
Plains and valleys outside Africa (traditional agriculture)
Forest and forest fringe
Desert fringe and highland fringe
Coastal and marshland
Urban slums
Agricultural developments
Socio-political disturbances

ingly in epidemiology. They allow the handling of large, related data sets linked through spatial co-ordinates – longitude and latitude. Extensive ground-station weather data sets have been constructed for many parts of the world using methods of interpolation between weather stations. Given that climate is a strong determinant of the distribution of malaria risk, applications of GIS using meteorological data have been used to develop provisional risk maps in Africa (Plate 1; Craig *et al.*, 1999).

GIS provides a powerful means of capturing large amounts of information and modelling spatial risks. However, the map shown in Plate 1 only uses rainfall and temperature and consequently ignores many of the other spatial determinants of infection risk described above. Other sources of high-resolution spatial data can now be derived from geo-stationary and earth-orbiting satellites. In concert with developments in GIS, new approaches to interpreting remote-sensed imagery of the earth provide new opportunities to capture additional information on population settlement, land-use patterns and rivers and permanent water sources. These data can now be obtained on a real-time basis for $1 \times 1$-km resolutions. This provides a comparative advantage over ground-station data in that it does not depend upon interpolation across wide geographical areas.

The full applications of remote-sensed imagery and GIS in predicting risk, malaria seasons, epidemics and population distribution have yet to be realized. However, it is hoped that proposed developments in this area over the next few years will provide new epidemiological tools for mapping malaria risk.

## HEALTH IMPACT OF *P. FALCIPARUM* MALARIA

The definition of infection risk is an important first step to understanding the local epidemiology of malaria in any community. The previous sections consider the measurement and determinants of these risks. The relationships between the frequency of parasite exposure and disease outcome are complex. It is notable from most texts on the epidemiology of malaria that greatest attention is given to parasite exposure and its measurement, but very little to the epidemiology of disease. The following sections attempt to redress this by providing some background to the measurement and epidemiology of morbidity and mortality from malaria.

## Measuring malaria morbidity

Malaria, as a clinical presentation, is often difficult to diagnose uniquely. Fever is common to almost every infectious disease and the severe pathology caused by *P. falciparum*, such as acidosis, anaemia and altered consciousness, is also a complication of other infections. Demonstrating the presence of malaria infection during a clinical event increases the likelihood that symptoms are directly due to the infection, but the high prevalence of asymptomatic infections makes it difficult to exclude other diagnoses. Increasing parasite densities in the peripheral blood increases the statistical chances that a fever is attributable to infection, and the sensitivity and specificity of definitions of morbid events are improved by the use of population-attributable fractions (PAFs). The PAF can be calculated as shown in Table 5.5 using data derived from cross-sectional surveys. Given that relative changes in

geometric parasite densities occur with increasing age, it is important to ensure that PAFs are derived for different age groupings. It is difficult to derive PAFs under conditions of very intense transmission where there are multiple, independent parasite populations within a single peripheral blood sample. Under these conditions, logistic regression methods have been used (Smith *et al.*, 1994).

Defining rates of malaria morbidity usually involves passive and/or active case detection of fevers accompanied by microscopic examination of thick blood smears taken from all fever cases. Fever can be defined as a measured axillary or rectal temperature and/or a history of fever. Both active and passive case detection usually relates to fixed cohorts of children identified through census enumerations. Active case detection involves household visits to obtain histories of illness during the preceding week, month or 24 hours. Passive case detection at health facilities better reflects what the local community perceives as ill-health, although, by definition, will not detect all mild, transitory clinical events. The frequency with which active surveillance is undertaken during a year or a malaria season will determine the number of clinical events detected; monthly surveillance tends to detect only one quarter of the events detected through weekly surveillance. Weekly surveillance detects

**Table 5.5** *What proportion of fever may be attributable to malaria?*

Suppose that the incidence of fever among children without parasite is $i_0$, and that among children with parasites is $i_1$. The relative risk of fever in those with parasites compared to those without is denoted by $R$, and thus $i_1 = Ri_0$. Among those with parasites, the proportion of fevers due to malaria is $(i_1 - i_0)/i_1$, or $(R-1)/R$. Among those without parasites, none of the fevers is due to malaria. Among all cases of fever, therefore, the proportion due to malaria, the attributable fraction (AF), is $p(R-1)/R$, where $p$ denotes the proportion of fever cases with parasites. The AF is also known as the attributable proportion, the aetiologic fraction or the attributable percentage. Data on the parasite prevalence among febrile cases and suitably chosen controls can be used to estimate $R$ and $p$, and hence the AF. Case–control data collected in a study of malaria in The Gambia during 1989 illustrate the method. An approximate confidence interval (CI) for the AF can easily be found.

**Cases**  Approximately 900 children aged 1–5 years living in 26 villages were visited weekly from October to mid-November 1989, and axillary temperatures were measured. Fever cases (temperature ≥37.5 °C) had a thick blood film taken, and *P. falciparum* parasite density was recorded.

**Controls**  A cross-sectional survey on a simple random sample of these children was carried out in mid-November 1989, and a blood film was taken from all these children.
55% of cases (41/74) but only 26% of controls (86/333) had parasitaemia. Thus $p = 0.55$ and $R = 3.568$ (the estimated odds ratio, $41 \times 247/86 \times 33$). Thus, AF = (0.55) (2.568/3.568) = 0.399, so about 40% of fever cases during this period at the end of the rainy season were due to malaria. The approximate 95% CI for the AF is (21%, 54%).

Directly abstracted from Schellenberg *et al.* (1994).

approximately 75 per cent of events detected through daily surveillance. Increasingly, studies use combinations of both active and passive detection.

In some areas of the world, routine case detection is maintained by the health services as part of their control strategy. Examples of these active surveillance approaches can be found in South Africa, Ethiopia, Thailand and China. Sub-national statistics of combined active and passive case detection in these areas may not be comprehensive definitions of risk, but do allow for comparative evaluations aimed at targeting resources.

## Severe and complicated malaria

Malaria is a complex disease whose pathogenesis is still incompletely understood (see Chapter 10). However, for epidemiological purposes, it is convenient to define two major syndromes, cerebral malaria and severe malarial anaemia. Patients with cerebral malaria present in coma, which may have a variety of underlying causes, ranging from a primarily neurological condition to being the result of a systemic metabolic disturbance.

Severe malarial anaemia is arbitrarily defined as a haemoglobin of less than 5 g/dL in association with malaria parasites. There are potential problems in that, in malaria-endemic areas, there are many, often interacting, causes of anaemia, and also in areas of high-intensity transmission it may be the norm to be parasitized. Nonetheless, in many settings, children presenting with an acute febrile disease, peripheral parasitaemia and very low haemoglobin concentrations form the majority of inpatient admissions during the malaria season, and thus the rather arbitrary and approximate definition proves useful.

Most hospital settings in malaria-endemic areas have a system of recording patients' admission diagnoses. Invariably, these diagnoses are made in the absence of microscopy or strict clinical criteria and rarely altered on discharge. Nevertheless, these data can be obtained from a review of admission ward registers to provide a crude approximation of:

- the periods of a year in which the greatest clinical burden is experienced,
- case fatalities as a marker of changing therapeutic success in the periphery or in hospital,

- a rough estimate of the relative age distribution of complicated malaria as a crude indication of the community's immune status (see below).

It is possible to instigate an upgraded system of admission surveillance that captures all demographic details of the patient, including residence, strict clinical examination protocols, blood film examination for malaria infection and haematology. Such surveillance systems have been used during a series of epidemiological studies to define risks of severe malaria from fixed populations to examine the age and clinical presentation of disease among African children.

## Measuring malaria mortality

Defining malaria-specific mortality rates poses several additional problems for field epidemiologists. Most deaths in developing countries occur outside the formal health service, and national government systems of civil registration are notoriously incomplete. Consequently, epidemiologists interested in defining malaria-specific mortality use detailed demographic surveillance systems (DSS) of large populations (between 20 000 and 100 000 people).

The DSS is a methodology developed, and refined, by French demographers in West Africa and the United Nations (UN) in Bangladesh. Detailed descriptions of how to undertake a DSS are provided elsewhere (Smith and Morrow, 1996). Briefly, the critical components include the following:

- *Community sensitization*. DSS methodologies are intrusive upon communities and require complete co-operation with investigators. Careful preparation and dialogue are required with the community and its leaders before they begin.
- *Mapping*: detailed maps and numbering of households within a fixed geographical area, divided into manageable or ecological distinct zones. Combinations of hand-drawn maps and hand-held global positioning systems (GPSs) are used to provide spatial maps showing the positions of households in relation to other physical, environmental and health service features. These maps are used to locate households during

follow-up visits. In addition, longitudes and latitudes can be used within a GIS platform to explore environmental and health service determinants of malaria risk.

- *Census.* A full census is undertaken of the entire population, recording, as a minimum, name, relationship to other household members, age and sex. These data are stored on a computer and used for subsequent population monitoring.
- *Multi-round household visits.* Combinations of methods have been used to prospectively record migration, birth and death events of the enumerated population. Village or community reporters can be used to report all vital events to project staff. Field workers visit each household periodically to define events from computerized household schedules since the last visit, or tri-annual or bi-annual re-enumerations of the entire population are undertaken. In practice, the more frequent the contact with households, the fewer the missed vital events. Given the rapidity of early neonatal mortality events and the social constraints associated with discussing these events in many communities, an additional system of pregnancy monitoring is recommended.

Post-mortem interviews are used to define the causes of deaths that occurred without contact with a clinical service and are conducted as soon as is culturally appropriate after the event. This verbal autopsy technique requires careful development for each local setting, ensuring that disease descriptions are appropriate for the local common diseases and vernacular. Both closed and open questions are recorded onto pro formas, and it is common for at least three independent reviewers to assess probable causes of death. Algorithms have also been adopted that first exclude easily defined causes of death such as trauma, measles, kwashiorkor or those with a definitive diagnosis from hospital. Thereafter, symptoms and signs solicited from interviews with bereaved relatives, which include fever lasting between 1 and 28 days linked to various combinations of convulsions, inability to follow with the eyes, difficulty in breathing or pallor, have previously been used to define a possible malaria death.

Validations of the verbal autopsy have demonstrated sensitivities between 45 per cent and 72 per cent and specificities between 77 per cent and 89 per cent for malaria mortality (Anker *et al.*, 1999). The accuracy of a verbal autopsy estimate of the cause-specific mortality fraction for different levels of sensitivity, specificity and cause-specific mortality have been calculated (Table 5.6). It indicates that algorithms with only moderate levels of sensitivity and specificity are not suited for measuring rare causes of death, whereas they could provide approximate values for relatively common causes of death. Less common causes of death require very high rates of specificity (but can tolerate low levels of sensitivity).

## THE EPIDEMIOLOGY OF *P. FALCIPARUM* MORBIDITY AND MORTALITY RISKS UNDER STABLE TRANSMISSION

Congenital infection may be common, but is probably transient and the resultant disease risks may be rare, although it is fair to say that the clinical outcomes of congenital infections have not been well described. Young infants enjoy a period of protection from the clinical consequences of infection, due essentially to the passive transfer of maternal antibody *in utero* and the presence of fetal haemoglobin. From infancy to adulthood, the relative rates of infection, mild morbidity, severe complicated disease and mortality are best shown in Figure 5.2, recorded during a series of studies at Kilifi on the Kenyan coast among children aged 0–15 years. The risks of a fatal outcome decline during early childhood, and the frequency of clinical attacks declines sometime later in childhood. These declining risks of disease and death occur against a constant risk of infection throughout childhood until adulthood. It is reasonable to assume that these declining adverse health risks associated with age are related to the development of functional immunity. It appears that at least three levels of immune acquisition occur, beginning with protection against severe and fatal outcomes, followed by protection against mild, self-limiting clinical disease and, much later, followed by an ability to regulate peripheral infection.

Studies undertaken in stable endemic areas of Africa on the incidence of mild, transitory clinical events attributed to infection with *P. falciparum*

**Table 5.6** *Differences between the verbal autopsy estimate and the true cause-specific mortality fraction for different levels of specificity and sensitivity and for different cause-specific mortality fractions*

| Sensitivity | True cause-specific mortality fraction | Specificity 0.60 | 0.70 | 0.80 | 0.85 | 0.90 | 0.95 | 0.99 |
|---|---|---|---|---|---|---|---|---|
| 0.60 | 0.01 | +0.392 | +0.293 | +0.194 | +0.145 | +0.095 | +0.046 | +0.006 |
| | 0.05 | +0.360 | +0.265 | +0.170 | +0.123 | +0.075 | +0.028 | −0.010 |
| | 0.10 | +0.320 | +0.230 | +0.140 | +0.095 | +0.050 | +0.005 | −0.031 |
| | 0.20 | +0.240 | +0.160 | +0.080 | +0.040 | +0.000 | −0.040 | −0.072 |
| | 0.30 | +0.160 | +0.090 | +0.020 | −0.015 | −0.050 | −0.085 | −0.113 |
| | 0.40 | +0.080 | +0.020 | −0.040 | −0.070 | −0.100 | −0.130 | −0.154 |
| 0.70 | 0.01 | +0.393 | +0.294 | +0.195 | +0.146 | +0.096 | +0.047 | +0.007 |
| | 0.05 | +0.365 | +0.270 | +0.175 | +0.128 | +0.080 | +0.033 | −0.005 |
| | 0.10 | +0.330 | +0.240 | +0.150 | +0.105 | +0.060 | +0.015 | −0.021 |
| | 0.20 | +0.260 | +0.180 | +0.100 | +0.060 | +0.020 | −0.020 | −0.052 |
| | 0.30 | +0.190 | +0.120 | +0.050 | +0.015 | −0.020 | −0.055 | −0.083 |
| | 0.40 | +0.120 | +0.060 | 0.000 | −0.030 | −0.060 | −0.090 | −0.114 |
| 0.80 | 0.01 | +0.394 | +0.295 | +0.196 | +0.147 | +0.097 | +0.048 | +0.008 |
| | 0.05 | +0.370 | +0.275 | +0.180 | +0.133 | +0.085 | +0.038 | −0.001 |
| | 0.10 | +0.340 | +0.255 | +0.160 | +0.115 | +0.070 | +0.025 | −0.011 |
| | 0.20 | +0.280 | +0.200 | +0.120 | +0.080 | +0.040 | +0.000 | −0.032 |
| | 0.30 | +0.220 | +0.150 | +0.080 | +0.045 | +0.010 | −0.025 | −0.053 |
| | 0.40 | +0.160 | +0.100 | +0.040 | +0.010 | −0.020 | −0.050 | −0.074 |
| 0.90 | 0.01 | +0.395 | +0.296 | +0.197 | +0.148 | +0.098 | +0.049 | +0.009 |
| | 0.05 | +0.375 | +0.280 | +0.185 | +0.138 | +0.090 | +0.043 | +0.005 |
| | 0.10 | +0.350 | +0.260 | +0.170 | +0.125 | +0.080 | +0.035 | −0.001 |
| | 0.20 | +0.300 | +0.220 | +0.140 | +0.100 | +0.060 | +0.020 | −0.012 |
| | 0.30 | +0.250 | +0.180 | +0.110 | +0.075 | +0.040 | +0.005 | −0.023 |
| | 0.40 | +0.200 | +0.140 | +0.080 | +0.050 | +0.020 | −0.010 | −0.034 |
| 0.99 | 0.01 | +0.396 | +0.297 | +0.198 | +0.148 | +0.099 | +0.049 | +0.010 |
| | 0.05 | +0.380 | +0.285 | +0.190 | +0.142 | +0.095 | +0.047 | +0.009 |
| | 0.10 | +0.359 | +0.269 | +0.179 | +0.134 | +0.089 | +0.044 | +0.008 |
| | 0.20 | +0.318 | +0.238 | +0.158 | +0.118 | +0.078 | +0.038 | +0.006 |
| | 0.30 | +0.277 | +0.207 | +0.137 | +0.102 | +0.067 | +0.032 | +0.004 |
| | 0.40 | +0.236 | +0.176 | +0.116 | +0.086 | +0.056 | +0.026 | +0.002 |

For example, if the sensitivity and specificity of a verbal autopsy algorithm are both 70% for a fairly common cause of death (e.g. one which is responsible for 30% of deaths), the verbal autopsy estimate will be approximately 12 percentage points off (i.e. the verbal autopsy would classify 42% of the deaths as due to that particular cause, whereas, in fact, only 30% of the deaths were really due to that cause). Even if the specificity were as high as 80% and sensitivity still 70%, the size of the error would be off by 5 percentage points (35% vs 30%).
Anker *et al.* (1999).

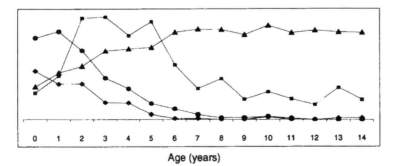

**Figure 5.2** *Relative risks of infection (triangles), morbidity (squares), severe disease (circles) and mortality risks (diamonds) among a population aged 0–15 years located in a stable endemic area of the Kenyan coast.*

Age (years)

suggest that children less than 5 years old experience, on average, 1.2 clinical attacks every year. Sometimes, parasitaemia with or without associated fever can continue for several months, resulting in a fall in the haemoglobin level (Figure 5.3). Children aged 5–9 years will experience a clinical attack every 18 months and children aged above 10 years and adults will experience one attack of clinical malaria every 3–4 years.[1]

From recent DSS studies[1] under a range of stable transmission conditions in Africa, the average mortality rate among children aged 0–4 years is 8.3/1000 per annum, or 20 per cent of all childhood mortality outside the neonatal period.

Mortality rates among children aged 5–9 years are, on average, 1.2/1000 per annum. Given the focus on child survival programmes in Africa, we know relatively little about the risks of mortality outside childhood. However, several studies suggest that malaria-specific mortality among populations aged 10 years or older could be in the order of 0.1/1000 per annum.

The most obvious consequences of living in a high-intensity transmission setting are that children are exposed to malaria at a younger age and develop immunity at a younger age than is the case in lower transmission areas. This is reflected in lowering of the mean age of patients presenting with severe malaria

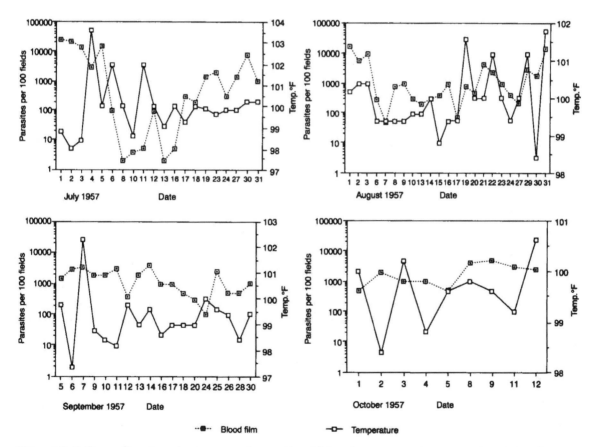

**Figure 5.3** *Daily parasitaemia and temperature of a Gambian child aged 1 year 2 months. The parasitaemia lasted 106 continuous days. The child did not appear ill and was not given antimalarials. However, his haemoglobin level dropped to 8 g/dL and the parasitaemia was cleared with chloroquine. A similar drop of haemoglobin would occur if children were repeatedly treated with chloroquine in areas where RII resistance is common, despite remaining asymptomatic.*

[1] Unpublished data (RW Snow) derived from the Burden of Malaria in Africa Project.

with increasing transmission intensity (i.e. the pattern shown in Figure 5.2 for mortality and severe disease is shifted towards the left). These observations suggest that the development of functional immunity may be dependent upon an ill-defined amount of parasite exposure from birth. In general, it is also true that severe malarial anaemia tends to dominate the clinical picture in areas of high transmission, whereas cerebral malaria assumes increasingly greater importance in areas of lower transmission.

What is important for disease control is whether the cumulative risks of disease or death decline with declining parasite exposure. Clearly, at one end of the transmission spectrum, where the risks of infection are very low, there will be a very slow acquisition of immunity and all age groups are likely to be at risk of both disease and death following parasite exposure. Under these conditions, the risks of a disease outcome or death will simply be a function of the chance encounters with the parasite. As transmission intensity increases, it would appear from recent studies among African childhood populations that rates of severe disease or death vary very little, despite log-order increases in transmission intensity ranging from 3 to 300 infectious bites per person per annum (Trape and Rogier, 1996; Snow *et al.*, 1997; Marsh and Snow, 1999).

In areas where the intensity of transmission is high, what remains uncertain is whether artificially reducing the rate of natural parasite exposure through sustained vector control or personal protection will lead to new epidemiological conditions typical of intermediate transmission. The net result would be a change in age-specific risks but not cumulative risks.

These initial epidemiological observations need to be explored further as they have important implications for understanding the impacts of various targeted interventions. Perhaps what these recent debates have highlighted is our rather poor understanding of the epidemiological basis of clinical malaria and immunity.

## CONSEQUENTIAL HEALTH IMPACTS OF MALARIA

It has long been recognized that the relationships between *P. falciparum* infection, morbidity and disease outcome are complex. What we do know is that individuals born into areas of stable *P. falciparum*

transmission frequently move between periods of being infected with the parasite and states in which the individual remains uninfected. Most individuals will, at some stage in their lives, develop an overt clinical response to an infection, often manifesting itself as a febrile event. These clinical events may progress to severe pathological clinical states, which may resolve naturally or the patient survives through medical intervention.

This simplistic view of infection to death provides only part of the overall public health equation. There are morbid and fatal consequences allied to each step of the infection and disease process. Chronic subclinical infections may render an individual anaemic. It has also been argued that subclinical infections predispose to the severity and outcome of other infectious diseases. A far greater body of evidence supports the view that asymptomatic infection of the placenta of a pregnant woman significantly reduces the weight of her newborn child, reducing its survival chances. Patients seek treatment and treatments often carry their own risks of fatal or morbid outcomes. Patients who survive the severe pathological consequences of infection may be left with debilitating sequelae, such as epilepsy, spasticity or blindness, or more subtle behavioural or cognitive impairments. To summarize the direct and indirect health consequences of *P. falciparum* infection, a schematic representation is shown in Figure 5.4.

The overall health impact of *P. falciparum* infection on any community may extend beyond the direct effects of disease and mortality risks. It is important to define additional health effects of infection and disease as they may be relevant in the overall balance between changing immunity, intervention and community health. Nevertheless, our understanding and quantification of the consequential health impacts of infection shown in Figure 5.4 remain poorly defined. Defining these risks, how they change from birth through adulthood and how these changes vary according to the risks of repeated infection from birth are the challenges facing the modern malariologist.

## DETERMINANTS OF RISKS OF DISEASE AND DEATH

Perhaps the single most important factor that influences the risk of a poor health outcome following

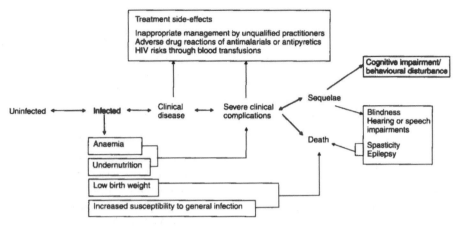

**Figure 5.4** *Direct and indirect health consequences of malaria infection.*

infection is immunity (see above and Chapter 11). However, the risks of a severe complication or fatal outcome following infection are dependent upon a wide range of other factors, including host genetics, behavioural features related to early management of the illness, nutrition and variation in parasite phenotypes. This section considers some of the factors responsible for protection from and susceptibility to the severe and fatal consequences of infection, derived essentially from two recent, large, case–control studies of severe life-threatening disease compared to mild disease and those asymptomatically infected in The Gambia and Kenya.

## Host genetics

A striking feature of studies of risk factors for malaria is the number of host genetic polymorphisms that have been shown to confer protection from severe disease: these include sickle-cell trait, beta- and alpha-thalassaemia, glucose-6-phosphate dehydrogenase (G6PD) deficiency, human leucocyte antigen (HLA) class I and II alleles, Band 3, spectrin, Lewis and Kid Js(a) red cell types. The variety and number of these protective traits also suggest that others await description (Hill, 1992). Only a limited number of susceptibility genes have been identified, e.g. homozygotes for the TNF2 allele (a variant of the TNF-alpha promoter region) have a relatively

higher risk of death or severe neurological sequelae due to cerebral malaria. Together, these genetic characteristics of human populations constitute the polygenic control over Africa's leading cause of parasite-related death and may profoundly influence the micro-epidemiology and macro-epidemiology of severe disease.

## Parasite phenotypes and polyparasitism

There has been particular interest in the genes regulating the expression of proteins on the surface of the infected red cell, some of which demonstrate adhesion properties linked to cerebral malaria (see Chapter 2).

## Nutrition

Autopsy studies undertaken during the 1950s and 1960s in Ghana and Nigeria noted that it was most unusual for the marasmic or kwashiorkor child to be found at necropsy to have had either cerebral malaria or malarial anaemia. These observations and other experimental data using animal models led to a widely held view that undernutrition protects against *P. falciparum* disease. However, more recent work in Kenya supports a view that malnutrition does not protect against severe malaria and, in fact, is a risk factor for it. These apparently disparate views are not necessarily incompatible, because it is possible that there are, as yet, unknown subtle differences in the host – parasite relationship between undernutrition and extreme starvation. These relationships need to be tested further through detailed prospective studies.

## Socio-economic factors

Environmental, behavioural and socio-economic risks have so far appeared to have little influence over an individual child's risk of developing severe disease under the stable endemic conditions common in The Gambia and Kenya. These results reflect the homogeneity in these features within the populations studied, as it would be hard to argue that the total absence of first-line treatment, whether through physical isolation, poverty or behaviour, would not influence the risks of developing severe disease.

## Drug resistance

Recent observations by Trape et al. (1998) in three rural populations in the sahel, savannah and forest areas of Senegal have noted a temporal increase in malaria-specific mortality (between 1.2- and 5.5-fold) co-incidental with the emergence of chloroquine resistance. These studies demonstrate the role that effective therapy of disease has upon the risks of mortality in communities.

## EPIDEMIC MALARIA

## Defining epidemics

The term epidemic may be applied to a sharp rise of the incidence of malaria among a population in which the disease was unknown. Mathematical models have focused on whether malaria transmission has the potential for epidemics, using the relationships described earlier for the stability index, basic reproduction rate and vectorial capacity.

However, just who is exposed to epidemic conditions and how best to define these conditions are much debated and often hard to quantify. Strict mathematical definitions do not capture the complex nature and public health significance of changes in factors affecting local transmission, which lead to the popular notion of 'epidemics'.

Perhaps the best definition of epidemic malaria was proposed by MacDonald (1957) as follows: 'An epidemic is an acute exacerbation of disease out of proportion to the normal to which the community is subject.' There is a proposal to restrict the term to the narrower sense of outbreaks in places where the disease is rare, but *RWS has found this a restricted definition unworkable in practice and prefers the wider and more colloquial term.* Epidemics occur only in zones of unstable malaria, where very slight modification in any of the transmission factors may completely upset equilibrium, and where restraining influence of immunity may be negligible or absent, and they therefore show a very marked geographical distribution.

In an epidemic of malaria, three periods can be distinguished, although they cannot be easily separated from one another. Following a pre-epidemic increase of transmission due to the higher gametocyte rate and the greater density and infectivity of the *Anopheles* population, there is a sharp rise in the incidence of the disease. This is the epidemic wave, which is also accompanied by an increase of mortality, directly due not only to malaria but also to the intercurrent diseases. The severity of an epidemic of malaria cannot be easily related to the increase of transmission that has caused it; even small increases of transmission may produce quite dramatic epidemics. The rise of the epidemic wave is usually faster in *P. vivax* outbreaks than in those due to *P. falciparum*, although the severity of the latter is far greater. During the post-epidemic period, the incidence of malaria falls to its usual low levels.

One of the greatest epidemics of malaria in modern times struck the former USSR after the First World War; more than 10 million cases were reported in 1923–26, and there were at least 60 000 deaths. The Sri Lankan (or Ceylon) epidemic of 1934–35 caused nearly 3 million cases of malaria and 82 000 deaths. In 1938, the invasion of Brazil by *A. gambiae* was followed by an epidemic with over

100 000 cases and at least 14 000 deaths. In 1963, there was an epidemic of malaria in Haiti, in the wake of the typhoon Flora. In 1967, a serious resurgence of malaria in Sri Lanka greatly handicapped progress towards eradicating malaria from the island. Africa has also witnessed several devastating P. falciparum malaria epidemics: during the early 1930s in South Africa, 1958 in Ethiopia, 1986 in Madagascar and 1997 in north-eastern Kenya. These African epidemics resulted in between 1 per cent and 14 per cent of the population dying during the epidemic period.

These epidemics have had varied aetiologies. Authors have variously attributed epidemics to changes in the El Niño phenomena, environmental management, population migration, breakdown in health service provision, drug resistance and global warming. Common to nearly all malaria epidemics has been the observation that the clinical burden has overwhelmed the health services and the childhood and adult populations have been equally at risk of both clinical disease and death.

Defining epidemic-prone areas is pragmatically and conceptually difficult. New approaches to combined GIS and remote sensing may provide new tools. Currently, 'expert-opinion' approaches may constitute the best possible means of defining epidemic risk areas for targeted control and resource allocation.

## Epidemic forecasting, early warning and early detection

There are basic distinctions between the concepts of epidemic forecasting, early warning and early detection. Forecasting and early warning are both intended to warn of environmental conditions that are suitable for the occurrence of an epidemic. As yet, there are no good models based on medium-range weather for epidemic forecasting and models would have to be developed for each geographical setting. This is one of the likely applications of long-term remote-sensed imagery data from satellites. Early warning, on the other hand, consists of monitoring environmental risk factors directly and locally, in order to detect when conditions suitable for an epidemic have appeared at a given time and place.

Early detection is the monitoring of epidemiological data in order to detect the actual occurrence of an epidemic as soon as it begins. Such data usually include weekly or monthly assessment of health facility data. Historical malaria data (e.g. outpatient attendance or severe malaria admission) can be summarized in simple graphical form. This would show, for each week or month, the mean or median figures over recent years (e.g. the last 5 years), together with an estimate of the upper limit of the 'normal range' (e.g. the 75th percentile) over this period. Current data would be plotted onto the graph as they are collected. Figures in excess of the historical 'normal range' would signal an early detection of an epidemic.

Each of these functions has an important role in an integrated strategy signalling warning flags at different time scales. Epidemic forecasting provides the longest lead times, but is likely to be the least specific and reliable. It will allow heightened surveillance and some initial precautionary measures in the danger areas. Early warning should provide greater reliability and local specificity, and therefore a lower frequency of false alarm, but will allow less time to prepare a response. Early detection will be even more reliable and geographically specific, but at the cost of much reduced lead times.

## THE EPIDEMIOLOGY OF P. VIVAX

It is opined that, among the malaria parasites of humans, P. malariae is the most ancestral, followed by P. vivax/P. ovale, with P. falciparum being the most recent from an evolutionary point of view.

P. vivax sporozoite polymorphism has been proposed to explain the mechanism of latency.

The epidemiology of P. vivax malaria and its impact on P. falciparum in areas where the two parasites co-exist are variable.

### Unstable P. vivax malaria

Studies in Italy in the 1930s demonstrated that P. vivax malaria is characteristically a disease of infancy and early childhood. However, this early exposure to

*P. vivax* did not protect adults from acquiring severe clinical attacks when *P. falciparum* infections developed in later life.

In the well-documented epidemic in Ceylon in 1934–35, it was reported that *P. vivax* played a predominant part during the early stages of the epidemic, but gave way to *P. falciparum* towards its close. The toll of life was approximately 100 000, and probably one-third to one-half of the total population of the island was clinically infected. During the acute stages of the epidemic, infants and children were mainly involved, whereas during the decline of the epidemic, the mortality was almost exclusively confined to people over 40 years of age. Virtually all deaths were due to *P. falciparum*.

The effects of *P. falciparum* and *P. vivax* in Sri Lanka seem inconsistent. In an endemic region where *P. vivax* accounts for more than 95 per cent of malaria cases and where the incidence of *P. falciparum* is low (although severe epidemics occur at 7–10-year intervals), both adults and children have low clinical tolerance to *P. falciparum* and develop acute symptoms of malaria (Mendis *et al.*, 1990).

In contrast, Gunewardena *et al.* (1994), also reporting from Sri Lanka, noted that whereas infection with *P. vivax* did not prevent patients from developing subsequent infections with *P. falciparum*, the subjective symptomatic scores of such patients were lower than those of patients who had not suffered from *P. vivax* infection.

Based on hospital data, the incubation period of patients with *P. vivax* malaria in Sri Lanka ranged from less than 28 days up to 40 weeks and relapses developed between 8 and 44 weeks. Paroxysms were relatively mild when compared to non-immune individuals experiencing their first infections. As with *P. falciparum*, mathematical models have been developed that simulate the incidence of malaria satisfactorily in Kataragama, and a strong association between malaria and house construction, vicinity to breeding sites and mosquito densities was found.

## Stable *P. vivax* malaria

On Espiritu Santo, Vanuatu, there has been a long established stable co-existence of *P. vivax* and *P. falci-*

*parum* in the population. Studies in the 1990s by Maitland *et al.* (1996) found that there was a reciprocal relationship between *P. falciparum* and *P. vivax*, indicating that infection with the former species may inhibit infection or relapse of *P. vivax* disease, while cerebral malaria and malaria-specific morbidity were low. It was also found, paradoxically, that the incidence of uncomplicated *P. falciparum* malaria and the prevalence of splenomegaly were most marked in children with alpha-thalassaemia and that the effect was most marked in the youngest children and for *P. vivax*.

As a result of these observations, it has been postulated that early exposure to *P. vivax* modulates the outcome of subsequent infections with *P. falciparum* and protects against severe disease and morbidity. In support of this hypothesis is evidence of cross-species immunity in animal models.

Recent studies have confirmed that symptom-free cases of *P. vivax* are not uncommon in the western border of Thailand, among native Amazonians and in Sri Lanka (Luxemberger *et al.*, 1996; Camargo *et al.*, 1999; Gamage-Mendis *et al.*, 1991). Of particular importance are the recent observations on the morbid consequences to the mother and newborn of *P. vivax* infections during pregnancy (Nosten *et al.*, 1999).

The studies in Vanuatu are in marked contrast to most of the findings in Italy and Sri Lanka, where, despite a long exposure to *P. vivax*, *P. falciparum* causes substantial morbidity and mortality among the population whenever it cyclically reappears. Whether this difference is merely the result of differences in *P. vivax* transmission – 'unstable' in Sri Lanka and 'stable' in Vanuatu – or whether there are additionally other factors involved remains to be elucidated.

## IMPORTED MALARIA

Given the rapid growth in international travel over the last 50 years, it is not surprising that imported malaria has grown. This has been compounded by the emergence and spread of drug resistance. Labels such as 'airport malaria', 'baggage malaria' and 'taxi-rank malaria' are the result of infected vectors transported from endemic areas in aircraft, suitcases and taxis, biting non-immune individuals who had not journeyed to malarious areas. In Britain, around 1200 cases of *P. falciparum* are notified yearly. Deaths have varied from four in 1989 to 13 in 1997. In 2000, there were 15 deaths (PHLS Malaria Reference Laboratory, London School of Hygiene and Tropical Medicine, 2000).

## BIBLIOGRAPHY

Anker M, *et al.* A standard verbal autopsy method for investigating causes of death in infants and children. ANb WHO/CDS/CSR/ISR/99.4. Geneva, World Health Organization.

Camargo EP, Alves F, Pereira de Silva LH. Symptomless *Plasmodium vivax* infections in native Amazonians. *Lancet* 1999; **353**: 14–16.

Craig MH, Snow RW, le Sueur D. African climatic model of malaria transmission based on monthly rainfall and temperature. *Parasitol Today* 1999; **15**: 105–11.

Gallup JL, Sachs JD. Geography and economic development. Paper presented at the World Bank's annual bank conference on development economics, April 20, 1998. http://www.hiid.harvard.edu/research/newnote.htm1#geogrowth

Gamage-Mendis AC, Rajakaruna J, Carter R, Mendis KN. The infectious reservoir of *Plasmodium vivax* and *Plasmodium falciparum* malaria in an endemic region of Sri Lanka. *Am J Trop Med Hyg* 1991; **45**: 479–87.

Gamage-Mendis A., Rajakaruna J., Carter R., Mendis KN. Transmission blocking immunity to human *Plasmodium vivax* malaria in an endemic population in Kataragama, Sri Lanka. *Parasite Immunol* 1992; **14**: 385–96.

Gunewardena DM, Carter R, Mendis KN. Patterns of acquired anti-malarial immunity in Sri Lanka. *Mem Inst Oswaldo Cruz, Rio de Janeiro* 1994; **89** (Special Issue): 61–3.

Hay SI, Toomer JF, Rogers DJ, Snow RW. Annual entomological inoculation rates (EIR) across Africa. I. Literature review. *Trans R Soc Trop Med Hyg* 2000; **94**: 113–27.

Hill AVS. Malaria resistance genes: a natural selection. *Trans R Soc Trop Med Hyg* 1992; **86**: 225–6.

Lindsay SW, Martens WJM. Malaria in the African highlands: past, present and future. *Bull World Health Organ* 1998; **76**: 33–45.

Luxemburger C, Thwai KL, White NJ, *et al.* The epidemiology of malaria in a Karen population on the western border of Thailand. *Trans R Soc Trop Med Hyg* 1996; **90**: 105–11.

MacDonald G. *The epidemiology and control of malaria.* Oxford, Oxford University Press, 1957.

Maitland K, Williams TN, *et al.* The interaction between *Plasmodium falciparum* and *P. vivax* in children in Espiritu Santo island, Vanuatu. *Trans R Soc Trop Med Hyg* 1996; **90**: 614–20.

Marsh K, Snow RW. Malaria transmission and morbidity. *Parassitologia* 2000; **41** (1–3) 241–6.

Mendis C, Gamage-Mendis AC, Zoysa DE, *et al.* Characteristics of malaria transmission in Kataragama, Sri Lanka: a focus for immunoepidemiological studies. *Am J Trop Med Hyg* 1990; **42**(4): 298–308.

Molineaux L, Gramiccia G. *The Gharki project: research on the epidemiology and control of malaria in the Sudan savanna of West Africa.* Geneva, World Health Organization, 1980.

Nosten F, McGready R, Simpson JA, *et al.* Effects of *Plasmodium vivax* malaria in pregnancy. *Lancet* 1999; **354**; 546–9.

Nosten F, van Vugt M, Price RN, *et al.* Effects of artesonate–mefloquine combination on incidence of *Plasmodium falciparum* malaria and mefloquine resistance in western Thailand: a prospective study. *Lancet* 2000; **356**: 297–302.

Price RN, Nosten F, *et al.* Effects of artemisinin derivatives on malaria transmissibility. *Lancet* 1996; **347**: 1654–8.

Schellenberg JRMA, Smith T, *et al.* What is clinical malaria? Finding case definitions for field research in highly endemic areas. *Parasitol Today* 1994; **10**: 439–42.

Smith PG, Morrow RH. *Field trials of health interventions in developing countries: a tool box*, 2nd edition. London, Macmillan Education, 1996.

Smith T, Schellenberg JRMA, Hayes R. Attributable fraction estimates and case definitions for malaria in endemic areas. *Stat Med* 1994; **13**: 2345–58.

Snow RW, Craig MH, *et al.* Estimating mortality, morbidity and disability due to malaria among Africa's non-pregnant population. *Bull World Health Organ* 1999; **77**: 624–40.

Snow RW, Omumbo JA, *et al.* Relation between severe malaria morbidity in children and level of *Plasmodium falciparum* transmission in Africa. *Lancet* 1997; **349**: 1650–4.

Trape JF, Pison G, *et al.* Impact of chloroquine resistance on malaria mortality. *C R Acad Sci Paris, Sciences de la Vie* 1998; **321**: 689–97.

Trape JF, Rogier C. Combating malaria morbidity and mortality by reducing transmission. *Parasitol Today* 1996; **12**: 236–40.

WHO. A global strategy for malaria control. Geneva, World Health Organization, 1993, 12–14.

# 6

# Rationale and technique of malaria control

PETER F BEALES AND HERBERT M GILLES

Malaria control cannot be a campaign; it should be a policy, a long-term programme. It cannot be accomplished or maintained by spasmodic effort. It requires the adoption of a practical programme with the reasonable continuity that will be sustained for a long time. (Boyd, 1949)

To be successful, malaria control must be based on a sound understanding of the local epidemiology of the disease and of the facilities and resources available, or that can be made available for its control. This may be accomplished by conducting a thorough situation analysis as a first major step in the planning process. The epidemiology of malaria is described in Chapter 5 and the principles and issues discussed therein need to be applied in the context of the local ecological, social and economic conditions. The life cycles of the parasite and vector species, and human social and cultural practices need to be examined to determine the most effective points of intervention. These will form the basis of the approaches (measures and means) to be used for malaria control in that situation.

Thus, malaria control is a dynamic process, which necessitates a thorough understanding of the epidemiology of the disease under different prevailing conditions. Unlike malaria eradication, a greater awareness of epidemiology is needed at the periphery for successful control. Health workers at different levels of the health care system need to be well trained in malaria epidemiology, or some aspects of it, depending on their responsibilities for malaria control.

# PRINCIPLES OF MALARIA ERADICATION

Soon after the Second World War, the World Health Organization (WHO) recognized that malaria not only killed more people than any other disease, but also interfered with the development of agriculture and industry, especially in the newly emerging independent countries. The intensive control methods carried out in some Western countries and in certain tropical territories gave satisfactory results, but could not be applied in many rural, tropical areas. The advent of dichloro-diphenyl-trichloroethane (DDT) presented the world with a new method of reducing, and eventually interrupting, the transmission of malaria infection. This was by attacking the adult *Anopheles* vector during its epidemiologically most important stages, when it feeds on humans in their dwellings and when it shelters indoors in the nearest house or animal shelter.

The epidemiological concept of the interruption of malaria transmission by residual insecticide spraying is simple. After taking her blood meal, the female *Anopheles* usually rests on a nearby indoor surface such as a wall or ceiling for several hours while the blood meal is digested and the batch of eggs matures. Spraying of all inside surfaces of dwellings with a long-lasting insecticide creates conditions in which the life span of a substantial proportion of *Anopheles* would be reduced before they could transmit the disease (see Chapter 5).

This concept proved to be correct, as shown in several examples of early campaigns in Italy, Cyprus, Greece, Guyana and Venezuela. It appeared that the widespread use of DDT and other residual insecticides was the most reliable, feasible and economical method for the interruption of transmission. Any remaining foci of malaria could be detected by proper surveillance and eliminated by the distribution of antimalarial drugs and the local application of insecticides.

This simplified description of the principle of malaria eradication gives only a perfunctory idea of the operational complexity of a large-scale programme (Pampana, 1969).

A malaria eradication programme has been defined as an operation aimed at the cessation of transmission of malaria and the elimination of the reservoir of infected cases in a campaign limited in time and carried to such a degree of perfection that, when it comes to an end, there is no resumption of transmission.

Three main epidemiological principles of malaria eradication can be summarized briefly as follows:

1. Female *Anopheles* of vector species feed preferably on humans, who are the only host of human malaria parasites. Frequency of feeding is related to the gonotrophic cycles of mosquito (usually every 2–3 days). After feeding, the female mosquito rests on a surface inside the house to digest the blood.
2. The duration of the cycle of development of malaria parasites in the mosquito depends on the temperature. For *Plasmodium falciparum* at 26 °C, it takes about 12 days. During that period there are four to six mosquito feeds on a human being and this increases the chance of mortality of female mosquitoes alighting on indoor surfaces covered by an insecticide deposit.
3. Residual insecticides maintain their toxicity for several months and, as a result of this, the local population of *Anopheles* decreases its mean longevity to a point at which maintenance of transmission becomes impossible and the malaria infection of the community is gradually eliminated. Case detection and treatment deal with any remaining foci of infection.

The substantial differences between malaria control and malaria eradication are given in Table 6.1.

Because of the size and cost of the undertaking, a malaria eradication programme is usually organized on a national scale. The planning of a full-scale programme presupposes that its practical feasibility has been assured. If there is doubt that the proposed attack measures will stop transmission, it must first be tested in a well-designed pilot project on a limited scale in each epidemiological stratum.

The programme is usually carried out over 8 or more years, in four phases (Figure 6.1). The phases of the programme are described below:

1. *A preparatory phase*: 1 or 2 years are devoted to geographical reconnaissance of the area, training

**Table 6.1** *Differences between malaria control and eradication*

| | Control | Eradication |
|---|---|---|
| Objective | Reduction of mortality and disease incidence until no longer a major public health problem | Cessation of malaria parasite transmission and elimination of the human reservoir of infection |
| Duration | Indefinite | Limited in time |
| Area of operation | Only where mortality and disease incidence are high or where the disease has a major impact on economic development | All areas where transmission occurs |
| Total coverage (by spraying and surveillance) | Not necessary | Indispensable |
| Operational standards | Good | Perfect |
| Cost | Recurring | Capital investment; after completion, no recurring annual cost except for surveillance |
| Assessment of results | Sampling of population for malaria mortality, disease incidence and prevalence, parasite rates and spleen rates (malariometric surveys) | Case detection (active and passive) in advanced stages; surveillance procedure |
| Imported cases | Not relevant | Of concern in advanced stages of the programme |
| Health systems | Essential public health systems in place and functioning for the delivery of control measures and disease surveillance on a sustainable basis | A perfectly organized and managed campaign structure and surveillance system required for eradication; maintenance of eradication ensured by careful vigilance by public health services |

of field staff, identification and numbering of sprayable houses and structures, assignment of office accommodation and storage facilities and procurement of equipment, vehicles and supplies.

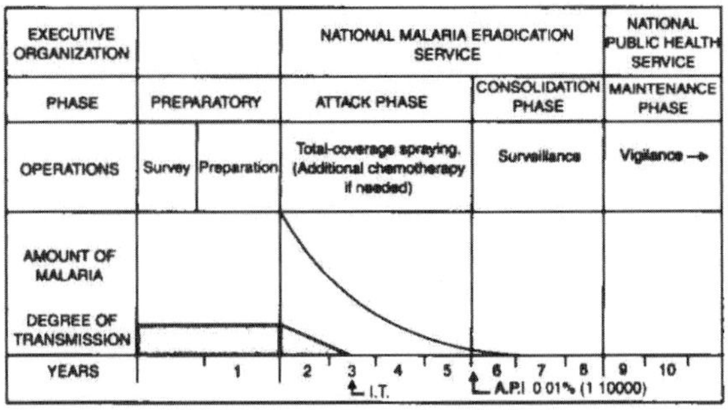

**Figure 6.1** *Diagram of theoretical sequence of phases in malaria eradication programmes. I.T., interruption of transmission; A.P.I., annual parasite incidence.*

2. *The attack phase*: residual house spraying and other measures aimed at the vector population are instituted, so that the principle of 'total coverage' of all premises and areas is observed. The dosage and frequency of spraying depend on local epidemiological conditions. Spraying may be supplemented by chemotherapy. The duration of the attack phase is 4 years or longer.

The decrease of transmission is followed by taking blood slides from samples of the population to determine the parasite rate according to age groups. When the parasite rates reach a level of 5 per cent, the evaluation methods must be changed to measure the amount of malaria, not in samples of the population, but in all possibly infected individuals.

This basic process of surveillance is case detection, in which the presence or recent occurrence of fever is used as a screening device, to be confirmed by blood examination. Active case detection is carried out by house-to-house visits at fortnightly intervals; passive case detection is based on reporting from static medical units such as malaria clinics, health posts, dispensaries, health centres and hospitals. The number of blood slides examined from fever cases in any given area should be not less than 1 per cent of the population for each month of transmission. As the parasite reservoir falls, full surveillance is instituted; this comprises, besides case finding, epidemiological investigation and remedial measures. If the transmission is interrupted, the parasite rate of infants born after the start of the attack phase should be zero, while the successive parasite rates in population age groups over 3 years should decline annually to the value of less than 22 per cent of the previous annual figure. The remedial function of surveillance is the treatment of cases by the administration of a 'presumptive' (single) dose of antimalarial drugs having both schizontocidal and gametocytocidal action, at the time of blood examination, followed (in confirmed cases) by full (radical) treatment (Figure 6.2).

3. *The consolidation phase*: this phase of malaria eradication begins when the surveillance activity shows that the annual parasite incidence (API), which is the proportion of positive slides per 1000 population, is below 0.1/1000. Cessation of complete coverage by residual spraying is allowed when there is no more transmission of malaria throughout the area. Experience of successful programmes showed that surveillance operations alone should be effective to mop up the remaining foci of infection. However, the receptivity and vulnerability of the area to introduced infections must be considered.

Receptivity is the degree of probability of resumption of transmission, largely dependent on the presence and abundance of local vectors of malaria and climatic or other conditions favouring the infectivity. Vulnerability is the probability of importation of the sources of infection, either from abroad or from nearby malarious areas, through immigrants or through infected mosquitoes.

4. *The maintenance phase*: this begins at the end of the consolidation phase and the entry into it demands that, during three consecutive years, there is no evidence of transmission of malaria after the cessation of anopheline control by residual spraying. The preventive activities during the maintenance phase are known as vigilance, which consists of watchfulness for any occurrence of any imported or indigenous cases of malaria, and the application of appropriate measures. Thus, normally, the maintenance of malaria eradication is the responsibility of general health services.

Certification of malaria eradication by the WHO was requested by several countries, and given. The inspection and review of the accomplishments of the programme were vested in a special certification team acting on behalf of the WHO and subject to confirmation of its findings by the WHO Expert Committee on Malaria.

## VALIDITY OF THE MALARIA ERADICATION STRATEGY

The strategy of malaria eradication described above remains valid today if the objective is to eradicate malaria as a parasitic infection of humans. However, its success was dependent upon several factors and

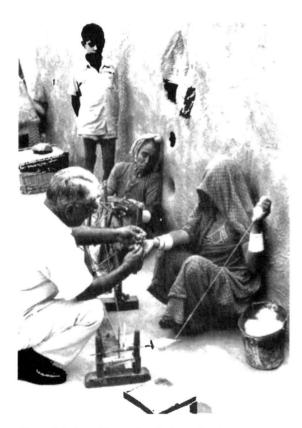

**Figure 6.2** *Surveillance of malaria eradication programme in Rajastan, India. (WHO photograph by AS Kochar.)*

**Table 6.2** *Progress of malaria eradication and control in 1961 and 1976, in terms of millions of population according to the WHO*

| Description of area | Population in millions (approx.) | |
| --- | --- | --- |
| | 1961 | 1976 |
| Areas freed from endemic malaria (under vigilance) | 317 | 436 |
| Areas under surveillance | 75 | 809 |
| Areas under mosquito control or protected by drugs | 576 | 451 |
| Areas without specific antimalarial measures | 452 | 352 |
| Grand total of the population in originally malarious areas | 1420 | 2048 |

must be seen in the light of the social, economic and development status that existed at the time the campaign was launched by the WHO in 1956.

The achievements of the WHO Malaria Eradication Campaign were quite remarkable at a time when no form of health services whatsoever penetrated into most endemic villages and there were no roads, bridges, railway lines, airports, electricity or telephones and, therefore, very limited population movements. Much of the work was carried out on foot, by boat, by donkey, horse or camel back where vehicles could not penetrate. Millions of people were freed from the burden of this disease (Table 6.2) and large areas of land were opened up to agriculture and industrial development because of it, principally in southern Europe, southern USA, Latin America, the Middle East and Asia. It was the first form of health care to reach millions and the spin-off from the campaign included the control of leishmaniasis and yaws. The smallpox eradication campaign was able to reach remote areas by using the malaria eradication campaign information, maps, population census, vehicles and personnel in many countries.

Some examples of the outcome of country-wide malaria eradication programmes are illustrated in Figures 6.3, 6.4 and 6.5. It should be noted that the information system developed during this campaign was extremely thorough and reliable.

These vertical information systems were dismantled in most countries on the advice of the WHO in the early 1980s, in the anticipation that the primary health care systems being developed would provide comprehensive health information. Thus, any statistical comparisons of global data beyond 1980 are not valid. In addition, during the 1980s, many countries changed their malaria-reporting criteria, which generally down-played the seriousness of the malaria problem (Figure 6.6).

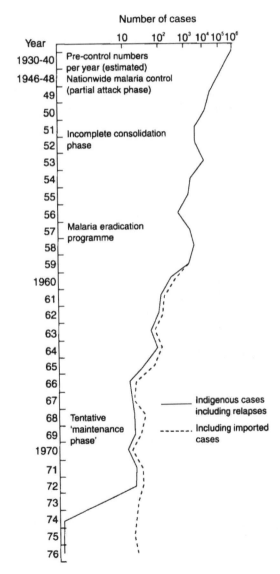

**Figure 6.3** *Progress and achievements of malaria eradication in Greece. (Reproduced from Bruce-Chwatt and de Zulueta, 1980.)*

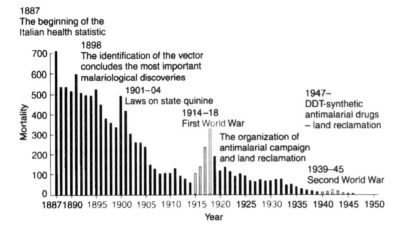

**Figure 6.4** *Progress and achievements of malaria control in Italy between 1900 and 1950. (Reproduced from Bruce-Chwatt and de Zulueta, 1980.)*

There are several basic assumptions inherent in the malaria eradication strategy that were relevant at the time, but that may not be today in most rural endemic areas. Principally, during the normal biting hours of the vector, the human population is to be found inside houses, the vectors are endophilic or, if not, at least endophagic, and the only available resting place for mosquitoes after the blood meal is the sprayed wall.

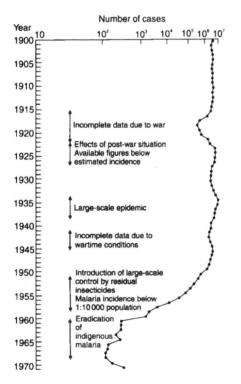

**Figure 6.5** *Progress and achievements of malaria eradication in USSR. (From Bruce-Chwatt and de Zulueta, 1980.)*

It has been often said that the mosquitoes have changed their behaviour to become exophilic and exophagic. This may be so in some cases. However, major changes have occurred in the behaviour of the human population and there has been comparative economic improvement in malaria endemic areas. Rural communities were usually farming communities, with the population returning to their homes early in the evening, eating an evening meal and then retiring early and waking early. Now, the provision of electricity and a move away from an agricultural economy have changed this. Early and late evening outdoor activities have increased (humans have become 'exophilic') and communal and individual television has compounded this. Furniture and household belongings have increased, which provide alternative resting places for mosquitoes. There is also now increasing public resistance to the nuisance and mess of residual spraying and public and political concerns for the environment.

The feasibility of malaria eradication today, even if technically justified, may be considerably reduced for economic, technical, programmatic, organizational, political and other reasons. Costs have increased considerably, both for commodities and for labour. Alternatives to DDT are more costly to purchase and to apply, are shorter acting, more unstable and more toxic. Alternative drugs to chloroquine bring additional problems and constraints. On the other hand, all forms of communication have advanced, but this has brought additional difficulties of increasing local, national and international population movements.

Accepting that malaria eradication may not be achieved in a number of countries, the only reason-

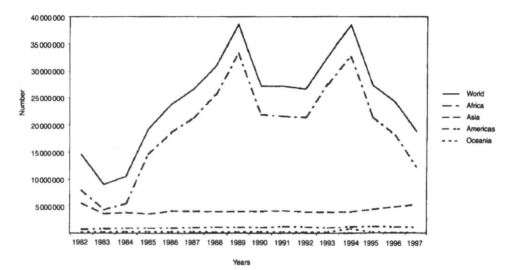

**Figure 6.6** *Numbers of malaria cases reported to WHO during the period 1982–97.*

able course of action is malaria control, which may be defined as follows (WHO, 1979):

> A malaria control programme is an organized effort to institute, carry out and evaluate such antimalarial measures as are appropriate for achieving the greatest possible improvement of the health situation of a population living in given epidemiological and socioeconomic conditions and subjected to the burden of this disease or exposed to the risk of its resurgence.

As the resurgence of malaria in many parts of the world gives cause for anxiety, a number of countries are intensifying their efforts by adapting their health policies to the epidemiological situation and mustering their resources. The aim is to merge antimalarial activities at the peripheral level with the work of expanding health services. The promotion of international and bilateral assistance for the application of environmental methods of malaria control and stimulation of training courses for all cadres of medical and health personnel are long-term programmes which are closely related to the pace of socio-economic advance of developing tropical countries where malaria will remain a serious health problem for many years.

## PRINCIPLES OF MALARIA PREVENTION AND CONTROL

The control of malaria may be an individual matter, i.e. for the protection of one person or one house, or a community. It may have to be undertaken at short notice in the middle of an epidemic, or may be planned and arranged during the off-season; it may be necessary for a short period only, or for a long season throughout most of the year. In each of these cases, different approaches are necessary (Table 6.3).

Generally speaking, the measures for the prevention of malaria in individuals and for larger scale control of the disease can be divided according to the classification proposed by Russell (1952):

1. Measures designed to prevent mosquitoes from feeding on humans (human–vector contact).
2. Measures designed to prevent or reduce the breeding of mosquitoes by eliminating the collections of water or by altering the environment.
3. Measures designed to destroy the larvae of mosquitoes.
4. Measures designed to destroy (reduce the longevity of) adult mosquitoes.
5. Measures designed to eliminate the malaria parasites in the human host.

Protecting people from the bites of *Anopheles*, or curing the person from whom the mosquito gets its infection, is sound in theory, and as much as possible should be done to achieve this end in practice. However, experience has shown that, despite the high hopes once vested in the latter method, it can never be relied upon to give complete control of the infection in a community. With the high-endemic types of malaria, many infected people are free from

**Table 6.3** *Principles of comprehensive malaria control*

| Type of control | Effect |
|---|---|
| *Individual protection*[a] | Reduction of human–mosquito contact |
| Mosquito repellents | |
| Insecticide-treated mosquito nets | |
| Insecticide-treated curtains | |
| Protective clothing | |
| Treated clothing | |
| House screening | |
| House siting | |
| Use of pyrethroid aerosols | |
| Antimosquito fumigants | |
| Deviation to animals | |
| | |
| *Vector control*[a] | |
| Environmental modification and manipulation | Reduction of vector breeding habitats |
| Chemical and biological larvicides | Reduction of vector densities |
| Insecticide outdoor space spraying | Reduction of vector densities |
| Indoor residual insecticide spraying | Reduction of longevity of vector population |
| | |
| *Antiplasmodial measures*[b] | |
| Early diagnosis and treatment of acute cases of malaria | Elimination of malaria parasites and prevention of transmission |
| | |
| Chemoprophylaxis and suppression of malaria infection | |
| Radical treatment of relapses | |
| Mass treatment (epidemics) | |
| | |
| *Social participation* | |
| Health education | Motivation for personal and family protection |
| Social mobilization | Stimulation of community action for prevention and control |
| | |
| Information, Education and Communication (IEC) | Modification of human attitudes and behaviour |
| | |
| *Health systems* | |
| Health systems | Essential for delivery of malaria control |
| Management effectiveness | Sustain gains achieved |

[a]Factors reducing the vectorial capacity.
[b]Factors reducing the parasite reservoir.

symptoms and are not discovered or treated. Protection from mosquito bites should always be put into practice, and may be expected to yield valuable results, particularly in the presence of acute epidemic malaria, but can rarely be relied upon exclusively.

The classification proposed by Russell regards malaria principally as a parasitic infection, which must be eliminated, and not as a disease that must be controlled. The critical premise of malaria eradication was to consider malaria as a parasitic infection, whereas, for malaria control, malaria is first and foremost a disease. This means that we must add to the five measures listed above:

1. Measures designed to prevent and reduce mortality from malaria, especially in high-risk groups.
2. Measures designed to reduce malarial morbidity.
3. Measures designed to reduce malaria transmission (alter the epidemiological equilibrium).

## ESSENTIAL FEATURES OF MODERN CONTROL PROGRAMMES

Modern long-term control programmes should incorporate the following major priniciples:

- Precise formulation of objectives, approaches to achieve the objectives, and operational targets to be achieved each year.
- Operational flexibility appropriate to the local situation and available resources.
- Selection of appropriate antimalarial measures based on stratification of the malaria problem and geographical areas, taking into consideration epidemiological, operational and socio-economic criteria and administrative and financial capabilities of the country or territory.
- Ready access to antimalarial treatment based on total coverage in space and time for every inhabitant of malarious areas.
- Methods applied for monitoring interventions and carrying out impact assessment of the control approaches in relation to the objectives, approaches and targets.
- Appropriate diagnostic and treatment activities conducted through the primary health care delivery system.
- Preventive activities carried out through primary health care and specialized antimalarial epidemiological services within the overall structure of the health care delivery system.
- Epidemiological services, with applied research and training components, which are capable of identifying and defining problems, planning control activities and monitoring and evaluating operations based on the principle of appropriate selective coverage in time and space.
- A peripheral structure of epidemiological services that corresponds to the malaria status and its potential instability, including the risk of epidemics and the re-establishment of transmission in areas where it has been interrupted.
- A built-in response capability to meet emergency situations (a reserve for outbreaks).
- Community participation in antimalarial operations.

## PROTECTION AGAINST THE BITES OF MOSQUITOES

### Nets

The use of mosquito nets as a protection from mosquito bites during the night has been practised from very early times. They still remain one of the most important of all measures of personal protection, not only from mosquitoes but also from flies, beetles and other creatures. The size of the mesh is determined not only by the number of holes to the square unit of the material, but also by the thickness and the type of thread of which the netting is made. A netting suitable for protection against most vector *Anopheles* is one of 25/26 mesh. The number of holes to the square inch would be about 150. A band of cloth about 300 mm wide should form the lower part of the mosquito net at the mattress level to protect arms and legs in contact with the net during sleep, as this will make it more difficult for the mosquito to bite through it.

Nowadays, mosquito nets are made of nylon, a mixture of nylon and polyester or some other synthetic material, which is lighter, easy to wash and preferably forms a bond with certain chemicals when applied as insecticides or insect repellents. The mean size of holes of nylon nets is usually 1.2–1.5 mm; there should be six to eight holes to 10 mm.

The preferred and traditional pattern is the rectangular net with a reinforced lower end and no openings in the side for the purpose of entering the net. There should be no tears or holes; if there are, they should be mended immediately. When in use, the net should be tucked all round under the mattress or sleeping mat (Figure 6.7). It should be let down before dark in the evening and, when going to bed, a thorough search should be made for any mosquitoes that may be inside it, preferably using an electric torch. A useful precaution is to spray the inside and outside of the net with an aerosol dispenser or a hand-sprayer using an appropriate insecticide preparation. Attempts are now being made to produce cheap and effective mosquito nets for wider use by the populations in developing countries. Also, different sizes and different types are being made, such as round nets that suspend from a single point and even special nets to use when sleeping in a hammock.

During the last 10 years, several field trials have demonstrated that the protective effect of mosquito nets can be greatly enhanced by treating them with a repellent or insecticide. The insecticides that are most commonly used for mosquito-net impregnation are the pyrethroids, especially permethrin (0.2–0.5 g a.i.[a]/m$^2$), deltamethrin (15–25 mg a.i./m$^2$) and lamdacyhalothrin (20–30 mg a.i./m$^2$), because of their low toxic hazard and good residual effect. Others are being tested and some may prove to be good alternatives.

[a] a.i. = active ingredient.

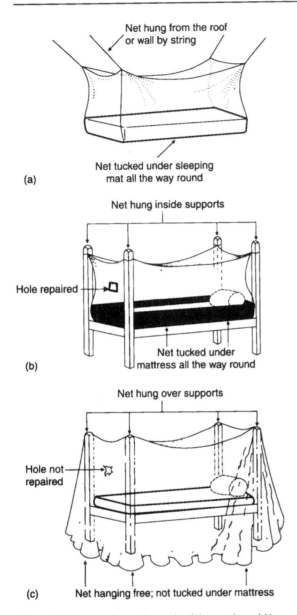

Net hung from the roof or wall by string

Net tucked under sleeping mat all the way round

(a)

Net hung inside supports

Hole repaired

Net tucked under mattress all the way round

(b)

Net hung over supports

Hole not repaired

Net hanging free; not tucked under mattress

(c)

**Figure 6.7** *A mosquito net hung the right way (a and b) and the wrong way (c).*

Good results have also been reported using curtains on doors and windows and eaves strips impregnated with permethrin (1.0 g a.i./m²). Good reviews of this type of approach are given by Curtis *et al.* (1990), Rozendaal (1989) and WHO (1989).

In some countries, such as the People's Republic of China, mosquito netting is permanently nailed to four posts attached to the bed, with a crossover opening in the front to allow entry. The top of the net is made from fine linen and the sides are made from mosquito netting or even coarsely woven muslin. The nets are sprayed by a member of the community twice a year with a pyrethroid solution, using a plastic knapsack sprayer. This has formed part of a very successful strategy for malaria control, with many millions of nets being used by the at-risk population.

## Protective clothing

'Mosquito boots' made of soft leather or canvas are useful to protect the ankles in the evening. Alternatively, a pair of thick socks may be pulled up outside the bottoms of trousers. Colour is important: dark colours tend to be more attractive to mosquitoes than light colours. Sleeves should be rolled down and trousers substituted for shorts or skirts after sunset. Mosquitoes may pierce through clothing that is in contact with the skin. Special hoods and gloves are sometimes used for military personnel to protect them while on guard duty at night.

A considerable amount of research has been carried out by the military on impregnating clothing with repellents or insecticides to protect frontline troops against mosquito bites, body lice, fleas, mites, ticks and other insects. This has proved to be very effective, especially as new chemical products have become available. There is some evidence from Afghanistan that impregnating clothing such as shadoors worn by Afghan women (and Muslim women from other countries) is beneficial as protection against malaria.

## Repellents

These are substances applied to the skin, clothing or mosquito nets to repel mosquitoes and prevent them from biting. In the past, citronella or eucalyptus oil was used on the skin, but its effect is very short, not exceeding 15–20 minutes. Other botanical products with demonstrated insect-repellent activity include cedarwood, geranium, nutmeg and peppermint (Barnard, 1998).

Later, a number of synthetic repellents were developed, with a duration of protection of 2–4 hours. The most useful of these are indalone, Rutgers 612, dimethyl phthalate (DMP), dibutyl phthalate (DBP) and a mixture known as 6-2-2. The most effective against *Anopheles* is DBP (average protection 4 hours) and DMP (average protection 3 hours). Several newer compounds are now available and among these N,N-diethyl-3-methylbenzamide (DEET) appears to be the best repellent against many blood-sucking arthropods. It can be active for as long as 10 hours. It is frequently used in the form of a 50 per cent solution in alcohol, but is available in a wide range of concentrations and formulations such as lotions, creams, gels, aerosols, pump sprays and towlettes. It is a major ingredient in 90 per cent of commercial repellents.

Two synthetic repellent compounds 1-(3-cyclohexen-1-ylcarbonyl) piperidine and 1-(3-cyclohexen-1-ylcarbonyl)-2-methyl piperidine are equally as effective as DEET. Toxicity studies indicate no adverse effects, but more tests are required before registration. Two other promising synthetic repellents are ethyl butylacetylaminopropionate and 1-methylpropyl 2-(2hydroxyethyl)-1-piperdinecarboxylate (WHO, 1998a).

Whatever preparation is used, it should be applied liberally, especially about the neck, ankles and wrists. Eyelids and other sensitive skin surfaces or mucous membranes are irritated by these substances and should be avoided. Generally, repellents are applied at dusk or dawn when *Anopheles* are most active. Synthetic repellents are solvents of plastic materials and when spilled or carelessly spread they may damage plastic eyeglass, or watch lenses, stockings, fingernail polish, plastic pens, varnish and similar objects. For added protection, repellents may be applied to clothing (especially socks) or to mosquito nets; in the latter case, mosquito nets sprayed with pyrethrum solutions or diethyltoluamide will retain repellent action for a few days and may be particularly welcome for protection against midges, which can pass through ordinary nets. Special wide-mesh netting impregnated with repellents for use as head nets has been widely used in the former USSR. Mosquito coils or joss sticks containing pyrethrum are useful as a type of repellent. Their value varies greatly, because it depends on the amount of the active substance that the smoke emits when the coil smoulders. In more common use today, based on the mosquito-coil principle, is the small semi-porous rectangular mat impregnated with a synthetic pyrethroid compound, with the addition of perfume and a blue dye. It is inserted in a small electrical heater, whereupon the mat slowly releases the insecticide and perfume by vaporization. The amount of insecticide released is sufficient to prevent mosquitoes from entering the room and biting for several hours. Once spent, the mat loses or changes its colour.

## Screening

Mosquito-proofing of dwellings, especially where electricity is also available for light and fans, has made a great difference to the health and comfort in the tropics and its popularity is on the increase. There is no doubt that this type of protection is a practical and effective method of malaria control.

The building to be screened must be well constructed and in good repair. Door frames should be made of seasoned wood with metal brackets at the corners and should not sag on their hinges. They should open outwards and be made to fit against a batten all round; they should have a strong spring to ensure tight closing. It is an advantage to have double doors, with a porch at least 2 m in length between them. Every aperture in the building must be screened. Outside privies should also be made mosquito-proof.

The size of aperture in the screening material will vary with the diameter of the wire used. As there are several different gauges in use, it is best to specify sizes of wire. It has been found that 16–18 mesh (16–18 holes along the linear inch/2.5 cm) and 28–30 standard wire gauge (SWG; 0.025–0.03 mm) is the optimum for general use; the aperture of such wire gauze is 1.2–1.3 mm, sufficient to protect from most mosquito species and leaving about 70 per cent of free area for ventilation.

Many materials have been used for screening, such as zinc-coated steel, brass, aluminium, monelmetal and plastic. A salt-laden atmosphere is very destructive to wire screening and under such conditions it is ultimately an economy to install the most resistant screen available. Certain plastic screens are of good quality, fairly durable and not expensive. Frequent inspection is necessary for the detection of rents or holes in the screen and defects in the wooden framework, the latter being especially likely to develop where there is extreme variation in humidity between the dry and wet seasons.

## Site selection

The selection of a suitable site for new housing (temporary or permanent) may avoid much subsequent difficulty. The principles are simply to place the housing upwind from the nearest water source and to ensure that there is the minimum possible breeding of mosquitoes within a radius of half a mile (0.8 km), and only a little within a mile (1.6 km); local specialist advice may enlarge on or modify these general points.

It may be less expensive to pump water some distance from the pond or river than to site the buildings near the water and then incur the heavy expense of some special methods of mosquito control. At one time, such site selection was literally vital to the success of many projects, and it still considerably affects their prospects, although the availability of better methods of control nowadays makes it less important. Systematic malaria control measures should be practised in any malarious village within 1 mile of the periphery of the new housing site or temporary camp.

## MOSQUITO CONTROL

The control of mosquitoes is undoubtedly the best method of protecting a community against malaria. Original attempts early in the twentieth century were by 'source reduction', namely, the prevention of breeding, the only means then available.

The spectacular achievements of sanitary measures employed during the building of the Panama Canal were linked to large engineering projects; other equally successful projects were seen in Brazil, Cuba, Holland, Italy and the USA. Much pioneer work was carried out in Malaysia, where Malcolm Watson identified the characteristic breeding habits of the main vectors, the type of water in which they lay their eggs and the best methods to change their habitat in such a way that the vectors avoid these areas. This naturalistic approach, known as 'species sanitation', was not attempted as widely as it should have been. In many countries, the majority of water types were dangerous; moreover, during the period 1955–75, the development of residual insecticides offered more promise. However, since then, environmental management for vector control has regained its popularity and is now widely advocated by the WHO.

## Insecticides directed against the adult mosquitoes

Insecticides directed against the adult mosquitoes (imagicides) were first used on a large scale in about 1935. Pyrethrum was the first, and good results were

achieved with it in southern Africa and in parts of India, but the new insecticides such as DDT, known as residual compounds, replaced it after the Second World War. They have had brilliant success, incomparably greater than many of the older methods, which they soon almost entirely replaced throughout most of the world. Despite their general adoption, it would be wrong to conclude that the prevention of breeding has now outlived its usefulness. Each of the two main methods of mosquito control has its place, according to the epidemiological conditions of the area and other factors.

In places where malaria is of high endemicity, control by the prevention of breeding cannot be effective unless it is very near perfect, the smallest observable density of adult anophelines being enough to keep the disease going on a substantial scale. Perfection, or near perfection, may be attainable where the breeding places are limited and of a distinct, easily recognizable type; it is not attainable where the breeding places are diffuse and various. High epidemic potential in areas of low endemicity offers conditions for easier control of malaria and the same perfection of technique is less important.

The pattern of amenability to control by residual insecticides is the same in principle, but very different in degree. The object is not to kill all *Anopheles* at once, but to prevent a large proportion of them surviving for 12 or 14 days. Even with the most potent vectors, this can be achieved if the daily mortality inflicted on them is of the order of 40 or 50 per cent. This is about the upper range of efficiency of insecticides applied using present techniques, but it can always be exceeded by a more thoughtful and generous application, which secures absolute control in most of the highly malarious places. In those places described as of low endemicity and high epidemic potential, malaria is very sensitive to changes in the factors controlling it. A daily mosquito mortality of perhaps 20–25 per cent will achieve the objective, and this is well within the range of purely routine applications. Insecticides directed against the adult mosquito can therefore be prescribed to control the epidemic degrees of malaria, and routine applications by standard techniques will easily control the transmission of infection.

Another consideration is strictly economic. The prevention of breeding demands attention to a large area of ground around inhabited places, and varies little with the number of people in the area. It is therefore more costly per person in sparsely populated areas. On the other hand, insecticides against the adult mosquitoes are applied in the house, at a cost per house that varies only a little with the density of population. They are therefore very much preferable in rural areas, but may lose some of their advantages in thickly populated places and where the main vectors are highly exophilic and bite early in the evening.

The techniques of larval control require real skill and discrimination on the part of the worker. Those involving insecticide spraying against the adult mosquito require skill, but of another sort, which can be acquired by routine drill and which does not demand the same degree of understanding or discrimination.

As a general principle, the residual insecticides are faster in their effect than the methods of prevention of breeding. There are, however, exceptions to their superiority, wherever the breeding places are few and easily accessible; in such places, environmental management measures are preferable.

## Antilarval control measures

Antilarval measures of control are of particular value when employed in conjunction with other means such as environmental management. The use of larvicides should be governed by technical, operational and economic considerations. Technical considerations include:

- very brief seasonal activity of mosquito vectors,
- behaviour characteristics (exophily) of the vector that make residual spraying ineffective,
- cultural or other objections to indoor/house spraying,
- at least one other vector of another endemic vector-borne disease will also be controlled by the same method (comprehensive vector control).

Operational reasons refer to situations in which the breeding areas of *Anopheles* vectors are limited and well known. Obviously, the advantages of antilarval measures are greater, particularly in urban areas, unless permanent environmental measures are feasible.

Economic reasons are related to operational conditions and the co-existence of malaria and another vector-borne disease that could also be controlled by the same method. Generally, operational convenience is also more economical. Permanent measures, although more expensive at first, may be much more economical in the long run, especially when repetitive maintenance and supervision are not required. Antilarval operations of any but the smallest-sized projects should be based on technical requirements and on the assessment of the administrative and financial feasibility of the proposed method. Major items that should be considered are: personnel (permanent and temporary employees), equipment, chemical compounds and transport; supervision of field staff is essential, as is their training. Entomological evaluation of the effectiveness of the methods used is indispensable. Among various ways of evaluating the results of antilarval control methods, the use of capture stations is most advisable. Capture stations are selected shelters suitable as resting places for *Anopheles* mosquitoes and are located in various quarters of the area to be protected. They are visited regularly and the mosquito collector sprays them with pyrethrum insecticide and picks up the killed mosquitoes from a sheet previously placed on the floor. This is a valuable means of testing the efficacy of control measures; the presence of adult mosquitoes is the most reliable test of antilarval work, and often leads to the detection of breeding places that would otherwise be overlooked.

The control of existing breeding places by any method must be carried out within the radius of flight of the local vector, commonly 1 mile (1.6 km) and throughout the entire transmission season, which usually starts a month or so before the first clinical cases occur. It must be based on a knowledge of the local vector and particularly of its breeding habits, and depends on a detailed survey of the area, showing all water surfaces of the potentially dangerous type within the radius prescribed. The collection of this information based on a preliminary survey demands knowledge and the use of skilled labour. All of these may be available or possible in advanced communities or in highly organized industrial undertakings, but they are not features of the general rural conditions in developing countries.

One cannot overemphasize the cardinal principle, true in both the urban and the rural areas, that one should avoid the creation of conditions in which the breeding of mosquitoes does occur or can do so during the rainy season. Man-made malaria is a curse of the tropics, and much of it can be avoided. The breeding places may be created by:

- digging large holes in the ground to obtain earth for road-making or house-building

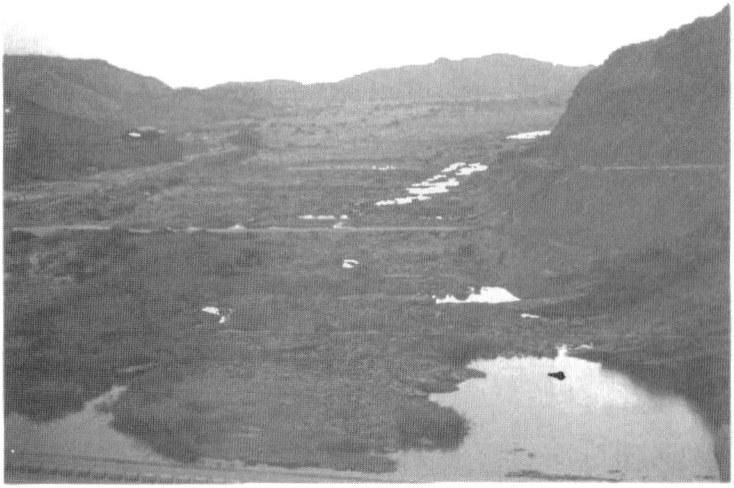

**Figure 6.8** *Man-made malaria. Typical breeding sites in Iran caused by road and dam construction. Earth and stones have been taken from the river bed, leaving large pits which retain water in the hot summer months providing ideal conditions for mosquito breeding. (Photograph by Hamedi, 2000).*

- the lack of, or poor, maintenance of roads, allowing 'pot holes' to persist
- faults in irrigation systems
- the lack of, or poor, maintenance of drainage systems
- leaking taps in water pipes
- engineering works that interfere with the natural lines of land drainage
- individual and large-scale exploitation of natural resources such as gem, gold and tin mining.

The correction of all these errors is usually much more difficult and costly than their prevention (Figure 6.8).

The rising problem of the resistance of mosquitoes to the insecticides used in public health programmes and in intensive agriculture, together with the growing concern for the environment exposed to repeated applications of potentially toxic compounds, has been responsible for the present interest in other less hazardous measures. Moreover, the high cost of new insecticidal compounds has increased the competitiveness of alternative techniques as components of integrated control strategies. Details of the use of chemical and other larvicidal methods are given below.

## ENVIRONMENTAL MANAGEMENT FOR MOSQUITO CONTROL

This section provides the basic information about environmental management for mosquito control. Those who are interested in the many engineering and technical details of the environmental control of malaria vectors will find exhaustive information in the *Manual on environmental management for mosquito control*, published by the WHO (1982a). The WHO has also produced a more recent publication outlining individual and community vector control (WHO, 1997b).

As mentioned above, the importance of measures against the aquatic stages of malaria vectors has now been emphasized. The relatively new term of environmental management has been defined as the 'planning, organization, implementation and evaluation of deliberate changes of environmental factors, with the view to preventing the propagation of vectors and reducing the human–vector pathogen contact'. Any long-lasting or permanent changes of land, water or vegetation aimed at the reduction of the habitat of the vector are often referred to as 'environmental modifications'; similar temporary or recurrent activity may be known as 'environmental manipulation'. The often-used term 'source reduction' refers to any measure that will prevent or eliminate the breeding of mosquitoes in their natural or man-made habitats.

## Environmental modifications

Many engineering works greatly influence the amount of mosquito breeding. In the past and also at the present time, highway and road construction, irrigation systems, agricultural drainage and flood control or impoundment have greatly increased the amount of malaria wherever proper study of the presence and habits of the vector species has been neglected or adequate preventive measures have not been taken. Apart from the health problems created by an increase of mosquito breeding, other water-related diseases may be a consequence of the bad management of impounded water.

## IMPOUNDMENTS

Impoundments are reservoirs for the storage of water behind dams and its subsequent release for power generation, irrigation and other uses. The flooding of a large area following the construction of a dam may have a beneficial effect in controlling the mosquito population if, instead of innumerable, scattered breeding foci, there is a large, well-defined water surface, more amenable to supervision and control. In the absence of floating vegetation, mosquitoes do not breed in the deep water, far from the edges of the reservoirs. The usual habitats of mosquitoes generally (and *Anopheles* in particular) are along the indentations of the shoreline, in shallow water covered with floating vegetation.

Thus, mosquito control related to impoundments should be based on the following considerations:

- proper preparation of the reservoir site and particularly the clearance of trees and other vegetation at all levels between high and low water;
- provision for fluctuating water levels of the reservoir;
- appropriate marginal drainage to avoid pools along the margins of the reservoir;
- the maintenance of shoreline vegetation control and drift removal.

This method of water management has been carried to perfection by the Tennessee Valley Authority in the USA. After the preparation of a clear shoreline, and dyking of shallow areas, the water levels of the main reservoirs were subjected to periodic fluctuations (intermittent sluicing) to strand the mosquito larvae and pupae.

In deltaic regions such as Lower Bengal, the annual flooding of the land by the rise of water level in the great rivers provides a striking example of the natural control of malaria. The silty floodwaters are inimical to the breeding of the local vectors, the extent of breeding edge is reduced, and the raising of the water level above that of the aquatic vegetation exposes the larvae to the attacks of fish and other predators.

## FILLING

Filling is a permanent measure of mosquito control, resulting in complete elimination of waterlogged areas, if the source of fill material can be obtained without creating borrow pits that cannot drain. The filling of small holes, abandoned ditches, borrow pits, ponds and similar water pockets is a simple operation, which can be carried out by unskilled labour and with simple equipment consisting of shovels, picks, wheelbarrows or animal-drawn carts. It can be greatly speeded up when a tractor or motorized earth-moving machinery is available; at times, road contractors, public works departments or industrial firms may be requested to provide this equipment (with the driver) for a few hours.

It is evident that the potential breeding places of *Anopheles* mosquitoes are more dangerous the nearer they are to human settlements. Moreover, some discrimination in their recognition is needed. Thus, an old overgrown, water-filled ditch may be more likely to breed malaria vectors than a stagnant pond containing heavily polluted water. When the depression is on sloping land and filled with ground water, the filling should start at the upper slope, so that the water runs towards the natural outlet.

Sanitary land-fills using refuse disposal for depressions of the ground are acceptable as a method of mosquito control, provided that nuisance and fly-breeding are avoided by compaction and earth cover. Filling on a large scale makes use of the spoil from such operations as harbour dredging, demolition, mining etc. Access to such material is extremely valuable because whole swamps and vast mosquito breeding areas can be converted into dry land. A special type of filling is that of 'hydraulic fill', when a slurry of silt or sand mixed with water is pumped from estuaries, lagoons and creeks into the coastal swamp, which is gradually filled and converted into valuable land.

## DRAINAGE

Drainage is the removal of unwanted water from the land surface or below it. The purpose of a drainage system is the opposite to that of irrigation, but otherwise the hydrological concepts and techniques of the two systems are the same. Whereas a well-constructed drainage system greatly reduces or prevents mosquito breeding, a system that is inadequate to cope with the excess water or that is technically faulty may contribute to the proliferation of mosquitoes. The straightening and deepening of channels of natural streams, and the maintenance of their margins free from pockets and vegetation, allow the water current to exert its greatest effect and to ease the access of larvivorous fish and other natural enemies. This has a marked effect in reducing the breeding of mosquitoes.

Surface drainage involves the shaping of the land surface, the improvement of natural watercourses and the construction of open ditches. It is particularly effective on flat, gently rolling lands, overlaying less permeable clay or hard rock. The planning and construction of a major surface drainage system are a matter for the specialist. However, small drainage schemes may be attempted by less experienced people and carried out by unskilled personnel with simple equipment. An important condition is a good topographical survey of the area, so that lines of drainage will follow the natural discharge flows (Figure 6.9).

Open earth drains are the oldest and simplest structures for surface drainage. The cross-section of an earth drain is usually trapezoidal, with the sides sloping at an angle that depends on the type of soil that will withstand the flow of water. The ratio of horizontal to vertical projection of the drain varies between 3:1 and 1:1 (Figure 6.10). Earth drains rarely maintain their original shape, because the rapid flow damages the channel, while slow water movement

**Antimalarial drains**

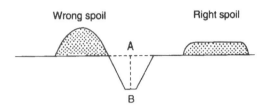

**Normal soils**

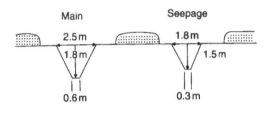

**Sandy soils**

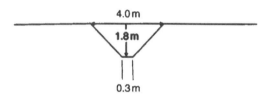

**Figure 6.10** *Characteristics of earth drains in relation to the type of soil and the disposal of spoil.*

deposits silt. If the flow of water is very swift, undermining of the banks may occur or, if there is some temporary obstruction, excessive local scouring may ensue, removing soil from below the grade line of the bottom of the drain and causing a pot-hole. Subsequently, if the rest of the drain becomes dry, as in storm-water drains, pools will remain, which may become *Anopheles* breeding sites. A small, temporary channel should then be made to connect these pools and drain off the water.

As a general rule, the drains should be narrow and deep rather than broad and shallow; their banks should be kept clear of vegetation and sloped to an angle of 45–60°; and tributaries should enter at wide angles and not at right-angles, in order to lessen the deposit of silt and debris at the point of junction. The bottom of a narrow drain should be rounded and not V-shaped, but in broad drains a shallow V is preferable to a flat bottom. A few simple precepts concerning the uniform shape of drains and the disposal of spoil are indicated in Figures 6.11, 6.12 and 6.13.

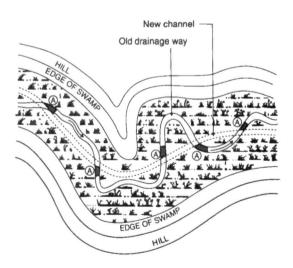

**Figure 6.9** *Lay out drains as straight as possible, following the low land so that deep drains will not be needed. When a new channel cuts across an old, winding watercourse, an earth dam (A) should be built to prevent water from flowing into the old channel.*

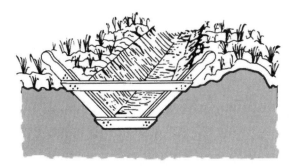

**Figure 6.11** *The use of a wooden template facilitates the completion of a uniformly shaped slope of an earth drain.*

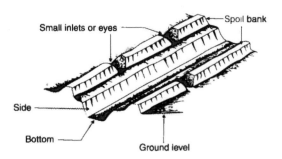

**Figure 6.12** *When a drain is dug, the removed 'spoil' is used to fill low spots near the drain or is spread or piled up evenly on each side at least 1–2 m from the edge of the drain. Such piles must be separated by small inlets to let the water run into the drain. If the drain crosses sloping ground, the spoil should be piled up on the low side.*

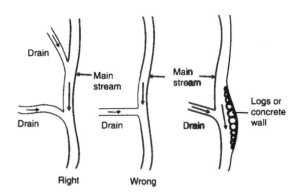

**Figure 6.13** *Where two drains or a drain and a stream join, the smaller drain should enter the main stream at an angle of about 30° in the direction of the flow. When a drain must enter the main stream directly, the bank opposite the flow should be reinforced with stones, logs or concrete.*

In the case of foot-hill seepage, the best method is to construct a system of contour drains at right-angles to the direction of flow, to intercept the seepage at the point at which it arises.

Drains should be as few and as short as possible, and their gradient should be carefully considered before starting work. The excavation for drainage should start at the outfall end. Sharp bends should be avoided wherever possible. The main drain should be constructed first and the tributaries afterwards.

Fieldwork should start by locating the centre line of the ditch by driving pegs at intervals of 25–50 m, and at some distance (2–3 m) from the actual ditch centre line. A guiding frame made up from two posts and a horizontal batten should be fixed at each point marked by a peg. A cord stretched from the centre of each batten to the next few will give a line above the ground parallel to a fixed height over the bottom of the ditch. Staffs (grade rods) marked to show the standard distance between the cord and the bottom of the ditch give the depth of the proposed excavation, which should be checked often (Figure 6.14).

Manual ditching is generally used in tropical countries where labour costs are moderate. The width at ground level of trapezoidal earth drains ranges between 1 m and 2.5 m. An average good worker can dig about

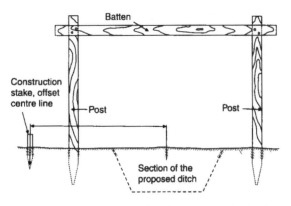

**Figure 6.14** *A guiding frame for alignment and depth of earth drains. The height of the horizontal batten when the frame is fixed over the centre line of the proposed drain gives the depth of the bottom of the drain when measured by grade rods. A cord stretched over a line of several guiding frames from the centre of the battens serves as a guide above the ground, parallel to the desired depth of the drain. The location of the centre line of the drain is given by its distance from the indicator pegs, driven into the ground every 30–50 m. (Reproduced from* Manual on environmental management for mosquito control, *WHO, 1982.)*

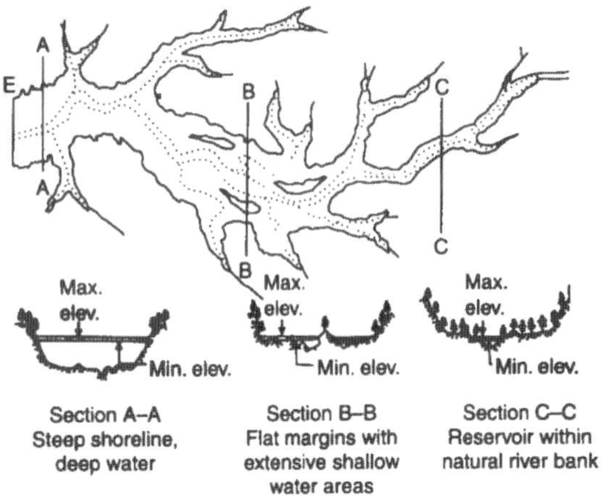

**Figure 6.15** *Diagram of a water impoundment with different degrees of mosquito breeding potential. The section B–B is of greatest importance, as the shallow water and extensive vegetation provide the best habitat for pond-breeding Anopheles. (Reproduced from* Manual on environmental management for mosquito control, *WHO, 1982.)*

$2 \, m^3$ daily in not too compacted soils, at a depth of about 1 m; at depths greater than 1.5 m, the output per worker drops rapidly because of the need to lift the spoil to the surface. However, ditching by machines is now becoming more common in developing countries despite high initial costs and the price of fuel.

Although some mosquito breeding may be expected in any part of the drainage system, the greatest amount usually occurs in the minor channels, where maintenance is neglected. If the water flow is sluggish, and the banks of drains eroded and covered by vegetation, mosquito breeding is at its most prolific (Figure 6.15). Furthermore, drains with sharp bends are liable to erosion and silting, forming pockets of standing water. Erosion of the banks is accelerated by turbulence as it occurs downstream of culverts, bridges etc. Thus, wherever there is a change of water velocity, the cross-section should be protected against the scouring action.

## THE 'LIDO SYSTEM'

The 'Lido system', also known as filling and deepening, is useful if for any reason it is difficult to drain an extensive shallow water area covered with vegetation. In such circumstances the circumscribed shallow area may be widened and deepened below the depth of tolerance of emergent plants and the spoil used for an

embankment. Providing that the side slopes are steep and stable, mosquito breeding rarely occurs and can be easily dealt with by the use of larvivorous fish. In this manner, the shoreline can be greatly shortened and a public amenity may result. This technique is also applicable to fish ponds or similar water reservoirs.

Lining of earth drains is the best way of improving their performance and decreasing the cost of their maintenance. Open drains can be lined with cement concrete, asphalt concrete, stone or brick. When well constructed and looked after, lined drains allow for faster flow of water, less silting and reduce the growth of weeds. Concrete lining can be made on site, but the use of connecting precast slabs is more common. The slabs for the bottom of the lined drain should have a central narrow invert (cunette) to give free water flow when its level is low. Stone lining may be used where this material is plentiful and the cost of labour low. Recently, membrane lining made of asphalt felt sheeting or of butyl rubber has been introduced. However, this type of lining is more affected by weather conditions and has a life expectancy of a few years only, as opposed to the much longer duration of cement concrete. A lined drain should never be constructed without first making an earth drain to determine the requisite depth of the drain, and to see whether the flow is satisfactory.

At the point of junction with a side channel, the opposite side of the drain should be strengthened and raised to prevent overflow. Weep-holes should be made in the sides of the lined drain so that the subsoil water may get into it; these should slope downwards towards the bottom of the drain. It is also an advantage to construct key-walls at right-angles to the drain at intervals, especially where there is a curve in its course, to prevent water from outside from tearing away the earth supporting the sidewalls (see Figures 6.12 and 6.13).

The necessity of repeated regrading, cleaning and oiling of open earth drains makes their upkeep expensive. However, lined drains that are more easily cleaned also require frequent inspection.

## SUBSOIL DRAINS

Subsoil drains (also known as 'subsurface drains') are widely used for irrigated areas; they prevent water-logging and improve aeration and leaching out of salts. There are many varieties of underground drains and the simplest of them, known as 'French drains', are made by half filling a deep trench with rocks, rubble, gravel etc., which present little resist-

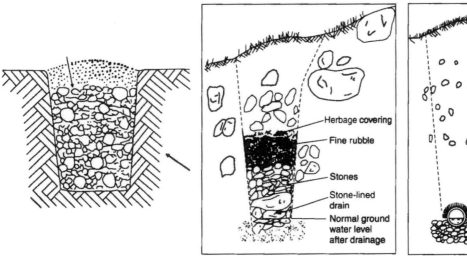
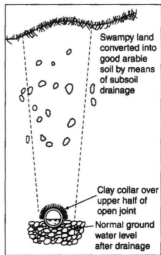

**Figure 6.16** *Three types of subsoil drains.* Left: *Common 'French' drain filled with rock, rubble or gravel and covered with a layer of thatch, palm leaves or long grass.* Centre: *Stones used for lining a drain provide a cheap and reasonably good subsoil system.* Right: *Typical deep subsoil drains using fired clay pipes. (Reproduced from* Manual on environmental management for mosquito control, WHO, 1982.)

ance to water flow. The best way is to place three or four flat stones at the bottom of a deep trench to form a triangle or a square; this construction, when continued, will result in a stone-lined, underground channel. This may be covered by coarse sand, palm leaves or straw to prevent the silt and clay from clogging the pervious sections of the drain (Figure 6.16).

A variant of primitive subsoil drains is that in which wooden poles, coconut husks, bamboo or faggots are used. The last-mentioned type refers to large twigs or tree branches being laid at the bottom of a trench, the water draining through the interstices when the ditch is filled in with layers of coarse grass.

A successful type of subsoil drainage evolved in Malaysia consists of using 'tile pipes'. The drain in this case is formed by a series of earthenware pipes laid end to end in trenches beneath the ground, the water entering from below at the joints between the pipes. If soft spots are found in the bottom of the trench (which must be properly graded), stones are rammed into place until a solid foundation is obtained. The laying of the pipes should commence at the outlet of the drain and continue upwards as the trench is made. Greasy water and house waste must not be allowed to discharge into any part of the system. Where pipes come near the surface, proper bridge crossings are necessary, to protect them from being crushed by wheeled vehicles. The pipes should

be laid in an absolutely straight line, with as few changes in gradient as possible. Periodic inspections should be made to see that the outlets do not become clogged with silt or other deposits (Figure 6.16).

It has been claimed that subsoil drainage is self-cleaning, permits a rapid inspection, needs little attention and requires no oiling. However, experience gained during the past 30 years has shown that it has many drawbacks; its main disadvantage is its high initial cost, added to the upkeep.

## DESIGN OF DRAINAGE SYSTEMS

The design of drainage systems may be quite simple for a small area, but its complexity increases with the size of the area and its topography. Moreover, the climatic characteristics, type of soil, height of the water table and other factors must be considered. The layout of the drains is also determined by natural and artificial features such as lakes, roads, buildings etc. The most common layout in a flat land is that of a herring-bone or gridiron pattern (Figure 6.17).

The herring-bone drainage system consists of a main drain with a series of parallel laterals set at an angle to the main drain. This system, although suitable for draining flat land, is often erroneously employed for swampy valleys, where water running from the surrounding higher contours collects

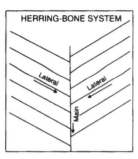

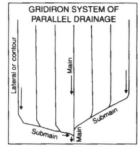

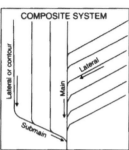

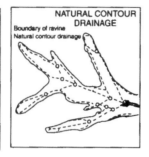

**Figure 6.17** *Some typical layouts for surface drainage systems. The general principles are to assure efficient flow of water without exceeding a water velocity that will erode the drains. This refers particularly to earth drains, but even concrete-lined drains may be subject to some erosion and silting. (Reproduced from* Manual on environmental management for mosquito control, *WHO, 1982.)*

between the lateral drains and creates new breeding places for mosquitoes. The alternative system of gridiron design intercepts most of the water from the surface and underground. The use of the gridiron system avoids the multiplicity of junctions at which blockage may take place. Moreover, its advantage lies in the possibility of using each drain at the outer end as a contour drain aiding in the removal of seepage water (see Figures 6.15 and 6.17). Lateral drains are connected to a main disposal drain, which discharges into a stream, river, lake etc. Interceptor ditches (contour drains) are needed to protect the sloping land from the flow produced by heavy rainfall. These drains run along the contour of the area, with little gradient, or along the foot of hills where the land is flatter; they should also intercept seepage, which may cause heavy breeding of some species of *Anopheles*. Water collected by interceptor drains is carried away to the lateral and main drain.

Coastal swamp drainage presents special problems related to the topography of the shoreline, tidal levels, outflow of rivers, climate, coastal vegetation and

many other factors. The silt carried by rivers tends to settle and forms deltas with lagoons that turn into swamps. Sand carried by tides and waves forms river bars, behind which brackish water is retained and where several species of important malaria vectors (e.g. *A. melas*, *A. sundaicus*) breed profusely. Some coastal swamps may be drained by constructing embankments (bunds) to prevent the inflow of seawater at high tides. Fitting large pipes into the bunds with an automatic outflow gate allows for the removal of water from the lagoon into the sea (Figure 6.18). In other conditions, large sluices (tide gates) operated manually or mechanically, let out the water from the bunded area. When the land slope or low tides make it impossible to operate drainage by gravity, pumping may be necessary (Figure 6.19).

## VERTICAL DRAINAGE

Vertical drainage is sometimes used to drain swamps or marshes. The bed of the marsh is probably of silt or clay, which retains the water, but beneath this there may be permeable or fissured rock, which will afford drainage. A shaft is sunk down to the permeable rock, the exposed surface of which is blasted. A vertical pipe surrounded with stone or gravel is inserted to the level of the marsh bottom. A strainer is placed at the mouth of each sink-hole and a certain amount of grading is required in the marsh leading up to the holes.

## EXPLOSIVES

Explosives have been successfully used in drainage and ditching operations, with great saving of time

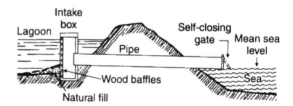

**Figure 6.18** *Bund and gravity pipe-drain from a lagoon into the sea. The upper end of the pipe is at the level near the bed of the lagoon and is fitted with an intake box. Grooves at the open side of the box are provided to use wooden boards to adjust the silt height when the lagoon becomes filled with sand. The lower end of the pipe-drain is equipped with a self-closing gate, to stop the inflow of water at high tides. (Reproduced from* Manual on environmental management for mosquito control, *WHO, 1982.)*

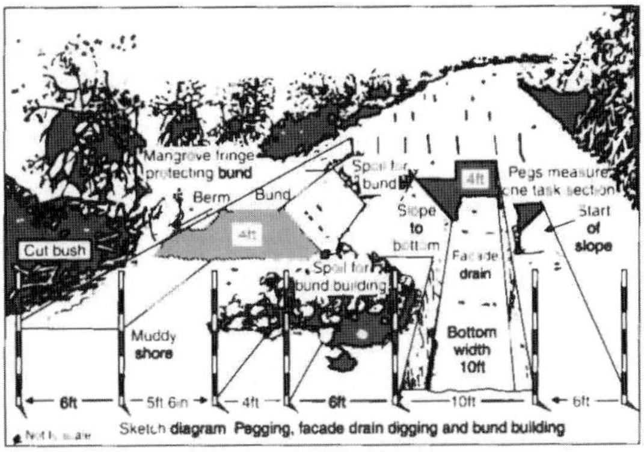

**Figure 6.19** *Diagram of the method of coastal swamp drainage as carried out in Nigeria. (Gilroy, 1948.)*

and cost. Ditches, varying from 1 m to 10 m wide and from 0.75 m to 3.5 m deep, can be blasted using an appropriate amount of explosive and a precise method of placing the sticks of dynamite.

## ENVIRONMENTAL MANIPULATION

This recurrent activity aims at producing local conditions unfavourable for the breeding of mosquito vectors in their usual habitats. Many measures described below were classified as naturalistic methods of control. As they are usually directed against known species of local malaria vectors, they were often referred to as 'species sanitation'. The success of such practices depends largely on the behaviour characteristics of local *Anopheles*. No general advice as to the use of a particular method can be given; thus, field trials are the best way of applying methods that were successful with regard to another vector of similar behaviour pattern.

### Changing water levels

Changing water levels has been mentioned before as one of the methods used in impounded reservoirs. A variant of this practice, known as 'intermittent drying', is of particular value for the control of mosquitoes in rice-growing areas, where the terraced or dyked fields are flooded during the planting and growing season. The basic practice is to drain the flooded plots periodically for a few days, to strand and kill the aquatic stages of mosquitoes without any damage to

the plants. The periodicity of such wet and dry cycles depends on the species of mosquitoes present, on the type of irrigation, soil texture, variety of rice and other factors. Field trials of this method should be carried out in consultation with agricultural experts. Some mosquitoes (*Psorophora*) may deposit masses of eggs on the dry soil, so that flooding may be followed by an emergence of swarms of fiercely biting pests. Culicine mosquitoes, including *Aedes aegypti*, breed in various water containers. Enforcement of a 'dry pot day' when all exposed containers must be emptied and allowed to dry out is the usual method of control of peridomestic mosquito vectors of diseases such as dengue and of nuisance mosquitoes.

### Stream sluicing or flushing

Stream sluicing or flushing methods are similar in principle to changing water levels. They were used extensively in tea gardens and rubber estates of South-east Asia, where *A. minimus* and *A. maculatus* prefer the edges of gently flowing streams. A periodical discharge into the stream of a large volume of water, behind a dam after opening a hand-operated sluice or released from an automatic self-priming siphon or tipping bucket, will carry the larvae and pupae from the edges of the stream and strand them on the banks. This method may also be used for the control of other stream-breeding malaria vectors such as *A. fluviatilis*, *A. maculatus*, *A. superpictus* and others (Figure 6.20).

### Changing water salinity

Changes of water salinity in coastal marshes or lagoons through increasing the flow of seawater, banked up by automatic tide gates or other devices, has been attempted with some success in several countries. In Albania, *A. sacharovi* was eliminated by this method from a large coastal marsh. This measure may be of value if the major local vector cannot breed in seawater, especially if the salt content in the lagoon increases as a result of evaporation. However, in areas with heavy seasonal rainfall, the measure is less likely to succeed, unless the area is properly drained. On the other hand, desalination of coastal swamps and irrigation with fresh water for growing wet crops may prove to be a risky procedure if there is an alternative, more dangerous

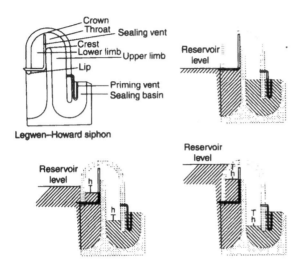

**Figure 6.20** *Design of an automatic self-priming siphon for stream flushing as a method of mosquito control. The water level in the reservoir rises until it reaches the lip of the upper limb and seals the siphon, when the priming cycle begins. (Reproduced from* Manual on environmental management for mosquito control, *WHO, 1982.)*

vector. This was the case with the replacement of *A. aquasalis*, a secondary vector in Guyana, by *A. darlingi*. The same may be true in West Africa, where the salt-water-breeding *A. melas* would be replaced by the equally dangerous *A. gambiae* or *A. arabiensis*. On the other hand, in South Vietnam, as a result of defoliation and forest destruction in the 1970s in the central part of the country, the subsequent reduction in rainfall has allowed the seawater to encroach inland as far as 80 km, thereby expanding the breeding places of the salt-water malaria vector *A. sundaicus* and reducing the arable land along the coastal region.

## Shading of stream banks

Shading of stream banks was used in Assam, India, and elsewhere to deter *A. maculatus* and *A. minimus*, which prefer more open breeding spaces. Various shrubs, and especially the thorny *Duranta*, were planted to provide dense shade; this may be useful for the partial control of other sun-loving species such as *A. gambiae*, *A. quadrimaculatus*, *A. fluviatilis* and *A. sundaicus*. A large number of other plants appear to have been used for this purpose with a variable degree of success. Under dense shade, no vegetation can grow along the margins of a stream,

so that the influence of the current extends right up to the bank and there are no longer any pockets of still water where mosquitoes can deposit their eggs.

## Clearing vegetation

Clearing of vegetation in densely shaded areas has been used with success for the control of *A. b. balabacensis* in Sabah, and could be employed on a small scale in other parts of South-east Asia where this elusive vector is important. Large-scale clearing of the forested areas may be dangerous, however, as it may favour the breeding of the sun-loving *A. minimus*. This has been demonstrated in Myanmar and Thailand, where large forested areas have been denuded by exploitation, with the disappearance of *A. dirus* and its replacement by the equally efficient malaria vector *A. minimus*. Generally speaking, clearing of scrub vegetation removes the sheltering places of adult mosquitoes; it promotes evaporation and therefore speeds up the drying of water collections and discloses breeding places that otherwise may be overlooked. Indiscriminate clearing of jungle may, however, favour the breeding of various vector species that lay their eggs in water exposed to bright sunlight. Afforestation by planting eucalyptus and other trees has been introduced for the partial drying up of waterlogged lands.

Some plants have a reputation for preventing mosquito breeding. Among these are musk grass (*Chara*), floating leaf (*Brasenia*) and especially bladderwort (*Utricularia*); the last-mentioned is a carnivorous plant that may trap a few larvae in its specialized structures. All these plants grow preferentially where anopheline breeding is not heavy, in deeper waters. The duck-weeds (*Lemna*, *Wolffia*) occasionally form dense mats where mosquito larvae may be less numerous. However, in practice, the use of plant growth for mosquito control is not recommended.

## Deliberate water pollution

Deliberate water pollution has been used in India and Malaysia for the control of *A. fluviatilis* and *A. maculatus*. *Anopheles* generally are clear-water breeders, but some species, such as *A. gambiae* and *A. stephensi*, may also breed in muddy waters, often containing organic waste. This is also the case for many culicine mosquitoes, and for this reason this method of control cannot be universally recommended. The technique consists simply of filling the large pool or pond with freshly cut grass, leaves and garden refuse, which, on decomposition by anaerobic bacteria, may deter some species of *Anopheles* from egg laying and may kill larvae or pupae. Although this method may appear attractive, it does not offer any permanent solution and is often the source of pest mosquitoes. The use of any industrial waste for the deliberate pollution of water should be strongly condemned.

## Biological methods

These methods of mosquito control are based on the introduction into the environment of various pathogens and predators of insect vectors of disease. Such agents range from viruses, bacteria, protozoa, fungi, plants and nematodes to natural predators such as larvivorous fish.

The effective use of biological methods of control requires a good knowledge of the bionomics of the vector species, as well as of local ecological conditions. The great potential of these methods lies in their use together with environmental manipulation, with agricultural practices and even with some insecticides. This is the essence of combined attack on multiple factors of disease transmission implied in the concept of 'integrated control'.

Several viruses (cytoplasmic polyhydrosis, baculovirus) have been isolated and studied in mosquitoes, but have shown little practical applicability. On the other hand, considerable attention has been given to two bacteria and their products. *Bacillus israelensis* (Bti), also known as *B. thuringiensis* serotype H-14, forms spores and produces a toxin that can be isolated; it is a potent gut poison when ingested by mosquitoes and other aquatic insects, but harmless to plants, animals and humans. The crystalline toxin, now produced industrially in large quantities as a wettable powder or an emulsion under various proprietary names (Baktimos, Teknar'), can be easily applied as a biological larvicide in waters for domestic supply or for the irrigation of food crops. It is biodegradable and frequent periodic treatments are necessary. Bti products have been used for more than 15 years and there is no documented evidence of any resistance of mosquitoes to them. Genes coding for the toxic component of the toxin have now been transferred to other bacteria and more potent compounds may be developed.

*B. sphaericus* (Bsph) also produces a toxin in its spore envelope. This toxin, harmless to animals and humans, is also more potent and more specific to various mosquitoes. Because *B. sphaericus* can multiply even in polluted waters, it has a longer action than *B. israelensis*. Much field research on this method is now in progress. A good review of both these bactericides is given by de Barjac and Sutherland (1990). The principal active ingredient of Bsph is a single toxin (unlike Bti) and resistance has already developed in some populations in India, Brazil and France (WHO, 1999d).

Fungi of the genera *Coelomomyces*, *Culicinomyces* and *Lagenidium* have been studied as a means of mosquito control. *Coelomomyces* have a complex life cycle with an alternate crustacean host. Some species, such as some varieties of *C. iliensis*, are capable of causing massive mortality in the larvae of *Anopheles*. This parasite of mosquito larvae and adults has a high infectivity for *Anopheles* and decreases their ability to transmit malaria. However, field trials have not demonstrated the economic practicability of using microsporidia.

Nematodes of the family Mermithidae are now being studied as biological control agents. Three species of these parasites received some attention, but the most interesting of them is *Romanomermis culicivorax*, which can greatly reduce larval populations and survives in a variety of habitats. Field trials showed certain limitations of the value of this type of mosquito control. Predatory mosquitoes of the genus *Toxorhynchites*, the larvae of which feed voraciously on other mosquito larvae, have been investigated recently. They may be useful for the destruction of container-breeding species, but not for species breeding in ground water.

Of all biological mosquito control methods, the use of larvivorous fish has been the most successful in many parts of the world. Larvivorous fish are natural enemies of mosquito larvae and have been utilized with advantage for malaria control in Spain, Italy, Greece and other countries in southern Europe and northern Africa, and also in Georgia, India, Papua New Guinea, Malaysia, Madagascar and many other countries. Naturally, the use of larvivorous fish is limited to some special situations where the water and other conditions are suitable. Cisterns, shallow ponds, small streams, ornamental pools and wells are ideal places for mosquito control by fish. The main indications for the selection of fish as a method of mosquito control are their preference for insect larvae over any alternative sources of food, their small size (less than 6 cm long), which makes for access to shallow waters, their rapid maturation and high fecundity, a degree of tolerance to salinity or pollution and harmlessness to other valuable species of the aquatic ecosystem. The most promising species belong to the family Cyprinodontidae of the genera *Aphanius*, *Valencia* (Mediterranean region and western Asia), *Aplocheilus*, *Oryzias* (southern Asia), *Epiplatys*, *Aphyosemion*, *Roloffia* (West Africa), *Nothobranchius*, *Pachypanchux* (East Africa), *Rivulus*, *Cynolebias* and *Fundulus* (the Americas). In principle, indigenous fish should be selected in preference to imported species, if possible. The most important and best known are the top-feeding minnow *Gambusia affinis*, the guppy (*Poecillie reticulate*) and several others of the families Poecilidae, Cyprinidae and Cyprinodontidae. Of the latter, several species of 'annual fish' (genera *Nothobranchius* or *Cynolebias*) have been described and seem to hold some promise for the control of mosquito larvae in certain situations. The special merit of these small fishes lies in their capacity to survive and multiply in non-permanent waters, where other species would perish. Annual fish occupy tropical habitats with a wide range of temperatures, where surface water disappears during the dry season. They survive until the next rainy season in the form of eggs buried in the soil. These eggs may be collected and transported in damp peat. Ripe eggs hatch within a few hours after being introduced into the water. The voracious young are hardy, mature rapidly and show high fertility.

The most popular among larvivorous fish is still the *Gambusia affinis* of the family Poecilidae, because it is small (30–65 mm), breeds rapidly (a single female may produce 200–300 offspring in a year) and its rearing and transport are easy. It adapts itself to a wide range of waters, warm and cold, fresh and brackish. Such adaptation is slow and it is advisable to transport the fish in water taken from an original source and gradually adjust them to the type of water in which they are expected to thrive. There is now a considerable amount of technical literature on the breeding and introduction of larvivorous fish.

The disadvantages of the use of fish as a mosquito control measure are that they are only effective if pre-

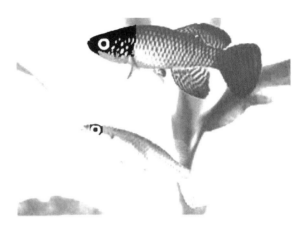

Figure 6.21 *Larvivorous fish used in some malaria control programmes. This species of 'annual fish', Nothobranchius guentheri, male and female (×c. 1/3), is of the family Cyprinodontidae. (Hildemann and Walford, 1963.)*

sent in very large numbers; they are less effective for the control of *Anopheles*, especially in the presence of weeds and floating debris; and constant inspection is necessary to see that the fish are flourishing and are in sufficient numbers and that the water is free from horizontal vegetation. Occasionally, *Gambusia* may become a predator of other ecologically useful aquatic animals. For this reason *Gambusia* fish should preferably not be introduced into areas where they are not already indigenous. The favoured approach is to use the most effective indigenous mosquito larvae-eating fish.

For any mosquito control programme utilizing fish, the operational problems related to their rearing, transport and stocking must be solved. Rearing can be done in artificial tanks or natural bodies of water; the depth of water is a critical factor as the fish must be protected from the cold during winter months. For the transportation of fish, several methods are in use. In Afghanistan, *Gambusia* were successfully carried for up to 12 hours in open containers holding 1500 fish, at temperatures between 13 °C and 18 °C. In the Islamic Republic of Iran, the fish were transported in double-walled, polyethylene bags of 30–40 L capacity, packed in wooden boxes, each bag half filled with water and inflated with oxygen (Figure 6.22). Some 300 fish were transported in each bag for distances of over 2000 km. Plastic churns of 25 L capacity or metal tanks equipped with an aerator have also been used. Release of fish to the breeding place must be done so

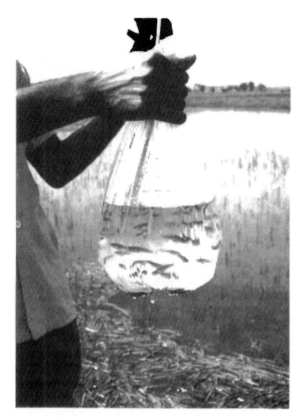

**Figure 6.22** *Larvivorous fish* (Gambusia affinis) *are widely used for mosquito control in many parts of the world. (WHO photograph by P Almasy.)*

that the temperature of the water is balanced. It has been found that effective larval control requires two to five fish per m$^2$ of water surface.

Some species of fish have been found to have secondary uses for reducing the rooted aquatic vegetation and floating algae. These are the carp (*Cyprinus carpio*) and a species of *Tilapia*. Both species benefit larvicidal operations by ensuring a greater open water area in ponds and streams and to enhance the effectiveness of compatible species of mosquito larvae-eating fish for the control of *Anopheles* vectors.

Genetic control is a special type of biological control. It has been defined as the use of any method that can reduce the reproductive potential of insects by altering the hereditary material of the vector species. Attempts at mass sterilization of insect pests have been the subject of much research since the early 1950s, when the eradication of the screw-worm in the southern states of the USA was largely successful.

Various methods of genetic control have been used, but the release of males sterilized by ionizing irradiation or chemical compounds has received most attention. The principle of this method is that the sterilized males seek out and mate with the wild females in the natural population, thus preventing the hatching of their eggs and lowering their reproductive potential.

Chemosterilant compounds fall into two main categories: the alkylating agents (e.g. apholate) and the antimetabolites (e.g. methotrexate), used for treatment of tumours in humans. A large number of compounds in the two groups have been tested during the past few years in order to find the lowest concentration that produces complete sterility in male mosquitoes without causing excessive mortality, so that they should be able to compete with normal males. Various compounds have given promising results, but the toxicological and mutagenic implications for mammalian species, including humans, present an additional difficulty. In a field trial in El Salvador some 4.3 million adults of *A. albimanus* were released after the sterilization of their pupae in a solution of an alkylating agent. In further releases, the treatment of pupae by a juvenile hormone (methoprene) was also employed. Although the results seemed to be promising at first, the rapid influx of normal anophelines from the periphery of the area was a setback.

Another method of genetic control is based on crossing two sibling species of *Anopheles*. This leads to hybrid male sterility and, when very large numbers of sterile males are released, their competition with fertile males is so great that eventually the size of the succeeding generation decreases below the threshold at which the transmission of malaria is possible.

The third method is that of incompatibility, in which the release of one sex of a certain species, infertile with the opposite sex of another population of the same species, achieves the same effect.

The introduction of mass hybrid sterility for control of the *A. gambiae* complex was tried in Burkina Faso, West Africa, but little mating between sterile males and wild females occurred. The main and difficult requirement for the success of all genetic methods of mosquito control is the production of very large numbers of healthy, competitive, though genetically different, mosquitoes and their release in the right place and at the right time to mate successfully with wild insects.

Finally, a new concept of genetic control involves the mass release of mosquitoes carrying genes that prevent the development of malaria parasites in female *Anopheles* or genes imparting greater susceptibility to some insecticides.

## ZOOPROPHYLAXIS

In describing the behaviour pattern of *Anopheles* and their feeding preferences (see Chapter 5), it has been pointed out that several species of *Anopheles* are equally attracted to humans and animals and some species prefer feeding on the blood of domestic cattle, but will bite humans when they find no other source of blood. On the other hand, even such seemingly anthropophilic mosquitoes as *A. gambiae* may be diverted to cattle and horses if these animals are easily accessible. Such diversion of vectors to animal hosts has been used deliberately in some parts of the world, including the People's Republic of China and the former USSR, as an auxiliary method of malaria control. Indeed, it is likely that progressive deviation of the local *Anopheles* vectors was partly responsible for the decrease of malaria from northern Europe and much of North America. Many of the important vectors of malaria in India, Indonesia and Malaysia have zoophilic tendencies. Although it may not be feasible to employ zooprophylaxis as a practical antimalarial measure, the beneficial effects of deviation of some *Anopheles* species to cattle may have a bearing on agricultural practices in integrated vector control. The converse has occurred in recent years where cattle and buffalo have been redeployed in areas destined for new economic development. For example, in Vietnam, the depletion of animals from the areas from which cattle and buffalo were taken resulted in a dramatic increase in malaria transmitted not only by *A. sundaicus* but also by *A. campestris*, which was previously feeding almost entirely on animals.

## CHEMICAL METHODS

Chemical insecticides are still the mainstay of most vector control programmes, but the growing problem of the resistance of many insects to insecticides and the present concern with the effect of some of these compounds on the environment have stimulated an intensive research programme co-ordinated by the WHO to develop a number of candidate insecticides and to test their activity and safety (WHO, 1997a).

The specifications for pesticides used in public health are part of the WHO Pesticide Evaluation Scheme (WHOPES). One of the mandates of WHOPES is to collect, consolidate and disseminate information on the use of pesticides for public health use. There are four phases to the scheme and the fourth is the establishment of the final specifications by WHO Expert Committee meetings. The efficacy of chemical control measures depends on a number of factors: the species of vector involved; efficacy of the insecticide; type of its formulation; thoroughness of its application; nature of the surface treated and climatic conditions; acceptability to the inhabitants; and management of the control programme. A detailed description of various chemical insecticides must be preceded by some knowledge of their classification.

## Classification of insecticides

Insecticides can be classified as follows:

1. according to their chemical composition
2. by way of their entry into the body of the insect
3. by the method of their application
4. by the stage of the life cycle of the insect against which they are used.

Classified by their chemical characteristics, the most common insecticides applied in public health practice are:

- petroleum oils and their derivatives;
- active constituents of flowers of pyrethrum (pyrethrins) or some newer synthetic compounds of this group (pyrethroids);
- chlorinated hydrocarbons: dichloro-diphenyl-trichloroethane (DDT), hexachlorocyclohexane (HCH) and dieldrin;
- organophosphorous insecticides: malathion, temephos etc.;
- carbamates: propoxur, carbaryl etc.;
- insect growth regulators: diflubenzuron, methoprene, pyriproxyfen.

Insecticides may be absorbed by the insect as follows:

- by introduction into the plant or animal which is to be protected: these systemic insecticides are used mainly in agriculture and to some extent in veterinary medicine;

- by ingestion through the mouth (e.g. Bti) of anopheline larvae: this is also the mode of action of various insecticides employed in agriculture (stomach poisons);
- by inhalation through the tracheae: all highly volatile insecticides (e.g. methyl bromide, dichlorvos) act in this way; some contact insecticides (HCH) also have this type of 'fumigant' action;
- by contact with the cuticle and penetration into the body of the insect: such contact insecticides are DDT, HCH, diel\drin; some of them may exert 'particulate' action through minute airborne particles without direct contact with the insect.

According to the method of application, insecticides may be:

- released into the surrounding air space (space spraying) in the form of vapour or aerosol such as fog, smoke etc., so that they are absorbed by inhalation or contact;
- deposited on a solid surface, such as indoor walls and ceilings, for eventual contact with the insect: these long-acting or residual insecticides are generally used for the control of malaria and other mosquito-borne infections and include a wide range of compounds from DDT to the newer organophosphates and pyrethroids;
- released on the surface of water or into it in the form of floating film, powder, granules, briquettes etc.

Insecticides may also be classified according to their action on the life cycle of mosquitoes into larvicides and imagicides. (The use of the term adulticides for the latter is not recommended.)

In selecting a suitable insecticide the following factors should be taken into consideration:

- its effective toxicity towards the target insect (the problem of specific resistance to a particular compound must be considered);
- the duration of action on a surface to which it will be applied at a given dosage;
- the ease of application in existing topographical and climatic conditions;
- toxicity towards humans, domestic or wild animals or fish;
- the cost of insecticide and of transport and labour involved;
- the acceptability to the population/community at risk of the disease;
- minimal environmental hazard.

In the following section, a simple classification by chemical composition is used for convenience, although reference to the methods of application of these compounds is unavoidable. In addition, reference is made to the WHO recommended classification of pesticides by hazard (WHO, 1992c). In this regard, the hazard referred to is the acute risk to health (that is, the risk of single or multiple exposures over a relatively short period of time) that might be encountered accidentally by any person handling the product in accordance with the directions for handling by the manufacturer or in accordance with the rules laid down for storage and transportation by competent international bodies. The classification is based primarily on the acute oral and dermal toxicity to the rat because these determinations are standard procedures in toxicology. Toxicity is expressed in $LD_{50}$, which is a statistical estimate of the number of milligrams of toxicant per kilogram of body weight required to kill 50 per cent of a large population of test animals (Table 6.4 overleaf).

## Petroleum oils

Petroleum oil fractions, which include various paraffinic and other hydrocarbons, have played an important part in mosquito control as larvicides since the beginning of the twentieth century. These oils are applied on the water in such a way as to produce a continuous, thin film on the surface. When larvae come up to the water surface to breathe, the oil penetrates into their tracheae and kills them, either by suffocation or by poisoning. For larvicidal work, the mineral oil selected should have high toxicity to larvae and pupae, should spread easily and evenly over the water surface to form a stable film, should penetrate quickly into the tracheal system of larvae, have no offensive odour, and be harmless to fish, waterfowl and livestock.

The addition of 1–2.5 per cent of vegetable oil, such as castor or coconut oil, may increase the spreading power considerably. However, it is usually more satisfactory to use one of the proprietary oils (such as Malariol), which are specially designed for larvicidal work, as they contain surface-active agents that increase their spreading property and toxic action. The approximate amount of oil to use in practice is between 200 mL and 600 mL for each 100 m$^2$ of water surface or 20–60 L per hectare.

**Table 6.4** *Toxicity and degree of hazard related to chemicals used as insecticides in agriculture and public health practice*

| Common name | Chemical type | Toxicity to rats LD$_{50}$ (mg/kg) | | Degree of hazard |
|---|---|---|---|---|
| | | Oral | Dermal | |
| *Larvicides* | | | | |
| Chlorpyriphos | OP | 135 | 2000 (rabbit) | MH |
| Diflurobenzuron | IGR | 4640 | — | UH |
| Fenthion | OP | 250 | — | MH |
| Iodphenphos* | OP | 2100 | >1800 | UH |
| Methoprene | IGR | 34 600 | — | UH |
| Temephos (Abate) | OP | 8600 | >4000 | UH |
| *Imagicides* | | | | |
| Alpha-cypermethrin | Py | 79 | — | MH |
| Bendiocarb | C | 55 | — | MH |
| Carbosulfan | C | 250 | — | MH |
| Chlorphoxim* | OP | 500 | — | SH |
| Chlorpyrifos-methyl | OP | >3000 | — | UH |
| Cyfluthrin | Py | 250 | — | MH |
| Cypermethrin | Py | 250 | — | MH |
| DDT | Ocl | 113 | 2510 | MH |
| Dichlorvos | OP | 100 | >500 | MH |
| Dieldrin | Ocl | 37 | 60 | MH |
| Deltamethrin | Py | 135 | — | MH |
| Etofenprox | Py | >10 000 | — | UH |
| Fenitrothion | OP | 503 | 350 | MH |
| HCH | Ocl | 88 | 900 | MH |
| Lambda-cyhalothrin | Py | 56 | — | MH |
| Landrin | C | 119 | >2500 | MH |
| Malathion | OP | 210 | >4000 | SH |
| Parathion | OP | 3 | 6.8 | HH |
| Permethrin | Py | 4000 | — | UH |
| Pirimiphos-methyl | OP | 2018 | — | MH |
| Propoxur | C | 95 | >2400 | MH |
| Pyrethrum | Py | 200 | >1800 | UH |

C, carbamates; IGR, insect growth regulators; Ocl, organochlorines; OP, organophosphates; Py, pyrethroids; HH, highly hazardous; MH, moderately hazardous; SH, slightly hazardous; UH, unlikely to present hazard; HCH, hexachlorocyclohexane. The list of imagicides contains those in common use and also some compounds (*) recommended for testing in the field by the WHO.

Oils are usually applied from a knapsack sprayer, which is preferable to and less wasteful than a compression sprayer. All spraying requires careful supervision and regular (usually once a week) application. Oil may also be applied from a garden watering can or garden syringe, by using cotton waste soaked in oil and pegged into the ground for seepages and small pools, by means of a long stick with a bundle of old sacking attached, by balls of sacking tethered to the banks of streams or pools, by brushing over the surface with a sweeper's broom, by drip cans placed over streams and drains, by oil booms fixed across streams or irrigation channels, or they may be mixed with sawdust and thrown over breeding places in a manner similar to that of sowing grain.

The disadvantages are that: the product will not easily penetrate a barrier of grass and, to make it thoroughly effective, all vegetation and floating debris must be removed; wind will break up an oil film and carry it to one side of a sheet of water; it is cumbersome and costly for transportation; it may kill fish and render them unfit for human consumption; and it renders water unfit for drinking purposes. On the other hand, it kills the eggs and pupae of mosquitoes and it is easy to see whether it has been properly applied.

Mineral oils are not cheap and are not environmentally acceptable. An alternative is the synthetic monolayer films (aliphatic amines and polyoxyethylene stearyl alcohols), which have been used with good results when the mosquito breeding activity has been limited to a few, large water surfaces.

## Pyrethrins and pyrethroids

Pyrethrum is the oldest effective insecticide known and its main advantage is its high immediate toxicity to insects while it is harmless to humans, although classified in class II 'moderately hazardous' ($LD_{50}$ 500–1000 mg/kg). It is obtained from the flowers of the plant *Chrysanthemum cinerariaefolium*, which is grown commercially in many parts of the world and cultivated on a large scale in Kenya, Zaire, Japan, India and South America.

Pyrethrum is used mainly in the form of a 10–25 per cent extract of crushed dry flowers in kerosene or other organic solvents. This extract can be used when further diluted to 0.1–0.5 per cent with kerosene. If a suitable emulsifier is added, this extract can be diluted with water. Pyrethrum contains from 0.7 to 3.0 per cent active principles. These are mainly esters of pyrethrins I and II, which are rapidly oxidized and inactivated in sunlight, with a loss of insecticidal activity.

Pyrethrins are nerve poisons, acting through the insect cuticle, which is permeable to them. When sprayed, the droplets come into contact with the insect and their toxic action is fast. The addition of certain synergists increases the toxicity of pyrethrins to insects. Among these synergists, piperonyl butoxide is most commonly used.

Pyrethrins in crude form have been used for the control of various insects for many years. Their rapid 'knock-down' effect is of particular importance, although this action is relatively short-lived and frequent applications are necessary. There is no significant evidence of mosquito resistance. Their use has greatly increased recently because of the popularity of aerosol dispensers for rapid insect control at home and for the disinfestation of aircraft. Pyrethrum was also the first insecticide used for large-scale malaria control by attacking the adult *Anopheles*.

In malaria control programmes, the common formulations of pyrethrum are: 0.2–0.4 per cent dusts; 0.1–0.4 per cent solutions in kerosene or petroleum distillate; as aerosol insect sprays (synergists are included in the formulations). The pattern of use of pyrethrum is very wide. It is applied as thermal fogs, mists for non-residual control by repetitive application in kitchens, food stores, factories etc. where toxic residual insecticides cannot be used. Thermal fogs of 0.02 per cent pyrethrins with 0.4 per cent piperonyl butoxide are used for fly control. Ultra-low-volume (ULV) sprays are used against mosquitoes, houseflies and tsetse flies. Pyrethrum is repellent to mosquitoes; thus, it is used in insect repellent creams and mosquito coils. Pyrethrins have a very low toxicity for warm-blooded animals, but are toxic to fish; however, their persistence in water is brief.

Recently, a number of synthetic compounds have been developed. They are as potent as pyrethrins and some of them present definite advantages over the natural products.

The first useful synthetic pyrethroid came from the USA in 1969; it was given the generic name of allethrin. Allethrin has eight possible isomers, depending on the position of the hydrogen atoms on the one (*cis*) or other (*trans*) side of the cyclopropane ring.

The chemical names of the new compounds now available commercially are: allethrin, cismethrin, dimethrin, resmethrin, tetramethrin, deltamethrin, permethrin, lambda-cyhalothrin and others. The toxicity data for pyrethroids are highly variable according to Lisomer ratios, the vehicle used for oral administration and the husbandry of the test animals. The single $LD_{50}$ value now chosen for classification purposes is based on administration to test animals in corn oil and is much lower than that in aqueous solution. These compounds are more stable when exposed to sunlight and are less volatile than the natural product; they are equally safe in use, because their acute toxicity to mammals is generally low.

The insecticidal activity (knock-down and kill) of synthetic pyrethroids is high, but each compound has a specific range of action, which is influenced by the formulation and the degree of synergism with other compounds. Synthetic pyrethroids are used as coarse space sprays, aerosols and smokes in mosquito coils. The exceptional toxicity of synthetic pyrethroids against mosquitoes and other insects is important because they are expensive and must be used at dosage rates much lower than those of other insecticides. The new compounds are now available as usual formulations of solutions, emulsion concentrates and even as water-dispersible powders.

Deltamethrin, which has a fairly high mammalian toxicity (moderately hazardous; $LD_{50}$ 135 mg/kg), was used at a dosage of 0.05 g/m$^2$ in a field trial in Africa and was safe and effective as a residual spray for at least 2 months. Permethrin, a safer pyrethroid (moderately hazardous; $LD_{50}$ 500 mg/kg), when employed at a dosage of 0.5 g/m$^2$ was fairly effective as a residual spray for about 3 months. The latest synthetic pyrethroid, discovered in the early 1980s and developed as an insecticide for agricultural and public health applications, is lambda-cyhalothrin. The formulations available for residual spraying are 2.5 per cent and 5 per cent emulsifiable concentrate and 10 per cent wettable powder. Application rates are typically in the range of 10–25 mg/m$^2$ or, for prolonged action (6 months), 25–30 mg/m$^2$ are suggested. It is classed as a 'moderately hazardous' insecticide, with an $LD_{50}$ of 56 mg/kg.

As already mentioned, the pyrethroids are being used increasingly for the impregnation of mosquito nets and curtains (Figure 6.23). Comparative studies, which included deltamethrin, permethrin and lambda-cyhalothrin (Miller *et al.*, 1991), showed a 40 per cent loss of permethrin after 12 weeks' use, compared with no loss and a 38 per cent loss for deltamethrin and lambda-cyhalothrin, respectively. Each insecti-

cide, especially lambda-cyhalothrin, caused significant mosquito mortality; permethrin-treated nets reduced the number of *A. gambiae s.l.* entering the experimental hut by 60 per cent. Sleepers using the nets had no medical symptoms. Permethrin tends mainly to deter mosquitoes from house entry at a high dose of 0.67 g/m$^2$, thus enhancing personal protection, whereas the other insecticides kill higher proportions of the endophilic mosquitoes, which would give better community protection aganst malaria transmission.

## Chlorinated hydrocarbons (organochlorines)

Insecticides of this group employed in public health practice are DDT, HCH and dieldrin; the last two are collectively known as cyclodienes. However, only DDT and HCH are still in use in some countries today and the manufacture of these products is limited to only a few places in the world.

DDT (known also under the name of **dicophane** or **chlorophenothane**) was originally synthesized in 1854, but its insecticidal properties were discovered in 1939 by Paul Muller of Switzerland. The first field trials of DDT took place during the Second World War. The abbreviated name DDT was given to this compound by the British Ministry of Supply.

Until the last decade of the twentieth century, DDT was still the most widely used insecticide in public health practice. The chemical structures of DDT and other organochlorine insecticides are shown in Figure 6.24. The two chlorine atoms attached to the benzene rings may be linked with other carbon mole-

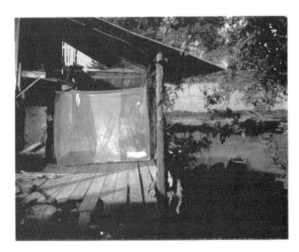

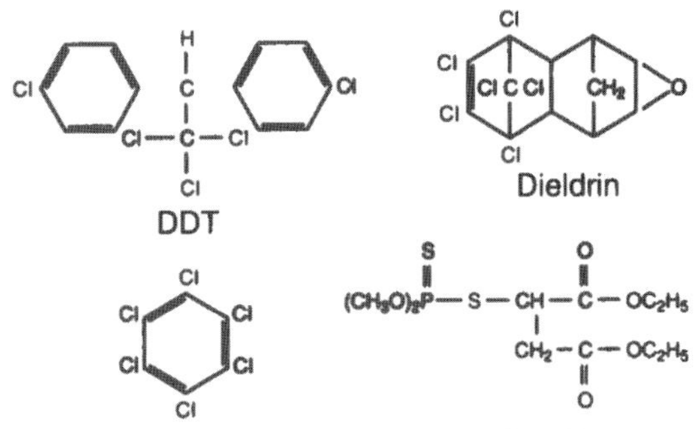

**Figure 6.23** *Mother and child protected by an impregnated mosquito net at sundown in Thailand.*

**Figure 6.24** *Chemical structure of four common insecticides used for malaria control.*

cules, giving different isomers of the compound, but the most effective of these is the para-para isomer of DDT. Technically, DDT is a mixture of isomers, but it must contain at least 70 per cent of para-para isomer to be acceptable. The content of the para-para isomer is usually stated on the container.

DDT is a white, amorphous, waxy powder with an aromatic smell. It is soluble in oils and organic solvents, but not in water. It is very stable and, on suitable impervious surfaces, it may remain active for as long as a year, but normally, if the DDT deposit is not rubbed off or covered up, it is applied twice a year. On sorptive surfaces such as mud (adobe), DDT loses its insecticidal effect somewhat faster. It has a certain irritant effect on insects, causing some of them to leave the treated surface soon after alighting on it, but its toxicity to most species of insects is high. Its toxicity to humans is very low and there is no evidence that the millions of people whose houses were treated with DDT are at any risk from exposure to it. It is classed as a moderately hazardous insecticide, with an $LD_{50}$ of 113 mg/kg. On the other hand, it is true that DDT may adversely affect some animals, including cats, chickens, predatory birds and fish. For this reason, the use of DDT outdoors, when gross environmental contamination is likely, should be avoided. The amount of DDT for the residual spraying of indoor surfaces is usually given in terms of technical DDT and the standard dosage is 2 g/m² of the treated surface every 6 months. DDT has also been used for its larvicidal properties, mainly as an additional compound to fortify the toxic action of oils; the required dosage is very small. Two methods were used: a 2–5 per cent solution of DDT in 'high-speed' oil employed at 0.3–0.6 L to 1000 m² of water surface, and an emulsion concentrate, to be diluted with water so that the final concentration of DDT is 0.1–0.15 per cent, to be sprayed at a rate of 10–20 L per 1000 m² (about 10–20 gallons per hectare) of water surface.

Like all chlorinated hydrocarbons, DDT has a short effect when used as a larvicide: the insecticide is diluted or washed away or absorbed by mud and vegetation. Today, the use of all chlorinated hydrocarbons as larvicides is frowned upon because of their persistence in the environment due to low biodegradability. The water-dispersible powder of DDT for the residual spraying of houses contains 50–75 per cent of active substance; the higher content of the insecticide is preferable for a number of reasons, mainly economic.

HCH, formerly called benzene hexachloride (BHC), was synthesized in 1825, apparently by Faraday. Its insecticidal action was discovered in the UK in 1942, when it was first known under the code name 666; it became widely used during the 1950s in agriculture, veterinary medicine and public health.

Its chemical constitution is remarkably simple ($C_6H_6Cl_6$), because it consists of a benzene ring with a chlorine atom attached to each carbon. The arrangement of the hydrogen and carbon atoms in space may vary, so that a number of optical isomers exist, the most active of which is the gamma isomer. This isomer, when pure, or at least 99 per cent pure, is called lindane. Technical HCH must contain at least 12 per cent of the gamma isomer. It is soluble in organic solvents, and is a whitish or light-brown, granular or flaky substance with a characteristic musty smell. It is relatively volatile and may kill insects fairly rapidly by fumigant action. However, because of this volatility, its residual action is generally half as long as that of DDT, although its toxic action is faster. It is classed as a moderately hazardous insecticide, with an $LD_{50}$ of 100 g/kg based on the cumulative properties of the beta isomer. HCH may be used in the form of a water-dispersible powder, containing 6.5 per cent gamma isomer, as a residual insecticide for indoor spraying of walls; other formulations (solutions, emulsions) exist for use as larvicides or as insecticidal smoke. The usual dosage of HCH for residual spraying is 0.3 g/m² every 3 months or 0.5 g/m² every 4–6 months.

Dieldrin, together with aldrin, belongs to a small group of compounds obtained by the cyclodiene synthesis discovered by Diels and Alder, whose names were given to the first two products.

Dieldrin is more toxic than DDT and HCH to insects, to other animals and to humans (highly hazardous; $LD_{50}$ 37 mg/kg). It has two main disadvantages: fairly high toxicity to humans and other animals, and proneness rapidly to produce resistance to cyclodiene compounds and to HCH. Dieldrin has been responsible for poisoning spray operators, domestic animals and poultry. Because of this and other factors, its use in public health practice has now virtually ceased.

## Organophosphorous compounds

This group of insecticides, widely used in agriculture (e.g. parathion), is now commonly employed in public health practice, mainly because the chlorinated hydro-carbons have fallen out of favour due to their comparatively low biodegradability and because some insect vectors of disease have become resistant to them.

Most of the organophosphorous insecticides are esters or amides of organically bound phosphoric or pyrophosphoric acid. Their general mode of action is due to the inhibition of the enzyme cholinesterase in arthropods as well as in mammals. The normal mechanism of transmission of nerve impulses is through the liberation of acetylcholine, which acts on the effector cells of a muscle or a gland. Cholinesterase present in the nerves stops the effect of acetylcholine by hydrolysing it; organophosphorous compounds neutralize the enzyme and cause an accumulation of acetylcholine. This results in a blockage of the nervous system, with consequent muscle paralysis, excessive gland secretion and finally death. Atropine is a specific antidote, which counteracts these effects of organophosphorus poisoning. The suitability of organophosphates for use in public health programmes depends on their toxicity to the target insects and their danger to humans, but also on their properties of persistence, tendency to produce resistance in mosquitoes, ease of formulation and cost. Generally speaking, these insecticides are more volatile than chlorinated hydrocarbons and their activity is shorter, which also increase the cost of application of these compounds. The following organophosphorous compounds are in use for malaria control as imagicides or larvicides.

## MALATHION

Malathion was widely employed in the 1970s, 1980s and early 1990s. It is an ester of dimethyl phosphorodithioate. The technical product is a brownish liquid with an unpleasant, garlicky smell that can be masked by various additives. Its chemical structure is shown in Figure 6.24.

Its formulation consists of emulsifiable 60–90 per cent concentrates or of water-dispersible powders containing 50 per cent of the active compound. Thus, malathion can be used either for outdoor space spraying or for indoor residual applications. The duration of residual action of malathion depends on the substrate on which it is used, but averages about 2–3 months when the dosage of the active substance is at the standard 2 g/m² of sprayable surface.

Because of its higher cost and shorter residual action, the application of malathion is about three times as expensive as that of DDT at the same dosage. Whereas most of the organophosphates are very toxic to humans, the toxicity of malathion is relatively low (slightly hazardous; $LD_{50}$ 2100 mg/kg) and this compound has been widely used for indoor spraying of human dwellings and animal shelters. However, some formulations undergo rapid chemical degradation on storage in tropical conditions, and their toxicity can be much higher than expected. Thus, even with malathion, very strict safety precautions should be observed.

## FENTHION

Fenthion (Baytex), another derivative of phosphorothioate, has a higher toxicity to insects and to mammals than malathion (highly hazardous; $LD_{50}$ 330 mg/kg) and it was used with some success in Africa and Iran as a water-dispersible powder at a target dosage of 1.5 g/m². However, because of its toxic hazards to sprayers, fenthion is not suitable for routine indoor spraying, although it is of some value as a larvicide for the control of culicine mosquitoes.

## FENITROTHION

Fenitrothion is an ortho-dimethyl-nitro-tolylphosphorothioate known under the proprietary names of Sumithion or Folithion. It has been widely used in agriculture. Trials in Kisumu, Kenya, showed that it can be of value for residual control of malaria vectors when used as a water-dispersible powder for house spraying. At a dosage of 2 g/m² this insecticide gave good results for about 3–4 months. This insecticide can be used for spraying houses provided that various precautionary measures are observed for protection of sprayers and domestic animals.

## DICHLORVOS

Dichlorvos (DDVP), a dichlorovinyl dimethyl phosphate, is a liquid product with a high volatility; the vapours thus produced are highly toxic to flying insect pests and of low toxicity to humans. The compound is now widely used when incorporated into various plastic resins (e.g. Vapona) for the control of domestic flies. Despite many field trials carried out in Africa and elsewhere, dichlorvos has not found its place in the control of malaria vectors, but has been employed for the disinsectization of aircraft, although this practice fell out of favour due to corrosion problems in the ventilation systems. In the People's Republic of China, it has been used in houses for family protection on a communal basis. It is classed as highly hazardous, with an $LD_{50}$ of 56 mg/kg.

## TEMEPHOS

Temephos (Abate) is a tetramethyl-thiodiphenylene phosphorothioate, highly active against the aquatic larvae of mosquitoes and other insects. It has been formulated as an emulsifiable concentrate or in the form of fine granules impregnated with 1–5 per cent of the compound. The granules are applied on water surfaces at monthly intervals, in doses aiming at one part per million of the active product. This compound is highly effective against various species of mosquito larvae, including those resistant to other insecticides. Its toxicity to fish, birds and mammals is very low (unlikely to present acute hazard: $LD_{50}$ 8600 mg/kg). It is also used in liquid form as an emulsion at a rate of 37–100 mL per hectare and in granular form of 2 per cent concentration at between 5 kg and 20 kg per hectare, depending on the type of water and the amounts of aquatic vegetation. This treatment can be repeated at intervals of 2–3 months, i.e. much less frequently than any other larvicide.

## CHLORPHOXIM

Chlorphoxim, at active ingredient $2g/m^2$, gave a satisfactory reduction of A. gambiae and A. funestus hut-resting populations for 3 months in Africa and of A. aconitus for 24 weeks in Indonesia, but had a less satisfactory impact on indoor and outdoor human-biting rates. These conflicting results make it difficult to assess the potential effectiveness of chlorphoxim in malaria control. It is unlikely to present an acute hazard in normal use, with an $LD_{50}$ of less than 2500 mg/kg.

## PIRIMIPHOS-METHYL

Pirimiphos-methyl is a broad-spectrum, non-cumulative organophosphorous insecticide. It is a cholinesterase inhibitor with fast-acting fumigant contact and stomach action. It is slightly hazardous to mammals ($LD_{50}$ 2018 mg/kg). This insecticide has now been used successfully for a number of years. Studies conducted between 1979 and 1981 in Indonesia showed that the 50 per cent emulsifiable concentrate was as effective as the 25 per cent water-

dispersible powder at $2 g/m^2$ and had the advantages of not leaving a brown deposit on the walls or causing rapid erosion of the nozzle tips. At a dosage of $2 g/m^2$, it controlled DDT-resistant A. aconitus for about 12 weeks; at a dosage of $1 g/m^2$, mosquito mortality in houses remained above 50 per cent for 5 weeks by contact exposure and for less than 2 weeks by airborne exposure. It was as effective or even better against A. culicifacies and A. stephensi in Pakistan, especially at $2 g/m^2$ or sprayed twice with $1 g/m^2$.

# Carbamates

This comparatively recent class of carbamic acid esters resembles in some ways the organophosphorous insecticides because they also affect the enzyme cholinesterase.

## CARBARYL

Carbaryl (Sevin) is an alpha naphthyl methylcarbamate and is in use as an agricultural insecticide. Field trials carried out in Haiti showed some promise at a dosage of 1–2 $g/m^2$, but the persistence of the compound was not as long as expected. It is classified as moderately hazardous, with an $LD_{50}$ of 300 mg/kg.

## PROPOXUR

Propoxur (Arprocarb) is an isopropoxy-phenyl methylcarbamate and underwent a number of field tests in various parts of the world. The results showed that, at the dosage of $2 g/m^2$ in the form of a water-dispersible powder, propoxur remains highly active against Anopheles for up to 3 months; it also has an airborne effect, which extends to about 20 m from sprayed houses. It has moderate toxicity to humans ($LD_{50}$ 95 mg/kg) and can be used with ordinary precautions in the field. However, its relatively high cost has limited the application of propoxur.

## BENDIOCARB

Bendiocarb, although applied at low dosages (active ingredient 0.4 $g/m^2$) because of its high insecticidal activity, has a high mammalian toxicity. However, it is classed as a moderately hazardous insecticide with an $LD_{50}$ of 55 mg/kg. This is minimized by providing the 88 g/kg (80 per cent) water-dispersible powder formulation in preweighed sachets: one sachet added to the water in the spray pump gives the required 10 g/L (1.0 per cent) spray suspension. Because bendiocarb is virtually odourless and does not leave an unsightly deposit, it is acceptable to householders. In a study in Zimbabwe, the insecticide remained active for up to 8 weeks (96 per cent mortality) on thatch, and in southern Mexico for up to 3 months on most common indoor house surfaces.

## Insect growth regulators

These are synthetic compounds that interfere with the larval growth and moulting of insects. These chemicals mimic the natural juvenile hormone and prevent the formation of chitin during the pre-pupal stage. An isoprene compound (methoprene) and a chitin-inhibiting substituted urea (diflubenzuron) are now available, the former as slow-release briquettes and the latter as a 25 per cent wettable powder or as 0.5 per cent granules. However, their use is limited by high cost and restricted availability. They are fairly rapidly decomposed in water, but as granules or microcapsules they may last several weeks or even several months.

## Formulations of insecticides

Formulations of chemical compounds for mosquito control are numerous, ranging from fogs to fluid oils to solid and floating briquettes.

### SOLUTIONS

Solutions are either in oil or kerosene, solvent naphtha or white spirit, with concentrations of 10–15 per cent. Aromatic hydrocarbons such as benzene and cyclohexane permit higher concentrations, up to 25–40 per cent, which can be diluted to the required spray concentration.

Insecticide solutions can be used either for larviciding or as imagicides for the control of adult mosquitoes by space spraying and residual spraying. The latter method has been used when spraying some types of houses in which the staining of walls by unsightly deposits of water-dispersible powder had to be avoided. For this reason, the introduction of water emulsion concentrates found greater favour.

### EMULSIONS

Emulsions are made up from two immiscible liquids, one of which is broken up into globules and scattered in the other liquid. To prevent the separation of the two, various emulsifying agents are added. Emulsions are prepared from various concentrates containing 10–35 per cent of a chemical compound by dilution with water. Pastes are special types of emulsion concentrates.

### WATER-DISPERSIBLE POWDERS

Water-dispersible (or wettable) powders are composed of an active insecticide diluted with an inert carrier, to which various wetting, suspending and anti-caking agents are added. Commercially available water-dispersible powders contain between 50 and 75 per cent of the technical product. When mixed with water and stirred, these powders form a suspension, i.e. a mixture of the liquid and of the insoluble small particles, which tend to settle more or less rapidly. The rate at which the particles settle depends on various physical factors related to the composition of the water-dispersible powder, its amount, the type of water used and, naturally, the agitation of the suspended powder. Particle size and suspensibility are important factors in residual insecticide spraying. In standard formulations of water-dispersible powders, the WHO specifications require that at least 50–70 per cent of the insecticide content should have a particle size of less than 10–20 μm.

Solutions and emulsions are readily absorbed by porous surfaces of very rough walls in rural dwellings in the tropics; as a result, the toxic effects on mosquitoes may be decreased. Highly volatile compounds (HCH, propoxur, fenitrothion) still exert their action, especially at higher doses. Water-dispersible powders in suspension leave most of the active, crystalline particles of the insecticide on the surface. However, some particles penetrate beneath the surface and, during the rainy season, when the humidity is high, an increase of the insecticidal effect takes place.

### SOLID FORMULATIONS

Solid formulations of insecticides are powders, microcapsules, granules, pellets or briquettes. All of these preparations used as larvicides are designed to disintegrate slowly in the water while releasing the toxic agent.

Because *Anopheles* mosquitoes are surface feeders, floating slow-release preparations have been formulated. These can be placed in small bodies of water (temporary or permanent breeding sites) and remain there even when the water dries out; they then float to the surface and release the insecticide when the sites fill up with water again after rain.

A new type of formulation is that of granules. These are produced from inorganic materials such as clays or organic polymers. The choice of carrier, solvent and binder provides some control over wetting and break-up, with subsequent release of the active ingredient. The granules are safe to handle, convenient and with little hazard of drifting away from the target.

Another new procedure is that of microencapsulation. The tiny capsules containing the insecticide can be stored as suspension in water and diluted for spraying. Like the granules, microcapsules are designed to provide controlled release of the insecticide.

## SPACE-SPRAYING FORMULATIONS

Space-spraying formulations range from fumigants, through fogs, mists and other aerosols, to fine droplets.

Some insecticides (such as dichlorvos) have a low vapour pressure and volatilize spontaneously. This fumigant action has been proposed for aircraft disinsectization. However, this insecticide is no longer recommended for this purpose. Instead, aerosol applications of resmethrin, bioresmethrin, *d*-phenothrin or permethrin, each with 2 per cent active ingredient in dichlorodifluoromethane (Freon 12) and chlorotrifluoromethane (Freon 3), have been recommended either before take-off (blocks away) or upon arrival. The use of chlorofluoromethanes as aerosol propellants is now questioned on environmental grounds. Recommendations have been made for the use of permethrin at a rate of 0.2 g a.i./m² on exposed surfaces of the aircraft cabin and cargo holds and at the rate of 0.5 g a.i./m² on the floor covering in the passenger cabin. The insecticide usually remains effective for up to 8 weeks and retreatment can be carried out to fit aircraft maintenance procedures.

Coarse sprays, which consist of droplets over 400 μm volume median diameter (VMD), have a space-spraying effect if the relevant liquid evaporates.

Fine sprays, in which the droplets are between 100 and 400 μm VMD, also have this effect, in addition to a direct impact on flying mosquitoes. When the droplets are between 50 and 100 μm VMD, they are classified as mists. Finally, true aerosols or fogs have particles less than 50 μm VMD; the latter type of aerosol remains suspended in the still air for about 1 hour.

Aerosols are produced from containers through the action of a compressed, liquefied, inert gas; for large-scale use, various thermal or rotary generators are available.

## LARVICIDAL METHODS OF MOSQUITO CONTROL

The technique of application of larvicides to water surfaces depends on both the type of compound used and on the type of mosquito breeding place (Table 6.5). Liquid larvicidal compounds such as oils may be applied from a simple garden watering-pot or a hand sprayer on small pools or drains. Alternative simple methods such as using an ordinary sweeper's broom dipped into oil, drip cans improvised from tins with a hole in the bottom, sawdust mixed with oil and broadcast by hand etc. have been employed with reasonably good results provided the water surfaces are stationary and not too extensive. However, more commonly, knapsack sprayers are used, as by this means the oil can be distributed 5–10 m from the operator. Various designs of knapsack or shoulder-sling larvicide sprayers exist, but their general design is the same, consisting of a container with a 7–9 L capacity, with a lever-operated plunger or diaphragm pump, connected by a rubber or plastic hose to a cut-off valve, lance and nozzle. The pressure developed by the hand-operated lever is low and the semi-continuous pumping can be maintained without much effort while the operator points the lance towards the target of the spray.

Various hand-operated or motor-driven modifications of these sprayers, mounted on wheels, on boats or now on small hovercraft, are available, but their description exceeds the bounds of this book.

Larvicidal dusts may be broadcast by hand, small bellows-operated blowers, pump-type hand dusters, knapsack-carried or front-carried rotary blowers and power-operated, wheel-mounted dusting machines.

Gelatine capsules containing an emulsifiable concentrate of pyrethrins with piperonyl butoxide (Tossits), when tossed into the water, will disintegrate and release the contents within minutes, each capsule spreading over an unobstructed water surface of 5–9 m² (60–100 ft²).

**Table 6.5** *Selected insecticides for larvicidal application in mosquito control*

| Insecticide | Dosage of active ingredient per hectare | Duration of effective action (weeks) | Remarks |
|---|---|---|---|
| Diesel oil (fuel oil) and other petroleum oils[a] | 142–190 L in open ponds to cover water surface | 1–2 | With an addition of a spreading agent the amount can be reduced five times or more; even so, their effect on the environment must be carefully considered |
| Larvicidal oil[a] | 19–47 L (with special spreading agents) | 1–2 | Various proprietary formulations available; effect on the environment must be carefully considered |
| Malathion[b] | 224–1000 g | 1–2 | As emulsion concentrate or granules; avoid overdosing, which may injure fish |
| Temephos (Abate)[c] | 56–112 g pure compound | 2–4 | As emulsion concentrate or granules; higher dosages are used in polluted waters |
| Fenitrothion[b] | 100–1000 g | 1–3 | Not to be applied to waters containing fish or crustaceans (prawns, crabs); caution in use |
| Fenthion[c] | 22–112 g | 2–11 | As above |
| Pirimipos-methyl[b] | 50–500 g | 2–11 | As emulsion concentrate |
| Chlorphoxim[b] | 100 g | 2–7 | As emulsion concentrate |
| Chlorpyriphos[c] | 11–25 g | 3–17 | As emulsion concentrate, granules or water-dispersible powder |
| Permethrin[b] | 5–10 g | 5–10 | As emulsion concentrate; the lowest levels are recommended for fish-bearing waters |
| Deltamethrin[b] | 2.5–10 g | 1–3 | As above |
| Diflubenzuron[c] | 25–100 g | 1–4 | As granules or water dispersible |
| Iodofenphos[c] | 50–100 g | 7–16 | As emulsion concentrate or granules |
| Methoprene[c] | 100–1000 g | 4–8 | As slow-release suspension |
| Phoxim[c] | 100 g | 1–6 | As emulsion concentrate |
| *Bacillus thuringiensis*[c] | 500–5000 g | 1–2 | Varies from liquid to granular formulation |
| *Bacillus sphaericus*[c] | 10 000–20 000 g | 8 | Against *culicinae* in pit latrines |
| Mononuclear film (oil)[a] | 3–5 L | 2–10 days | A very rapidly spreading oil, greatly affected by wind movements |

See also Table 3, page 21, in *Chemicals, methods for the control of arthropod vectors and pests of public health importance.* (WHO, 1984, 1997c.)
[a] To be used in special and suitable situations when recommended larvicides are not available
[b] To be used in emergency situations when other more suitable products are not available.
[c] Recommended for use provided target organism is susceptible to it

Briquettes containing 8 per cent methoprene, an insect growth regulator (Altosid), have been devised to release an effective larvicide for 30 days on small bodies of water or for shorter periods in small streams.

For the application of granulated compounds, several modifications of standard equipment have now been developed and are increasingly used.

For the large-scale application of larvicidal measures, either in the form of large droplet sprays or as granulated insecticide formulations, fixed-wing aircraft and helicopters are the best solution. In general, aerial spraying using rotary atomizers produces a broad spectrum of droplets, so that the resulting effect is due to direct action on the larvae and adults of mosquitoes as well as to some residual action on the vegetation.

Applications of larvicides must be repeated at intervals corresponding to the development cycle of the *Anopheles* species. Generally, the relevant period is between 7 and 14 days; longer periods are possible with some newer compounds.

## IMAGICIDAL MEASURES AIMED AT CONTROL OF ADULT MOSQUITOES

Although individual protection from bites of adult mosquitoes by smoke or various fumigant devices ('joss-sticks') was well known in the past, large-scale malaria control projects by indoor spraying with pyrethrum solutions proved to be unexpectedly successful some 50 years ago in southern Africa and India. However, the introduction of DDT and other synthetic insecticides resulted in the revolutionary concept of malaria control by residual action of the new compounds. In contrast to the immediate knock-down effect of pyrethrum, which lasts only for a short time, the new synthetic insecticides retain their toxic action for a considerable period when applied to a surface with which adult *Anopheles* (and other mosquitoes) may come into contact.

Residual insecticides are almost invariably applied in some liquid form, which, on drying, leaves a crystalline deposit on the wall. Some wall surfaces absorb the original fluid that is put on and, if this is a solution or an emulsion, some of the active insecticide is drawn into the inner part of the wall where the insect cannot come into contact with it. This causes some loss of insecticidal power on mud and porous plaster walls. Surfaces such as wood may not absorb much of the insecticide that remains on the surface in an active form for many months.

These insecticides act slowly and some of them irritate the mosquitoes, leading to their flight towards the light out of the house. The fate of the mosquitoes after that depends on whether or not they take away a small quantity of insecticide on their legs (tarsi). Crystals formed after the evaporation of the solvents used in solutions and emulsions vary in size, but the range of insecticide particles in a wettable powder formulation is determined in the course of manufacture and is standardized to a specification that can be checked by suitable suspensibility tests to ensure optimum size for biological effectiveness. Volatility is important because a volatile product disappears in time whatever the quality of the wall, but exerts some fumigant effect, which will kill insects not in actual contact.

The irritant effect, which occurs with DDT, nullifies the value of counts of mosquitoes in treated houses as an index of efficacy because it always leads to the mosquito avoiding the house as a shelter, although it may still use it as a feeding place. The only reliable checking mechanism consists of trapping mosquitoes leaving the house and noting the proportion of them dying in the next 12 or 24 hours. This demands the use of special traps and a rather elaborate technique that cannot be universally applied.

Obviously, the large-scale application of residual insecticides will have a particularly marked effect on those species of mosquitoes that feed preferentially on human beings inside their dwellings or that shelter in human houses or animal sheds. A good residual insecticide should have the following characteristics:

- high biological activity against the vector species, with a lethal effect for at least 3 months after application and without (or with minimal) irritant reaction on the mosquito, to assure the full toxic action;
- fairly rapid kill, after a brief contact with the toxic surface;
- low acute or chronic toxicity to humans and domestic animals;
- good stability on storage, easy formulations and application;
- economy in use and low cost;
- acceptability to the at-risk human population.

The duration of residual activity of insecticidal compounds and their formulations depends not only on the intrinsic persistency of the chemical, but also on its effectiveness, i.e. the biological action on the target insect. The latter varies considerably in relation to the type and composition of the sprayed surface. Thus, on porous walls made of unbaked clay or mud (adobe), the phenomenon of sorption interferes with the effectiveness of some insecticides incorporated into water-dispersible powders. This is the case for DDT, which lasts much longer on non-porous surfaces (e.g. wood) than on mud. On the other hand, HCH may be effective even after sorption through its fumigant action. Organophosphorous insecticides formulated as water-dispersible powders may be less effective on sorptive walls after a few weeks.

All houses within the area to be protected should receive the appropriate dose of the insecticide before the start of the transmission season and at agreed intervals. The usual doses of insecticides (e.g. DDT at 2 g/m$^2$ every 6 months), although widely applicable, may vary somewhat depending on local conditions. The insecticide must be applied to the indoor walls and ceiling surfaces of all inhabited rooms and also animal shelters. Heavy furniture in the rooms must also be sprayed, particularly the back of furniture close to the walls. Where wall surfaces and furniture are of good quality, emulsions or solutions of insecticides should be used rather than suspensions of water-dispersible powders, which leave a whitish deposit (Table 6.6).

## Space spraying

Despite the tremendous success of the technique of residual insecticide spraying, the method of space dispersion of fast-acting compounds is still of value. A degree of local control of mosquitoes (and other flying insects) may be achieved by 'space spraying', i.e. by releasing the insecticides into the air as smoke or as fine droplets. Naturally, such measures of pro-

tection must be frequently repeated to result in any significant effect.

In epidemics of insect-borne diseases, the 'space-spraying' technique can be a valuable method to rapidly reduce the numbers of mosquitoes not only in dwellings, but also temporarily in outside breeding grounds. It is also generally well accepted by the community as it has a broad action against mosquitoes in general. It is, however, expensive in terms of the insecticide itself, the special equipment needed and vehicle or aircraft resources, and poses a problem of accessibility. Moreover, it is less effective against *Anopheles* than against *Aedes* and *Culex*. *Aedes* are normally active during the day and *Culex* can become so if disturbed, and both are generally fully active at dusk. This contrasts with the most efficient malaria vectors, which are active in the middle of the night. Furthermore, they are widely dispersed in daytime resting places and thus are less likely to be affected when fogging is carried out while there is still daylight.

The critical feature of space spraying is the size of the droplet, which determines the time the insecti-

**Table 6.6** *Insecticides as residual indoor spray for the control of* Anopheles *vectors of malaria*

| Insecticide | Dosage (g a.i./m$^2$) | Effectiveness (months) | Chemical type | Remarks |
|---|---|---|---|---|
| DDT | 2.0 | 6 or more | OC | In some conditions 1.0 g/m$^2$ may be used |
| γ-HCH | 0.2–0.5 | 3 or more | OC | Some sorption by mud; used in some areas to control DDT resistance in the absence of dieldrin resistance |
| Fenitrothion | 2.0 | 3–6 | OP | Reasonably safe when precautions are observed, but expensive; airborne toxicity |
| Malathion | 2.0 | 2–3 | OP | Less used now due to odour and toxicity if not stored properly; sorption by mud |
| Pirimiphos-methyl | 1–2 | 2–3 or more | OP | Long-lasting airborne toxicity |
| Bendiocarb | 0.1–0.4 | 2–6 | C | High mammalian toxicity |
| Carbosulfan | 1–2 | 2–3 | C | |
| Propoxur | 1–2 | 3–6 | C | Rather expensive; sorption by mud |
| Alpha-cypermethrin | 0.02–0.03 | 4–6 | Py | Considered moderately hazardous |
| Cyfluthrin | 0.02–0.05 | 3–6 | Py | |
| Cypermethrin | 0.5 | 4 or more | Py | There may be cross-resistance with DDT |
| Deltamethrin | 0.01–0.025 | 2–3 | Py | High costs which are partially neutralized by low dosage |
| Etofenprox | 0.1–0.3 | 3–6 | Py | Low oral toxicity LD$_{50}$ > 10 000 mg/kg |
| Lambda-cyhalothrin | 0.02–0.03 | 3–6 | Py | Proved to be effective; high cost offset by low dosage |
| Permethrin | 0.5 | 2–3 | Py | Low mammalian toxicity |

OC, organochlorine compounds; OP, organophosphorous compounds; C, carbamate; Py, synthetic pyrethroids

cide remains suspended in the air and penetration. Space sprays are measured by VMD in micrometres. A course spray has a VMD of more than 400 $\mu$m, fine between 100 and 400 $\mu$m, mists 50–100 $\mu$m and fogs or ULV sprays below 50 $\mu$m.

## Treatment of mosquito nets

Numerous studies over the years have demonstrated that, if mosquito nets are kept in good condition and are used correctly, they afford good protection against mosquito and sandfly bites. However, if they are treated with an insecticide, they afford even better individual and family protection against the bites of flying insects. They can also reduce bedbug, flea and lice problems, as long as these insects are susceptible to the insecticide used. If used on a large scale within a community, this technology could have some impact on the epidemiological equilibrium of malaria transmission. Studies have shown clearly an impact on malaria morbidity and mortality rates in children (Snow et al., 1987, 1988).

The new synthetic pyrethroid insecticides are the most common and practical substances used to treat mosquito nets for personal protection against malaria and leishmaniasis. These are short-acting insecticides and their residual effect is usually sufficient for only 3–4 months. Thus, depending on the length of the main transmission season, nets have to be treated regularly once or twice a year to maintain their effectiveness. Insecticides with a low toxic hazard, such as permethrin, deltamethrin and lambdacyhalothrin, are generally used at present, but new products may be appearing on the market soon. In addition, there are reports of resistance of malaria vectors to the synthetic pyrethroids; thus, alternatives are being sought.

## EQUIPMENT FOR VECTOR CONTROL OPERATIONS

Equipment for the control of mosquitoes can be classified in many different ways. The following classification is convenient and relevant to the malaria control strategy. It was followed by the WHO Expert Committee on Vector Biology and Control (WHO, 1990).

- Insecticide application equipment
  —hand compression sprayer
  —motorized knapsack mist blowers
  —thermal foggers
  —aerosol generators
  —dusting equipment
  —household equipment
  —aircraft
- Equipment for biological control
  —equipment for the application of insect pathogens
  —equipment for rearing, transporting and distributing larvivorous fish
- Equipment for environmental management
  —light machinery
  —heavy machinery
  —domestic equipment
  —water management devices.

The choice of equipment depends on the size of the control operation and knowledge of the vector involved, and it must be consistent with the recommended method of control. Moreover, one has to bear in mind:

- the frequency and duration of control measures
- the extent and accessibility of the target area
- the ease of use of the equipment by the operator
- the amount of maintenance
- initial and recurring costs.

Only the briefest description of conventional equipment can be given here (see WHO, 1990, 1997).

## INSECTICIDE APPLICATION EQUIPMENT

Evaluation according to standard specifications is necessary for appropriate selection and purchase of insecticide application equipment for use in programmes for the control of disease vectors, disease reservoirs and pests. Evaluation is also needed to ensure that equipment is suitable for a specific application, and that it is durable, reliable and easily maintained. To achieve this, the WHO established the WHO Insecticide Application Equipment Evaluation Scheme (WHO, 1977).

The selection of properly designed equipment for the recommended method of control is an important part of any vector control programme (WHO, 1990). Routine maintenance is essential and personnel need to be properly trained to do this.

Most vector control programmes continue to give preference to properly designed hand-operated equipment, with the compression sprayer being the most commonly used for various control operations such as residual treatment and the application of larvicides and insect pathogens.

The operation and maintenance of motorized equipment need additional skills, and problems will occur unless specially trained personnel are placed in charge.

Aerosols are used to apply insecticides for the temporary control of adult mosquitoes and other flying insects, especially during epidemics of mosquito-borne diseases such as malaria, yellow fever, dengue, or dengue haemorrhagic fever.

## Hand compression sprayer

Most of the residual insecticidal spraying for control of *Anopheles* is carried out now by means of hand compression sprayers. However, in some parts of the world, the much simpler and cheaper stirrup pumps or bucket sprayers have been extensively used in the past and may still be of value. These pumps consist of a bucket containing the liquid to be sprayed and a pump with a double-acting piston operated manually. A hose attached to the pump leads to the spraying lance, ending with a nozzle (Figure 6.25). Obviously, this equipment must be operated by two people: one working the pump and the other directing the spray lance. Moreover, the pressures are erratic, which does not allow even application. Nevertheless, stirrup pumps are adequate for use in malaria control if no other sprayers are available.

Coffee (1979) announced a revolutionary new concept of electrodynamic spraying. As the name suggests, this sprayer operates on electrodynamic energy, capable of atomizing liquid insecticide into evenly sized droplets, which are attracted by the surface being sprayed. The sprayer runs on four torch batteries (60 hours' operation), generating an electric charge of 25 000 volts at the sprayer nozzle, thus atomizing the insecticide packed in a special disposable container. The resulting spray cloud, because it is electrically charged, is attracted by the surface, giving perfect coverage. Electrical attraction, in addition to increasing the spray efficiency, prevents insecticide wastage and losses. This sprayer was designed for use in agriculture, and especially for cotton. Its use for

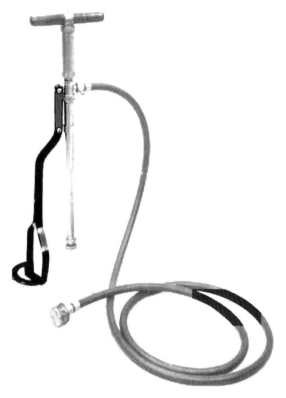

**Figure 6.25** *A stirrup pump, a simple and robust type of sprayer used for residual indoor spraying of insecticides. (Wellcome Museum of Medical Science.)*

malaria control has yet to be evaluated, especially from the point of view of cost efficiency. It is very safe, light and easy to use.

The hand compression sprayer is universally regarded as standard equipment for residual insecticide spraying (Figure 6.26). This type of sprayer (e.g. Hudson Expert) consists of a cylindrical tank made of stainless steel and of about 13 L (2–3 gallons) capacity, in which the liquid insecticide formulation (usually a suspension of water-dispersible powder) is contained. The internal pressure in the tank is raised by a hand-operated pump incorporated in the sprayer; the cover is of the 'inner seal' type, which tightens when the pressure is high. It is fitted with a hose, a cut-off valve, a lance and a nozzle. Some types of sprayers also have a constant pressure valve and a pressure gauge. One or more straps are attached for carrying the sprayer. This equipment is designed to produce a uniform insecticide dosage on sprayed surfaces and to be simple, robust and durable so that it can be used by sprayers with elementary technical

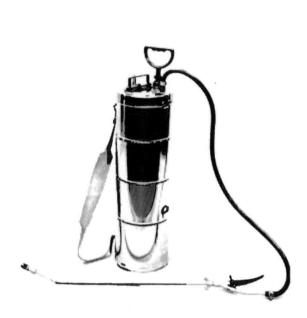

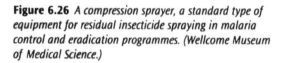

**Figure 6.26** *A compression sprayer, a standard type of equipment for residual insecticide spraying in malaria control and eradication programmes. (Wellcome Museum of Medical Science.)*

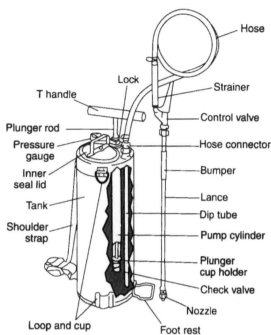

**Figure 6.27** *A cutaway diagram of a compression sprayer.*

knowledge. The important requirement is a controllable and uniform nozzle discharge rate. Nozzle spray patterns of different forms have been tried, the flat-fan shape being favoured because it facilitates the application of parallel, vertical spraying swaths on interior surfaces.

In practice, the rate of application of an insecticide is regulated by three controlling factors: its concentration in the liquid carrier, the nozzle discharge rate and the speed of spraying.

The generally recommended operating pressure in the delivery lance and nozzle to give the most efficient application is 2.8 kg/cm$^2$ (40 lb/in$^2$). Maintaining this pressure until the sprayer is empty after a single filling and pumping involves a constant pressure in the tank and a pressure-control valve in the lance. The required cylinder pressure may be achieved by a given number of strokes of the pump or more accurately read from a pressure gauge (Figure 6.27).

The ideal nozzle to ensure uniformity of application is the Tee-Jet Nozzle 8002, delivering a fan-type spray, with a spray angle of 80° and an output of 0.76 L (0.18 gallons) per minute at the standard

pressure. Held at a distance of 45 cm (18 inches) from the surface to be sprayed, such a nozzle will deposit a swath of spray 75 cm (30 inches) wide, of which the middle half is effective. In practice, therefore, the marginal 18–20 cm of one swath should be overlapped by the margin of the next swath to produce a uniform deposit.

Irregularities in spraying and uneven dosage are due in part to faults of the operator, and in part to faults of the apparatus. The first can be overcome by thorough training, in which the operator is taught how to apply a standard dose, usually 4.5 L to 100 m$^2$ (1 gallon to 1000 ft$^2$), with complete regularity. The training having been given, supervision must continue to ensure its maintenance. The principal faults in maintenance are wear in the nozzle and fall of pressure as the quantity of fluid in the tank decreases. The ordinary brass nozzle may wear very quickly, particularly when wettable powders are used, because their composition may be abrasive. The nozzle should be made of very hard material, for which various metal alloys and ceramic materials are used.

Important from the standpoint of spraying efficiency is the frequent and regular maintenance of sprayers, in particular the replacement of worn washers, pressure hose, nozzles and hose clips.

Essential requirements of spraying equipment are that it should be of a standard type, constructed of durable materials, with a standard lance and a cut-off valve that does not leak, thus ensuring the uniform application of insecticide with minimal risks of toxicity to sprayers. Specifications of hand-operated compression sprayers have been established by WHO (1971) and later revised (WHO, 1977). It is also important to make provision in advance for sufficient supplies of equipment and for ample spare parts and replacements to be available at all field depots. At least one person in each spraying team should be trained in the maintenance of equipment.

## Motorized knapsack mist blowers

Motorized knapsack mist blowers, powered by a small two-stroke (two-cycle) internal combustion engine, produce a high-velocity airstream (0.5 m³ air/minute) to a hand-directed, vertical nozzle. An airflow sucks the spray from a 1 L plastic container to the nozzle via a metering restrictor. The volume of liquid insecticide applied can be up to 350 mL/minute. These mist blowers are widely used in mosquito and tsetse fly control as they are the only type of portable equipment that can project spray into the eaves of houses or thickets around villages where exophilic vectors can occur. They are useful for areas that are difficult to access by road.

The vast majority of these machines have a recoil starter; however, some new machines are equipped with an electrical starter, which makes the engine easier to start. The main difficulties in starting occur because fuel mixture (oil and petrol) left in the engine after use evaporates, leaving an oily residue over the ignition plug, which prevents ignition. Also, the use of an incorrect fuel mixture can rapidly cause wear, especially when the engine is left idling. When sprayers are used without full air output, poor atomization of the spray liquid occurs. With poor atomization, droplets are generally far too large to be effective for vector operations, and there is increased fall-out of spray, contaminating the ground.

Constant output is dependent upon positive pressure in the tank, but this will not be achieved if, as often happens, the lid gasket has been affected by the insecticide formulation and no longer fits properly. Other components can also be adversely affected by some insecticide formulations, especially those used in ULV applications.

The spray operator walks along the street, directing the lance of the mist blower through the doors or windows. People working with these generators for long periods must wear ear protectors because of the high level of noise. There is a risk of burns from unguarded exhausts with some types of these machines, and proper precautions should be observed.

## Thermal foggers

These machines (Figure 6.28) are preferred in many vector control programmes, despite the extra cost, because the highly visible fog is psychologically more acceptable to the user and to those who wish to see that control operations are being carried out. Where thermal foggers are used, consideration should be given to increasing the concentration of insecticide and decreasing proportionally the flow rate, in order to reduce formulation costs. A reduction in flow rate will decrease fuel consumption in the combustion chamber as less heat is required to atomize the lower volume. Manufacturers of thermal foggers should be consulted on appropriate insecticide flow rates and combustion chamber temperature settings.

There is a potential fire hazard when thermal foggers are used, especially when the pulse-jet-type foggers are carried indoors. It is important that they are operated only by well-trained personnel using appropriate insecticide formulations and with access to a fire extinguisher. When manufacturers' instruc-

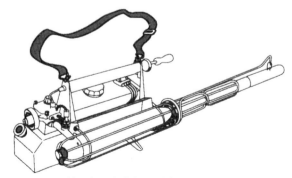

Hand-carried thermal fog generator.

**Figure 6.28** *A hand-carried thermal fog generator.*

tions are followed carefully, the fire risk with equipment that meets WHO specifications is minimal, because safety devices on the machines are designed to stop the flow of insecticide if the engine stops. The main advantage of the pulse-jet-type fogger is its simplicity of design and construction, as there are no rotating parts and no lubrication is required, but its loud noise can be objectionable and harmful to hearing unless suitable ear protection is used. Large pulse-jet-type foggers may be vehicle mounted, but it is usual, when treating extensive areas with fog, to use equipment with a rotary blower to move more hot gas through the nozzle and thus vaporize higher volumes of insecticide diluted in kerosene or a similar refined oil.

## Aerosol generators

Insecticidal aerosols are used for both indoor and outdoor space treatments for the control of adult vectors. The optimum droplet size range is 8–18 μm VMD. Some residual effectiveness may be achieved with high doses of persistent insecticides applied indoors because the small droplets eventually deposit on surfaces. Ground applications of aerosols alone may provide satisfactory vector control on a temporary basis for the interruption of disease transmission, but they are used principally as a supplement to other vector control methods.

Aerosol generators used to disperse insecticides are designed for the control of flying insect pests and vectors with ULV applications. One type uses a high volume of air at low pressure in a vortex nozzle to atomize concentrated or technical formulations of insecticide; other aerosol generators use high-pressure, low-volume airflow to atomize the insecticide, or a rotary nozzle driven by an electric motor. ULV applications, in which the minimum volume of liquid insecticide formulation is applied per unit area, provide maximum effectiveness against target vectors. Most organophosphorous insecticides can be applied as technical formulations, but other insecticides, such as carbamates and pyrethroids, must be formulated with compatible solvents for ULV application. These non-volatile formulations permit improved control of droplet size. (In contrast, thermal foggers may present a fire hazard and can contribute to environmental pollution through the production of exhaust gases. They also require

costly oil diluents and increased insecticide storage capacity, and entail higher formulation costs.)

Vehicle-mounted aerosol generators (Leco, Micro-Gen) are particularly useful in reducing the numbers of adult mosquitoes in urban and suburban areas with adequate access roads. Where roads are inadequate, hand-carried or knapsack-type aerosol generators are available. For adequate coverage inside open houses and other buildings, the vehicle-mounted equipment should be capable of discharging an aerosol cloud on either side of the vehicle; this discharge should extend more than 8 m from the vehicle. For outdoor space treatment, a swath at 100-m intervals should be achieved by wind dispersal of the cloud.

Although portable ULV aerosol generators are used primarily indoors or for small-scale applications outdoors, large-scale treatments can be carried out when several machines and operators are used in a team. In some circumstances, portable ULV aerosol generators are more efficient because the aerosol can be placed precisely into a dwelling, whereas virtually none of the aerosol cloud from vehicle-mounted equipment may penetrate the interior of dwellings.

The smaller hand-carried and shoulder-slung machines are usually powered by a two-cycle internal combustion engine, as on the knapsack mist blowers. These require more care in operation and maintenance than four-cycle engines, which are more reliable and convenient to use. The larger machines have a solvent-flushing system and remote control in the vehicle cab; thus, the operator has less direct contact with the insecticide.

Factors that need to be considered when choosing a method for the ground application of aerosols include: cost; efficiency; convenience and safety of operation and optimum timing of the spraying to obtain maximum impact on the target species; environmental impact; reliability, ease of maintenance, durability and availability of the equipment; insecticide formulations; fuel-oil diluents; and the availability of trained staff.

The ULV technique of applying insecticides proved to be a particularly useful and economical method of temporary control of adult mosquitoes. This method is based on the production by special machines (Buffalo Turbine and others) of insecticide droplets of 10–20 μm diameter for ground aerosols and 20–50 μm diameter for aerial sprays. The great advantage of the ULV technique is that the total amount of insecticide distributed per unit area is the same as or slightly less than that in thermal fogging, whereas the total volume of the carrier is very much less. Thus, about 0.5–1.0 L of the liquid carrier per hectare is sufficient and this results in great savings in the materials and labour involved.

Both thermal fogging and ULV spraying should be undertaken preferably at dawn or in the late evening because of thermal currents that build up during the day. The area to be treated should be divided into sections related to the desired frequency of spraying. ULV methods can cover a much greater area in a given time than any fogging units.

For indoor fogging, the usual formulation consists of 0.5 per cent pyrethrins, 1 per cent piperonyl butoxide in high-grade deodorized kerosene; the dosage is 25–30 mL/100 m³ of space. For outdoor application, 6 per cent malathion or 1 per cent DDVP in number 2 fuel oil is commonly used. Some liquid proprietary concentrations (e.g. Cythion) used for ULV sprays in populated areas may permanently damage paint on houses, boats, motorcars etc. To avoid this, the droplet size produced by the machines must be accurately determined and not exceed the VMD range of 50 μm.

It must not be concluded that the ULV methods briefly described in this section represent the best techniques for mosquito control, although they have been used in some projects in India, Indonesia, Venezuela and, more widely, in the USA. The difficulties encountered are: lack of uniformity of dosage of the insecticide and of coverage; high initial and recurrent costs; shortage of trained staff for maintenance and repair; and contamination of non-target areas.

## Dusting equipment

Although dusts contain only a small proportion of active ingredient, the main concern in the field is the risk of inhalation of insecticide particles smaller than 10 μm in diameter. This problem is accentuated if the equipment is carried in front of the operator, or if the operator walks into a cloud of dust. Nevertheless, in some situations, the application of dusts is considered to be important, particularly in emergencies such as epidemics.

The trend has been away from the use of heavy, well-constructed metal dusters to those made of plastic components. So far, there has been no feedback on the reliability of these machines in vector control.

With all the dusters that use a rotary blower, there are problems of metering the dust accurately.

One of the oldest types of dust and granule applicator is the 'horn seeder', originally used for sowing seeds. Early commercial versions used a metal horn fitted to a bag container, but new plastic versions have recently been marketed. Simple equipment of this type is useful for spreading larvicides on water surfaces, especially to control mosquito larvae.

## Household equipment

The simplest hand-operated atomizers (e.g. Flit guns), used for space spraying of pyrethrum solutions of bedrooms in the evening, need no elaborate description. They are composed of a pump, container and nozzle; they are often crudely made and easily damaged. The spray they produce is usually coarse and much of the insecticidal solution is wasted. Some better sprayers have a continuous (instead of an intermittent) action, which produces finer droplets, and are more effective. In using the simple sprayers, it is important to keep the nozzle upward during the operation and to start with the corners of the room, finishing in the centre. If there is a mosquito net for the bed of the treated room, it should be fitted over the bed before spraying; a few strokes should also be directed over the sides of the mosquito net. Moreover, one should be certain that the solution of insecticide (usually about 0.05–0.1 per cent of pyrethrum extract in kerosene with various synergists) is of good quality. The number of strokes required depends on the size of the room and the type of insecticide solution, but, on average, about 10 mL/30 m³ (about 1000 cubic feet) of space are generally adequate. To obtain the best effect of space spraying, the room should be closed during application and for 10–15 minutes afterwards.

### PRESSURIZED AEROSOL DISPENSERS AND SMOKES

At the present time, the hand-operated pumps have been largely replaced by aerosol dispensers that contain liquid insecticides under pressure of a liquefied gas. The amount of pressure and the size of the orifice of the container determine the rate of discharge of the liquid and its droplet size. The time required to produce an effective dosage of the insecticidal solution for a given volume of space is indicated by the manufacturers, although it averages 3–5 seconds/30 m³. The aerosol dispensers must always be operated in an upright position and kept away from excessive heat. There is increasing concern about the effect of the propellant gas on the ozone layer, and aerosols are being replaced increasingly by pump-action sprayers.

Smokes are special types of aerosols produced by a chemical mixed with an insecticide compound. Mosquito coils containing pyrethrum are produced in large numbers in eastern Asia. Each coil consists of a flat spiral of material that will smoulder slowly when lit; it releases smoke, which deters mosquitoes from entering the room and prevents them from biting. These coils are made of a vegetable filler, a starch-binding agent, and contain 0.1–0.4 per cent of natural or synthetic pyrethrins. More recently, electrically heated fumigation mats have become available, which last from 6 to 8 hours.

Other smoke generators, such as 'HCH bombs' for outdoor use, are of limited value because a proportion of the insecticide is decomposed by the heat.

## NETS AND SCREENS

In addition to household applications of insecticides by use of mosquito coils, fumigation mats and hand sprayers, and the use of nets and screens, there has been a recent trend towards the treatment of household materials such as wallpaper, plaster, mosquito nets and curtains. Pyrethroids have been widely tested in recent years for impregnating mosquito nets.

The treatment of mosquito nets is particularly suitable for community action within an integrated strategy for malaria control. The chemical treatment of netting is simple and can be conducted seasonally under the supervision of community health workers. There is potential for large-scale local manufacture of treated nets in areas where malaria is a major public health problem, particularly when nets can be made from local fibre. The use of treated mosquito nets should be integrated with other available methods, on the basis of comparisons of the cost effectiveness of each method in the particular epidemiological situation.

# Aircraft

Aerial space sprays are commonly used in agricultural practice and also occasionally in malaria control.

There are a number of aircraft especially suited for this purpose. Two different principles are employed. The solution of insecticide may be pumped or gravity-fed into a boom with nozzles along it. The spray so produced is further broken up by the slipstream of the aircraft or by a rotary atomizer. An alternative system, in which the insecticide is introduced into the exhaust of the aircraft's engine to produce a thermal aerosol, is less favoured because of some decomposition of the active compound. At the present time, the use of ULV atomizers has been generally adopted. Helicopters are increasingly used because of the down-draught of this type of aircraft and better distribution of the spray. As mentioned above, aerosol-generating machines and aircraft are of particular value when rapid elimination of mosquitoes from a relatively small area is needed, as in the case of epidemic outbreaks of a vector-borne disease.

Several types of atomizers are used for aerial ULV spraying. The most widely employed consist of a metal gauze cylinder rotating around a fixed spindle, which is attached to a bracket on the aircraft wing or to a boom designed for helicopter operation. The rotating power comes from the slipstream through a fan clamped in a hub that carries the bearing assembly. The pitch of the fan blades is adjustable, which controls the particle size of the insecticide solution, introduced through the hollow spindle under pressure and dispersed by a diffuser tube over the rotating gauze of the cylinder. Normally, four to six such units are mounted on the aircraft.

Another type of ULV atomizer uses an electrically driven, rotating multidisc. In this type, the particle size is independent of the speed of the aircraft; such atomizers are particularly suited for low-speed helicopter operations.

Aircraft have been used for the aerial application of insecticides for the past 50 years, but only recently on a larger scale. The early aircraft used occasionally for anti-mosquito spraying were standard military (such as the USA Air Force C-123 cargo) or commercial planes, equipped with a range of D2–13 nozzles on a boom at a 45° downward angle. This produced a 170-m swath at the flight altitude of 50–60 m. In some anti-mosquito spraying programmes, Twin Beech aircraft equipped with a boom carrying four Teejet 8004 nozzles, spraying at a pressure of 100 psi, and producing a 100-m swath at a height of 50–60 m were used. More commonly, in the USA the Stearman (PT-T7), in the UK and Canada the DHC-2 (Beaver), and in the former USSR the Antonov (AN-2M) were employed. Except in an absolutely flat country, four-engined, piston-driven aircraft have to fly much higher than twin-engined planes. Spraying at high altitudes produces a wide but uneven dispersion of insecticides, and a relatively small aircraft designed specifically for insecticide spraying is greatly superior. The Piper Pawnee (PA25) is now the most popular, but further developments in this field are in progress. The present technique of aerial spraying tends to decrease the size of the spray drops while maintaining the concentration in order to allow the spray to drift across wide swaths (ULV drift spraying). For large spraying programmes such as for tsetse and locust control, the Avro Anson was widely used, but now Piper Aztec, Beechcraft Baron, Cessna 310 and Britten-Norman Islander are increasingly popular. For vector control, aircraft need higher operating speeds than for agricultural work and thus must have special navigational instruments, flow meters and a 'black box' to record all the information on airspeed and height. The spraying equipment should be an integral part of the aircraft.

Helicopters have been used in some field projects, but they require special equipment such as a rotary nozzle that must be mounted behind and below the boom to minimize the effect of air turbulence.

Generally speaking, fixed-wing aircraft are to be preferred when high payload and speed are more important for the planned task. They are also less expensive to operate than helicopters, the latter have the advantage of good manoeuvrability, better delimitation of the coverage in population areas and safety of unprepared landing in any emergency.

Large-scale and emergency vector control programmes often benefit from the use of aircraft to apply chemicals. Aircraft are especially well suited for the rapid treatment of large areas or areas where wet soil, water, rough terrain or dense, woody vegetation prohibit or render impractical the use of ground or hand-carried equipment. The use of aircraft over or near populated areas, especially during daylight hours when adult insects are most vulnerable to chemical control, may create concern about safety and requires co-ordination with governmental agencies responsible for aviation safety.

Accurate placement of sprayed chemicals is usually more difficult from aircraft than with ground or hand-carried sprayers because many interacting factors affect the trajectory of the spray particles after

they are released. Therefore, the decision to use aerial sprays, as opposed to alternative methods, should be carefully considered, including safety, timeliness, cost, meteorological conditions, vector habitat and biological effectiveness, as well as the availability of suitable equipment, operational sites and trained crews.

Both fixed-wing aircraft and helicopters have been used successfully to apply larvicides rapidly to large and remote breeding areas. Such applications require precise targeting of the chemical, in either granular or liquid form, to ensure thorough coverage of the treated area and a high level of effectiveness. The remote location and inaccessibility of many of the breeding areas often make the use of ground personnel for flagging aircraft swaths impossible or impractical. There is a need for affordable electronic swath guidance systems for use on small fixed-wing aircraft and helicopters to increase the precision of application. Because breeding sites are often covered by dense canopies of vegetation, penetration by either liquid or dry particles to the breeding sites is often critical to the success of the application.

## Equipment for biological control

The biological agents considered over the years for malaria control are:

- fish, e.g. *Gambusia affinis*, *Poecilia reticulata* and *Tilapia* spp.
- bacteria, e.g. *Bacillus thuringiensis* serotype H-14 (*B.t.* H-14), *B. sphaericus*
- nematodes, e.g. *Romanomermis culicivorax*, *R. jingdeensis*, *R. iyengari*, *Octomyomermis muspratti*
- predatory mosquitoes, e.g. *Toxorhynchites* spp.

The most promising have been bacteria and fish. Nematodes have a potential use in specific situations, but their use requires mass rearing facilities and mass handling of live parasites. The use of predatory mosquitoes has not been particularly useful because the breeding habits of the predators rarely coincide with those of anopheline vectors.

### EQUIPMENT FOR THE APPLICATION OF INSECT PATHOGENS

The use of formulations of *B. thuringiensis* in operational programmes is limited due to its short residual effect. However, improved formulations with longer residual effect are being developed. *B. sphaericus*, on the other hand, can multiply in polluted habitats rich in organic matter, giving extended periods of mosquito control, but its value for *Anopheles* has not been well demonstrated. All the bacteria for vector control form spores and potent, stable toxins and can be stored for long periods. They can be formulated as suspensions, wettable powders and dusts for easy application with conventional equipment.

The equipment required for application of *B.t.* H-14 and *B. sphaericus* will vary according to the formulation used. Compression sprayers or other sprayers used for chemical control can be used to apply particulate suspensions. Granular formulations, including those using corn cob as a base, are usually applied by hand, although the horn seeder and knapsack dusters can be used. Briquettes can be applied by hand, but where there is running water, especially in rice fields, the larvicide may be introduced using a constant-flow dripping device. Such a device can be connected directly to the formulation container and the rate of application adjusted either by a stopcock or a flow control with different sized holes. The aerial application of *B.t.* H-14 to large bodies of water has been carried out in the USA for mosquito control. For this operation, light planes were fitted with a hydraulic spray system and cone nozzles (D6 and D12 type).

In the Onchocerciasis Control Programme in West Africa, special formulations have been developed for the aerial application of *B.t.* H-14 to large rivers for the control of blackflies. The latest formulations are applied by helicopter (cross-river) or by fixed-wing planes, with a discharge of up to 200 m$^3$/second, during the dry season in rivers by dropping predetermined quantities of the formulation upstream of the target area. The river's current disperses the formulation to the breeding sites.

## EQUIPMENT FOR REARING, TRANSPORTING AND DISTRIBUTING LARVIVOROUS FISH

Larvivorous fish have been used extensively. Indigenous species should be selected wherever feasible as they are adapted to local conditions and are less likely to have an adverse ecological impact. Laboratory evaluations of indigenous larvivorous fish have shown that they can be highly effective in mosquito control. Fish can also be employed at low cost and can be used at the village level, with community participation.

*Gambusia affinis, Tilapia* spp. and *Poecilia reticulata* are most often used for larval control, mainly against *Anopheles* and, to some extent, against *Culex* and *Aedes* spp.

The advantage of biological vector control is that the predators that are used can be produced and reared within the local community. The equipment needed for production and rearing, i.e. tanks, aerators and nets, is simple and can be manufactured or bought locally.

Wherever possible, suitable local fish species should be utilized for larvicidal programmes. Because transport distances and times will then be relatively short, the need for sophisticated equipment is reduced.

Fish should preferably be reared in their natural habitats or, if this is not practicable, in specially prepared breeding ponds, which can be simply constructed according to accepted fish farming practices. Where the soil is pervious, a plastic sheet or cement lining may be necessary.

Fish can be collected using conventional netting techniques, involving a 'butterfly' net of 60–90 cm in diameter, a sweep net stretched between two sticks, or other traditional methods. Care must be exercised to avoid injury to the fish. The fish can be transported in any convenient carrying device, e.g. buckets with provision to avoid spillage, or plastic bags about half full with water. Containers should be protected from heat and bright sunlight. No other special measures are necessary for journeys lasting for less than about 4 hours. Beyond this time, the container should be insulated, the water may be chilled by the addition of ice and provision must be made for aeration or oxygenation. Naturally occurring water should be used for transport and topping up. The fish can be dispersed manually.

## Equipment for environmental management

Environmental management, using appropriate equipment, is a principal measure in integrated disease control. The major modifications and manipulations are land filling, land clearance, drainage, waterway construction and maintenance, land forming, weed control, pumping, reservoir operation and salt-marsh management. Such activities should not preclude community planning and collaboration with government or private agencies.

The advantages of environmental management are that they are long-lasting and not damaging to the environment, and that they minimize the need for the application of insecticides. Environmental management measures in vector control vary from regular maintenance of small-scale, existing schemes to large-scale or emergency activities. The equipment required may range from simple, easily available, hand-held, lightweight tools to heavy, sophisticated machinery. The selection of the appropriate equipment must be based on the needs and resources of the programme. Local leaders, professionals and community representatives should participate in establishing the selection criteria.

The main criteria to be considered when specific equipment for environmental management for vector control is being selected include (but are not necessarily limited to): durability of equipment; reliability; operation and maintenance costs; the capability of local technicians or residents to operate and maintain the equipment; environmental compatibility; effectiveness; safety; and cost effectiveness.

## LIGHT MACHINERY

Members of local communities can contribute a wide range of skills and equipment of great potential value in environmental management. Skills in carpentry, ironwork and farming will usually be available. Equipment will include a range of agricultural tools and machines, which, depending on the local farming system, may be operated by hand, by animals or by tractor. The use of available equipment and skills will encourage local understanding and participation in environmental management, and will also bring economic benefits to the community. The infrastructure to support the continuing use of the equipment will already exist in large measure. Through the use of local skills, equipment and services, the community will realize that it is able to execute and maintain environmental management works from its own resources. This process is an important advantage of community-based methods and is the basis for the pride of community ownership and understanding that make such programmes long-lasting.

The equipment available will mostly be light agricultural machinery, ranging from hand tools to equipment drawn by tractors of up to about 50 kW (65 hp). In many rural communities, the hoe is the most widely available tool and is used in a wide range of operations such as land clearance, soil preparation, formation and maintenance of ditches and bunds etc. Other widely available hand tools include the machete, spade, sickle and various forms of rakes or levelling boards. A hand-operated winch, which may have to be purchased, is able to clear large trees at lower cost than heavy tractor-driven land-clearing machines and with less environmental disturbance.

There is a wide range of activities to which animal-drawn equipment might be able to contribute. Equipment that can be used with tractors of low to medium power, much of which may already be in use locally, includes the bulldozer blade, heavy-duty cultivator (which may be used as a light ripper), land leveller, scraper, bund former, trailer and various types of cultivation equipment such as the plough or rotary hoe. Other tractor-drawn equipment of a more specialized nature, which may not be in local use but is readily obtainable through commercial channels, includes ditch formers, ditch cleaners and trenchers used for laying underground drainage pipes.

The applications for which this equipment would need to be used include land clearance, drainage, soil preparation, soil movement, land forming, waterway construction, waterway maintenance and vegetation control.

## HEAVY MACHINERY

Community environmental management programmes should use to the fullest extent the equipment and human resources available locally. However, when local resources are not sufficient, there may be a need to look beyond the community.

Major construction and maintenance work requiring the use of large machines should be considered only after careful planning and design of the project and in the light of a complete understanding of the vector ecology. Some large machines that have been used successfully are backhoes, draglines, excavators, bulldozers, rotary ditchers and mowers.

## DOMESTIC EQUIPMENT

Several simple measures for the improvement of housing, such as plastering of walls, screening of houses, installation of roof and wastewater drains, collection of solid waste and proper disposal of refuse, should be included in the basic community approach to vector control.

Many mosquitoes, particularly some *Aedes* species, which are vectors of arboviral diseases, breed in a wide variety of water storage tanks and vessels, discarded containers and other scrap materials. Screens and other materials have been used successfully to cover water storage containers to prevent mosquitoes breeding in them. In both urban and rural communities, only an efficient refuse collection and disposal service can reduce the tremendous number of discarded containers that provide sources of mosquito production. Refuse can be disposed of by burial, incineration or composting, using hand tools such as shovels, picks and wheelbarrows. Community vehicles such as donkey carts can be used for the collection and disposal of refuse.

## WATER MANAGEMENT DEVICES

Technical devices that have been successfully used in water management as part of vector control programmes are diesel and electric pumps, pipes and culverts, gates, gate valves and weirs, siphons, artesian wells and porous drains.

## TECHNIQUE OF RESIDUAL SPRAYING

In view of the importance of correct technique for the application of residual insecticides, some details of the relevant practice may be of value. Knowledge of the number, location and accessibility of the houses and field shelters is of great importance and this is the real aim of geographical reconnaissance or, more currently, geographical information systems (GIS), which should be carried out during the preparatory phase of the programme and kept up to date as much as possible.

The main data to be provided by geographical reconnaissance or GIS are as follows.

- The extent of the area must be clearly known: maps showing the location of villages, roads and other features must be available; if not, they should be prepared by a properly trained team.
- The number, type and size of dwellings and other sprayable structures must be identified and recorded.
- The mean sprayable surface per dwelling must be calculated, in order to know the amount of insecticide needed for one spray round. This is done by measuring the walls and ceilings of a sample of dwellings.
- The maps are useful for preparing itineraries and for plotting the location of villages, houses and roads for the squad leaders to follow. Each dwelling should receive a reference number, painted on the

wall or on the door, to enable the spraying-squad leaders to check the work done.

- Information on the population in each locality is important, for epidemiological evaluation of the prevalence of malaria and any subsequent changes.
- The timing of spraying operations is important: in areas with a short transmission period, the spraying should be planned so that it is completed before the onset of the high activity of the vector. Certain customs and cultural patterns of the local population must be taken into consideration. Replastering of indoor walls, whitewashing, smoke deposits, re-thatching etc. may greatly decrease or nullify the insecticidal effect and require changes of spraying routine or additional spraying.
- Population movements related to seasonal migration, planting, harvesting and cattle grazing may result in locked houses or the building of temporary shelters away from the locality; this would often require special insecticide applications.

The spraying is done at stated intervals. The operation of spraying in one locality is known as the spraying round; the spraying of all houses in a given area, repeated at regular intervals, is known as the spraying cycle. Focal spraying is limited to a group of houses forming a distinct focus of transmission. The progress of spraying operations is measured by comparing the number of houses sprayed and localities, with the totals included in the programmes. Special measures are put into action to ensure the complete spraying of all houses, localities and the area involved.

## Dosage

The dosage is the amount of insecticide applied to a unit of indoor surface of the inhabited or other premise; it is expressed in terms of grams of active compound per square metre of surface ($g/m^2$). Dosages and cycles must be determined according to local conditions and depend on the results of an entomological study of the habits of the vector species. Each type of residual insecticide requires an optimum dosage, depending on the toxicity of the compound to the mosquito, the type of surface to which it is applied (wood, adobe, thatch), climatic conditions and the transmission season. If the last-mentioned is of short duration (3–4 months), one spraying cycle per year may be sufficient. Dried-mud (adobe) surfaces usually decrease the duration of insecticidal effect, whereas wood increases it markedly.

The total amount of the insecticide formulation required for each spraying round depends on the dosage. For example, if a group of villages had 10 000 houses, each averaging 200 $m^2$ of sprayable surface, requiring a dosage of DDT at 2 $g/m^2$, the total amount of the active compound needed would be 4000 kg. However, if the formulation consists of 75 per cent water-dispersible powder, then 6000 kg of the formulation will be required. Usually, about 10 per cent of the product is added to cover possible waste or spillage; thus, the total amount to be supplied would be 6600 kg per spray round (Table 6.7).

## Personnel

The personnel required for a spraying operation depend on the size of the proposed activity and on the intended degree of supervision and evaluation. Normally, the whole area is divided into sectors, with a sector chief in charge. The sector chief's responsibilities include the preparation of work schedules, maintenance of personnel rosters, checking on performance, filling in spraying reports, ordering of supplies, co-ordination of transport, public relations etc. The squad leaders should be responsible to the sector chief.

The basic field unit for carrying out a spraying operation is a spraying squad, which consists of two to six spraypersons and a squad leader. The predetermined area of work and itinerary must be

**Table 6.7** *Quantities of formulations for standard spraying*[a]

| Insecticide | Formulation | Active content (%) | Dilution for field use[b] | Remarks |
|---|---|---|---|---|
| DDT | WDP | 50 | 90 g/L (14 oz/gallon) | Imperial gallons (4.5 L) throughout |
| DDT | WDP | 75 | 60 g/L (9.5 oz/gallon) | |
| DDT | LC | 20 | 1 part to 3.5 parts kerosene or water | Kerosene for solutions, water for EC |
| HCH | WDP | 25 | 40 g/L (6 oz/gallon) | |
| HCH | WDP | 50 | 20 g/L (3 oz/gallon) | |
| HCH | LC | 20 | 1 part to 22 parts kerosene or water | Kerosene for solutions, water for EC |
| Malathion | WDP | 50 | 90 g/L (14 oz/gallon of water) | For dosage 1 $g/m^2$ double the water |
| Malathion | WDP | 25 | 180 g/L (28 oz/gallon of water) | For dosage 1 $g/m^2$ double the water |
| Malathion | EC | 20 | 1 part to 4 parts of water | For dosage 1 $g/m^2$ double the water |
| Lambda-cyhalothrin | WDP | 10 | 7.5 g/L | |
| Lambda-cyhalothrin | EC | 2.5 | 1 part to 50 parts water | |
| Bendiocarb | WDP | 80 | 10 g/L | One preweighed sachet added to water in standard spray-pump gives required dosage as spray suspension |
| Pyrimiphos-methyl | EC | 50 | 1 part to 10 parts water | For dosage 1 $g/m^2$ double the water |
| Fenitrothion | WDP | 40 | 112 g/L | |
| Fenitrothion | EC | 20 | 1 part to 4 parts water | |
| Permethrin | WDP | 25 | 45 g/L | |
| Permethrin | EC | 25 | 1 part to 20 parts water | |
| Deltamethrin | WDP | 6 | 22 g/L | |

[a] This table indicates the quantity of different formulations required to prepare 1 gallon (4.5 L) of diluted spray for application using a sprayer with an average spraying rate of 1 gallon per 1000 $ft^2$ of surface (4.5–5.0 L/100 $m^2$) to obtain the usual application rates of DDT 2 $g/m^2$, dieldrin 0.5 $g/m^2$ and malathion 2 $g/m^2$.
[b] The generally used standard type of sprayer operating at the recommended pressure and with the usual nozzle aperture allows the sprayman to cover 1000 $ft^2$ or close to 100 $m^2$ of treated surface in the time required to deliver 1 gallon (4.5 L) of diluted spray.
WDP is water-dispersable powder; LC is liquid concentrate; EC is emulsion concentrate.

established in advance. The task of the spraypersons consists of proper application of the insecticide formulation to all sprayable surfaces of all the dwelling units and other premises in the locality. This must often include animal sheds and temporary field shelters away from the centre of the village. The number of spraying personnel required depends on the number of houses that one sprayman can deal with in a day, but also on many other factors, such as accessibility, number of rooms, distances between villages etc. As an average, it can be stated that one sprayman can treat eight to 10 houses, with a 200 m$^2$ surface, in a day. Therefore, in a month of 22 working days, some 500–600 houses can be sprayed by a squad of three spraypersons with one squad leader. In addition to the squad leader, a squad often has a mixer to prepare the spray, to fill the sprayers, to help with moving the furniture, stored water and food out of the house, to clean up at the end of the day etc. A tentative calculation for spraying 10 000 houses every 4 months is that it would require five to six squads, each with a squad leader and one sector chief, making a total of 25–30 people, not counting drivers of vehicles.

## Spraying

Although residual insecticides may be applied by a variety of spraying equipment, the hand-operated compression sprayer continues to be the most effective and commonly used method. The five factors governing the application of a uniform dosage rate are:

1. the insecticide concentration in the liquid
2. the air pressure in the sprayer
3. the nozzle aperture
4. the distance from the nozzle tip to the sprayed surface
5. the speed of application to the surface.

The need for total coverage was of particular importance in malaria eradication campaigns, for which it was rigidly observed. However, in malaria control projects, a more flexible approach can be adopted, adjusting the type of coverage by residual insecticides to epidemiological conditions and entomological assessment of results. The following modifications may be considered:

- Selective spraying of ceilings, parts of the walls and other parts of the house where *Anopheles* mosquitoes rest may be effective, with a consequent saving of insecticide.
- Focal coverage of villages, groups of buildings or parts of the area closest to the main breeding places of vectors will give a measure of control while at the same time reducing the workload of available staff.
- Barrier spraying of groups of houses or of a concentric zone of dwellings at the perimeter of the protected area may intercept the influx of vector mosquitoes from the non-controlled outer area. It may be preferable to spray the inner area if there is evidence of a marked influx from outside. Partial coverage may exclude from spraying those buildings that are not inhabited, such as grain stores, shops, schools, etc.

## Involvement of the population

Involvement of the population is essential. The people in an area to be treated should be involved in the planning of the spray programme, be given adequate warning of the day and time of spraying, be asked to ensure that as many houses as possible are open, foodstuffs removed or covered, and furniture pulled out into the middle of the rooms (Figure 6.29). Spraypersons must be accompanied by a responsible local resident whose main function is to secure co-operation and vouch for the safety of people and property in the houses treated, as without their support future work may be hampered by misunderstandings. After spraying, a printed form should be left on the indoor wall of the house, with the date of spraying and the date of the next visit, which gives needed information to inspectors checking the work and to the householder about provision for the next spraying.

The public response may be that of suspicion in the early stages, but this soon gives way to active collaboration when they are genuinely involved in the programme and the benefits become apparent. For the most part, such schemes run smoothly if well planned, organized and implemented.

## Transport

Transport facilities for moving equipment, materials and personnel play an important part in most vector control programmes. In developing countries, vehicles

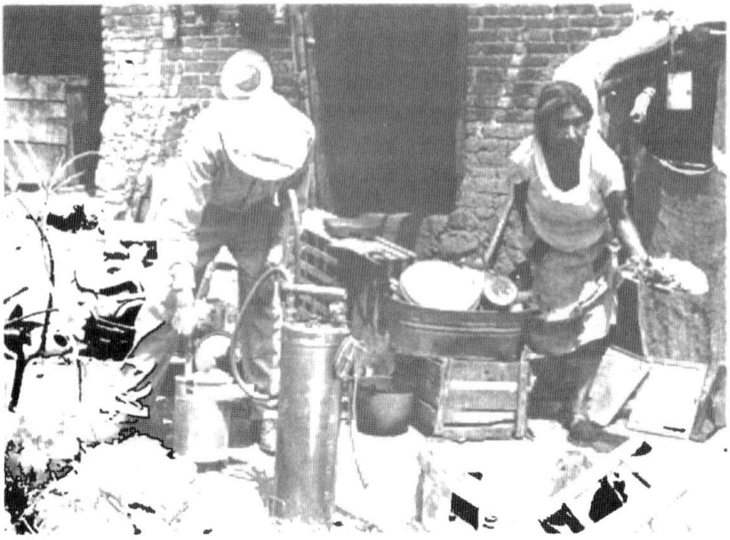

**Figure 6.29** *Temporary removal of part of the furniture and food supplies from dwellings before residual spraying begins. The involvement of local inhabitants in this procedure is an important factor. (WHO photograph by E Schwab.)*

must generally be imported and delays in receiving them can seriously impede the planned operations, which are timed to coincide with an appropriate season of the year. Several months may occur between placing the orders and the arrival of the vehicles, but even then, the delivery may be delayed by various customs formalities. Similar delays may occur in the delivery of spare parts. It is essential that all vehicle service centres have an experienced mechanic and are provided with workshop manuals and proper tools. Drivers should receive adequate training and perform simple maintenance tasks. The type of transport facilities required in developing countries may range from bicycles to four-wheel vehicles and boats. Detailed assessment of the type of transport and quantities needed must be made at an early stage of planning so that the specific needs of the programme are taken into account (Figure 6.30).

## Entomology

As the residual spraying aims specifically at the adult anopheline vectors of malaria, it is evident that the role of entomological methods in measuring the impact on the target insect is of importance. The choice and interpretation of the results of sampling of the vector population are the responsibility of an experienced professional entomologist, with the aid of auxiliary personnel. Baseline data collected before the start of control will have provided information

on the vector species concerned, its distribution, behaviour, susceptibility to the insecticide etc.

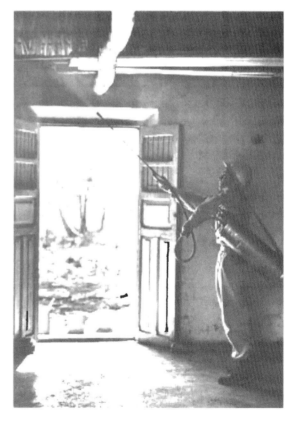

**Figure 6.30** *Residual house spraying as carried out in the state of Yucatán in Mexico. (WHO photograph by P Almasy.)*

After the first and subsequent spray rounds, entomology provides information on:

- the impact of the spraying on the vector population
- the duration of the insecticidal effect
- the need for alteration in the spray cycles and rounds
- the need to change the insecticide dosage
- the need to change insecticides because of incipient resistance or other problems
- changes in mosquito behaviour induced by insecticidal exposure
- incidental effects on domestic animals and insects such as bedbugs, cockroaches, fleas and flies
- harmful effects on beneficial insects (honey bees, silkworms).

Many sampling methods for *Anopheles* have been used, and only the briefest mention of them can be given here. They vary from the measuring of indoor resting densities (by the spray-sheet method), through outdoor resting densities (collections in natural or artificial resting places), to the use of window-exit traps, indoor and outdoor biting collections on human or animal bait, bioassay tests (exposing samples of 20–25 mosquitoes in a plastic, conical chamber held against the treated wall), to testing vector susceptibility in contact with a known dosage of insecticide (WHO, 1976).

## RESISTANCE OF MOSQUITOES TO INSECTICIDES

### General considerations

Resistance to insecticides has been defined as the 'ability of a population of insects to tolerate doses of an insecticide which would prove lethal to the majority of individuals in a normal population of the same species'. It is understood that this biological phenomenon develops as a result of selection pressure by the relevant insecticidal compound or its analogue.

The above definition refers to what is known as physiological resistance affecting the direct mortality of a proportion of a population of insects exposed to the toxic compound. Another, different, aspect of this phenomenon is the change of behaviour pattern of a population of insects, so that they acquire the ability to avoid contact with the insecticide. This

phenomenon is known as 'behaviouristic resistance' or 'insecticide avoidance'.

Both types of resistance may interfere with the results of malaria control measures, especially when the main method comprises residual insecticide spraying. Although 'physiological resistance' is by far the most important of the two and more easily measurable, 'insecticide avoidance' can become an obstacle to malaria control. The efficacy of indoor residual spraying depends, among other things, on the feeding and resting habits of the vector. Obviously, any changes in the house-entry pattern, a shift to outdoor biting to avoid insecticide-treated surfaces, and exophilic and exophagic tendencies will affect the result of the control programme. This has been observed in some species of the *A. gambiae* complex in Africa, in *A. nuneztovari* in Venezuela, *A. punctulatus* in New Guinea, *A. farauti* in the Solomon Islands, *A. dirus* and *A. minimus* in Thailand, *A. balabacensis* in Bangladesh and *A. philippinensis* in India. It is not certain that this change of behaviour is due to a specific selection pressure of the insecticide.

Changes in the environment have also been shown to alter the ecology of various vector species. For example, urbanization development activities and insecticide use have led to a decline in the density of *A. culicifacies* in India; other studies have shown that *A. stephensi* has assumed importance in areas where water is stored in tanks and wells and, although essentially endophilic, this species was found to rest outdoors in southern Iran and southern India.

In Afghanistan, agricultural development led to the replacement of *A. pulcherrimus*, an established vector, by *A. hyrcanus*, which was found to be resistant to DDT and also exophilic and exophagic. Observations in Kisumu, Kenya, revealed that, before spraying with the insecticide fenitrothion, *A. gambiae* was the dominant species and was more endophilic than *A. arabiensis*, although the two species did not differ in infectivity and host preferences. After spraying, the density of both species was reduced, but there were increases in the degree of exophily and the relative proportion of *A. arabiensis*. In Ethiopia, *A. gambiae s.l.* and *A. funestus* have been shown to be partly exophilic, whereas *A. pharoensis* and *A. nili* were strongly exophilic. *A. aconitus* in Central Java or Indonesia was found mostly resting outdoors and the endophilic fraction rested only on the lower parts of walls, so that effective control could be achieved by selective spraying of the lower portion of the walls only.

Although the physiological resistance of *Anopheles* to DDT was recognized as a potentially serious problem 55 years ago, the impact of this phenomenon on malaria control and eradication has only become fully obvious during the past two decades.

The extension of resistance from DDT to other chlorinated hydrocarbons (HCH and dieldrin) led to the use of these compounds being abandoned in many parts of the world. The alternative use of organophosphorous and carbamate insecticides proved to be expensive, and few developing tropical countries are able to afford it without external help. Moreover, mosquito vectors have developed a degree of resistance to several newer insecticides, and particularly those widely used in agriculture. Research on and development of new insecticidal compounds are expensive and increasingly difficult, and therefore the possibility of having a vast array of valuable compounds in the immediate future is not very likely. Nevertheless, even in the present, less than satisfactory, situation, the available insecticides, if properly selected and used, can still decrease malaria transmission.

## Nature and cause of resistance

Much research in the laboratory and in the field has been devoted to our understanding of the nature and mechanism of the development of resistance. Only the briefest review of this complex problem can be given here.

The multiple factors that influence the development of resistance to insecticides in a population of mosquitoes can be classified into genetic (e.g. the presence of specific genes and their frequency), operational (e.g. the type of insecticide and its method of application) and biological (e.g. the size and characteristics of the insect population). Resistance to insecticides does not arise through a process of gradual adaptation of mosquitoes to a toxic compound. It is a speeded-up process of Darwinian selection, which can occur when, in the original population of mosquitoes, there was a small proportion of mutant individuals genetically endowed with the capacity to withstand (at least partly) the toxic action of the insecticidal compound (Table 6.8).

Such a protective mechanism may depend on a single genetic factor, which is recessive, partially dominant or dominant in the process of inheritance. Resistant individuals are rare when they first appear in the heterozygous state in a mosquito population. Heterozygotes that survive the contact with the insecticide (which gradually eliminates the susceptible mosquitoes) mate with other heterozygotes and produce a proportion of homozygotes, with a higher degree of resistance. If the resistance gene is dominant, it will spread rapidly through the whole population.

Some types of resistance are due to a single gene, whereas other types are related to several genes. Studies that revealed that certain types of resistance can be assigned to specific loci on the chromosomes of relevant mosquitoes allowed us to distinguish between different biochemical mechanisms of resistance. Whereas some such mechanisms involve detoxification by enzymatic processes of the chemical compound, other mechanisms are due to the change of the site of the toxic action or reduced penetration of the toxicant. These largely unknown protective mechanisms may be specific for a particular compound or active against several compounds. They probably depend on the reduced penetration and increased detoxification of the given chemical poison.

When resistance due to the selection of one or more genes by a certain insecticide extends to other chemical compounds, we are dealing with the phenomenon of cross-resistance. The spectrum of cross-resistance may be narrow, as in the case of the cyclodiene group (HCH, dieldrin), or it may be wide, also covering other groups (e.g. organophosphate compounds). It has been known for some time that resistance to DDT caused by the action of the *kdr* gene also imparts cross-resistance to pyrethroid insecticides. It was subsequently demonstrated that selection of mosquitoes by pyrethroids confers or enhances resistance to DDT.

Resistance to carbamates and organophosphorous compounds in *A. albimanus* in Central America is primarily caused by the selection of acetylcholinesterase that is less sensitive to the action of these chemicals. The mechanism was later also found in *A. sacharovi*, *A. atroparvus* and *A. nigerrimus*. In most instances, it has produced a broad spectrum of resistance to many organophosphorous and carbamate insecticides. The low levels of resistance to fenthion of *A. albimanus* and of *A. sacharovi* to malathion are notable exceptions.

A distinction between monogenic resistance and the more complex polygenic type is important, as the former is more amenable to countermeasures such

**Table 6.8** *Insecticide resistance in 34* Anopheles *that play an important role in malaria transmission, as reported by the WHO*

| Species | DDT | Organophosphate compounds | Other compounds |
|---|---|---|---|
| *A. aconitus* | Bangladesh, India, Indonesia, Nepal, Thailand | — | — |
| *A. albimanus* | Belize, Colombia, Costa, Rica, Cuba, Dominican Republic, Ecuador, Guatemala, El Salvador, Haiti, Honduras, Mexico, Nicaragua, Panama | Costa Rica, El Salvador, Guatemala, Honduras, Mexico, Nicaragua | Costa Rica, El Salvador, Ecuador, Guatemala, Haiti, Honduras, Panama |
| *A. albitarsis* | Brazil, Colombia | — | — |
| *A. annularis* | Bangladesh, India, Myanmar, Nepal, Pakistan, Thailand | Sri Lanka | — |
| *A. arabiensis* | Ethiopia, Mauritius, Saudi Arabia, Senegal, Sudan, Swaziland, United Republic of Tanzania (Zanzibar) | Sudan | Sudan |
| *A. atroparvus* | Portugal, Roumania, Spain, Portugal, UK, former USSR | Portugal, Spain | Portugal, Roumania, Spain |
| *A. barbirostris* | Myanmar, India, Indonesia, Sri Lanka | Sri Lanka | — |
| *A. coustani* | Egypt, La Reunion, Saudi Arabia | Egypt | — |
| *A. culicifacies complex* | Afghanistan, Bhutan, India, Islamic Republic of Iran, Myanmar, Nepal, Oman, Pakistan, Sri Lanka, Thailand | India, Oman, Pakistan, Sri Lanka, United Arab Emirates | India, Oman, Sri Lanka,United Arab Emirates |
| *A. darling* | Colombia, Venezuela | — | — |
| *A. d'thali* | Islamic Republic of Iran | Egypt, Jordan | Egypt |
| *A. farauti* | Solomon Islands | — | — |
| *A. fluviatilis* | Afghanistan, India, Nepal, Pakistan | — | Nepal |
| *A. funestus* | Sudan | — | — |
| *A. gambiae sensu stricto* | Benin, Burkina Faso, Cameroon, Central African Republic, Congo, Ghana, Liberia, Mali, Niger, Nigeria, South Africa, United Republic of Tanzania (Zanzibar), Togo, Zaire | — | Nigeria (only in the laboratory) |
| *A. hyrcanus* | Afghanistan, Myanmar, Pakistan, Turkey, former USSR | Turkey | Turkey |
| *A. labranchiae* | Algeria, Morocco, Tunisia | Italy | — |
| *A. maculatus* | Bhutan, India, Myanmar, Nepal, Pakistan, Thailand | — | — |
| *A. maculipennis* | Bulgaria, Greece, Islamic Republic of Iran, Roumania, Turkey, former USSR | Turkey, Greece, Roumania | Bulgaria, Greece, Roumania, Turkey |
| *A. minimus* | Thailand | — | — |
| *A. nigerrimus* | India, Indonesia, Myanmar, Pakistan, Sri Lanka, Thailand | India, Sri Lanka | Sri Lanka |
| *A. pharoensis* | Angola, Egypt, Ethiopia, Sudan | Egypt | Egypt |
| *A. philippinenesis* | Myanmar, Thailand | — | — |
| *A. pseudopunctipennis* | Bolivia, Guatemala, Honduras, Mexico, Panama, Peru | Guatemala, Honduras | Guatemala, Honduras |
| *A. pulcherrimus* | Afghanistan, Iraq, Pakistan, Saudi Arabia, former USSR | — | — |
| *A. punctimacula* | Colombia, Ecuador | — | — |
| *A. quadrimaculatus* | Mexico, USA | USA | USA |
| *A. sacharovi* | Bulgaria, Greece, Islamic Republic of Iran, Lebanon, Syrian Arab Republic, Turkey, former USSR | Bulgaria, Greece, Lebanon, Syrian Arab Republic | Bulgaria, Lebanon, Syrian Arab Republic |

**Table 6.8** *(Continued)*

| Species | DDT | Organophosphate compounds | Other compounds |
|---------|-----|---------------------------|-----------------|
| *A. sergentii* | Egypt | Egypt, Jordan | — |
| *A. sinensis* | China, Japan, Nepal, Vietnam | China, Hong Kong, Japan, Republic of Korea | — |
| *A. stephensi* | Afghanistan, India, Oman, Iraq, Pakistan, Islamic Republic of Iran, Yemen, United Arab Emirates | India, Iraq, Islamic Republic of Iran, Pakistan | Dubai, India, Pakistan |
| *A. subpictus* | Afghanistan, Bangladesh, India, Indonesia, Myanmar, Nepal, Pakistan, Sri Lanka, Vietnam | India, Sri Lanka | Sri Lanka (only larvae) |
| *A. sundaicus* | Indonesia, Malaysia, Thailand, Vietnam | — | — |
| *A. superpictus* | Afghanistan, former USSR | — | — |
| *A. vagus* | Bangladesh, India, Indonesia, Malaysia, Myanmar, Nepal, Sri Lanka, Thailand, Vietnam | Sri Lanka | Sri Lanka |

*Note.* This list, based on data provided by the WHO in the Technical Report Series Nos 737 (WHO, 1986c), 813 (WHO, 1991) and 818 (WHO, 1992d), refers only to the most important vectors of malaria. It should be remembered that in each of the species quoted the phenomenon of resistance and its degree do not cover the whole geographical area of distribution of the species concerned. Information on the latter point will be found in the reports quoted above.

as the addition of synergists or change to a different insecticide.

The insecticide selection pressure depends also on the relative toxicity of the compound, the degree of coverage of the area, the developmental stage and density of the mosquito population, the number of generations exposed, the behaviour characteristics of the respective species of mosquitoes, and many genetic factors. Resistance to dieldrin (and HCH) is more common and develops more rapidly than DDT resistance, because the former is of a higher degree and because the gene for dieldrin resistance is fully or partially dominant. On the other hand, the DDT resistance is of a lower degree and recessive in its genetic expression. Even if DDT resistance in *Anopheles* is confirmed, its development may be slow and the continued use of DDT may still have a sufficient impact on the mosquito population to achieve a fair degree of control.

Insecticide resistance often develops within a small part of the population of one species of *Anopheles* and assumes different patterns, depending on the type of selection pressure. Thus, *A. funestus* populations in a few parts of Africa show only dieldrin – HCH resistance, without any other chemical group being involved.

A multiple resistance pattern covering organochlorines, organophosphates and carbamates is rare, but has been described in some populations of *A. albimanus*, *A. atroparvus* and *A. sacharovi*. This is generally due to the widespread use of various insecticides for the control of agricultural pests in neighbouring areas and severe contamination of anopheline breeding places. Knowledge of the genetic factors involved in insecticide resistance allows one to make some predictions about the speed of its selection and the ways to avoid it, if possible.

## Determination of resistance

The standardized WHO method entails a comparison of the mortality of a number of female *Anopheles* of a known species exposed in special tubes to filter papers impregnated with various concentrations of a given insecticide dissolved in mineral oil (Figure 6.31). Some comments on the criteria and interpretation of tests for vector resistance to insecticides will be of practical value.

The detection and measurement of this phenomenon are based on the comparison with a strain of the *Anopheles* species of normal susceptibility, tested under similar conditions. Preferably, the response of the susceptible strain should be known before the control campaign, but it may be possible to compare the results of tests in treated and untreated areas.

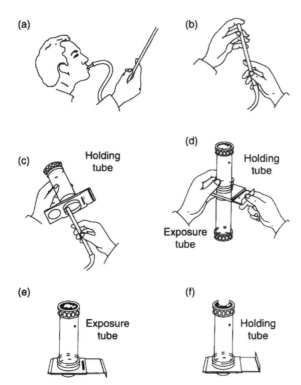

parallel to the line seen in susceptible strains, the sample exhibits only a higher tolerance, due to the physiological condition of the mosquitoes (gravid) or to microclimatic factors of the test.

A simpler test has been widely used. It consists of exposing samples of *Anopheles* to a single diagnostic concentration of a given insecticide on impregnated papers prepared by the WHO. These diagnostic concentrations, which kill all susceptible *Anopheles*, are: DDT 4 per cent, dieldrin 0.4 per cent, malathion 5 per cent, propoxur 0.1 per cent and fenitrothion 1 per cent. They require the exposure of mosquitoes in special plastic tubes for 1 hour, with the exception of fenitrothion, which needs 2 hours' exposure. The proportion of surviving mosquitoes after the 24-hour period of recovery indicates the development of resistance and its degree in the vector population. Another method is applicable to anopheline larvae. Appropriate test kits for the determination of resistance are issued by the WHO, which also periodically

**Figure 6.31** *A method for determining the susceptibility of resistance of adult mosquitoes. Note: mosquitoes are collected by means of an aspirator (a and b); they are then transferred to a special plastic holding tube (c). A plastic exposure tube lined with insecticide-impregnated paper is then connected to the holding tube and the mosquitoes are transferred to the exposure tube through a hole in the slide between the two tubes (d). The slide is closed and the exposure tube is allowed to stand upright for the determined period of time (e). After the exposure period, the mosquitoes are transferred back to the holding tube, which should stand upright for 24 hours, with a piece of moist cotton wool on the gauze end (f). Counts of dead mosquitoes killed by contact with the insecticide are made at the end of this recovery period. (WHO, 1970, Technical Report Series, No. 443.)*

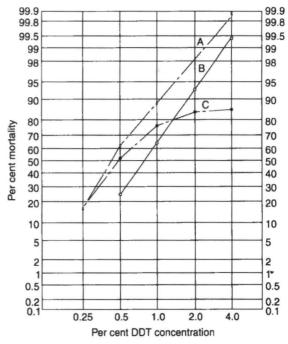

**Figure 6.32** *Dosage mortality regression lines for DDT indicating susceptibility of a sample of vectors to the insecticide (A); (B) seasonal fluctuation or tolerance; (C) presence of resistance in the vector population. (Reproduced from WHO, 1976, Technical Report Series, No. 585.)*

The more elaborate test consists of exposing samples of female *Anopheles* for a standard time (usually 1 hour) to a forced contact with a range of three concentrations of a given insecticide on impregnated filter papers. The mortality after 24 hours' recovery of exposed mosquitoes, when plotted on a logarithmic probability graph, gives a dosage/mortality regression line (Figure 6.32). If the regression line flattens out at high concentrations of the insecticide-impregnated papers, this indicates a resistance in the mosquito population. If the regression line remains

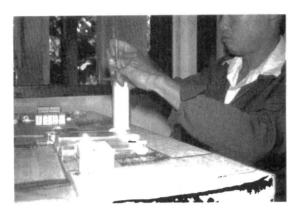

**Figure 6.33** *Testing* Anopheles *mosquitoes collected in the field for insecticide resistance in Thailand. (Photograph by PF Beales.)*

circulates the latest reports on findings in the field (Figure 6.33).

Recently WHO has produced two documents relating to insecticide resistance. One includes test procedures for insecticide resistance monitoring based on an informal consultation (WHO, 1998b) and the other is a field and laboratory manual on techniques to detect insecticide resistance mechanisms (WHO, 1998c).

In any malaria control programme based on a wide use of residual insecticides, one should attempt an early detection of resistance. Once the presence of resistance has been established, its progress should be monitored; this means the assessment of its operational importance and planning of countermeasures. The chances of an early detection of resistance are greater if the surveillance operations concentrate on areas where agricultural insecticides have been widely used. A suitable policy for detection of resistance in vector control programmes should provide for investigation of 5–10 per cent of villages or groups of houses over the entire control area. When the presence of resistance is confirmed, the operational significance of it requires studies of vector density as well as epidemiological appraisal of the origin of human infections. If it is established that a low degree of insecticide resistance is the cause of increased transmission, then insecticide spraying at shorter intervals or at higher dosage of the active compound combined with better detection of cases and their treatment may be a temporary solution. However, when the degree of resistance is high and transmission continues, a change of insecticide becomes imperative, together with other

attack measures to decrease the amount of transmission. Detailed discussion of these problems can be found in the WHO Technical Report Series No. 585 (WHO, 1976) and No. 655 (WHO, 1980).

New biochemical and immunological resistance assays have now been developed. These methods detect resistance mechanisms in single insects in the field and are both cheap and simple to use. Resistance can be detected at very low frequency, allowing efficient monitoring of vector populations.

As biochemical insecticide susceptibility assays are more widely used as diagnostic procedures, there is a need for standardization. Criteria should be set for good practice in applying methods, allowing their consistent use anywhere, and encouraging a more careful use of the new techniques in the field.

## PRESENT STATE OF RESISTANCE TO INSECTICIDES IN MALARIA VECTORS

In 1946, only two species of *Anopheles* were resistant to DDT, but by 1991 a total of 55 species showed resistance to one or more insecticides. Of the 55 species, 53 show resistance to DDT, 27 to organophosphorous compounds, 17 to carbamates and 10 to pyrethroids; 16 species show resistance to three or four chemical compounds.

Twenty-one of the 55 resistant species are very important vectors of malaria, namely: *A. aconitus, A. albimanus, A. albitarsis, A. annularis, A. arabiensis, A. culicifacies, A. darling, A. fluviatilis, A. gambiae, A. labranchiae, A. maculatus, A. pharoensis, A. pseudopunctipennis, A. pulcherrimus, A. sacharovi, A. sergentii, A. sinensis, A. stephensi, A. subpictus, A. sundaicus* and *A. superpictus*. They are listed in Table 6.8, which has been taken from a table reported by WHO in 1986 (WHO, 1986c), which showed the insecticide resistance of 51 anopheline species in countries or areas, and adjusted following later information contained in two subsequent reports in 1991 (WHO, 1991) and 1992 (WHO, 1992d).

The following findings of resistance in malaria vectors are of particular significance. *A. aconitus* is resistant to DDT in central and western Kalimantan, Bangladesh, India, Nepal and Thailand. *A. albimanus* is resistant to organophosphoruos compounds and carbamates in most of Central America and in some parts of Mexico. *A. annularis* is resistant to DDT in

Bangladesh, Myanmar, India, Pakistan and Thailand, to DDT and cyclodienes in Nepal, and to DDT and organophosphates in Sri Lanka.

It seems that nearly all members of the *A. gambiae* complex are resistant in various degrees to DDT and other organochlorine insecticides over most of tropical Africa, but *A. arabiensis* (formerly *A. gambiae* B) in the Sudan has become resistant also to malathion. *A. culicifacies* is resistant to DDT and HCH in several countries of the Middle East and in the Indian sub-continent; it has developed resistance also to malathion, especially in the Gujarat and Maharastra states of India and in Oman, Sri Lanka and the United Arab Emirates. *A. minimus* has shown a decrease of susceptibility to DDT in Thailand. *A. sacharovi* is now resistant to DDT, organophosphates and carbamate in certain areas of Bulgaria, Greece, Turkey and the former USSR and to fenitrothion in parts of Lebanon and the Syrian Arab Republic. *A. sinensis* has been found to be resistant to DDT, cyclodienes and malathion in southern China and partly in Vietnam. *A. stephensi* is resistant to malathion in Afghanistan, India, Iraq, the Islamic Republic of Iran, Oman, Pakistan, Saudi Arabia and the United Arab Emirates, and has shown resistance to permethrin in India and the Islamic Republic of Iran.

The method formerly employed to meet the problem of insecticide resistance to a specific compound was to use an alternative insecticide. However, this is now less feasible. A WHO Programme for the Evaluation of Insecticides has been in operation since 1957 and by 1982 over 1800 compounds were screened for their activity and safety. Only a small number of some 20 compounds passed the stringent tests and a few of them were tentatively tried in the field.

In 1982, the programme was revised to cover a wider range of vectors and formulations, and was renamed the WHO Insecticide Evaluation Scheme. It now comprises four progressive phases: laboratory examinations, small-scale and large-scale field trials and, if all other phases have successfully passed, specifications for purchase.

The aim of the revised programme is the same as that of the original, namely, the assessment of new candidate insecticides and formulations in order to provide suitable alternatives for insecticides used for all types of vector control to which resistance has appeared or is likely to appear.

In recent years, however, there has been a decline in the number of compounds submitted by industry, primarily because of the high cost of insecticide development, and particularly the cost of mounting large-scale field trials.

DDT still remains the cheapest and probably the most widely employed insecticide for malaria control. Its use is expected to continue, with a preference for emulsifiable instead of water-dispersible powder formulations. The demand for malathion is also expected to remain high, as it is still effective against many malaria vectors. Fenitrothion may be used instead of malathion in some countries; however, its cost is higher than that of malathion and resistance to it is most likely to include resistance to malathion, whereas the converse is not the case. This implies that malathion should be used before fenitrothion for malaria vector control. Permethrin, deltamethrin, pirimiphos-methyl and propoxur may be used in special circumstances, especially in view of the increasing resistance of vectors to organochlorine and organophosphorous compounds.

## OPERATIONAL APPROACHES FOR MALARIA CONTROL TO COUNTERACT INSECTICIDE RESISTANCE

As mentioned before, the development of insecticide resistance is related to two main factors:

1. the biological characteristics of the species and of the local population of the respective vector,
2. the type and degree of the selection pressure of the insecticide.

Research carried out in the past has improved our capacity to judge the relative speed with which a specific resistance pattern may appear under certain circumstances. However, it is still impossible to predict the time when the resistance gene will attain a certain frequency and present operational problems. It is now clear that the selection pressure is related to the degree and time of action of the toxic compounds on the heterozygote individuals within the insect population and on the house-haunting habits of *Anopheles*. Thus, the appearance of resistance might be slower with less persistent residual deposits and, if the susceptible mosquitoes enter the target area from the outside, cross-breeding with the resistant ones would lower the frequency of heterozygotes. In practice, it would mean that, in an area where new houses have been built after the last spraying cycle, it may be preferable to leave the new houses unsprayed and to respray only the houses that were sprayed before. However, these considerations may not be acceptable in practice when prolonged residual activity is required for an acceptable degree of control.

In order to prolong the useful life of the insecticides currently available for public health use, methods need to be devised to minimize or counteract the selection pressure exerted on vector populations by insecticide applications. This would involve both close co-ordination in insecticide use by health and agricultural authorities and the introduction of a new practical rationale of insecticide application based on vector population genetics.

In view of the fact that the contamination of mosquito breeding sites by the extensive use of agricultural insecticides often leads to marked resistance of *Anopheles* vectors, the co-ordination of antimalaria activities with other schemes, based on the outdoor use of insecticides, is imperative.

The results of susceptibility tests alone may be misleading if the sample size is small; these tests should be supplemented by studies of vector density, survival rates from window traps and malaria prevalence. All these indices provide a more precise picture of the extent of the problem. Collaboration between entomologists and malariologists will make it possible to continue adequate monitoring and provide early warning of any deterioration of the situation.

Monitoring vector resistance is essential in assessing its operational importance. This monitoring can be limited to its simplest form, namely, the continuation of entomological vigilance without any change of the diagnostic concentration of tests of resistance to determine the distribution and proportion of susceptible vectors. In its more complex form, it may involve the longitudinal determination of the phenotypic composition of the vector population, with a periodic assessment of cross-resistance characteristics and detailed epidemiological studies to correlate resistance levels with possible failures of control operations. However, the substitute compound may not remain useful for very long, especially in areas where various insecticides are widely applied in agriculture. This has happened already in cotton-growing areas of Central America and in other parts of the world.

Other solutions have been proposed, although not often used on a realistic scale. One of them is to use, sequentially or in rotation, two or three unrelated insecticides, thus maintaining an overall insecticide coverage of the whole operational area. The other is to use combinations of various compounds, on the assumption that the genes of resistance to each chemical compound exist in such low frequency that they are not likely to occur within a given population of the vector. These methods have a number of logistic or economic constraints in residual insecticidal programmes, but present some advantages in larvicidal control.

When the presence and degree of resistance of malaria vectors in the area have been confirmed, often the only solution is to change to a different insecticide, taking into account the operational and financial consequences of this decision. Should resistance to both groups of chlorinated hydrocarbons occur, it may be necessary to change either to one of the organophosphate compounds or to a carbamate. Although there are some cases of cross-resistance between these two groups, this is uncommon and usually one may employ one or the other of these compounds as an alternative solution, although operational and financial consequences may be serious. This is particularly important in areas of socio-economic importance, where residual house spraying needs to be maintained, using either DDT or a suitable alternative insecticide wherever DDT is no longer effective. Where insecticidal attack is not feasible, large stocks of antimalarial drugs should be made available for the protection of at least the most vulnerable group of the human population and for the prevention of morbidity and mortality in general. It is understood that any insecticidal attack should be considered as a temporary measure until more permanent environmental control measures become feasible.

## Integrated vector control

The development of resistance to insecticides as well as the growing concern about environmental contamination, human safety and the increased costs of alternative chemical compounds led to the present emphasis on the value of integrated vector control. This has been defined as the utilization of all appropriate technological and management techniques to bring about an effective degree of vector suppression, in a cost-effective manner. In fact, this is the nineteenth-century concept, revived and improved through the use of appropriate new chemical and biological compounds.

The essential requirement for integrated vector control is the ability to use one method that favours (or at least does not interfere with) another method. Thus, in several countries, such as Italy, Hawaii and Japan, larvicidal treatment of ponds with an insecticide is combined sequentially with various source-reduction methods and the use of larvivorous fish. An adequate knowledge of the biology, ecology and behaviour characteristics of the vector, of some agricultural practices and of aquatic animal life is necessary to avoid costly mistakes. Naturally, human safety must also be taken into account. The trend of integrated vector control is in the direction of community involvement through well-planned, sustained measures, related to socio-economic conditions. Generally speaking, personal protection, better sanitation, skilful agriculture and water management, source reduction, waste disposal and acceptable insecticides will remain the major components of integrated mosquito control schemes.

## SAFE USE OF INSECTICIDES

### General principles

All insecticides are, to some degree, harmful to animals and to humans, but there is a major difference between the toxicity of a given compound and the hazard that it presents. Highly toxic compounds are excluded from use in vector control because of the difficulty of reducing human exposure to them. A measure of potential toxicity of a given insecticide to humans or other mammals is the oral or dermal $LD_{50}$ value, i.e. the estimate of the amount of toxicant per kilogram of body weight required to kill 50 per cent of experimental animals (usually rats) used for testing (see Table 6.4). According to this table, parathion (an agricultural insecticide) is the most toxic and temephos the least toxic organophosphorous compound if taken by mouth. The apparently low toxicity of malathion may be misleading because some formulations may become toxic in tropical conditions, especially if not stored properly. Such an

unexpected change in an insecticide with a previous good safety record was seen in 1976 in Pakistan, where about 2500 cases of illness occurred among spraypersons, five of whom died. An investigation showed that the major toxic component was isomalathion, formed in malathion dispersible powder during prolonged storage in tropical conditions. This unfortunate episode, while revealing a new problem, indicated ways for the improvement of insecticide formulations.

During the past few years, there have been few changes in the use of insecticides for public health purposes, except for the introduction of pyrethroids and insect growth regulators. A number of operational field trials provided information on the safety precautions concerning malathion, fenitrothion, chlorfoxim, pirimiphos-methyl, landrin, some pyrethroids and insect growth regulators. It appears that, although the acute mammalian toxicity of permethrin and deltamethrin is quite high, no serious problems have been encountered in the field.

The degree of hazard is estimated by the dangers involved when the insecticide is used under the particular conditions of usage. Thus, the factors relevant to hazard depend not only on the intrinsic toxicity of the compound, but also on the type of formulation used, concentration of the insecticide, method of use, accidental exposure of food and drink, poor storage conditions, bad labelling of containers or improper use of contaminated barrels and tins. Illiteracy and lack of training are also important factors. The type of exposure is also of importance: people are generally aware of the danger of the ingestion or inhalation of insecticides, but many field workers are not aware that some compounds may be absorbed through the skin, particularly in hot climates.

### Precautionary measures

The safe use of insecticides depends on the availability of up-to-date information on the compounds and formulations selected for use, on their storage conditions and on the way they are going to be used. Naturally, both the compounds and the formulations must conform to the WHO specifications. Detailed instructions on the safe application of any insecticide have been prepared by the WHO. Only the main points of these instructions can be given here.

In the first instance, any vector control campaign must include provision for the safe transport and secure storage of insecticide concentrates. These should not be stored in rooms in which people live or in which food is kept. Protection against theft, misuse and accessibility to children must be provided. The safe disposal of empty insecticide containers must be taken care of. All insecticide containers should be adequately labelled in a form or language understood by the local operators. All equipment used for the distribution of insecticides should conform to the WHO recommendations with regard to design and manufacture. There should be regular systematic inspection of all equipment to ensure that it is adequate.

With careful handling, there is little real risk to the occupants of treated houses, but, as a safety measure, all foodstuffs should be removed or carefully covered before a house is sprayed. There is some risk to domestic animals, especially with dieldrin; casualties have occurred amongst cats, which lick their contaminated fur, and chickens, which have pecked along the floor near the sprayed walls. However, this insecticide is rarely, if ever, used in public health now.

The pre-packing of insecticides into small, labelled, plastic bags, containing enough material for a single tank charge, eliminates the need to measure the amount of the formulated compound in the field and this lowers the risk of contamination and ensures the correct application dose. It also reduces the spillage and wastage and minimizes the accidental poisoning of children.

Spraypersons, mixers and baggers should report any symptoms of illness promptly to the supervisor. A medical examination is advisable, including the determination of blood cholinesterase, of those applying organophosphorous compounds, and regular medical surveillance of spray operators should be enforced. Training in the safe use of insecticides should be provided for the supervisory medical and other personnel so that they are able to recognize the signs and symptoms of accidental poisoning and to give immediate treatment in an emergency. Equally important is the training of the foreman and other responsible field operators in the technique of proper spraying, safety precautions and maintenance of protective equipment.

Any extensive spraying should be carried out under adequate supervision. Spraypersons should wash, using soap or detergent, at the end of each working day and whenever the insecticide is spilled in quantity on the skin or clothes. They should not smoke or eat while on duty, or after duty unless they first wash their hands. Insecticide should be scooped out with proper implements and not by hand.

## Protective equipment

There are various items of protective equipment that should be used by field staff directly involved in insecticide spraying. The most important of these are the following:

- Hats: these should be of impermeable material with a broad brim to protect the face and neck.
- Veils: a plastic mesh net loosely attached to the hat will give protection from large drops of spray and permit sufficient visibility.
- Overalls: these should be of light, durable cotton fabric; they should be washed regularly with soap or detergent.
- Aprons: these should be made of rubber or plastic to provide protection from liquid concentrates.

Impervious gloves, capes, respirators and rubber boots are often advised, but they are seldom acceptable in tropical countries (Figure 6.34).

Greater risk occurs when handling oil solutions, such as concentrates or emulsions, which should be poured through threaded taps or by pumps arranged to prevent contact of the solution with the skin.

## Emergency treatment of poisoning by insecticides

As with all other types of poisoning, the emergency treatment of accidental ingestion or other contact with a toxic compound comprises:

1. action to deal with life-threatening symptoms
2. removal of the toxicant
3. administration of antidotes and alleviation of other symptoms.

### IMMEDIATE ACTION IN CASE OF LIFE-THREATENING EFFECTS

When vomiting and difficulty of respiration occur, lie the patient flat on the stomach with the head to one side, the lower jaw extended and tongue pulled forward. Clear the mouth and pharynx of vomit manually or by endotracheal intubation if necessary. Give

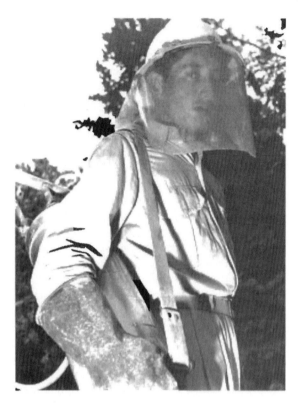

**Figure 6.34** *Sprayman employed by the Malaria Eradication Programme in Mexico wearing full protective clothing. (WHO photograph by E Schwab.)*

oxygen and apply artificial respiration if needed, but do not attempt mouth-to-mouth respiration to avoid further accidental poisoning. If the poisoning occurred by ingestion, gastric lavage is needed, except in the case of Paraquat, Diquat and zinc phosphide. Some toxic material may be present on the skin and clothing, from which absorption may continue. Clothing should be removed and the skin washed with soap and water. Contamination of the eyes must be dealt with by washing them with water. If several people show symptoms of poisoning, without any evidence of previous exposure, the most likely cause is contamination of food or water by the insecticide.

The symptoms of acute poisoning by chlorinated hydrocarbons such as DDT, HCH and dieldrin include convulsions followed by an adverse effect on the liver tissue. Acute poisoning due to ingestion (except Paraquat, Diquat and zinc phosphide) should be dealt with, if the person is unconscious, by inducing vomiting by tickling the back of the throat

with the tip of the finger. A doctor must be consulted as soon as possible. Chronic poisoning due to the continued intake of smaller quantities is heralded by nervous symptoms, which include hyperexcitability, anxiety and tremors. In addition, there is a very marked loss of appetite, which quickly leads to loss of weight. Convulsions should be controlled by doses of injectable phenobarbitones, diazepam or paraldehyde. Blood samples for organochlorine levels may be necessary for confirmation of the cause of poisoning, but this is a complex analytical procedure. Treatment must not be delayed pending the results of laboratory tests.

Any person who has suffered toxic effects due to handling chlorinated hydrocarbon insecticides should be removed from the risk of contact with the insecticide.

Symptoms of poisoning by organophosphate insecticides are similar in many respects to those of chlorinated hydrocarbon poisoning, but also include giddiness, nausea, vomiting and diarrhoea; excessive sweating and salivation may be present. In severe cases, cyanosis, respiratory difficulties, convulsions and loss of consciousness may follow. In such cases, artificial respiration by mechanical means may be necessary before the administration of atropine sulphate intravenously or intramuscularly (if the intravenous route is not possible) at 0.4–2.0 mg for adults and 0.05 mg/kg body weight for children under 12 years. The injections should be repeated every 15–30 minutes until signs of atropinization occur (dry mouth, flushing, mydriasis, tachycardia). There is no need to limit the dosage: signs of atropine toxicity need not be unduly alarming. A total of 25–50 mg or more may be necessary during the first day. Diazepam may be helpful in controlling intractable convulsions not controlled by antidotes. Atropine prophylaxis is not recommended. In addition, in severe poisoning, one might administer 1–3 g of a soluble salt of pralidoxime by slow intravenous injection for adults or 50 mg/kg body weight for children. Morphine and tranquillizers must *not* be given to people poisoned by anticholinesterase compounds. Organophosphorous insecticides inhibit cholinesterase (one of the vital body enzymes) and blood samples should be taken for cholinesterase determinations before and after the treatment of a case of poisoning.

Supplies of atropine should be available in first-aid kits when organophosphorous or carbamate insecticides are being applied, and the spraying supervisor should be trained to administer atropine in emergencies. Medical help should be sought immediately if poisoning is suspected. It is advised that people habitually handling these insecticides should have their blood cholinesterase levels checked periodically. Operators should be withdrawn from exposure if this level decreases by 25 per cent or more from a well-established pre-exposure value. The insecticidal carbamates give rise to a more rapidly reversible cholinesterase-inhibition complex. This makes it impossible to use estimates of cholinesterase activity as an accurate index of the levels of this enzyme in the tissues.

In cases of poisoning by *carbamates*, all the methods used for treating poisoning by organic phosphorous compounds are useful, with one exception: pralidoxime and other oximes are *not* recommended for routine use. Recovery from carbamate poisoning is usually quite rapid.

Generally, insecticides that are more toxic than DDT undergo faster degradation in the environment and are more acceptable to the ecologist. However, the hazard that they present to the operators is very much higher. The prevention and treatment of accidental poisoning should be given high priority in all spraying programmes.

## Insecticides and the environment

The application of residual insecticides and especially of DDT has been the main factor responsible for the eradication of malaria from large parts of the world and remains an important method for the control of this disease in the tropics. However, anxiety about the pollution of the environment by insecticides has increased during the past few years to such an extent that all the virtues of these compounds tend to be forgotten, while their disadvantages receive much sensational publicity. It has been estimated that during the period 1978–1982, the annual amount of DDT used for public health programmes all over the world was of the order of 30 000 tonnes, without any major adverse effect on the human population living in areas where this compound was employed. Studies carried out under the auspices of the WHO have shown that even high degrees of continued exposure to DDT of workers in industries that produce it have not led to any health problems when proper precautions are observed. The continued availability of DDT and other insecti-

cides is imperative until better methods of vector control are devised. There is no doubt that the indiscriminate use of organochlorines and organophosphates affects various species of wild fauna, especially birds. However, one should stress that the commonest method of malaria control, by the residual spraying of houses, has practically no effect on the environment, because the insecticidal compounds are confined within the house.

DDT and other more toxic insecticides (such as parathion) have been used in very large amounts, mainly for the protection of agricultural crops. It is the aerial spraying of fields that has been responsible for the contamination of mosquito breeding sites by run-off. This led to the phenomenon of multiresistance to a number of organochlorine and organophosphate compounds. The most complete study, carried out under the joint sponsorship of the United Nations Environment Programme and the World Health Organization, reported that the only demonstrated effects of DDT on the general population are the storage of this compound in the tissues and its excretion in urine and milk. No confirmed ill-effects of DDT have been reported in babies, even in the communities with the highest concentrations of the compound in human milk. There is no evidence that DDT is carcinogenic in humans; nor is there any indication that DDT affects human reproduction. DDT appears to have some depressant effect on the immune system, but the evidence for this is not conclusive.

Calls for the limitation of insecticides used in agriculture have not been very successful in many tropical countries, where food and cash crops are of great economic importance. Information on the adverse impact of such agricultural practices is often difficult to collect and to interpret. This was demonstrated in a much publicized controversy, in which the introduction into India of high-yield rice (which needs more irrigation and protection from pests) was alleged to be responsible for the spread of insecticide resistance and increase of malaria. A further complication arises from the widespread anxiety about the harmful effects of chemical compounds and very expensive screening of potentially valuable new candidate insecticides, so that many manufacturers are unwilling to invest in costly research and development.

Thus, in the final account, it seems that, for the immediate future, insecticides will continue to play a major role in agriculture and in the control of vector-borne diseases of humans and animals. Environmental contamination, accidental toxicity to humans, resistance and rising costs of insecticides are all serious problems. However, a solution may be found in devising, and applying, for each area concerned, appropriate methods of integrated control that will not preclude the use of chemical compounds, if they are effective and safe and applied at the right place and at the right time. All other methods, such as source reduction, water management, biological control, treatment and prevention of infection, will have to be used increasingly by well-informed and well-trained health service personnel. Although integrated control of malaria is still more of a concept than a practical reality, this is the present major trend.

# PLANNING MALARIA CONTROL

The strategy for malaria control approved by the WHO in 1979 stressed the need for flexibility of antimalaria programmes, namely, the adaptation of any and all available methods to realistic aims, set by national health authorities and feasible within the limitations of their human and material resources. Thus, a malaria control programme has been redefined as an organized effort to institute, carry out and evaluate activities that are appropriate in prevailing epidemiological and socio-economic conditions and are likely to achieve the greatest possible improvement of the health situation in the country concerned (WHO, 1979).

A realistic formulation of any control programme requires that the expenditure will be covered wholly from the government budget, with full commitment of the central and local authorities to a long-term programme. The cost of malaria control within an area will vary inversely to the density of its at-risk population.

Preference should be given to permanent measures of control rather than to those of a temporary character, unless the environmental conditions favour the latter methods. Permanent measures often require high capital expenditure in the short term, but the cost of their maintenance is low and the long-term benefits are great. Moreover, their impact may be of considerable economic importance if the land becomes suitable for agriculture or housing.

The objectives of any malaria control programme depend on the prevailing epidemiological situation, the effectiveness of available methods, the national commitment, the available resources of the relevant health authorities and the degree of support of the community.

Article VIII of the World Declaration on Malaria Control (WHO, 1992b), made at the WHO Ministerial Conference on Malaria held in Amsterdam on 26 and 27 October 1992, states: 'We commit ourselves and our countries to control malaria and will plan for malaria control as an essential component of health development and will incorporate health development as an essential component of national development.' This collective statement of political will may well prove to be a historic landmark in our quest to conquer this disease.

Planning for malaria control is clearly an intersectoral matter, which should be carried out carefully by an intersectoral team of responsible people. It is a dynamic process and follows a cycle of planning, implementation, evaluation and replanning.

Today, countries are faced with the difficult task of controlling malaria as a disease problem (not as a parasitic infection) in the face of rising costs, widespread population movement, varying degrees of *P. falciparum* malaria parasite resistance to some antimalarial drugs in some places, and resistance to some insecticides by some vectors in some areas.

Control programmes need to be developed which:

- have no time limit
- use available national resources or resources that can be mobilized
- are designed to ensure that the gains can be sustained
- take into account the local epidemiological conditions.

Malaria is naturally an acute clinical disease, not chronic; however, it may be a chronic parasitic infection. Its clinical manifestations may be modified by the inappropriate use of antimalarial drugs and by parasite resistance to them. Malaria disease control therefore means undoubtedly a continuing presence of infection in the community, maintained by mosquito transmission. Malaria transmission control implies keeping malaria transmission to a minimum by the effective use of the available resources and technology. It does not necessarily mean complete interruption of transmission, as in an eradication campaign.

Malaria control requires careful, pragmatic planning and replanning and necessitates frequent evaluation. It is inherently difficult in the sense that there are no general prescriptions that can be equally effective everywhere. Approaches have to be constantly modified to take account of local variability. This demands a greater epidemiological capability at the periphery than is necessary for the control of most other diseases and certainly more than was necessary for the malaria eradication campaign of the 1950s and 1960s.

In an attempt to standardize and simplify the approach to malaria control, a sequence of objectives and relevant actions was classified into four 'tactical variants' (WHO, 1979). The experience of countries in applying this approach was reviewed in 1985 and revealed a number of problems. The tendency was to view the variants as mutually exclusive compartments, to be selected and implemented according to the resources available, instead of planning antimalaria action based upon epidemiological stratification. Thus, the variants, while serving to highlight the need to view malaria more as a disease problem than as a parasitic infection, had not inspired countries to develop flexible approaches suitable to their individual needs through a process of planning (WHO, 1986a).

Antimalaria objectives need to be developed as part of the planning process relevant to each identified epidemiological stratum. However, it is possible to recognize that methods of attacking the problem can be graded according to their complexity, and that these methods require a range of different resources and development activities to ensure the long-term maintenance of any results obtained. One possibility is to begin malaria control with a sophisticated attack on malaria transmission, as attempted by eradication programmes, but this proved to be successful and sustainable in only a few areas. Thus, a hierarchy of objectives and activities can be envisaged as a broad spectrum of possibilities. This implies that a more complex plan of malaria control should not be adopted unless there is assurance that earlier objectives would be reached. Two substantially different approaches, aimed at attaining the objectives at the two extreme ends of the spectrum, can be identified:

• Improvement in the general health services to ensure adequate diagnosis, accessibility to health care, treatment for malaria cases, provision of adequate protection for the population at risk and the promotion of personal and community pro-

tection. This is aimed at obtaining objectives such as the reduction of morbidity and mortality and of the duration of sickness.
• Establishment of the capability for the long-term control of malaria transmission. This will require the planning of specific antimalaria actions designed to change the epidemiological equilibrium. It includes the objectives of preventing epidemics, reducing the foci of *P. falciparum* malaria and transmission control in selected areas or in the entire country.

At one end of the spectrum, as an absolute minimum, all countries would need to provide diagnosis and appropriate treatment for the sick, curative treatment and prophylaxis throughout pregnancy, and improved education to the population concerning the better use of health services, the non-tolerance of illness and the use of personal protective measures. At the other end of the spectrum, planned interference in malaria transmission on a large scale should only be considered if this will effectively change the epidemiological equilibrium and if this change can be sustained.

Intermediate approaches between these two extremes would be the progressive strengthening of the referral system and the development of a meaningful information system, as well as epidemiological surveillance with appropriate recognition of abnormal situations, delimitation of problem areas and the provision of an adequate response capability. This will progress from the control of epidemics to their prevention, and to the control of the most serious foci. It will include monitoring problems such as drug resistance and the evaluation of the response to control measures.

The art of planning is to identify which approaches should be implemented, where and when, to achieve and sustain desired objectives within the resources available, or that can be made available, based upon a sound scientific knowledge of the local epidemiological, sociological and environmental circumstances.

## The planning process

Planning involves identifying and analysing problems, examining solutions, setting priorities, making choices and decisions, setting objectives, developing approaches to achieve these objectives, allocating resources and organizing them into programmes for effective and efficient delivery and measuring progress towards those objectives. In an environment of scarcity, such as is found in many developing countries, planning takes on all the more importance in order to get as much accomplished with what little there is in the way of staff, supplies, equipment, drugs, transport, funds etc.

Planning is a systematic and continuous process for allocating resources to achieve objectives. It is a way to define why, how, when, where and by whom these objectives can be achieved. In health planning, we are concerned with extending coverage and improving the effectiveness and efficacy of health care services and systems. An integral part of this approach is intersectoral collaboration for programmes that will impact the total health environment of which malaria control is one component.

The aim of disease control is to reduce the impact of the disease on the health of the population to the lowest possible level that can be achieved within the available financial and human resources, in the context of other health priorities and according to existing technology and feasibility.

The intensity of the required disease control effort will depend upon the magnitude of the disease problem and the objectives being pursued and may vary from one situation to another. The required action will take the form of a co-ordinated set of activities, with targets and dates for their achievement designed to achieve well-defined objectives. These objectives should be regarded as intermediate steps towards the achievement of the ultimate goal. The objectives and the approaches decided upon will determine the form and the content of the national antimalaria action, which implies the expenditure of valuable resources.

It is difficult to establish meaningful objectives because of the complexity and uncertainty surrounding many of the factors that must be taken into account. Defining the objectives, formulating approaches and setting operational targets are closely interrelated and are best considered in a practical sequence. Setting the goal and priorities and deciding upon and supporting control approaches are primarily political decisions (political will). The planning process enables a logical approach to be taken to determine the appropriate combination of measures to use for control purposes, and where and when to use them, based upon an assessment of the local situation and the technical, operational and economic feasibility. It is suggested that the planning process should consist of an analysis of the malaria situation, stratification of the problem, formulation of objectives and approaches to achieve these objectives, the selection and definition of evaluation methods, establishment of the operational outputs and targets, programme budgeting and, finally, preparation of an implementation plan.

## The planning environment

There are certain characteristics of the planning environment in developing countries that should be recognized and taken into consideration. Health planners must work in an environment of scarcity, or at best inadequacy. Resources of all kinds may be in short supply: staff, staff accommodation, materials and supplies, facilities and equipment, drugs and vaccines, petrol, transport and communications, etc. Another aspect of the planning/management environment is the problem of organizing and managing health data. There is no lack of data, but rather the problem is in their collection and organization into a usable form. Also, much of the data collected is not used at all. Some of it could be eliminated; other data should be used closer to the source of collection for monitoring, evaluation and control at lower levels in the health system (e.g. at health centres, medical field units, mobile clinics, etc.).

This calls for intuition and creativity in approaching problems. The health planner manager must use judgement and educated guesses based on experience and an understanding of conditions that can contribute to the decision-making process. Furthermore, simple techniques should be used for sample surveys and field observation to set baseline data, and easily measured indicators should be applied to monitor, evaluate and control health programmes.

Health planners should be good observers; they should know what to look for and how to evaluate the information reaching their senses as they conduct field inspections, visit clinics and walk through the market place and villages.

## Analysis of the malaria situation

Analysis of the malaria situation is the essential basis for planning antimalaria action based upon the epidemiological characteristics. A complete analysis would include a description of the distribution of malaria (infection) and its consequences (morbidity, mortality, economic losses) and an explanation of that distribution in terms of its causal factors (geophysical, environmental, biological, social, political and economic). It is clear that a really complete analysis is practically impossible, and therefore malaria control will often have to be planned using imperfect knowledge. However, an important component of any plan should be to collect the additional, valid information necessary for replanning purposes, thereby improving the programme as it progresses. The analysis of the malaria situation has six major components:

1. The current malaria problem can be analysed by considering the impact of malaria on the health of the community, the economic and social effects of malaria, the economic and social effects on malaria, the infection in humans and the clinical manifestations, parasitological factors, the vector mosquito and other aspects of the environment.
2. The current malaria control activities and their effects on the malaria problem. This would include a critical review of individual current control activities, overall evaluation of the malaria control activities and current field research.
3. The health services resources that are available and that could be used for malaria control and the systems that are in place and the degree to which they are functioning.
4. Community involvement, which would include community structures and groups, the extent to which the community is involved in health matters and the potential for community involvement in antimalaria activities.
5. Intersectoral co-operation: the sectors that are associated with malaria transmission and/or its control will need to be identified. The analysis would also include the extent of intersectoral co-operation to date for malaria control and the mechanisms available at different levels.
6. The history of the problem, which would include past infection and especially the history of epidemics, major changes occurring over time in the epidemiology of the disease and identification of socio-economic changes over time, and the resulting amount of malaria.

Based upon the analysis of the malaria situation, certain key decisions need to be made. These include the relative importance of malaria in the politico-socioeconomic context warranting action; opportunistic resources for antimalaria action; the magnitude of the planning process necessary for malaria control (which parts of the country are more involved than others, what other agencies/organizations should be involved, how can resources be mobilized); the budgetary resources and limitations; and the extent of investment in infrastructure development.

## Stratification of the malaria problem

Very often, the same degree of malaria reduction cannot be achieved simultaneously all over the national territory due to administrative, operational, financial and technical constraints. Thus, it is necessary to proceed to a stratification of the country, with the definition of different objectives and consequently the selection of appropriate control measures in the different strata that have been defined. Stratification is a process intended to reduce and simplify a complex problem, to facilitate its understanding and to formulate solutions. Many factors contribute to the epidemiology of malaria, such as the distribution and relative prevalence of different *Plasmodium* species and their response to drugs, the distribution of vector species and their susceptibility to insecticides, the intensity of transmission etc. In addition, the ecological and geographical characteristics of different areas, socio-economic conditions of the populations, climatic and meteorological factors, which are not usually uniformly similar throughout a national territory, also play a major role.

In order to simplify this heterogeneity, it may be possible to identify common factors and to use this knowledge to delimit new areas, populations or situations that exhibit a relative similarity through specific characteristics which distinguish them from other areas dissimilar by the same characteristics.

An epidemiological stratification is essential and it should be considered as the preliminary step prior to arriving at an operational stratification of the country. Once the degree and distribution of the malaria problem have been assessed, and the interplaying climatic, geographical, logistical and socio-economic factors involved in the epidemiology of the disease have been analysed, homogeneous zones with similar epidemiological, socio-economic and ecological characteristics can be delineated. For each defined stratum, specific objectives and targets can then be formulated and the intervention methods selected for the objectives to be met.

## STRATEGY FOR MALARIA CONTROL

A strategy for malaria control was formulated by the WHO to address the serious worldwide malaria situation. It was presented to the Ministerial Conference on Malaria in Amsterdam in 1992. It is generally accepted that, with few exceptions, malaria eradication is not a realistic goal where it has not already been achieved. Reduction of malaria morbidity and mortality, with their consequences on human performance and socio-economic development, is a more modest and realistic goal. This will require an improvement in the capacity of existing health services and systems to provide diagnosis and early treatment within the umbrella of primary health care, and a reorientation of existing malaria control programmes to take into consideration epidemiological, ecological, environmental and social factors; as well as the primary goal of the new strategy.

The variability of malaria has already been pointed out and no uniform strategy applicable to all areas can be formulated. Nonetheless, four fundamental elements can be identified:

1. Early diagnosis and treatment.
2. Selective application of vector control, including human–mosquito barriers.
3. Development of epidemiological information systems.
4. Early detection or forecasting of epidemics and rapid application of control measures.

## Early diagnosis and treatment

Malaria is a curable disease and timely diagnosis and treatment are a basic human right of all populations in endemic areas, whatever their social or economic circumstances.

Because complications of *P. falciparum* in children, in particular, develop rapidly, children should ideally receive treatment within 12 hours after the onset of symptoms (fever); in adults, the antecedent history before severe manifestations occur is usually (although not invariably) longer (4–5 days).

In many of the highly endemic countries, the diagnosis of malaria is made on clinical grounds, because microscopy and other diagnostic tests are unavailable at the peripheral health posts; moreover, in these areas, a positive blood film does not necessarily mean a definitive diagnosis, although the density of infection can be a valuable index. Clinical diagnostic criteria should be defined according to the local epidemiology, bearing in mind, in particular, the transmission season, and the age and sex of the patient. Thus, any febrile illness in a child or in an individual of another risk group, for example primigravidae women, should be regarded as malaria; whereas, in partially immune adults, only fevers without symptoms suggesting another disease should be considered as malaria. This approach will reduce the wastage that is inevitable in these circumstances.

The choice of drugs will depend on a variety of factors, such as pattern of resistance, cost, side-effects, compliance and availability. At the first referral level, health personnel should be trained to have enough clinical competence to diagnose and treat malaria and to recognize severe anaemia, especially in children. An unusually large number of children with anaemia may indicate that RII resistance to the first-line drug such as chloroquine is occurring, and an alternative drug, for example sulfadoxine–pyrimethamine, may be indicated. National guidelines will determine which antimalarial drugs should be used as first-line and second-line treatments, the quantities required and their distribution. Patients with severe disease must be given parenteral treatment or a suppository preparation (if available) and referred to the next level of health care with greater facilities for diagnosis, monitoring and treating the patient.

Self-medication is increasingly common, almost universal, yet knowledge among those who provide or sell antimalarial drugs is abysmally low, resulting in inappropriate or incomplete treatment. People such as shopkeepers, teachers, priests, traditional birth attendants, traditional healers and mothers could be taught the importance of early treatment and the proper use of antimalarial drugs in different age groups at different times of the transmission season – using up-to-date and culturally acceptable means of communication. During the early 1990s, the WHO produced an excellent brochure for this purpose.

Evidence from several countries indicates that self-medication accounts for as much as half of all consumption of antimalarial drugs in rural areas.

Mass chemoprophylaxis against malaria is no longer recommended, except under special circumstances such as epidemics; for non-immune migrant labourers, soldiers and others living temporarily in endemic areas; special risk groups, such as pregnant women (especially primiparae); children with homozygous haemoglobinopathies; and immunosuppressed individuals.

Although early diagnosis and drug treatment are the first element of the malaria control strategy, it must be realized that neither the distribution nor the use of antimalarial drugs has hitherto followed a clear and tidy pattern, as is often assumed. An objective review of the situation is given by Foster (1991).

## Selective application of vector control including human–mosquito barriers

The aim is the progressive reduction of malaria transmission where this is sustainable and cost-effective. Decisions on whether to apply vector control and which methods to choose must depend on an assessment of the relevant epidemiological, ecological, social and operational determinants, including the local identification of epidemiological types. The various methods available have been described earlier and are aimed at (a) a reduction of mosquito breeding, (b) a reduction in the longevity and/or density of adult mosquitoes, and (c) reduction in human–mosquito contact. Residual spraying is now recommended for special situations, for example epidemic control or protecting particularly vulnerable populations. Impregnated mosquito nets or curtains are justifiably receiving considerable attention and their value in areas with different intensities of malaria transmission continues to be documented.

## Development of epidemiological information systems

The collection and handling of malaria data should be part of the general health service information system and is an essential prerequisite for the early detection and forecasting of epidemics. They are a means of monitoring the potential rapid changes in malaria transmission and disease. As much as possible, data should be analysed and appraised as peripherally as possible – at regional or even district level and below.

## Early detection or forecasting of epidemics

Throughout, and right up to the end of, the twentieth century, malaria continued to be the major cause of many devastating epidemics. In principle, an epidemic is a sudden increase in disease incidence beyond what is considered normal. This must be distinguished from seasonal increases in disease and newly discovered endemic areas. A requirement for an epidemic to occur is the presence of a large number of susceptible people who are likely to become clinically sick when suddenly exposed to infection. Thus, malaria epidemics do not occur in communities living in highly endemic areas where sufficient immunity is acquired early in life, provided this immunity is not interfered with. In some countries, epidemics tend to occur periodically over a number of years.

The impact of epidemics in terms of morbidity and mortality depends on the general health status of the affected population and the accessibility of facilities and services. Often, epidemics coincide with periods of famine, economic crisis, war, civil unrest and disturbances and natural disasters affecting impoverished populations who are often weakened by other diseases and conditions.

The aim, therefore, is the forecasting or early detection of epidemics in order to ensure rapid and effective control. The monitoring of meteorological data and population movements is useful because unusually heavy rains and/or increased temperatures are possible causes of malaria epidemics, as are man-made ecological changes often associated with the influx of many non-immune individuals. A relatively high rate of slide positivity among fever patients, or an increased demand for antimalarial drugs, could suggest an outbreak of malaria, and follow-up of therapeutic results could indicate that an alternative second-line medication may be required. Remote sensing may prove to be a useful tool in the future for the early warning signs, or the detection, of epidemic malaria.

Ideally, epidemics should be predicted and prevented. Failing this, they should be detected early and controlled rapidly. Thus, monitoring systems need to be established that monitor morbidity and mortality, population immunity (e.g. spleen rates), entomological variables, meteorological variables, socioeconomic variables and epidemic risk.

Once an epidemic occurs, the main objectives of control (Nájera et al., 1998) should be to:

- provide adequate relief to the affected population,
- contain transmission, if possible, in affected areas,
- prevent further spread of the epidemic,
- improve emergency preparedness in order to prevent future epidemics.

The first two objectives require the rapid use of effective control interventions using appropriate drugs and insecticides. Emergency action will include mass drug administration, mass fever treatment and space spraying with insecticides. Containment of transmission will include indoor residual spraying and the use of impregnated mosquito nets. The last two objectives require the assessment of risk and the application of preventive measures.

## PREVENTION AND CONTROL OF OUTBREAKS OF INTRODUCED MALARIA

Factors related to the origin of epidemics of malaria are discussed in Chapter 5. There is no doubt that the most important practical method for monitoring the malaria situation is a continued and regular surveillance of fever cases and examination of blood films from all, or a reasonable proportion of, such patients. An additional approach for determining the warning threshold of a possible malaria epidemic is the knowledge of the malariogenic potential, which is the product of receptivity and vulnerability of the area concerned. From the purely practical point of view, one may distinguish two different circumstances of an epidemic outbreak: (1) in a non-endemic area, and (2) in an endemic area. In both situations, one may take into account the ratio between indigenous and immigrant populations. Where the area is non-endemic, an outbreak would develop only when a large parasite reservoir has been imported. On the other hand, when there is an influx of a large number of non-immune people into an endemic area, an outbreak of malaria may occur rapidly, unless the new population is protected. Naturally, all the factors of the environment, as well as those related to the vector and the species of the parasite, will have to be considered. As mentioned before, P. vivax malaria is much faster in multiplying than P. falciparum and an outbreak due to the latter species reaches its epidemic peak when some 50 per cent of the population are infected. There is, in both cases, a stage of slow growth before a sudden rise. When secondary, locally

transmitted cases occur, the emergency insecticidal and chemotherapeutic measures cannot act as rapidly as they would if earlier action had been taken.

Two needs arise when dealing with a malaria epidemic: one is to recognize it at its earliest stage; and the other is to stop it by all the methods available. In planning control measures against a potential malaria epidemic, two degrees of prevention have been advocated:

1. first-degree prevention, in which measures are taken against the importation of vectors or suspected sources of infection,
2. second-degree prevention, in which measures are taken against the re-establishment of transmission.

If the infected vectors arrive from outside the area, there are no fully reliable defences, although protection of the border zone by residual spraying may be of some value. Protection against the influx of infected people comes under the vigilance mechanism, which should detect all cases of imported malaria and provide some information on the possibility of the introduction of drug-resistant strains of plasmodia. The activities required for second-degree prevention comprise the following: study of patterns of population movements, provision of diagnostic facilities, maintenance of case detection posts, epidemiological investigation of active foci of malaria, radical cure of patients with malaria, and re-introduction of residual spraying in the area involved. However, any such measures must be preceded by the wide use of antimalarial drugs, and especially those that can combine the treatment of acute malaria with good preventive properties. For most circumstances in which P. falciparum is the major species involved, 4-aminoquinolines are no longer the most appropriate drug to use due to widespread resistant strains of this parasite. Thus, other, more appropriate, drugs (preferably single dose) will have to be used, together with the wide use of primaquine as a gametocytocide. In the case of P. vivax epidemics, 4-aminoquinolines are still the most appropriate, except where highly resistant strains occur, together with primaquine for a radical cure of relapsing cases.

All necessary imagicidal measures of vector control should be instituted, including space spraying and aerial spraying if feasible. However, these measures have only limited impact and additional action is necessary.

A force of auxiliary health workers will have to be gathered and trained to search for malaria cases and apply the required remedial measures. It is important to follow up the foci from which malaria has been eliminated. It is doubtful whether the basic health services will be able to cope, unless they are of exceptional competence and can take appropriate and rapid action in cases of extensive or localized epidemics. It may be necessary to improve accessibility, acceptability and quality of care provided by the local health units that are responsible for detecting, managing and reporting malaria cases. The value of special epidemiological and epidemic detection and containment services as part of the health system may be particularly appreciated in areas prone to malaria epidemics.

## MALARIA CONTROL IN DEVELOPMENT PROJECTS

Development projects and industrial undertakings in the tropics are often a fertile ground for outbreaks of malaria, due to the fact that many among a large labour force, including newcomers to the area, are either non-immune to the local strains of plasmodia or introduce strains to which the local population is particularly susceptible. Moreover, the living conditions of the labour force may often be less than adequate and the construction activity contributes to environmental pollution. For detailed guidance on malaria control related to migration into development areas, see the WHO *Manual on personal and community protection* (WHO, 1974).

A point made in Chapter 5 concerning 'man-made malaria' deserves some amplification. It refers to the creation of breeding places of malaria vectors and other mosquitoes as a result of human activities. The list of such potential breeding places, which are usually close to human habitations, is very long. It comprises barrels, badly designed or blocked soakaway pits, garden pools, cisterns, disused wells, borrow-pits left by building projects, obstructed drains, etc. Much malaria has been due to bad handling of water in irrigation channels, poorly sited ditches, culverts, leaking sluice gates, seepages and fallow rice-fields. No major operations involving water supply should be undertaken without considering their possible impact on malaria and other water-related diseases

and requesting appropriate advice on the malaria situation of the area involved and on methods of prevention and control of the disease.

Three principles should be adhered to in all engineering projects in the tropics: the first is not to make additional breeding places for mosquitoes, the second is to know how to correct the errors once made, and the third is to involve the health authorities from the very beginning of the project.

The duty of the resident medical adviser is to foresee the potential dangers, to protect the health of the working force as well as of their families, and to be ready to act in an emergency.

Selection of a suitable site for new housing, temporary or permanent, may avoid much subsequent difficulty. The principles of this are described above. Such site selection may be vital to the success of many projects, though better methods of control, if available, should be fully used.

Existing breeding places may be dealt with by the use of larvicides, drainage, or modification of the water to make it unsuitable as a breeding place. The necessary steps must be taken within the radius of flight of the local vector, commonly a mile (1.6 km) but more in some places, and throughout the entire transmission season. They must be based on a knowledge of the local vector and particularly of its breeding habits, and on a detailed survey of the area showing all water sites of the potentially dangerous type within the radius prescribed.

The prevention of malaria among the non-immune labour force entails the provision of personal protection measures and regular chemoprophylaxis with an appropriate antimalarial drug.

If malaria is already prevalent on any scale among the labour force, the right policy is to eliminate the infection and thus reduce its transmission. The most practical way of doing this is to muster the work force and for each adult to be given and seen to swallow a single-dose radical treatment according to the national drug policy currently in force. This initial curative treatment should be followed by appropriate and regular chemoprophylaxis. 'Breakthroughs' should be promptly treated. Space spraying of insecticides is of limited practical value and the expense of this method is considerable. However, at times, noisy and clearly visible applications of thermal or other aerosols have some value, in addition to having a psychological effect, which may inspire confidence in the health authorities and increase the co-operation of the population and of administrative echelons.

The regular use of commercial, low-pressure aerosol containers for disinsectization of premises of the technical and managerial staff (usually at their own expense) should be encouraged.

For more permanent malaria control, residual insecticides should be used. This does not make great demands on personnel; several small schemes could be amalgamated into one. The most economical working unit is a population of between 10 000 and 20 000. Where amalgamation into units of such size is possible, one skilled assistant can be employed full time for organization and management. In smaller schemes, supervision may have to be part time, but should not be, for that reason, of minor importance. For the initial rounds of spraying, an appropriate insecticide will have to be selected based on clear-cut criteria. This application should be repeated as frequently as necessary to ensure an active deposit on the walls during the transmission period.

Workers should be carefully trained in the proper use of spray equipment in order to obtain a regular and even application of given quantities of fluid. Water can be used for training purposes. An even dosage of the spray can be attained by practice, provided that the supervisor has personally taken the trouble to become competent at it. All houses and animal sheds in the area should be sprayed, unless there is sufficient evidence or reliable experience to indicate that discrimination between different structures is possible.

After establishing full control by such means, a revision programme can be considered. The chief intention will be to prolong the interval between insecticide applications, but, before this is contemplated, the frequency with which walls are replastered should be carefully examined. If the walls are often whitewashed or replastered, frequent respraying is essential.

After the initial treatment has been operative, transmission of malaria within the treated area should decrease. The size of the treated area and the extent to which people move out of it at night will clearly affect the resulting incidence of malaria, but, in a labour group of 10 000 or more people, the amount of malaria should be reduced to negligible proportions.

Managerial and senior staff should also be protected by residual insecticide spraying. As they normally occupy houses in which the discoloration caused by wettable powders would be objectionable, solutions or emulsions of insecticides should be used. Such houses may well be screened or provided with some screened rooms, and for this purpose it is best to use plastic screen cloth. The use of mosquito nets, preferably impregnated, for labour forces and staff, even in screened houses, should be encouraged and the importance of regular drug prophylaxis emphasized.

## SUMMARY OF MAIN CONTROL MEASURES FOR SOME MAJOR MALARIA PROTOTYPES

1. African savannah malaria.
   (a) Provision of early diagnosis and treatment.
   (b) Impregnated mosquito nets or curtains may be useful.
2. Desert, highland fringe malaria.
   (a) Provision of early diagnosis and treatment.
   (b) Monitoring climatic and ecological changes.
   (c) Early detection and control of epidemics.
3. Malaria in plains and valleys outside Africa.
   (a) Provision of early diagnosis and treatment.
   (b) Sustainable vector control methods.
   (c) Early response to situations of increased risk.
4. Forest-related malaria.
   (a) Provision of early diagnosis and treatment.
   (b) Personal protection measures (repellents/impregnated mosquito nets).
   (c) Chemoprophylaxis.
5. Agricultural development malaria.
   (a) Provision of early diagnosis and treatment.
   (b) Personal protection measures (as above).
6. Urban malaria.
   (a) Provision of early diagnosis and treatment.
   (b) Environmental sanitation.
   (c) Personal protection measures (as above).
7. Coastal and marshland malaria.
   (a) Provision of early diagnosis and treatment.
   (b) Engineering methods.
   (c) Personal protection measures (as above).
8. War and socio-political malaria.
   (a) Provision of early diagnosis and treatment.
   (b) Temporary chemoprophylaxis.
   (c) Spraying of shelters.
   (d) Personal protection measures (as above).

A classification of malaria control measures is given in Table 6.9.

## COST OF MALARIA CONTROL

The cost of malaria control varies considerably in relation to a number of factors, such as the the prevalent parasite species and therefore the antimalarial drugs used, the type of insecticide used, the methods involved, the degree of surveillance, the cost of labour, transport, administration etc. Therefore, it is difficult, if not impossible, to give any idea of an average cost of a programme unless full information on it is available. Nevertheless, it should be possible to plan malaria control measures that are within the budgetary limitations of the programme and could be extended as economic development proceeds. Effective malaria control depends on the regular application of appropriate procedures. This can be assured only if a regular budget is provided and maintained over the whole duration of the programme, which should also be planned so that its eventual extension may be beneficial for the future development of the country.

The estimated cost, in 1999, of malaria control in an endemic area inhabited by a population of 1 million based on one round of spraying or a single full-dose treatment is shown in Table 6.10.

Generally speaking, the average expenditure in extensive programmes involving the protection of a million people is not comparable with the estimation of costs of antimalaria activities aimed at protection of a few thousand people over a limited period (e.g. construction phase of a development project). In the latter case, the overall costs may be lower if the degree of performance is adjusted to the temporary needs of the project over a relatively short time. However, such savings may be illusory if the degree of exposure to malaria is considerable. Normally, any measures of malaria control can be easily incorporated into the general medical and community health budgeting of an important development project. It is always preferable to involve the local population as much as possible in participating in all environmental methods of malaria control and to extend the benefits of them to the peripheral localities and villages.

Personal protection measures and the provision of mosquito-proof houses are important. Communal places such as hospitals and cafeterias should also be

**Table 6.9** *Classification of malaria control measures*

| Type of measures | Individual and family protection | Community protection |
|---|---|---|
| Prevention of human–vector contact | Repellents, protective clothing, impregnated mosquito nets, screening of houses | Site selection, screening of houses |
| Destruction of adult *Anopheles* vectors | Use of domestic space sprays including aerosols | Space spraying, ultra-low-volume sprays, residual insecticide spraying |
| Destruction of mosquito larvae | Peridomestic sanitation, intermittent drying of water containers | Larviciding of water surfaces, intermittent drying, sluicing, biological methods |
| Source reduction of mosquitoes | Filling, small-scale drainage and other forms of water management | Prevention of man-made malaria, environmental sanitation, water management, drainage schemes, naturalistic methods of control |
| Measures against the malaria parasites | Early diagnosis and treatment, chemoprophylaxis | Early diagnosis and treatment, chemoprophylaxis/intermittent presumptive treatment to primigravidae, mass drug administration (in epidemics) |
| Social participation | Motivation for personal and family protection | Community involvement, health education, expansion of rural health services, training of staff |

protected by screened windows and doors. It goes without saying that the proper organization of anti-malaria activities for a development project demands the availability of competent technical supervisory and executive personnel. Unreasonable budgetary restrictions on trained and experienced staff are a false economy as they jeopardize the very aim of some development projects.

## Cost-effectiveness and choice of interventions

Anne Mills (Mills, 1991) published a critical review of the economics of malaria control and studied the household costs of malaria in Nepal (Mills, 1993).

Clearly, the nature of the different epidemiological situations and the extent and management of the health systems will have an impact on the choice and cost of malaria interventions. Because chemotherapy is common to all the situations, it must be borne in mind that the cost of this intervention should take into account the comprehensive costs of the treatment itself to the provider and consumer as well as the costs of the patient seeking, or being referred for, treatment, which will vary from area to area. At 1999 prices, the approximate cost of one adult course of drug treatment alone for *P. falciparum malaria* was as follows: chloroquine $0.09; sulfadoxine–pyrimethamine $0.14; mefloquine $1.80; quinine and tetracycline $1.11; and artesunate monotherapy $6.54.

In evaluating the economics of malaria control Mills (1991) concentrated on the following five areas of concern:

1. The determinants of malaria transmission.
2. The resource costs of malaria.
3. The demand for malaria treatment and prevention.

**Table 6.10** *Estimated costs, in 1999, of malaria control in an endemic area inhabited by a population of 1 million, for one round of spraying and one full-dose treatment using the more commonly available products*

| Type of spraying | Requirements for one round or single dose | Price per unit (US$) | Total cost of insecticide or drug (US$) | Per capita cost of insecticide or drug (US$) |
|---|---|---|---|---|
| Residual spraying with DDT 75% water-dispersible powder (w.d.p.) at 2 g/m² | 147 tonnes | 3950 per tonne | 580 650 | 0.58 |
| Residual spraying with malathion 50% w.d.p. at 2 g/m² | 220 tonnes | 4300 per tonne | 946 000 | 0.95 |
| Residual spraying with deltamethrin 2.5% w.d.p. at 0.05 g/m² | 110 tonnes | 20 000 per tonne | 2 200 000 | 2.2 |
| Residual spraying with pyrimiphos-methyl 50% emulsion concentrate (e.c.) at 2 g/m² | 220 tonnes | 16 000 per tonne | 3 520 000 | 3.52 |
| Full 3-day treatment using chloroquine (25 mg base/kg) | 11.25 million tablets at 100 mg base | 6.05 per 1000 tablets | 68 063 | 0.08 |
| Full single-dose treatment with sulfadoxine–pyrimethamine (25 mg/kg) | 2.5 million tablets each 500 mg sulfadoxine and 25 mg pyrimethamine | 47.0 per 1000 tablets | 117 500 | 0.12 |
| Full-dose treatment with quinine (10 mg/kg) 8-hourly for 7 days | 31.5 million tablets each 300 mg sulphate | 41.25 per 1000 tablets | 1 299 375 | 1.30 |
| Full-dose treatment with artesunate (2 mg/kg) twice on the first day then daily for the next 4 days | 13.5 million tablets each of 50 mg | 365 per 1000 tablets | 4 927 500 | 4.93 |

*Note*: The annual number of spraying rounds depends on the endemicity of malaria and on the degree of control to be achieved. In order to obtain a good control in holoendemic areas, two rounds of DDT or three to four rounds of malathion would be required. The above figures do not include the cost of application of vector control measures or the distribution of drugs, that is to say that costs of transport, storage, salaries and travel of personnel have not been considered.

4. The characteristics of the supply of malaria control.
5. Economic evaluation, which includes cost analysis, cost-effectiveness analysis, cost-utility analysis and cost–benefit analysis.

Mills emphasizes the point that, in cost-effectiveness analysis, health effects are retained in natural units, whereas in cost–benefit analysis, they are converted into monetary terms.

The resource costs are two-fold: the costs of prevention and treatment, and the indirect costs expressed in terms of production. The latter have often been exaggerated and have not taken into consideration factors such as parasite species and immune status, frequency of proven attacks of malaria, efficacy and rapidity of treatment, time of year of alleged attacks and substitution by non-salaried members of the family, low value of labour at certain times of the year, and variation in productivity by age and sex.

Few studies on factors influencing the demand for drug treatment and mosquito nets have been carried out, and the supply role of the private sector has, until recently, been ignored. The often-observed waste in health centre prescribing practices has only occasionally been documented. Our knowledge about whether and how individuals adapt their behaviour to influence their malaria risk is rudimentary.

A review of the literature on treatment seeking for malaria prepared by McCombie (1994) reiterates that cost is an important consideration in the choice of treatment, and economic factors can be related to delays in seeking treatment. Such delays in areas highly endemic for *P. falciparum* will result in unnecessary malaria deaths, especially in children. There is some evidence that those who practise self-treatment begin treatments earlier than those who seek care in the official health sector.

With respect to prevention, the cost of impregnated mosquito nets varies considerably depending on importation taxes and whether they are locally manufactured or subsidized. Strange as it may seem, the cost of locally made nets may be higher than that of those imported and the quality may not be as good. The material, mesh and number of woven fibres all contribute to how long the nets will last and how long the applied insecticide will persist. In a review of the community-based malaria control programme in Tigray, northern Ethiopia (WHO, 1999a), mos-

quito net affordability and community willingness to buy the nets were assessed in a resettlement community with the highest malaria prevalence. It was found that 54 per cent of households had no secure source of regular monthly cash income and, in those that did, the mean monthly income was US$19, with considerable seasonal variation among agricultural workers. When asked, 61 per cent of interviewees said they would buy nets if they could afford them (meaning not more than US$1.80) and 17 per cent said they were too poor to buy nets. In this situation, the price of an imported net through the government was set at US$5.50 and the cost of treating with an insecticide at US$0.70.

This is an example of a well-proven beneficial technology for malaria prevention that is beyond the economic means of the populations who are most at risk. We should not lose sight of the fact that malaria is a major public health problem, affecting entire communities. Until governments accept total responsibility for its control as an essential public health function, and bring to bear upon it the latest technological advances in well-planned programmes, the unnecessary loss of life will continue unabated.

## THE FUTURE OF MALARIA CONTROL

The reasons for the reverses in global malaria status over the past few decades are complex. Technical obstacles, such as the exophilic habits of some anopheline species, resistance of malaria vectors to insecticides, resistance of plasmodia to antimalarial drugs, inaccessibility of outlying groups of houses, and the primitive structure of dwellings, are of undoubted importance. It has also been realized in recent years that failure to achieve or maintain control depends not only on the previous intensity of transmission, but also on new trends in agricultural exploitation and the distribution of rural populations. Extensive agricultural development projects attract large numbers of temporary workers, who are often concentrated in labour camps where inappropriate siting and quality of shelters, the shabbiness of the environment and the overcrowding create optimal conditions for malaria transmission.

Other serious difficulties are administrative, socio-economic (nomads, refusal to spray dwellings or extreme simplicity of their construction, replastering of sprayed walls), financial (increased cost of materials, equipment and transport), and political, which affect the improvement of health conditions in developing countries with inadequate basic health services, a shortage of trained personnel and uncontrolled development of irrigation and forest exploitation. The proper organization and country-wide coverage of public health services are necessary to sustain the gains achieved.

In 1979, the 31st World Health Assembly adopted a resolution on malaria control, stressing five principles, which remain valid to this day:

1. The national will to control the disease should be expressed through a government decision to support antimalaria activities on a long-term basis.
2. Malaria control should be an integral part of the country health programme.
3. The feasibility and practicability of reducing malaria to a low level should be demonstrated.
4. The participation of the community should be obtained because the success of various methods of control will greatly depend on this.
5. Wherever applicable, permanent measures for the control of malaria should be made an integral part of the relevant development programmes.

This resolution was in line with the general requirements for health development stressed at the International Conference on Primary Health Care held in Alma-Ata in 1978. Many national strategies for malaria control are now based in conformity with these principles.

The concept of primary health care, adopted by the World Health Assembly, on the basis of recommendations of the Alma-Ata Conference, includes as one of the priorities 'the prevention and control of endemic diseases, with the full participation of the relevant communities, at a cost that the community can afford and in the spirit of self-reliance and self-determination'. The report of the Alma-Ata conference stresses that primary health care should be based on 'practical, socially acceptable methods and technology, made universally accessible to individuals and families within the community'. According to this concept, one of the responsibilities of the system of primary health care is the control of malaria. The effective co-ordination of antimalaria activities with other responsibilities at various levels of the health system is of paramount importance.

The concept of primary health care provides the malaria control programme with a structure at the village level that is essential for securing community involvement, epidemiological information and application of control measures. However, insuffficient definition of the lines of competence, supervision and responsibility for an integrated programme is bound to affect the control of malaria. Thus, in planning country malaria control programmes, there still remains the need for expertise and responsibility at the central level of health authority. This is particularly evident when one must be flexible in adapting various control approaches to local epidemiological conditions in relation to all social, economic and political factors.

Where malaria is recognized as a major health problem and where its importance has been assessed in relation to other aspects of national health, the first responsibility of the relevant authorities is to provide access for the population to diagnosis and treatment of the disease, as well as to the means for its prevention. The primary health care approach requires the selection of feasible activities. Russell stressed more than 50 years ago that striving for continuity of a modest effort should be preferred to some spectacular attempts that are only of short-term value. The creation of a network of treatment units at the village level, with an appropriate referral system to more advanced health centres, may become a channel for further preventive activities. The main aim of primary health care is the projection of its possibilities to the community through the training and activities of health workers, whether volunteers or those in salaried employment. As the health systems develop and the participation of the community is stimulated, it may be possible to embark on, or further expand, specific vector control programmes.

One of the most important functions of those responsible for providing primary health care at the village level is the provision of health education aimed at encouraging community involvement in the planning, acceptance and implementation of antimalaria activities. Such community participation is part of the national culture in some countries, but in others it must be stimulated in order to produce the desired effect.

Present experience indicates that many problems of malaria control within the system of primary health care can be rapidly solved if, as a result of good planning of field activities, staff members and personnel of every grade have full knowledge of the tasks involved, of the expected degree of their competence, provision of supplies and equipment, system of supervision, and other administrative and technical details, including the support of the community.

All these and many other aspects of malaria control through integration with primary health care have been outlined in the Seventeenth, Eighteenth and Nineteenth Reports of the WHO Expert Committee on Malaria (WHO, 1979, 1986a, 1992a), in the report of the Seventh Asian Malaria Conference on Malaria Control and National Health Goals (WHO, 1982b), and in 1991 in *Malaria – obstacles and opportunities* (Oaks *et al.*, 1991).

## Socio-economic considerations

The important role of human behavioural, social and economic factors in the epidemiology of malaria has long been recognized. Several studies have been undertaken in recent years to improve our understanding of the burden of malaria and these have been reviewed by Nájera and Hempel (1996). Several types of impact have been studied, including economic loss due to malaria, malaria and productivity, impact of malaria epidemics, malaria as a major obstacle to collective enterprises, malaria as a remaining health problem in social and economically developed areas, the effects of malaria on the individual and family, and malaria and population pressure.

The economic impact varies with the different epidemiological characteristics: whether children are predominantly affected or all age groups; how much self-treatment is undertaken; the costs involved in reaching the local clinic; the costs to governments supplying the antimalarials and other protection against the disease; indirect effects of mortality; the cumulative effect on health by malaria superimposed on other infections that are commonly found in the same community; the knowledge, attitude and practices of the community.

Attempts have been made to calculate the burden of malaria and to express it as a single indicator. To accurately reflect the impact of this disease on the population by a single parameter, taking into account the enormous complexity of its epidemiology, would require a near-perfect knowledge of all the elements and their interaction in each epi-

demiologically specific situation. The use of Disability Adjusted Life Years (DALYs) has been advocated. However, as far as malaria is concerned, DALYs ignore several important factors (Nájera and Hempel, 1996). To disregard malaria as a significant health problem based on the DALY rating could prove economically disastrous. The analysis of the socio-economic impact of malaria is multifactorial and requires a cautious, multidisciplinary approach.

## The foundation for the future

The years 1992 to 1998 are among the most significant as far as the future of global malaria control is concerned. It was during this period that a very strong and growing political commitment in support of action against malaria, both in affected countries and among donor agencies, was actively developed by the WHO. The beginning was the Ministerial Conference on Malaria, held in Amsterdam in 1992, at which the Global Malaria Control Strategy was adopted. In addition at that meeting, a Declaration on Malaria Control was adopted by the Ministers of Health from more than 90 countries, committing them to developing and supporting malaria control programmes based on the Global Strategy. This strategy aims to control malaria disease through early diagnosis and prompt treatment, including improving the management of severe and complicated malaria, controlling epidemics and using preventive measures that are locally effective and sustainable.

This conference was followed in 1993 by a review of the global malaria situation by the Economic and Social Council of the United Nations (ECOSOC), which led to the endorsement of the Global Malaria Control Strategy by the 49th Session of the United Nations General Assembly in 1994 (Resolution 49/135). In the following year, the United Nations General Assembly called upon the Director General of the WHO (Resolution 50/128) and the international community to continue to mobilize all resources to provide the affected developing countries, especially African countries, with technical, medical and financial resources to implement national plans for malaria control.

The 1996 World Health Assembly responded by urging the re-establishment of an Action Programme against malaria and the Director General of the WHO provided US$10 million in each of the years

1997 and 1998 for an accelerated control programme in Africa. This laid the foundation for future action against malaria on that continent.

In June 1997, the Assembly of Heads of State and Government of the Organization of African Unity issued the Harare Declaration on Malaria Prevention and Control in the Context of African Economic Recovery and Development (AHG/Decl. 1 (XXXIII)). This was a major political step forward, because the Assembly pledged to fully support the implementation of the global and regional strategies and called upon all member states to take immediate action. In the year that followed, all endemic African countries strengthened their malaria control activities, supported by the accelerated programme.

During the Summit of the Group of Eight industrialized countries, held in Birmingham, UK, in May 1998, the leaders agreed to support the WHO-led antimalaria campaign as part of a larger plan to combat infectious and parasitic diseases.

Thus, by 1998, there had never been such a comprehensive political support for global action against malaria since the establishment of the WHO Global Malaria Eradication Campaign in 1956. All that remained to be done was to strengthen the support to the countries, particularly in the areas of planning, programme management, systems development, communications, surveillance and the introduction of more effective technologies. This augured well for the future success of malaria control, and economic development, in endemic countries as the world's population entered the third millennium.

## Roll Back Malaria

Roll Back Malaria is the title that has been given to a priority project of the WHO that was established on 23 July 1998. It is taken from the *Oxford English Dictionary* definition of 'roll back', which is 'to cause to retreat or decrease', which the project is intended to do globally to malaria, although it is concentrated in Africa. Its emphasis is on partnership, evidence-based action, political mobilization and participation of civil society. The core concepts are: to focus on results, to prioritize effective action, to stimulate attention, innovative approaches, evidence-based action, stronger emphasis on political context, a common platform for multi-disease action and fostering a social movement that puts concepts into practice. The movement is

expected to halve the global burden of disease associated with malaria by the year 2010, particularly deaths, and to reduce it further in succeeding years. In this regard, the WHO has now published its second edition of the practical handbook on the management of severe malaria (WHO, 2000b), which first came out in 1991 (Gilles, 1991). Both the first and second editions of this practical guide to managing severe disease were based on careful and painstaking reviews of the scientific evidence by the world's leading specialists in this field (WHO, 1986b, 2000a; Warrell *et al.*, 1990). In addition, the WHO has developed a set of learning materials consisting of a learner and tutor's guide, which is based on these publications together with practical experience in countries.

It is clear that we now have the scientific knowledge and the tools to prevent and manage severe malaria disease and thus to reduce the prevalence of malaria deaths anywhere in the world. However, it will only happen if health services are properly planned and effectively managed. This means that systems need to be in place and fully functioning for the timely delivery of both preventive and curative measures.

Strategies to manage malaria, both uncomplicated and severe, at the peripheral health level, and even in the home, are being developed by the Roll Back Malaria Project in collaboration with the Tropical Diseases Research Programme and various institutions, particularly in Africa.

## Essential systems for successful malaria control

For more than two decades, the WHO actively dismantled a vertical approach to malaria control and promoted an integrated approach. In that time, malaria became an increasing impediment to social and economic development in endemic areas, and the burden of death and disease continued unabated. It is clear that those responsible for national malaria control activities have not been able to influence the development of effective systems into which to integrate antimalarial activities for maximum effect. In fact, a systems approach to health services delivery, although advocated for many years, has yet to become a reality in the majority of tropical countries. The global efforts to eradicate and then to control malaria were far too premature to ensure that the gains achieved could be sustained by integration into health services.

As a prerequisite for effective integrated malaria control in highly endemic areas and as a basis to solving emerging problems, it will be essential to put in place various systems that will stand the test of time. Furthermore, because malaria is not just a health problem but a public health issue with social, economic and development components, governments need to accept responsibility for some very basic, critical and essential public health functions that transcend numerous ministries within government as well as the private sector.

A systems approach has the advantage of allowing long-range planning, both for the development of much needed human resources as well as for the development of the capacity to manage health problems. There are several systems that are essential for effective malaria control, and perhaps the most important, if the Roll Back Malaria initiative is to succeed, is to ensure that all families, especially the marginalized and poorest, have ready access to adequate doses of antimalarial drugs the moment they are needed and to appropriate preventive measures. Other systems that are needed include referral for severe cases, information, especially for early warning of epidemics, monitoring treatment failures, monitoring insecticide efficacy and environmental sanitation, just to mention a few.

However, systems are of little value unless they are appropriately managed. To address this, the WHO in 1999 developed a new programme called Management Effectiveness (WHO, 1999c). This is the beginning of the improvement in health services management emphasizing customer satisfaction and improved cost-effectiveness. Health managers will have to be quality-focused and committed to the continuous improvement of management processes and practices in health care. The challenges for institutional leaders will be to act on the whole system and for managers to constantly improve work processes. The Management Effectiveness Programme will function at country level and will be supported by Regional Learning Networks. The WHO Eastern Mediterranean Region countries have been the first to take up this programme, which has serious training and development components.

## MALARIA RESEARCH

Malariology is a well-defined discipline, aimed at increasing our understanding of all aspects of this disease and at forging better tools for fighting it. Malaria research was actively pursued throughout the entire twentieth century and well before that. It has provided the scientific evidence on which the Malaria Eradication and Global Malaria Control strategies have been based. In addition, governments, military and civil institutions and the pharmaceutical industry have conducted research from which new antimalarial drugs, insecticides and diagnostic tools have eventually been marketed.

In 1975, a Special Programme for Research and Training in Tropical Diseases was established jointly by the United Nations, the World Bank and the WHO. Its 20-year progress report covers the period 1975–94 (WHO, 1995) and provides a valuable insight into the development of the programme and what has been accomplished.

This programme (TDR) is still operational today, although since 1998 its programme management functions are dramatically different from what they were previously, according to the latest biennial progress report for the period 1997–98 (WHO, 1999b). However, the four main areas – of strategic research, product research and development, applied field research, and research capability strengthening – still remain.

Some of the TDR-supported ongoing applied field research into malaria includes community-based trials of artesunate suppositories for the coverage of children with severe malaria until they reach hospital; more feasible and effective ways to improve home management of uncomplicated malaria; drug packaging studies to improve patient compliance; iron supplementation versus intermittent treatment to prevent malaria anaemia in the first 5 years of life; and exploration of ways of stopping or delaying malaria parasite resistance to antimalarial drugs. Regarding the last-mentioned, it is encouraging to note that the work of Professor Wallace Peters carried out during the 1970s and 1980s is now being seriously pursued with respect to delaying resistance by the use of drug combinations, which he demonstrated in animal studies. Another very significant approach is the identification of markers of resistance for early detection and mapping.

## Drug development

The need for new drugs for malaria is particularly urgent as there are areas in the world where strains of

*P. falciparum* are showing resistance to almost all known antimalarials and many large industrial companies have stopped research in this area due to the very high costs and poor returns.

To help solve this crisis, public agencies have joined the pharmaceutical industry to create a unique mechanism for developing antimalarial drugs, which otherwise may never see the light of day. This is a major initiative that has been realized through dialogue on this subject between the WHO and pharmaceutical industry leaders, which began in October 1998 and culminated in agreement in November 1999. This new venture is called the Medicines for Malaria Venture (MMV) and has been established as an independent foundation operating as a non-profit business. Clearly, large sums of money are required for this to be successful. Three very large companies are already committed, along with universities that have the necessary capacity. Among the initial co-sponsors are the WHO, International Federation of Pharmaceutical Manufacturers Associations, World Bank, three government agencies and the Rockefeller Foundation.

It should be emphasized, however, that, unless comparable amounts of resources are invested in developing the means to deliver and use new drugs and tools properly – that is to say, effective and efficient health systems and national drug policies – this disease will continue to seriously burden populations and to impede social and economic progress.

The trioxane compounds derived from the plant *Artemisia annua* (qinghaosu, which was used in ancient times to treat fever in China) have continued to be the subject of trials and studies since they were first isolated by Chinese scientists in 1972. These and a series of synthetic derivatives are among the most potent antimalarial compounds known. Three compounds have been evaluated extensively: the parent compound artemisinin, the water-soluble artesunate and the oil-soluble ether artemether. Artesunate is unstable in solution and has to be made up immediately before intravenous injection. Artemisinin has been studied in oral and rectal formulations. Artemether is an oil-soluble methyl ether formulation for intramuscular injection.

TDR has been supporting research on a derivative related to artemether called arteether. It is approaching the manufacture and marketing stage and, so as not to confuse it with artemether, it has been proposed that the international non-proprietary name for arteether be changed to artenimol.

The search for approaches to manage, and to delay the emergence and propagation of, drug-resistant strains of *P. falciparum* continues. In this regard, there are many studies being conducted on different combinations of the available antimalarials. These include chlorproguanil and dapsone and various combinations with artemisinin and its derivatives.

## Vaccine development (*see also* Chapter 13)

It is expected that in the first part of this century, one or more malaria vaccines will be actively developed by the pharmaceutical industry. New techniques have become available and there is intensified political and financial support for research.

However, due to the antigenic diversity of the malaria parasite, the identification and development of vaccine candidate antigens are complex and high-risk undertakings. A multi-stage, multi-component vaccine that targets several antigens from several stages of the life cycle would have the best chance of controlling the growth of the parasite in the host and eventually the community. Asexual blood-stage vaccines, which prevent the merozoite from entering or developing within red blood cells, would directly impact disease morbidity and death. At present, more than 10 promising candidate vaccines for *P. falciparum* are in various stages of research. The adjuvant (a neutral substance that enhances the body's immune response to antigens) used with a vaccine is important and several novel adjuvants are also being studied.

A new formulation of the SPf66 blood-stage cocktail vaccine (which was developed in Colombia and underwent numerous field trials in the 1990s, with mixed results) combined with a new adjuvant is under clinical testing. Other vaccines being studied include an apical membrane protein, a combination B made up of three antigens, and a multi-stage, multi-component vaccine containing 12 B-cell, six T-helper cell and three CTL epitopes derived from nine antigens.

Pre-erythrocytic stage vaccines are designed to prevent the parasite's infective sporozoite stage from entering or developing within the liver cells. This would prevent infection in non-immunes. Four vaccines based on the circumsporozoite protein are in various stages of studies and trials in Africa, the USA and Europe.

Transmission-blocking vaccines aim at preventing the successful development of the malaria parasite in its mosquito host (WHO, 2000d). They would have an impact on transmission and drug resistance development. There is one major candidate vaccine antigen, PFs-25, being studied, but four others could eventually be included.

## Diagnosis

Several rapid diagnostic tests for malaria using immunochromatographic methods have now been developed. These have detection capabilities that are in general comparable to those commonly achieved by microscopy in health services. However, compared to microscopy, the main disadvantages are: lack of sensitivity at low levels of parasitaemia; inability to quantify parasite density; inability to differentiate among P. vivax, P. ovale and P. malariae as well as between the sexual and asexual stages of the parasite; persistently positive, despite parasite clearance by chemotherapy; and relatively high cost per test. Diagnostic tests, both the use of microsocopy and rapid tests, can contribute to improved and more cost-effective disease management, and reduce the unnecessary and irrational use of antimalarial drugs. The microscope is a key tool in integrated disease management and the optimum role of rapid diagnostic tests remains to be determined.

Recently, the WHO identified issues for further study (WHO, 2000c), which include further improvement of the technical characteristics of the rapid tests such as sensitivity, specificity, ease of use and robustness. It was also suggested that there should be a system of international quality control and quality assurance outside of the commercial sector, including the development of a bank of reference reagents and a network of field test sites.

## Other activities

Iron-deficiency anaemia, the main cause of nutritional anaemia worldwide, is a special problem in malaria endemic areas. In high transmission areas, malaria is the major contributor to severe anaemia in infants, accounting for 50 per cent of hospital admissions and episodes. Recent studies in Tanzania have demonstrated that daily oral iron supplementation prevented about 30 per cent of severe anaemia episodes in the first year of life and was not associated with any increased susceptibility to clinical malaria. On the other hand, weekly malaria chemoprophylaxis reduced the rate of severe anaemia by 57 per cent. Studies are now underway to compare the relative protection afforded by iron supplementation with that afforded by intermittent malaria treatment.

The above are the main thrusts of malaria research being conducted at the present time. However, there are numerous studies being carried out in institutions and national control programmes throughout the world in order to find better ways of managing the disease and changing the epidemiological equilibrium in favour of disease control and eventual elimination. The results of many of these studies may never be published, for various reasons, and the knowledge gained is often used to change the way in which countries approach the problem.

Thus, small-scale applied field research studies are essential in the malaria endemic areas in order to plan the most effective malaria control approaches based on the local epidemiological and economic situations. In addition, it is essential that health systems research be carried out in the context of malaria control to ensure the best possible use of the existing and new tools, and to meet the ever-changing and growing needs of the community.

## REFERENCES

Barnard D. Repellants/toxicants for application to skin/fabric for personal protection In Global collaboration for development of pesticides for public health – report of first meeting. Geneva, WHO/WHOPES/GCDPP/98.1, 1998.

Boyd MF. Malariology. Philadelphia, Saunders, 1949.

Bruce-Chwatt LJ, de Zulueta J. The rise and fall of malaria in Europe. Oxford, Oxford University Press, 1980.

Coffee RA. Electrodynamic energy – a new approach to pesticide application. Proc 1979 Crop Protection Conference – Pests and Diseases 1979; 22: 777–89.

Curtis CF, et al. Impregnated bed nets and curtains against malaria mosquitoes. In Appropriate technology in vector control. Boca Raton, CRC Press, 1990.

de Barjac H, Sutherland LJ. Bacterial control of mosquitoes and black flies, genetics and applications of Bacillus thuringiensis israelensis *and Bacillus Sphaericus*. New Brunswick, NJ, Rutgers University Press, 1990.

Foster SDF. The distribution and use of antimalarial drugs – not a pretty picture. In *Malaria – waiting for the vaccine*. Targett GAT, ed. Chichester, John Wiley, 1991, 141–68.

Gilles HM. *Management of severe malaria – a practical handbook*. Geneva, World Health Organization, 1991.

Gilroy AB. *Malaria control by coastal swamp drainage in West Africa*. 1948.

Hildemann WH, Walford RS. Annual fishes: promising species as biological control agents. *J Trop Med Hyg* 1963; **66**: 163–6.

McCombie SC. *Treatment seeking for malaria: a review and suggestions for future research*. TDR/SER/RP/94.1. Geneva, World Health Organization, 1994.

Miller JE, Lindsay SN, Armstrong JR. Experimental hut trials of bed nets impregnated with synthetic pyrethroid or organophosphate insecticide for mosquito control in the Gambia. *Med Vet Entomol* 1991; **5**: 465–76.

Mills A. Economics of malaria control. In *Malaria – waiting for the vaccine*. Targett GAT, ed. Chichester, John Wiley, 1991, 141–68.

Mills A. The household costs of malaria in Nepal. *Trop Med Parasitol* 1993; **44**: 9–13.

Nájera JA, Hempel J. *The burden of malaria*. WHO/CTD/MAL/96.10. Geneva, World Health Organization, 1996.

Nájera JA, *et al. Malaria epidemics: detection and control, forecasting and prevention*. Geneva, World Health Organization, 1998.

Oaks SC, Mitchell VS, Pearson GW, Carpenter CC, eds. *Malaria – obstacles and opportunities*. Washington DC, Institute of Medicine, National Academy Press, 1991.

Pampana EY. *A textbook of malaria eradication*, 2nd edition. Oxford, Oxford University Press, 1969.

Rozendaal JA. Impregnated mosquito nets and curtains for self-protection and vector control. *Trop Dis Bull* 1989; **86**: R1–R41.

Russell PF. *Malaria: basic principles briefly stated*. Oxford, Blackwell Scientific Publications, 1952.

Snow RW, Lindsay SW, Hayes RJ, Greenwood BM. Permethrin treated bed nets (mosquito nets) prevent malaria in Gambian children. *Trans R Soc Trop Med Hyg* 1988; **82**: 838–42.

Snow RW, Rowan KM, Greenwood BM. A trial of permethrin treated bed nets in the prevention of malaria in Gambian children. *Trans R Soc Trop Med Hyg* 1987; **81**: 563–67.

Warrell DA, Molyneux ME, Beales PF, eds. Severe and complicated malaria, 2nd edition. *Trans R Soc Trop Med Hyg* 1990; **84**(Suppl. 2).

WHO. *Insecticide resistance and vector control*. Seventeenth Report of the WHO Expert Committee on Insecticides. Technical Report Series No. 443. Geneva, World Health Organization, 1970.

WHO. *Application and dispersal of insecticides*. Technical Report Series No. 465. Geneva, World Health Organization, 1971.

WHO. *Manual on personal and community protection against malaria in development areas and new settlements*. WHO Offset Publications, No.10. Geneva, Offset Publications, 1974.

WHO. *Resistance of vectors and reservoirs of disease to pesticides*. Twenty-second Report of the WHO Expert Committee on Insecticides. Technical Report Series No. 585. Geneva, World Health Organization, 1976.

WHO. *Engineering aspects of vector control operations*. Technical Report Series No. 603. Geneva, World Health Organization, 1977.

WHO. *Seventeenth Report of the Expert Committee on Malaria*. Technical Report Series No. 640. Geneva, World Health Organization, 1979.

WHO. *Resistance of vectors of disease to pesticides*. Fifth Report of the WHO Expert Committee on Vector Biology and Control. Technical Report Series No. 655. Geneva, World Health Organization, 1980.

WHO. *Manual on environmental management for mosquito control, with special emphasis on malaria vectors*. WHO Offset Publications, No. 66. Geneva, Offset Publications, 1982a.

WHO. *Malaria control and national health goals*. Report of Seventh Asian Malaria Conference. Technical Report Series No. 680. Geneva, World Health Organization, 1982b.

WHO. *Manual on practical entomology in malaria*. Part I – Vector bionomics and organization of antimalaria activities; Part II – Methods and techniques. WHO Offset Publication, No. 13. Geneva, Offset Publications, 1982c.

WHO. *Chemical methods for the control of arthropod vectors and pests of public health importance*. Geneva, World Health Organization, 1984.

WHO. *Eighteenth Report of the Expert Committee on Malaria*. Technical Report Series No. 735. Geneva, World Health Organization, 1986a.

WHO. Severe and complicated malaria. *Trans R Soc Trop Med Hyg* 1986b; **80**. Suppl.

WHO. *Resistance of vectors and reservoirs of diseases to insecticides*. Technical Report Series No. 737. Geneva, World Health Organization, 1986c.

WHO. *The use of impregnated bednets and other materials for vector-borne disease control*. WHO/VBC/89.981. Geneva, World Health Organization, 1989.

WHO. *Equipment for vector control*, 3rd edition. Geneva, World Health Organization, 1990.

WHO. *Expert Committee on Insecticide Resistance*. Technical Report Series No. 813. Geneva, World Health Organization, 1991.

WHO. *Expert Committee on Malaria, Nineteenth Report*. WHO/CTD/92.1. Geneva, World Health Organization, 1992a.

WHO. *World Declaration on the Control of Malaria*, Ministerial Conference on Malaria, Amsterdam, 26–27 October 1992b.

WHO. *The WHO recommended classification of pesticides by hazard and guidelines to classification 1992–1993*. WHO/PCS/92.14. Geneva, World Health Organization, 1992c.

WHO. *Vector resistance to pesticides*. Fifteenth Report of the WHO Expert Committee on Vector Biology and Control. Technical Report Series No. 818. Geneva, World Health Organization, 1992d.

WHO. *Tropical disease research – progress 1975–94, highlights 1993–94*. Twelfth Programme Report. Geneva, World Health Organization, 1995.

WHO. *Specifications for insecticides used in public health*, 7th edition. WHO/CTD/WHOPES/97.1. Geneva, World Health Organization, 1997a.

WHO. *Vector control*. Geneva, World Health Organization, 1997b.

WHO. *Chemical methods for the control of arthropod vectors and pests of public health importance*. WHO/CTD/WHOPES/97.2. Geneva, World Health Organization, 1997c.

WHO. *Global collaboration for development of pesticides for public health – report of first meeting*. WHO/WHOPES/GCDPP/98.1. Geneva, World Health Organization, 1998a.

WHO. *Test procedures for insecticide resistance monitoring in malaria vectors, bio-efficacy and persistence of insecticides on treated surfaces*. WHO/CDS/CPC/MAL/98.12. Geneva, World Health Organization, 1998b.

WHO. *Techniques to detect insecticide resistance mechanisms (field and laboratory manual)*. WHO/CDS/CPC/MAL/98.6. Geneva, World Health Organization, 1998c.

WHO. *The community-based malaria control programme in Tigray, northern Ethiopia*. WHO/CDS/RBM/99.12. Geneva, World Health Organization, 1999a.

WHO. *Tropical disease research progress 1997–1998 – fourteenth programme report*. Geneva, World Health Organization, 1999b.

WHO. *Management effectiveness programme – a journey to improve quality for health*. WHO/EMR/EML/99.2. Geneva, World Health Organization, 1999c.

WHO. *Guideline specifications for bacterial larvicides for public health use*. WHO/CDS/CPC/WHOPES/99.2. Geneva, World Health Organization, 1999d.

WHO. Severe falciparum malaria. *Trans R Soc Trop Med Hyg* 2000a; **94**(Suppl. 1).

WHO. *Management of severe malaria – a practical handbook*, 2nd edition. Geneva, World Health Organization, 2000b.

WHO. *Malaria diagnosis – new perspectives*. WHO/CDS/RBM/2000.14. Geneva, World Health Organization, 2000c.

WHO. *Malaria transmission blocking vaccines: an ideal public good*. TDR/RBM/MAL/VAC/2000.1. Geneva, World Health Organization, 2000d.

# 7

# Clinical features of malaria

DAVID A WARRELL

## INTRODUCTION

Malaria is an acute febrile illness whose severity and course depend on the species and strain of infecting parasite and thus on the geographical origin of the infection; on the age, genetic constitution, state of immunity, general health and nutritional status of the patient; and on the effects of any chemoprophylaxis or chemotherapy that has been used. There may be no diagnostic clinical features of malaria, but some patients experience the classical periodic febrile paroxysms occurring every 48 or 72 hours, with afebrile asymptomatic intervals and a tendency to recrudesce or relapse over periods of months to many years.

The incubation period is the interval between infection and the first clinical sign, usually fever, of the primary attack. The prepatent period extends from the time of infection to the first discovery of malaria parasites in the blood (Table 7.1). The minimum incubation period (about 7 days in the case of falciparum malaria) is the earliest time after arrival in a malarious country when symptoms can be attributed to malarial infection. Theoretically, there should be no prepatent period and the incubation period

should be a few days shorter when infection is with blood stage parasites (as in the case of transplacental infections and those resulting from blood transfusions, organ/tissue transplants or needlestick injuries), because no preliminary hepatic cycle need occur before infection of erythrocytes. Shorter incubation periods have been observed in a large series of cases injected with infected blood (Covell and Nicol, 1951) but, usually, the non-mosquito routes of infection are associated with longer prepatent and incubation periods because of the relatively small inoculum of parasites. Because asexual erythrocytic cycle parasites cannot invade the liver, no true relapses will follow *Plasmodium vivax* and *P. ovale* infections by these unusual routes. Incubation may be prolonged by immunity, chemoprophylaxis or chemotherapy.

The best-known symptom of malaria is the febrile paroxysm, 'ague attack' or 'ague fit', which resembles, clinically and pathophysiologically, 'endotoxin reactions' in other infections (for example, lobar pneumonia, cholangitis and pyelonephritis), response to injections or infusions contaminated with bacterial components and the Jarisch–Herxheimer reaction to the treatment of syphilis, relapsing fevers and other infections. However, many patients do not

**Table 7.1** *Main features of the human malarias*

|  | *P. falciparum* | *P. malariae* | *P. vivax* | *P. ovale* |
|---|---|---|---|---|
| Prepatent period (days) | 5.5 | 15 | 8[a] | 9 |
| Incubation period, days (mean) | 9–14 (12) | 18–40 (28) or longer | 12–17 (15) or up to 6–12 months | 16–18 (17) or longer |
| Fever periodicity (hours) (duration of asexual erythrocytic cycle) | 24, 36, 48 (quotidian, tertian, sub-/bitertian) | 72 (quartan) | 48 (tertian) | 48 (tertian) |
| Erythrocytes parasitized | All | Mature | Reticulocytes | Reticulocytes |
| Merozoites per schizont | 8–32 | 6–12 | 12–24 | 4–16 |
| Relapses | – | – | ++ | ++ |
| Recrudescences | + | + | – | – |
| Invasion requirements | ? | ? | Duffy –ve blood group | ? |
| Drug resistance | + (multiple, widespread) | – | + (chloroquine, New Guinea) | – |

[a]Longer in some strains.

experience this 'classical' manifestation of malaria, but show a nondescript fluctuating fever without dramatic exacerbations.

For 2 or 3 days before the first malarial paroxysm, the patient may complain of prodromal symptoms such as malaise, fatigue and lassitude, with (according to Manson) a desire to stretch the limbs and yawn, headache, dizziness (especially on trying to stand up), pain or aching in the chest, back, abdomen and joints and bones, anorexia, nausea, vomiting, a sensation of cold water trickling down the back and slight fever (Manson, 1898). Fever may be detectable for 2 or 3 hours before the paroxysm. The patient looks ill, may be clinically anaemic and mildly jaundiced, with tender enlargement of the liver and spleen. The conjunctivae are suffused. There are no focal signs, lymphadenopathy or rash (except for cold sores – see Plate 2 – or drug reactions). The cold stage starts with a sudden inappropriate feeling of cold and apprehension. Mild shivering quickly turns into violent teeth chattering and shaking of the whole body. Patients try to cover themselves with all available bedclothes. Although the core temperature is high and rising quickly, there is intense peripheral vasoconstriction; the skin is cold, dry, pale, cyanosed and goose-pimpled. The pulse is rapid and of low volume. The patient may vomit and febrile convulsions may develop at this stage in young children. Rigors last for 15–60 minutes, after which the shivering ceases, the patient feels some waves of warmth and the

hot stage (flush phase) ensues. Patients quickly become unbearably hot and throw off all their bedclothes. A severe throbbing headache, palpitations, tachypnoea, prostration, postural syncope, epigastric discomfort, nausea and vomiting and thirst develop as the temperature reaches its peak of 40–41 °C (104–106 °F) or more. During this phase, the patient may become confused or delirious. The skin is flushed, dry and burning. The pulse is rapid, full and bounding. Splenic enlargement may be detected for the first time at this stage. The hot stage lasts from 2 to 6 hours. In the sweating stage (defervescence or diaphoresis), the patient breaks out into a profuse, drenching sweat. The fever declines over the next 2–4 hours, symptoms diminish and the exhausted patient sleeps.

The total duration of the typical attack is 8–12 hours. Most paroxysms start between midnight and midday or, at the latest, in the early afternoon.

The classical periodicity of febrile paroxysms develops only if the patient is untreated until the infection becomes synchronized, so that sufficient numbers of erythrocytes containing mature schizonts rupture at the same time. The interval is determined by the length of the asexual erythrocytic cycle: 48 hours in *P. falciparum*, *P. vivax* and *P. ovale*, producing febrile paroxysms on alternate days (or days 1 and 3, hence tertian, according to the ancient Roman system of counting); 72 hours for *P. malariae*, causing febrile paroxysms on days 1 and 4 (hence quartan). However, intermittent fever is usually absent at the beginning of the disease, when headache, malaise, fatigue, nausea, muscular pains, diarrhoea and slight increase of body temperature are the predominant and vague symptoms, which are easily mistaken for influenza or a gastrointestinal infection. Tertian periodicity is rarely seen in falciparum malaria. A high, irregularly spiking, continuous or remittent fever or a daily (quotidian) febrile paroxysm is more usual.

Relapses of *P. vivax* and *P. ovale* result from reactivation of hypnozoite forms of the parasite in the liver. Precipitants may include cold, fatigue, trauma, pregnancy, infections including intercurrent falciparum malaria and other illnesses. Recrudescences of *P. falciparum* and *P. malariae* result from exacerbations of persistent, undetectable parasitaemias in the absence of an exo-erythrocytic cycle.

## FALCIPARUM MALARIA ('MALIGNANT' TERTIAN OR SUBTERTIAN MALARIA)

Falciparum malaria is responsible for almost all of the 2 million or more deaths attributed to malaria each year worldwide. Those who live in endemic areas and have been frequently infected acquire some immunity so that they can tolerate *P. falciparum* parasitaemia with trivial or no symptoms (Chapter 11). However, in non-immunes, such as expatriate travellers in malarious regions, falciparum infection nearly always causes debilitating symptoms and is a potentially fatal disease. Experience with malaria induced for the treatment of neurosyphilis indicated that the shortest prepatent period following a mosquito bite was 5 days, and the shortest incubation period was 7 days (Covell and Nicol, 1951). These periods were inversely proportional to the dose of sporozoites. The incubation period is prolonged by immunity, chemoprophylaxis and partial chemotherapy. In Western countries, 65–95 per cent of patients with imported falciparum malaria develop symptoms within 1 month of arriving back from the tropics. A few present up to 1 year later, but none after more than 4 years. The classical febrile malarial paroxysm followed by an afebrile asymptomatic interval is unusual with falciparum infection. The illness starts with headache, which may be severe, dizziness, pains in the neck, back, limbs or joints, malaise, anorexia, nausea, vague abdominal pain, vomiting or mild diarrhoea and a feeling of chill. There are intermittent chills rather than a clearly circumscribed cold phase, and the fever is continuous or remittent, as in enteric fevers. When periodic febrile paroxysms do occur,

**Table 7.2** *Severe manifestations and complications of* P. falciparum *malaria in adults and children*

| | Frequency | |
|---|---|---|
| | Children | Adults |
| *Clinical* | | |
| Prostration | +++ | +++ |
| Impaired consciousness | +++ | ++ |
| Respiratory distress (acidotic breathing) | +++ | + |
| Multiple convulsions | +++ | + |
| Circulatory collapse | + | + |
| Pulmonary oedema (radiological) | +/− | + |
| Abnormal bleeding | +/− | + |
| Jaundice | + | +++ |
| Haemoglobinuria | +/− | + |
| *Laboratory* | | |
| Severe anaemia (Hb <5 g/dL, haematocrit <15%) | +++ | + |
| Hypoglycaemia (<2.2 mmol/L or 40 mg/dL) | +++ | ++ |
| Acidosis (bicarbonate <15 mmol/L) | +++ | ++ |
| Hyperlactataemia (>5 mmol/L) | +++ | ++ |
| Hyperparasitaemia (>4%)[a] | ++ | + |
| Renal impairment (creatinine > 265 μmol/L or 3 mg/dL) | + | +++ |

[a]Non-immune person.

they are daily (quotidian), every third day (tertian) or twice every three days (subtertian or bitertian). The physical findings, like the symptoms, are non-specific and include fever, prostration, postural hypotension, a tinge of jaundice and tender hepatosplenomegaly. One-third of patients are afebrile when first examined. The finding of a rash, other than febrile *Herpes simplex* of the lips (see Plate 2), lymphadenopathy and focal signs suggests a diagnosis other than malaria. In non-immunes, the disease can progress very rapidly to severe life-threatening malaria unless appropriate treatment is started, and in some cases despite treatment. Some patients have died within 24 hours of their first symptom.

During the past 15 years, new attempts have been made to describe and define more precisely the life-threatening manifestations and complications of falciparum malaria so that patients found to have these problems could be given special treatment (Table 7.2) (Warrell *et al.*, 1990; WHO, 2000a).

## Cerebral malaria

This is the most familiar presentation of life-threatening malaria. In most parts of the world, about 90 per cent of adult patients will become comatose sometime before dying of malaria (Lalloo *et al.*, 1996). In adults, there is commonly a preceding history of several days of fever and non-specific symptoms (see above) before gradual impairment of consciousness or a generalized convulsion followed by persisting coma. Drowsiness is always a worrying symptom, but

**Table 7.4** *Modified Glasgow Coma Scale: 'unrousable coma' is <10 (for children, see Table 8.3, p. 216)*

|  | Score |
|---|---|
| **Eyes open** | |
| spontaneously | 4 |
| to speech | 3 |
| to pain | 2 |
| never | 1 |
| **Best verbal response** | |
| oriented | 5 |
| confused | 4 |
| inappropriate words | 3 |
| incomprehensible sounds | 2 |
| none | 1 |
| **Best motor response** | |
| obeys commands | 5 |
| localizes pain | 4 |
| flexion to pain | 3 |
| extension to pain | 2 |
| none | 1 |
| Total | 3–14 |

because high fever alone can cause confusion, irritability, obtundation, delirium, psychosis and, in children, febrile convulsions, the term cerebral malaria, which implies an encephalopathy specifically related to *P. falciparum* infection, is restricted to patients with unrousable coma assessed by the Glasgow Coma Score (Tables 7.3 and 7.4) (Warrell *et al.*, 1982). Although this strict definition of cerebral malaria is important to allow the comparison of clinical and therapeutic findings in different studies, **in clinical**

**Table 7.3** *Cerebral malaria: definitions*

*Practical definition*
Any impairment of consciousness or convulsions in a patient exposed to malaria

*Research definition*
1. Unrousable coma (Glasgow Coma Score <10/14) (see Table 7.4) persisting for more than 6 hours after a generalized convulsion
2. Asexual forms of *P. falciparum* in the blood smear
3. Exclusion of other causes of coma (see Table 7.5, p. 204) by history, cerebrospinal fluid examination, cultures and serology
4. (Fatal cases only. Confirmation of typical brain histopathology, sequestered infected erythrocytes, by post-mortem needle necropsy) (WHO, 2000a, Annex 6)

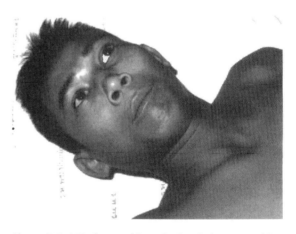

**Figure 7.1** *A Thai man with cerebral malaria: unrousable coma, open-eyed but not seeing. (Copyright DA Warrell.)*

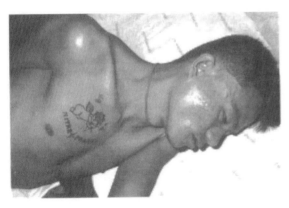

**Figure 7.2** *A Thai patient with cerebral malaria: unrousable coma, flailing and thrashing about. (Copyright DA Warrell.)*

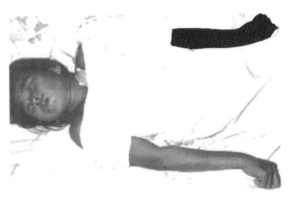

**Figure 7.4** *A Thai woman with cerebral malaria and profound hypoglycaemia showing extensor posturing (decerebrate rigidity). Note extension of the upper limbs and neck, with flexion of wrists and sustained upward gaze. (Copyright DA Warrell.)*

practice, patients with any degree of impaired consciousness and any other signs of cerebral dysfunction should be treated with the utmost urgency. Patients with cerebral malaria may be open-eyed but unseeing (Figure 7.1), may lie immobile or toss about restlessly, flailing their head from side to side (Figure 7.2) and grinding their teeth ('bruxism') (Figure 7.3). Spontaneous movement implies lighter coma and so its absence is a sign of poor prognosis. Various involuntary movements and muscular spasms are seen. Abnormal posturing may take the form of decerebrate (Figure 7.4) or decorticate (Figure 7.5) rigidity, with

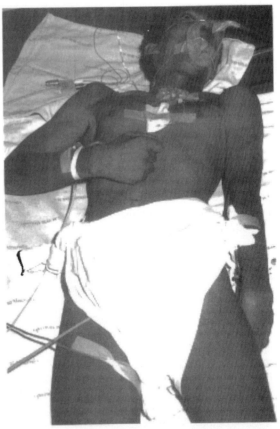

**Figure 7.5** *A Thai man with cerebral malaria uncomplicated by hypoglycaemia showing extensor posturing (decorticate rigidity). Note extension of the neck and sustained upward gaze, extension of the lower limbs and flexion of the elbows and wrists. (Copyright DA Warrell.)*

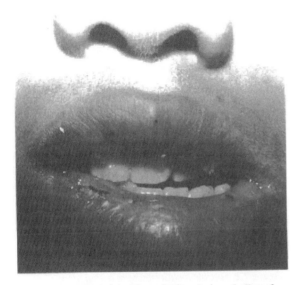

**Figure 7.3** *A Thai girl with cerebral malaria: grinding of teeth – bruxism. (Copyright DA Warrell.)*

extension of the neck and back, so that the patient assumes a position of opisthotonos, sustained upward deviation of the eyes and pouting with laboured, stertorous (grunting) respirations, or flexion of the limbs (flexor posturing). Abnormal posturing may occur spontaneously or be induced or accentuated by noxious stimuli. About one-fifth of adult patients and many more children experience convulsions. These are usually generalized, but Jacksonian-type or persistent focal seizures also occur. Subtle (covert) convulsions have been well documented in children. They may be detected clinically as nystagmoid eye movements, salivation, shallow, irregular respirations, or intermittent, minimal clonic movements involving a digit, eyebrow or mouth, or as stereotyped movements of one arm (Figure 8.3, p. 209). Electroencephalogram (EEG) monitoring confirms continuous spike-wave activity in the contralateral parieto-temporal region. There may be mild meningism and hyperextension of the neck, but neck rigidity and photophobia are unusual. Papilloedema is very rarely seen in cerebral malaria, but retinal haemorrhages (see Plate 3) are found in about 15 per cent of adults and are sometimes associated with exudates (Looareesuwan et al., 1983a). In Thai adults, but apparently not in African children, this retinopathy is associated with established or imminent coma and carries a bad prognosis.

Dysconjugate gaze is common (Figure 7.6) and convergent spasm (Figure 7.7), transient ocular bobbing, horizontal and vertical nystagmus and VIth nerve palsies are described. In adults corneal, eyelash, pupillary, oculocephalic ('doll's eye') and oculovestibu-

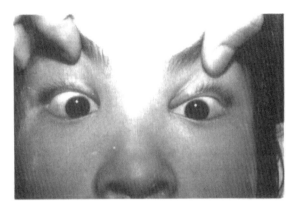

**Figure 7.7** *Convergence spasm in a Thai girl comatose with cerebral malaria. (Copyright DA Warrell.)*

lar (caloric) reflexes are usually normal, in contrast to the findings in African children (see Chapter 8). The mouth is often kept forcibly closed (Figure 7.8). The jaw jerk may be brisk. A pout reflex can usually be elicited, indicating frontal release, but a grasp reflex is rare. The gag reflex is normal. The usual neurological picture in adults is of a symmetrical upper motor neuron lesion with increased muscle tone, brisk tendon reflexes, ankle and sometimes patellar clonus and extensor plantar responses. However, muscle tone and reflexes are sometimes decreased. The brisk abdominal and other superficial reflexes usually found in younger people with fevers of other causes and with hysteria distinguish these conditions from cerebral

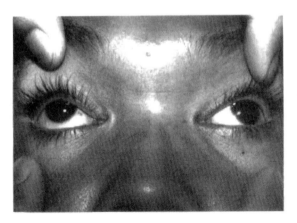

**Figure 7.6** *Dysconjugate gaze in a Thai girl comatose with cerebral malaria. The optic axes are divergent. (Copyright DA Warrell.)*

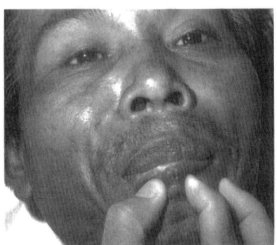

**Figure 7.8** *Forcible mouth closure in a Thai man, unrousably comatose with cerebral malaria. (Copyright DA Warrell.)*

malaria, in which these reflexes are absent. The clinical features of cerebral malaria in children are described in Chapter 8.

Patients who recover from cerebral malaria usually become rousable after about 40 hours of coma and are fully conscious within the ensuing 18 hours. Recovery after prolonged unconsciousness (for 1 week or even longer) has been observed, but is uncommon.

## PROGNOSIS OF CEREBRAL MALARIA

The mortality of cerebral malaria, as defined above, is about 15–20 per cent where good standards of hospital care can be provided (Hien *et al.*, 1996). However, patients with impaired consciousness alone, without other features of severe malaria, have a much better prognosis. In a series of 200 patients with severe malaria studied in eastern Thailand, the occurrence of 95 per cent of the deaths was evenly spaced over the first 4 days of hospital admission.

Complications of cerebral malaria include aspiration pneumonia, pressure sores and other consequences of unconsciousness. Their frequency depends on the quality of care, especially of nursing care.

Neurological sequelae are relatively common in African children (see Chapter 8), but are detected in less than 10 per cent of adults (Nguyen *et al.*, 1996). They include psychosis, extrapyramidal tremor, cerebellar ataxia (see below), cranial nerve lesions, polyneuropathy, mononeuritis multiplex, Guillain–Barré syndrome and focal or generalized convulsions.

## OTHER MANIFESTATIONS OF CENTRAL NERVOUS SYSTEM DYSFUNCTION

### Malarial psychosis

Acute psychiatric symptoms, as both the presenting feature and sequel to an attack of malaria, have been frequently reported, especially in the older literature (Anderson, 1927). However, in many cases, there were failures to confirm the diagnosis of malaria, to exclude a role for antimalarial and other drugs and to take into account the patient's previous personality. Mepacrine (quinacrine, atabrine), which was widely used for the prevention and treatment of malaria in the 1930s and 1940s, chloroquine, which was introduced in the 1950s, and mefloquine have been reported to cause psychiatric symptoms. Alcohol excess, stresses associated with life or military service in tropical countries and exacerbation of pre-existing functional psychoses may also have been implicated

in 'malarial psychosis'. Organic mental disturbances associated with malaria have been identified in some cases, usually during convalescence after the fever has subsided. Features have included apathy, amnesia, depression, atypical depression, acute psychosis, personality change, paranoid psychosis and delusions, such as the belief that family members had been killed. Brief reactive psychoses have been observed in patients recovering from cerebral malaria. These symptoms rarely persist for more than a few days, unlike those caused by functional psychoses.

### Cerebellar syndrome

Cerebellar ataxia has been described as a complication of a variety of infections, notably typhoid. The cerebellar syndrome of falciparum and vivax malaria may present as part of the acute illness in patients whose consciousness is unimpaired, in convalescence or after an asymptomatic interval of a few weeks. Most cases have been reported from the Indian subcontinent. In the late 1980s, a syndrome of delayed cerebellar ataxia was described in Sri Lanka (Senanayake, 1987; Senanayake and de Silva, 1994). Three to four weeks after developing transient fever attributable to falciparum malaria, patients presented with unsteadiness of gait and of the upper limbs, vertigo, dysarthria and headache. On examination, there was ataxia of gait, intention tremor, dysmetria, dysdiadochokinesis, nystagmus and cerebellar dysarthria. Symptoms progressed for up to 2 weeks, but resolved completely 3–16 (median 10) weeks after their onset. Corticosteroid treatment may have hastened recovery in one or two cases. Extrapyramidal tremor has been described as a sequel to cerebral malaria.

# Other features of severe falciparum malaria

## MALARIAL ANAEMIA

In parts of Africa, malarial anaemia (see Plate 4) kills as many children as cerebral malaria, its peak incidence being at the younger age of less than 2 years (see Chapter 8). It is also common in pregnant women (see Chapter 9). About 10 per cent of adult (Thai) patients with malaria are anaemic on admission to hospital (haemoglobin concentration <7 g/dL) (Phillips *et al.*, 1986). During the course of the attack, about one-third of these patients become anaemic. The severity of anaemia correlates with parasitaemia and schizontaemia. Clinical associations are with retinal haemorrhages, hepatic and renal dysfunction and secondary bacterial infections.

## MALARIAL HAEMOGLOBINURIA AND BLACKWATER FEVER

Blackwater fever was described as a common manifestation of severe falciparum malaria in long-term European expatriates, particularly in Africa in the earlier part of the twentieth century. Typically, the patient had lived in a malarious area for months or longer, had had previous attacks of malaria and was taking quinine sporadically for prophylaxis and treatment. The next attack of malaria began with the familiar symptoms, but after a few days the patient developed pain in the abdomen or loin, bilious vomiting, diarrhoea and polyuria followed by oliguria or anuria. The urine became mahogany coloured or even black. Physical signs included fever, tachycardia, tender hepatosplenomegaly, profound anaemia, jaundice and prostration. Renal failure was a common feature, as were hypotension and coma, but parasitaemia and fever were mild or absent. Severe intravascular haemolysis in the absence of hyperparasitaemia was usually attributed to immune haemolysis of quinine-sensitized erythrocytes, but this has never been proved (Hien et al., 1996). Older reports of blackwater fever among indigenous populations of malaria-endemic regions must be re-evaluated now that erythrocyte enzyme deficiencies such as glucose-6-phosphate dehydrogenase deficiency are known to be prevalent in these populations. These deficiencies render erythrocytes vulnerable to oxidant stress by antimalarial drugs such as primaquine or chloroquine (see Plate 5).

## JAUNDICE AND HEPATIC DYSFUNCTION
(Warrell and Francis, 1999)

Jaundice (see Plate 6) is far more common in adults than in children. Almost one-third of Thai patients become jaundiced during an attack of falciparum malaria (Wilairatana et al., 1994). Jaundice is associated with cerebral malaria, acute renal failure, pulmonary oedema, shock, hyperparasitaemia and other severe complications. Tender enlargement of the liver and spleen is a common finding in all human malarias, especially in young children and non-immune adults. Signs of hepatic dysfunction, other than jaundice, and altered handling of antimalarial drugs are unusual. Liver failure, with features of hepatic encephalopathy such as asterixis ('liver flap') and clinical and biochemical evidence of severe liver cell damage, does not occur in malaria unless there is concomitant viral hepatitis. Liver blood flow is reduced and intestinal absorption may be impaired (Molyneux et al., 1989).

## HYPOGLYCAEMIA

Anxiety, breathlessness, feelings of coldness, lightheadedness, tachycardia, impairment of consciousness, abnormal posturing and seizures – the classical symptoms of hypoglycaemia – are likely to be misattributed to the malaria infection itself. This may have been why hypoglycaemia in malaria was overlooked for so many years (White et al., 1983). Hypoglycaemia is now well recognized as a complication of falciparum malaria and its treatment. It is particularly common in children, pregnant women and patients with severe malaria and hyperparasitaemia. It is an important complication of treatment with the cinchona alkaloids, quinine and quinidine. In Thai adults, treatment with intravenous glucose usually results in an improvement in the respiratory pattern and often there is a lightening of coma. However, in children, this response is far less common.

## RENAL DYSFUNCTION

This is another of the complications of falciparum malaria that is much commoner in adults than in children (Trang et al., 1992). About one-third to one-half of non-immune adults with severe malaria develop biochemical evidence of renal dysfunction, which is associated with hypoglycaemia, jaundice, prolonged coma, pulmonary oedema, hypovolaemia, hyperparasitaemia and increased mortality. About one-third of cases fulfil a strict definition of acute renal failure and, of these, about one-half will require dialysis.

## HAEMOSTATIC ABNORMALITIES

Petechiae of the skin and mucosae (see Plate 7), spontaneous bleeding from the gingival sulci (see Plate 8), nose and gastrointestinal tract and subconjunctival haemorrhages (see Plate 9) are seen in less than 10 per cent of adults and rarely in children. Gastrointestinal haemorrhage has been associated particularly with corticosteroid and heparin treatment.

## SHOCK, 'ALGID MALARIA' AND OTHER CARDIOVASCULAR ABNORMALITIES

'The algide forms of pernicious attack, as indicated by the name, are characterised by collapse and extreme coldness of the surface of the body, and a tendency to fatal syncope. These symptoms usually co-exist with elevated axillary and rectal temperature' (Manson, 1898). This description by Manson of algid malaria is strongly reminiscent of bacteraemic shock and, in some patients with this clinical picture, Gram-negative rod bacteraemia can be detected by blood culture (Mabey *et al.*, 1987). However, in most patients with malaria, the blood pressure is at the lower end of the normal range. Mild supine hypotension with a postural drop in blood pressure is usually attributable to vasodilatation and hypovolaemia. Hypotension and shock are also seen in patients who develop pulmonary oedema, metabolic acidosis and haemorrhage into the gastrointestinal tract or from a ruptured spleen (de Aguirre *et al.*, 1998) (Plate 24). Cardiac arrhythmias and evidence of myocardial failure are hardly ever seen in malaria.

## PULMONARY OEDEMA (Figure 7.9)

This most dreaded complication of malaria may develop at any stage of the disease. When precipitated by excessive parenteral fluid therapy, it may present late when the patient appears to be recovering. It is a common terminal event and was found in all the patients in Spitz's autopsy series (Spitz, 1946). The earliest warnings are an increased respiratory rate, dyspnoea and detection of crepitations. Central venous pressure will be high when the mechanism is fluid overload, but in the majority of patients the clinical picture is that of adult respiratory distress syndrome (ARDS) with normal right heart pressures. A chest radiograph will help to distinguish bronchopneumonia and the hyperpnoea of metabolic acidosis ('respiratory distress syndrome' of childhood malaria) (Figure 7.10).

## Laboratory investigations in severe falciparum malaria

The microscopical diagnosis and measurement of parasite density and the use of rapid antigen detection are described in Chapter 3. Anaemia is common

and serum haptoglobins may be undetectable, indicating haemolysis. Neutrophil leucocytosis is associated with a bad prognosis and occurs whether or not there is a complicating bacterial infection. The presence of visible malarial pigment in more than 5 per cent of circulating neutrophils is associated with a bad prognosis. Thrombocytopenia is common in falciparum and vivax malarias and does not correlate with severity unless it is profound ($<20\,000/\mu L$). Prolonged prothrombin and partial thromboplastin times and other evidence of disseminated intravascular coagulation are found in less than 10 per cent

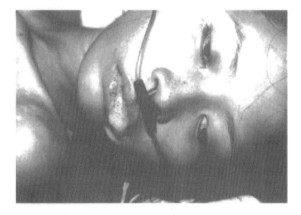

**Figure 7.9** *Acute pulmonary oedema developing immediately after delivery in a Thai woman with severe falciparum malaria. (Copyright Sornchai Looareesuwan.)*

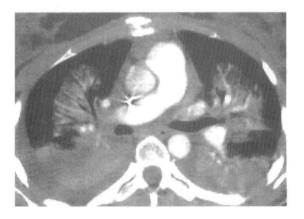

**Figure 7.10** *CT-PA (post-contrast) of a 20-year-old woman with* Plasmodium vivax *infection, showing bilateral pulmonary oedema with pleural effusions. (Copyright DA Warrell.)*

of patients. Plasma total and (van den Berg) indirect (unconjugated) bilirubin concentrations are increased consistent with haemolysis, but in some patients with very high total bilirubin concentrations, conjugated bilirubin predominates, indicating hepatocyte dysfunction. In some patients, there is evidence of cholestasis. Serum albumin concentration is reduced, reflecting catabolism and liver dysfunction. Serum aspartate and alanine transferases, 5' nucleotidase and glutamyl transpeptidase are moderately elevated (two to three times higher than normal) but not into the range seen in viral hepatitis. The International Normalized Ratio (INR) is prolonged to 1.2–1.5. Metabolic acidosis is usually explained by a lactic acidosis. Mild hyponatraemia is usually associated with increased plasma osmolality and so does not always imply inappropriate secretion of antidiuretic hormone. Mild hypocalcaemia and hypophosphataemia have been described, especially when the patient has been given blood or glucose infusions. Biochemical evidence of generalized rhabdomyolysis (elevated serum concentrations of creatine kinase, aldolase, aspartate transferase and other muscle-derived enzymes, myoglobinaemia and myoglobinuria) has been found in adults and children (Davis et al., 1999).

In cerebral malaria, the cerebrospinal fluid (CSF) shows a mild lymphocyte pleocytosis (rarely more than 15 cells/$\mu$L) and increased protein and lactate concentrations. In Thailand, CSF lactate concentration of more than 6 mmol/L was associated with a fatal prognosis (White et al., 1985). The CSF glucose concentration is appropriate to the blood glucose, but may be very low or undetectable in patients with profound hypoglycaemia. The urine may contain protein, erythrocytes, haemoglobin and red cell casts.

Gram-negative rod bacteria, including Escherichia coli and Pseudomonas aeruginosa, have been cultured from the blood of adult patients with severe falciparum malaria, some of whom had clinical features of bacteraemic shock ('algid malaria'). In African children, there is an association between malaria and non-typhoid Salmonella septicaemia (Mabey et al., 1987).

Cerebral CT and MRI scans in adults with cerebral malaria are usually normal. Rarely, in terminally ill patients, there may be evidence of cerebral oedema or even of brain herniation (Looareesuwan et al., 1983b, 1995).

## VIVAX MALARIA ('BENIGN' TERTIAN MALARIA)

The incubation period in non-immunes is usually between 12 and 17 days, but may be prolonged, to 8–9 months or even longer. Some strains of P. vivax, especially from temperate regions, show consistently long incubation periods of 250–637 days (for example, P. v. hibernans from Russia north of latitude 52°N, and P. v. multinucleatum in central and north China). Only about one-third of imported cases of vivax malaria present within a month of returning from the malarious area and, in 5–10 per cent, symptoms are delayed for more than a year after their return. The primary attack begins with headache, pain in the back, nausea and general malaise; these prodromal symptoms are mild or absent in relapses. The fever is irregular for 2–4 days, but soon becomes 'intermittent', i.e. with marked swings between the morning and the evening. At first there is no regularity in the pattern of fever because the several broods of the parasite are not synchronized, but soon the 48-hour periodicity becomes established. Febrile paroxysms occur chiefly in the afternoon or evening and the classical cold, hot and sweating stages become evident. The temperature may rise to 40.6 °C (105 °F) or higher. Nausea and vomiting may be distressing and herpes of the lips is common. Dizziness and mild impairment of consciousness may occur, but are transient. Cerebral vivax malaria has occasionally been reported, especially with the long incubation period of P. v. multinucleatum in China, but in none of the reported cases has mixed falciparum infection or another encephalopathy been adequately excluded. Severe vivax malaria has been described in the past (e.g. in Europe), possibly related to malnutrition and other intercurrent diseases. However, although the symptoms may be severe and temporarily incapacitating, especially in non-immunes, the acute mortality of vivax malaria is very low. For example, during the 1967–69 Sri Lankan epidemic of predominantly vivax malaria, there were more than 500 000 cases with a case fatality of only 0.1 per cent. A few cases of reversible pulmonary oedema have been described in patients with confirmed vivax malaria, reflecting increased pulmonary capillary permeability (Tanios et al., 2001) (Figure 7.10). Most people of West African origin are resistant to P. vivax infection because of the rarity of Duffy blood group antigen alleles $Fy^a$ and $Fy^b$ required for erythrocyte invasion. Mild anaemia is a common result of vivax malaria, but it may become severe and even life-threatening in children and debilitated patients after relapsing infections. Thrombocytopenia is common. Patients may become mildly jaundiced, with tender hepatosplenomegaly. Splenic rupture, which carries a high mortality, is as common with vivax as with falciparum malaria. It results from acute, rapid enlargement of the spleen with or without trauma. Chronically enlarged spleens are less vulnerable. Splenic rupture presents with abdominal pain and guarding, haemorrhagic shock, fever and a rapidly falling haematocrit, features which may be misattributed to malaria itself.

During the early phase of the primary attack, parasites are scanty in the peripheral blood, but they are common when the tertian rhythm of fever is established. Gametocytes appear in the blood about 1 week after the onset of the primary attack.

## Relapses of vivax malaria

A single untreated attack consists of a week or more of repeated febrile paroxysms. In about 60 per cent of untreated or inadequately treated cases, clinical symptoms recur after a period of quiescence, which depends on the strain of parasite. 'Short-term' relapses are seen during the first 8–10 weeks after the primary attack, 'long-term' relapses between the 30th and 40th weeks after the primary attack. Relapses are precipitated by an intercurrent attack of falciparum malaria. Vivax infections acquired in different parts of the world show striking differences in the duration of the incubation period and the occurrence of periods of latency. These differences have been broadly correlated with climatic zones. Prolonged latency has been observed chiefly in temperate regions.

In most temperate or subtropical areas, the incidence of vivax malaria shows a bimodal curve, with a peak in the spring and another in the summer. The first peak is composed of long-term relapses or of delayed primary attacks of those infections contracted in the previous summer; the second peak consists of primary attacks of recent infections. Prolonged primary latency must not be confused with the delayed appearance of the infection produced by the use of suppressive antimalarial drugs.

Tropical strains of vivax malaria show a different pattern of relapses, with short latencies.

## OVALE MALARIA (OVALE TERTIAN MALARIA)

The clinical picture closely resembles that of vivax malaria. The febrile paroxysms may be as severe, but spontaneous recovery is more common and there are fewer relapses. The parasite often remains latent and is easily suppressed by other more virulent species of plasmodia. It may appear in the blood when these have declined. Mixed infections in which P. ovale is found are common in people exposed to malaria in tropical Africa. Anaemia and splenic enlargement are less severe than in vivax and the risk of splenic rupture is lower.

## MALARIAE MALARIA (QUARTAN MALARIA)

The incubation period is never less than 18 days and may be as long as 30–40 days. The clinical picture of the primary attack resembles that of vivax malaria, but prodromal symptoms and rigors may be more severe. The febrile paroxysms are more regularly spaced and often occur in the late afternoon. Anaemia is less pronounced and, although splenomegaly may be particularly gross, the risk of splenic rupture seems to be lower than with vivax malaria.

P. malariae has no hypnozoite form or persisting hepatic cycle. However, undetectable parasitaemia may continue, with symptomatic recrudescences, frequent during the first year and then at longer intervals up to 52 years after the last exposure to infection. Asymptomatic parasitaemia may be detected in blood donors or as a result of transplacental spread to a neonate. All stages of asexual parasites are usually present in the peripheral blood at the same time, but parasitaemia rarely exceeds 1 per cent of the erythrocytes.

## Quartan malarial nephrosis (*see* Chapter 10)

In parts of East and West Africa, Guyana in South America, India, South-east Asia and Papua New

Guinea, there is strong epidemiological evidence that *P. malariae* is, or was, an important cause of nephrotic syndrome. Only a small minority of those exposed to repeated *P. malariae* infections develop the condition, suggesting that additional factors are involved. The histological appearances, which are not entirely specific, are of glomerulosclerosis with glomerular deposits of *P. malariae* antigen in about 25 per cent of the cases examined. Half the cases develop nephrotic syndrome before the age of 15 years. The prognosis is poor. Few patients respond to corticosteroids, but there is some response to azathioprine and cyclophosphamide in patients whose renal biopsies show coarse or mixed granular patterns of immunofluorescence. Antimalarial treatment does not reverse the lesion, but the condition can be prevented by antimalarial prophylaxis and has disappeared in countries such as Guyana following the eradication of *P. malariae*.

## MONKEY MALARIAS

Human erythyrocytes can be infected with strains of at least six species of simian malaria parasites (*P. brazilianum*, *P. cynomolgi*, *P. inui*, *P knowlesi*, *P. schwetzi* and *P. simium*). Zoonotic infections of humans and accidental laboratory infections are rare. High fever and other generalized symptoms have been described, but no cerebral or other severe complications. No human mortality has been reported. Parasitaemia may remain undetectable for 2–6 days after the start of symptoms. The periodicity of fever is quotidian for *P. knowlesi* and tertian for *P. simium* and *P. cynomolgi*. Infectivity and virulence may be enhanced by repeated passage in humans.

## TRANSFUSION, 'NEEDLESTICK' AND NOSOCOMIAL MALARIAS

Malaria can be transmitted in blood, blood products, bone marrow and transplanted organs from donors who may appear healthy. Exceptionally, donors may remain infective for up to 5 years with *P. falciparum* and *P. vivax*, 7 years for *P. ovale* and 4–6 years for *P. malariae*. Mean incubation periods are 12 (range 7–29) days for *P. falciparum*, 12 (range 8–30) days for *P. vivax* and 35 (range 6–106) days for *P. malariae*.

Whole blood, packed cells, leucocyte or platelet concentrates, fresh plasma, marrow transplants and haemodialysis have caused transfusion malaria. Diagnosis may be delayed and high parasitaemias can develop. Nosocomial outbreaks of malaria have been associated with the contamination of saline used for flushing intravenous lines, contrast medium and intravenous administration of drugs. Malaria has complicated parenteral drug abuse.

## TROPICAL SPLENOMEGALY SYNDROME (HYPERREACTIVE MALARIAL SPLENOMEGALY OR 'BIG SPLEEN DISEASE') (*see also* CHAPTER 11)

This syndrome is defined by the presence of gross splenomegaly (more than 10 cm below the costal margin) in a resident of a malarious area, elevation of serum IgM with malarial antibodies, hepatic sinusoidal lymphocytosis and clinical and immunological response to antimalarial prophylaxis.

In the malaria-endemic regions of Africa, Asia, South America and the western Pacific, some young adults show a progressive, sometimes massive, enlargement of the spleen instead of the usual reduction in splenic size after childhood. The prevalence of this condition reaches 80 per cent in some parts of Papua New Guinea. There is a past history of repeated attacks of fever or malaria, but parasitaemia is often not detectable when the patient presents with abdominal distension, a vague dragging sensation and occasional episodes of severe, sharp pain with peritonism, suggesting perisplenitis or splenic infarction. Anaemia, which may be exacerbated by haemolytic episodes, especially in pregnancy, may become severe enough to cause high output cardiac failure. The spleen may be enormous, filling the left iliac fossa, extending across the midline and anteriorly producing a visible mass with an obvious notch (Figure 7.11). In 80 per cent of patients there is non-tender hepatomegaly, especially of the left lobe. Patients may become cachectic and show chronic ulceration of the legs. The untreated mortality is high and is usually attributable to overwhelming infection arising in the skin or respiratory system.

The syndrome seems to be an abnormal immune response to repeated infections by any of the species of human malaria parasites with excessive IgM

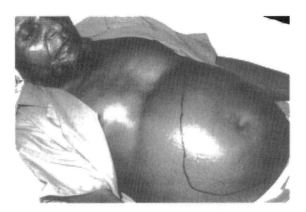

**Figure 7.11** *A Papua New Guinean man with tropical splenomegaly syndrome. (Copyright DA Warrell.)*

production, formation of macromolecular IgM aggregates and hypertrophy of the splenic reticuloendothelial system, which phagocytoses these immune complexes. In Africa, but not in Indonesia or New Guinea, peripheral lymphocytosis results from increased circulating B lymphocytes, whereas T-cell numbers are normal. Distinction from chronic lymphatic leukaemia may be difficult and there is some evidence from Ghana of evolution into a malignant lymphoproliferative disorder (Bates *et al.*, 1991). In Flores Island, Indonesia, CD8 lymphcoytes were reduced and there was no increase in B-cell numbers. In Africa and New Guinea, genetic determinants have been identified.

The blood picture is that of hypersplenism (normochromic, normocytic anaemia, reticulocytosis, thrombocytopenia, leucopenia and, especially in West Africa, peripheral lymphocytosis). There is a lymphocytic infiltration of the bone marrow. The raised serum IgM is polyclonal. Immune complexes, cryoglobulins, rheumatoid factor-like antiglobulins and other autoantibodies have been detected. Levels of both IgM and IgG antimalarial antibodies are raised.

## IMPORTED MALARIA (MALARIA IN TRAVELLERS) (*see also* CHAPTER 5)

The enormous increase in travel between Western industrialized and malarious tropical countries has resulted in many more cases of imported malaria in non-immune travellers. This important diagnosis is often overlooked and fatalities are not rare. For any patient with a short history of a feverish illness with any of the other features of malaria, this diagnosis must be considered until exposure to malaria can be excluded from the history or repeated examinations of thick and thin blood films and rapid malaria antigen tests have proved negative (at least twice daily for 72 hours or until another explanation for the patient's symptoms has been found). Antimalarial chemoprophylaxis that has failed to prevent infection may nonetheless reduce parasitaemia and alter the appearance of the parasites, making them more difficult to detect microscopically. To improve the chances of diagnosis in patients with suspected malaria, prophylactic antimalarial drugs should be stopped. If in doubt, a therapeutic trial of antimalarial chemotherapy should be started. When malaria is diagnosed in a traveller, other members of the tour group or expedition, who are likely to have shared the same exposure, should be checked to make sure they are not also unwell or parasitaemic.

## DIFFERENTIAL DIAGNOSIS OF MALARIA

The parasitological diagnosis of malaria is discussed in Chapter 3. **Malaria must be considered in the differential diagnosis of any acute febrile illness in a patient who could have been exposed to malaria.** Infection is most commonly acquired by a mosquito bite in a malarious tropical country, but the rare routes of transmission must also be considered: transplacental (in a neonate), blood transfusion, contact with blood-contaminated needles and organ/tissue transplants. Malaria can produce many different clinical features, none of which is specific. Patients with fever and prostration have often been misdiagnosed as having influenza; those with cerebral malaria presenting with altered behaviour, impaired consciousness or convulsions have been misdiagnosed as having viral encephalitis, psychosis or even alcohol withdrawal; those with jaundice as having viral hepatitis; those with bleeding and clotting abnormalities as having viral haemorrhagic fever; and those with gastrointestinal symptoms including diarrhoea as having travellers' diarrhoea.

The discovery of parasitaemia provides an explanation for symptoms in non-immune patients, but in those who are immune, parasitaemia may be incidental to the patient's current illness. Failure to discover parasites even after repeated examinations does not exclude the diagnosis of malaria and should not delay the start of a therapeutic trial, especially in patients with severe disease who could have been exposed to the infection.

Some of the more common and more important differential diagnoses of the various clinical syndromes caused by malaria are given in Table 7.5.

**Table 7.5** *Differential diagnosis of severe malaria*

| Symptom | Diagnosis |
| --- | --- |
| Acute fever | Fever due to other infections, heat stroke, drugs and other causes. In pregnant or post-partum women: infection of urinary tract, uterus, adnexa, breast |
| + Paroxysms (rigors) | Other infections, especially lobar pneumonia, ascending cholangitis, pyelonephritis and viral hepatitis; acute intravascular haemolysis |
| + Confusion, obtundation, coma ('cerebral malaria') | Viral, bacterial, fungal (e.g. cryptococcal), protozoal (e.g. African trypanosomiasis), helminthic meningoencephalitis<br>Cerebral abscess<br>Head injury, intracranial bleed/thrombosis/embolism<br>Intoxications and poisonings (e.g. antimalarial drugs, insecticides, herbicides)<br>Metabolic (diabetes, hypoglycaemia, uraemia, hepatic failure, hyponatraemia)<br>Septicaemias, 'cerebral' typhoid |
| + Convulsions | Encephalitides, metabolic encephalopathies, hyponatraemia, hyperpyrexia, heat-stroke, cerebrovascular accidents, epilepsy, drug and alcohol intoxication or withdrawal, poisoning<br><br>In pregnant women: eclampsia, listeriosis<br><br>In children: febrile convulsions, Reye's syndrome |
| + Bleeding/clotting abnormalities | Septicaemias (e.g. meningococcaemia), viral haemorrhagic fever, rickettsial infection<br><br>In pregnant women: post-partum defibrination syndrome |
| + Abnormal behaviour ('malarial psychosis') | Psychosis, alcohol intoxication/withdrawal, other drugs (including antimalarial drugs such as mefloquine) and poisons, viral encephalitis (e.g. *Herpes simplex*, rabies etc.) |
| + Jaundice | Viral hepatitis, yellow fever, leptospirosis, relapsing fevers, septicaemias, haemolysis, biliary obstruction, hepatic necrosis (drugs, poisons)<br><br>In pregnant women: acute fatty liver, cholestasis<br><br>In neonates: Rhesus incompatibility, other intrauterine infections (e.g. cytomegalovirus, *Herpes simplex*, rubella, toxoplasmosis, syphilis) |
| + Nausea, vomiting, diarrhoea ('bilious remittent fever') | Travellers' diarrhoea, dysentery, enteric fever, other bacterial infections, inflammatory bowel disease |
| + Abdominal pain | Ruptured spleen, enteric fevers, amoebic liver abscess, acute pancreatitis, perforation, peritonitis<br><br>In women of reproductive age: ruptured ectopic pregnancy |
| + Haemoglobinuria ('blackwater fever') | Drug-induced haemolysis (e.g. oxidant antimalarials in G6PD-deficient patient), favism, transfusion reaction, dark urine of other causes (e.g. myoglobin, urobilinogen, porphobilinogen) |
| + Acute renal failure | Septicaemias, yellow fever, leptospirosis, drug intoxications, poisonings, prolonged hypotension |
| + Shock ('algid malaria') | Septicaemic shock, haemorrhagic shock (e.g. massive gastrointestinal bleed, ruptured spleen), perforated bowel, dehydration, hypovolaemia, myocarditis |

G6PD = glucose-6-phosphate dehydrogenase.

# REFERENCES

Anderson WK. *Malaria psychoses and neuroses. Their medical, sociological and legal aspects.* London, Oxford Medical Publications, 1927.

Bates I, Bedu-Addo G, Bevan DH, Rutherford TR. Use of immunoglobulin gene rearrangements to show clonal lymphoproliferation in hyper-reactive malarial splenomegaly. *Lancet* 1991; **337**: 505–7.

Covell G, Nicol WD. Clinical, chemotherapeutic and immunological studies on induced malaria. *Br Med Bull* 1951; **8**: 51–5.

Davis TME, Pongponratan E, Supanaranond W, *et al.* Skeletal muscle involvement in falciparum malaria: biochemical and ulstrastructural study. *Clin Infect Dis* 1999; **29**: 831–5.

de Aguirre Z, De Droogh E, Van den Ende J, *et al.* Splenic rupture as a complication of *P. falciparum* malaria after residence in the tropics. Report of two cases. *Acta Clin Belg* 1998; 53–6.

Hien TT, Day NP, Nguyen HP, *et al.* A controlled trial of artemether or quinine in Vietnamese adults with severe falciparum malaria. *N Engl J Med* 1996; **335**: 76–83.

Hien TT, Day NP, Chuong LV, *et al.* Blackwater fever in southern Viet Nam: a prospective study of 50 cases. *Clin Infect Dis* 1996; **23**: 1274–81.

Lalloo DG, Trevett AJ, Paul M, *et al.* Severe and complicated falciparum malaria in Melanesian adults in Papua New Guinea. *Am J Trop Med Hyg* 1996; **55**: 119–24.

Looareesuwan S, Warrell DA, White NJ, *et al.* Retinal hemorrhage, a common physical sign of prognostic significance in cerebral malaria. *Am J Trop Med Hyg* 1983a; **32**: 911–15.

Looareesuwan S, Warrell DA, White NJ, *et al.* Do patients with cerebral malaria have cerebral oedema? A computer tomography study. *Lancet* 1983b; **I**: 434–7.

Looareesuwan S, Wilairatana P, Krishna S, *et al.* Magnetic resonance imaging of the brain in patients with cerebral malaria. *Clin Infect Dis* 1995; **21**: 300–9.

Mabey DC, Brown A, Greenwood BM. *Plasmodium falciparum* malaria and *Salmonella* infections in Gambian children. *J Infect Dis* 1987; **155**: 1319–21.

Manson P. *Tropical diseases. A manual of the diseases of warm climates.* London, Cassell, 1898.

Molyneux ME, Looareesuwan S, Menzies IS, *et al.* Reduced hepatic blood flow and intestinal malabsorption in severe falciparum malaria. *Am J Trop Med Hyg* 1989; **40**: 470–6.

Nguyen TH, Day NP, Chuong LV, *et al.* Post-malaria neurological syndrome. *Lancet* 1996; **348**: 917–21.

Phillips RE, Looareesuwan S, Warrell DA, *et al.* The importance of anaemia in cerebral and uncomplicated falciparum malaria: role of complications, dyserythro-poiesis and iron sequestration. *Q J Med* 1986; **58**: 305–23.

Senanayake N. Delayed cerebellar ataxia: a new complica-tion of falciparum malaria? *BMJ* 1987; **294**: 1253–4.

Senanayake N, De Silva HJ. Delayed cerebellar ataxia complicating falciparum malaria: a clinical study of 74 patients. *J Neurol* 1994; **241**: 456–9.

Spitz S. The pathology of acute falciparum malaria. *Milit Surg* 1946; **99**: 555–72.

Tanios M, Kogelman L, McGovern B, *et al.* Acute respira-tory distress syndrome complicating *Plasmodium vivax* malaria. *Crit Care Med* 2001; **29**: 665–7.

Trang TT, Phu NH, Vinh H, *et al.* Acute renal failure in patients with severe falciparum malaria. *Clin Infect Dis* 1992; **15**: 874–80.

Warrell DA, Francis N. Malaria. In *Oxford Textbook of Hepatology,* 2nd edn. Bircher J *et al.*, eds. Oxford, Oxford University Press, 1999, 1038–44.

Warrell DA, Looareesuwan S, Warrell MJ, *et al.* Dexamethasone proves deleterious in cerebral malaria. A double-blind trial in 100 comatose patients. *N Engl J Med* 1982; **306**: 313–19.

Warrell DA, Molyneux M, Beales PF (eds). Severe and complicated malaria, 2nd edn. *Trans R Soc Trop Med Hyg* 1990; **84**(Suppl. 2): 1–65.

White NJ. Controversies in the management of severe falciparum malaria. *Baillière's Clin Infect Dis* 1995; **2**: 309–30.

White NJ, Warrell DA, Chanthavanich P, *et al.* Severe hypoglycaemia and hyper-insulinemia in falciparum malaria. *N Engl J Med* 1983; **309**: 61–6.

White NJ, Warrell DA, Looareesuwan S, *et al.* Pathophysiological and prognostic significance of cerebrospinal-fluid lactate in cerebral malaria. *Lancet* 1985; **I**: 776–8.

Wilairatana P, Looareesuwan S, Charoenlarp P. Liver profile changes and complications in jaundiced patients with falciparum malaria. *Ann Trop Med Parasitol* 1994; **45**: 298–302.

World Health Organization. Severe falciparum malaria. *Trans R Soc Trop Med Hyg* 2000a; **94**, Suppl. 1.

WHO. *Management of severe malaria. A practical handbook,* 2nd edition. Geneva, World Health Organization, 2000b.

# 8

# Clinical features of malaria in children

TERRIE E TAYLOR AND MALCOLM E MOLYNEUX

## INTRODUCTION

Malaria infections produce the most severe disease in those with the least immunity. Ninety per cent of the world's malaria is transmitted in sub-Saharan Africa, and immunity is acquired over time, requiring repeated exposure to the bites of infective *Anopheles* mosquitoes. As a result, young African children are the group at highest risk of developing severe disease. Accurate statistics are scarce, but a current estimate of the annual paediatric death toll exacted by malaria in Africa is 1 million.

On average, each African child experiences one clinical attack of malaria per year. This represents about 200 million episodes of clinical malaria annually. Of these, approximately 4–6 million will be episodes of severe malaria (Figure 8.1). Why only some African children develop severe malaria is not known, although some interesting clues are beginning to emerge. Case fatality rates for children hospitalized with severe malaria are between 10 and 50 per cent. Rough estimates like these suggest that each clinical attack of malaria has a case fatality rate of 0.5–2 per cent. This figure will vary from area to area, depending on the health resources available, but serves to highlight the fact that the vast majority

of children infected with *Plasmodium falciparum* will experience a febrile illness of mild to moderate severity. The enormous annual mortality reflects the nearly continent-wide coverage enjoyed by this parasite.

## UNCOMPLICATED MALARIA

### Symptoms and parasitaemia

In endemic areas, many children with malaria parasitaemias are asymptomatic. Parasitaemic patients with symptoms such as fever or history of fever, headache, cough, rapid breathing, myalgias, vomiting and diarrhoea (in the absence of altered consciousness, respiratory distress, repeated convulsions, hypoglycaemia, acidosis, vomiting, prostration and severe anaemia) are defined as having uncomplicated malaria. The majority of these patients will respond to oral antimalarial chemotherapy (see Table 8.2, p. 214) and recover, but a proportion will, for reasons that are not clear, develop complicated (severe) malaria.

Although malaria is a common cause of fever in endemic areas, it is not the only cause. Determining

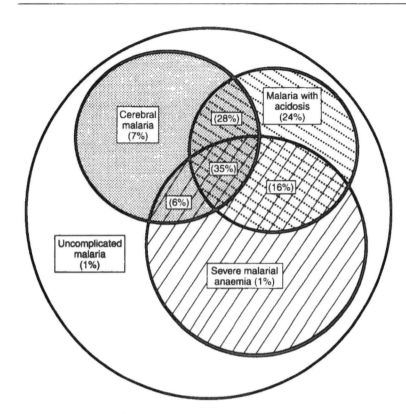

**Figure 8.1** *Overlapping clinical syndromes in fatal malaria. (After Marsh et al., 1995.)*

which fevers can be attributed to malaria is greatly simplified when a parasitological diagnosis can be made. The skill, experience and infrastructure required to collect, fix, stain and interpret malarial blood films are not trivial or inexpensive and are commonly not available at peripheral health centres in endemic areas. The practice of 'presumptive diagnosis and treatment', in which patients are assessed by their history and a physical examination, is common, but may, particularly in areas of low transmission, significantly overestimate the incidence of acute malaria.

However, even when a parasitological diagnosis of malaria infection has been made in a symptomatic individual, the attribution of those symptoms to the malaria infection is not straightforward. Much depends on transmission dynamics, underlying immunity and local patterns of drug use and susceptibility (Snow *et al.*, 1997). Efforts to develop clinical case definitions and to determine 'threshold parasitaemias' (parasite densities above which symptoms could be attributed reliably to malaria) have been successful in the individual study sites, but, because of the enormous variation in malarial

epidemiology, extrapolation from one site to others is unreliable.

Finally, a single negative blood film in a child suspected of having a malarial illness is not enough to exclude the diagnosis. Subpatent parasitaemias can still cause symptoms and, in patients with highly synchronous falciparum infections, the majority of parasites may be sequestered in deep tissues for 18–24 hours of the 48-hour life cycle. These parasites would not be detectable on a single peripheral blood film. For these reasons, several sequential blood films, repeated at 6- to 12-hourly intervals, are recommended to exclude the diagnosis of a malarial illness.

## Overlap with acute respiratory infections

There can be substantial overlap in the clinical presentations of acute uncomplicated malaria and acute respiratory infections (ARI), particularly in children (Dempsey *et al.*, 1993). Distinguishing between the two on clinical grounds alone is difficult, as fever, cough, chest pain, difficulty in breathing, rapid breathing, vomiting and diarrhoea are present in similar proportions of patients with malaria and ARI. Certain clinical signs are helpful, however: rapid, shallow breathing and auscultatory abnormalities are suggestive of pneumonia, whereas pallor and hepatosplenomegaly are strongly associated with malaria (Redd et al., 1992). Front-line health care workers are often forced to make clinical decisions rapidly, without the luxury of a physical examination. In these circumstances, distinguishing between malaria and ARI is difficult, but training in the recognition of a few important clinical signs can be helpful.

Children who require parenteral treatment (see Table 8.2, p. 214), but who are unlikely to progress to severe disease, are said to have moderate malaria (Newton and Krishna, 1998). They have none of the features of severe disease (see below), but require parenteral therapy because of a history of frequent/recent vomiting, drowsiness or prostration. In general, the case fatality rate in this group is low (less than 3 per cent), and most recover quickly. However, a small proportion will deteriorate. Because of the level of nursing care needed for parenteral therapy and the close observations required in this group of children, they should be cared for as inpatients, at least until they can take medicine by mouth.

## SEVERE MALARIA

Any malarial syndrome associated with a high mortality rate (more than 5 per cent), even with parenteral treatment, is defined as severe malaria. The common features of severe malaria in African children (altered consciousness, convulsions, hypoglycaemia, acidosis, anaemia) differ from those in adults, in whom renal failure, adult respiratory distress syndrome and jaundice are also common (Table 7.2, p. 193). Because of this diversity of features, research studies using 'severe malaria' as an entry point or outcome measure must base the diagnosis on clearly defined criteria that are appropriate to the population being studied.

## CEREBRAL MALARIA

'Cerebral malaria' represents part of the clinical spectrum in children with P. falciparum parasitaemia and altered consciousness. In research settings, where comparability is important and where estimates of expected mortality rates are necessary, a child has cerebral malaria if he or she is unable to localize a painful stimulus, has a detectable peripheral asexual falciparum parasitaemia, and has no other obvious cause (e.g. meningitis). Patients are excluded from this category if they improve within 1 hour of a convulsion or of being restored to normoglycaemia. Using this definition, case fatality rates range between 15 and 30 per cent. A consistent minority of survivors (9–12 per cent) are discharged with neurological sequelae (Brewster et al., 1990; Boele van Hensbroek et al., 1997), and half of these recover fully within 4–6 weeks (see below).

African children with cerebral malaria generally present in coma with a 1- to 3-day history of fever. The coma frequently develops quickly, is often immediately preceded by a convulsion, or series of convulsions, and is commonly attended with opisthotonos (Figure 8.2) or with abnormal posturing, altered respiratory patterns and conjugate gaze abnormalities (Molyneux et al., 1989) (Table 8.1).

## Neurological features of cerebral malaria

The neurological features of cerebral malaria in African children can differ from those in adults (Warrell, 1996). A generalized decrease in muscle tone is more common in children, as are abnormalities of corneal, oculocephalic ('doll's eyes'), oculovestibular and pupillary reflexes. Retinal changes are common in

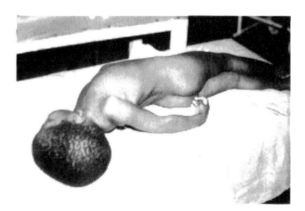

**Figure 8.2** Opisthotonos in an unrousably comatose child with cerebral malaria in Malawi; the cerebrospinal fluid cell count was normal. (Copyright ME Molyneux.)

**Table 8.1** *Clinical features in African children with cerebral malaria (from Newton and Warrell, 1998)*

| | |
|---|---|
| History of fever (median) (days) | 2 |
| Seizures | |
|    Before admission | 82% |
|    After admission | 24–62% |
| Deeply unconscious (Glasgow Coma Scale < 6) | 15% |
| Brainstem signs | 34% |
| Parasitaemia (log median) (per µL) | 5.2 |
| Hypoglycaemia (glucose ≤ 2.2 mmol/L) | 23% |
| Severe anaemia (Hb < 5.0 g/dL) | 46% |
| Metabolic acidosis | 42% |
| Duration of coma (median) (hours) | 18 |
| Sequelae | 9–11% |
| Death | 12–25% |

children with cerebral malaria. Appearances include retinal haemorrhages (see Plates 10a and b), papilloedema, retinal whitening (referred to as 'oedema' in earlier reports) and retinal vessel abnormalities (Lewallen *et al.*, 1999).

Papilloedema is seen in 8–10 per cent of patients, and cerebrospinal fluid (CSF) opening pressures at lumbar puncture are increased above the normal range in most African children with cerebral malaria (Newton *et al.*, 1991). There is evidence of brain swelling at post-mortem in many children dying of cerebral malaria. Cerebral herniation is not usually found at autopsy, however, and the relative contribution of raised intracranial pressure to the pathogenesis of cerebral malaria is debatable.

Examination of the CSF is important to exclude infections (e.g. bacterial meningitis) that may mimic cerebral malaria, but opinions are divided about the safety of lumbar puncture in these children. If raised intracranial pressure is contributing to malarial pathogenesis, a lumbar puncture might increase the likelihood of brain herniation. If the CSF is not examined for pleocytosis and pathogens, the child should receive presumptive antibiotic cover until a lumbar puncture can be performed.

Convulsions complicate the course of the illness in 50–80 per cent of children with cerebral malaria. Seizures can be generalized or focal; some are subtle or covert and can only be suspected by observing twitching of facial muscles, deviation of the eyes with nystagmus, salivation, irregular breathing and perhaps stereotyped posturing of one arm or, in some cases, only by electroencephalography (Figure 8.3)

(Crawley *et al.*, 1996). The cause of seizures in cerebral malaria is unclear; although some seizures can be attributed to hypoglycaemia or hyperpyrexia, these features are commonly absent in the convulsing child. Seizures, especially if repeated or prolonged, are associated with an increased risk of death or neurological sequelae. It is not known whether seizures damage the brain directly or whether they reflect severity of disease. Distinguishing between these alternatives has important therapeutic implications. Meanwhile, it is sensible to explore the best ways of preventing and controlling seizures safely.

Hypoglycaemia (blood glucose concentration of less than 2.2 mmol/L or 40 mg/dL) occurs in many

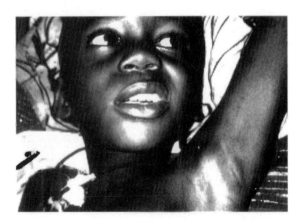

**Figure 8.3** *A Kenyan child with cerebral malaria, showing signs of a focal convulsion: deviation of the eyes, twitching of the left side of the mouth and stereotyped elevation of the left arm. (Copyright Jane Crawley.)*

paediatric illnesses (Figure 8.4); in falciparum malaria, it is associated with a poor outcome (White *et al.*, 1987; Taylor *et al.*, 1988). In adults with malaria, hypoglycaemia is occasionally a presenting feature; more commonly, it is a late complication of quinine treatment, especially in the pregnant woman. In children, pretreatment hypoglycaemia is more important and may contribute to the clinical picture in a child with severe disease. Hypoglycaemia should be considered in any comatose or convulsing child. Other non-specific neurological manifestations include opisthotonos, abnormal posturing, pouting and sustained upward deviation of the eyes (Figure 8.4). Quinine is a potent insulin secretagogue and, in African children, rapid infusions of quinine (more than 10 mg salt/kg over a 1-hour period) can precipitate hypoglycaemia associated with high plasma insulin concentrations. Slower infusion rates and the use of intravenous solutions with dextrose concentrations equal to or more than 5 per cent are safe and well tolerated (Taylor *et al.*, 1988). In pretreatment hypoglycaemia, plasma insulin levels are appropriately low. In most children, gluconeogenic precursors are present in sufficient concentrations to exclude starvation as an aetiology; recent evidence suggests that hepatic glycogen stores may be depleted and gluconeogenesis may be impaired.

Most cerebral malaria deaths occur within 24 hours of starting treatment, and most of those who survive recover fully within 48 hours of starting treatment. The rapidity of onset and of recovery is a striking feature of this syndrome and challenges many theories of malarial pathogenesis.

## Neurological sequelae

About 13 per cent of African children who survive cerebral malaria are left with neurological sequelae, of which the most common are ataxia, hemiplegia, speech disorders and blindness (Figure 8.5). Other sequelae include behavioural disturbances, hypotonia, generalized spasticity, tremors and auditory hallucinations. Among a group of Kenyan children

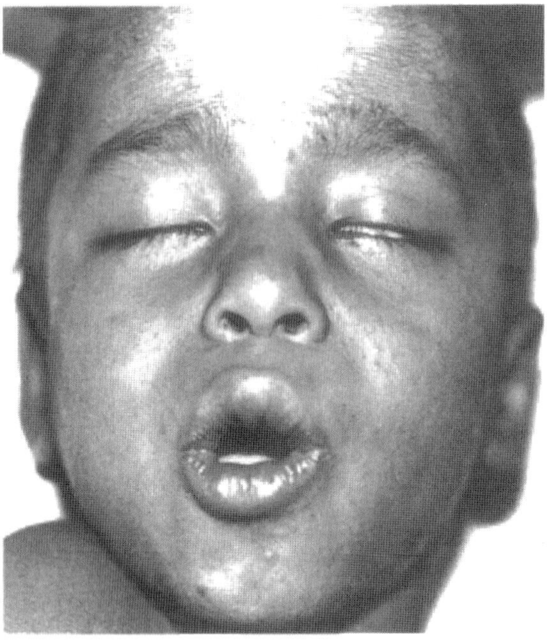

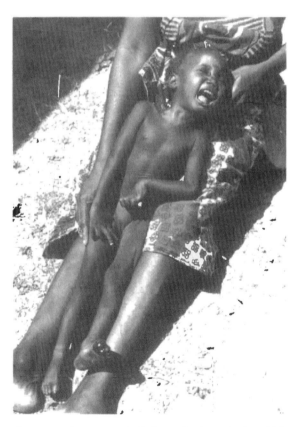

**Figure 8.4** *Neurological manifestations of profound hypoglycaemia. A Bangladeshi child with coma, pouting and upward deviation of the eyes associated with hypoglycaemia complicating dysentery. (Copyright RE Phillips.)*

**Figure 8.5** *Severe neurological sequelae in a Nigerian child who survived an attack of cerebral malaria but was left with cortical blindness, hemiplegia and irritability. (Copyright DA Warrell.)*

with sequelae after cerebral malaria, 14 per cent died as a direct result of severe sequelae. The sequelae most likely to persist are hemiplegia, speech and behavioural disorders, epilepsy and cerebral palsy. However, between 80 and 90 per cent of children with cortical blindness recover their sight fully. Studies from The Gambia and Papua New Guinea have shown negligible persistence of sequelae among children surviving for more than a year (Allen *et al.*, 1996; Boele van Hensbroek *et al.*, 1997). Some children show impairment of cognitive function. Brain computed tomography (CT) scans in Kenyan children with neurological sequelae have shown evidence of severe ischaemic damage (Figure 8.6) (Newton *et al.*, 1994).

## SEVERE ANAEMIA

Severe malarial anaemia (see Plate 4) is defined as a haemoglobin concentration less than or equal to 5 g/dL (or a haematocrit less than or equal to 15 per cent) in a patient with *P. falciparum* parasitaemia. In some communities with intense malarial transmission, it is necessary to stipulate a density of parasitaemia required for a diagnosis of severe malarial anaemia (e.g. more than 10 000 trophozoites/mm³ of blood), because incidental low-level parasitaemia is so common in the population. Children who have adjusted physiologically to low haemoglobin concentrations may decompensate rapidly when challenged by a febrile illness and, in this situation, the development of a life-threatening anaemia can occur at lower parasitaemias. Children with severe anaemia tend to be younger than those with cerebral malaria (Figure 8.7), but the two clinical conditions frequently coexist.

Overall, case fatality rates for children hospitalized for severe anaemia alone range from 5 to 15 per cent (Waller *et al.*, 1995). This has increased with the spread of chloroquine-resistant falciparum parasites across Africa (Bloland *et al.*, 1993; Trape *et al.*, 1998). Children may improve symptomatically following chloroquine treatment, but, unless the parasites are cleared completely, haematological recovery does not occur and, over time, with repeated infections, patients become increasingly vulnerable to life-threatening anaemia.

The characteristic physical findings of severe malarial anaemia are those of acidosis (deep Kussmaul respirations) and a hyperdynamic circulation. Blood can

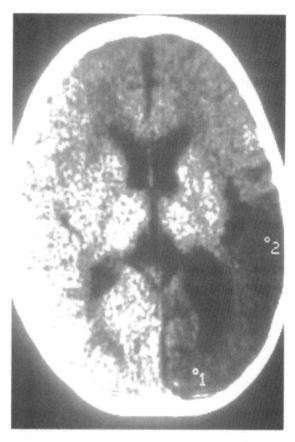

**Figure 8.6** *Cerebral CT scan in a Kenyan child with severe neurological sequelae after cerebral malaria. (Copyright K Marsh.)*

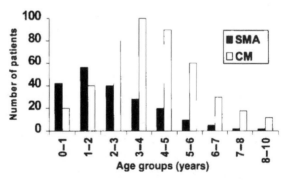

**Figure 8.7** *Age distribution of cases of severe malarial anaemia (SMA) and cerebral malaria (CM) in The Gambia. (After Gupta* et al., *1994.)*

be transfused fairly rapidly, particularly in children who are acidotic and volume depleted. As many malaria-endemic areas have a high proportion of human immunodeficiency virus (HIV)-positive blood donors, blood transfusions are potentially risky and most clinicians prefer to restrict transfusions (see below).

## METABOLIC ACIDOSIS

Metabolic acidosis carries a 24 per cent case fatality rate when it occurs alone, 35 per cent when associated with cerebral malaria and/or anaemia (Marsh et al., 1995). The most common clinical sign, deep (Kussmaul) breathing, occurs in nearly two-thirds of patients with acidosis. Acidaemia and hyperlactataemia may also be present, separately or together (Taylor et al., 1993; Krishna et al., 1994). Respiratory distress is not associated with abnormal pulmonary auscultatory or chest radiography findings, or with oxygen desaturation, and probably represents a compensatory response to the metabolic acidosis. Acidosis may be the sole presenting feature in a child with malaria; deep breathing (alar flaring, chest recession, indrawing of the bony structure of the lower chest wall on inspiration, the use of accessory muscles of respiration – see Plate 11) in this situation is a manifestation of falciparum malaria and not an indication of pulmonary pathology.

## OTHER FEATURES

Jaundice (see Plate 12) is uncommon in African children with malaria, but it is a risk factor for a poor outcome. Acute renal failure is a common complication of falciparum malaria in adults, but is rarely seen in children. Reversible elevation of the plasma creatinine concentration is found in a proportion of children with severe malaria, but this rarely progresses to acute tubular necrosis. The incidence of blackwater fever (malarial haemoglobinuria – see Plate 5) appears to be decreasing overall; it is seen occasionally in children, in whom it may contribute to anaemia but rarely to renal failure. Superimposed septicaemia can complicate malaria, particularly in anaemic patients. Thrombocytopenia is common, but a clinically significant bleeding tendency is rare. Moderate degrees of hyponatraemia and hypokalaemia are common at the time of presentation of severe malaria, but these appear to be rapidly corrected by fluid and drug treatment and rarely have any identifiable clinical significance (English et al., 1996).

## MANAGEMENT

The management of falciparum malaria infections begins with the administration of an effective antimalarial drug, delivered via an appropriate route (by mouth, intramuscular injection, intravenous infusion, or as a rectal suppository). The artemisinin derivatives are the most rapidly acting of all antimalarials, halving parasite clearance times when compared to quinine, the usual drug of first choice for patients with severe and complicated malaria (Hien et al., 1993). However, in studies designed to determine whether these drugs also reduce mortality when compared to existing standard treatment, there was no clear benefit of artemether (an artemisinin derivative formulated for intramuscular use) over quinine. This highlights the fact that a patient's survival depends not only on the removal of the parasites, but also on general supportive care, and on the recognition and prompt treatment of complications (Figure 8.8).

## Antimalarial treatment (Table 8.2)

The choice of antimalarial drugs is determined in part by the clinical condition of the patient: patients with uncomplicated malaria can be treated with oral drugs, whereas those with moderate or severe malaria require parenteral treatment. The known sensitivity of local parasites to various chemotherapeutic agents is important in the choice of antimalarial drugs to be used. Most endemic countries have national policies for antimalarial drugs, based on surveys of drug efficacies (see Chapter 2).

## Anticonvulsants and antipyretics

There are no studies demonstrating a reduction in mortality associated with the use of anticonvulsants, either as prophylaxis (Crawley et al., 2000) or as treatment, or with antipyretics (see Chapter 12). This dearth of evidence may reflect the difficulty of conducting large-scale clinical trials in malaria-endemic areas rather than accurately representing the potential value of these drugs.

### CONVULSIONS

Seizures are very common in children with malaria. Many convulsions are associated with hyperpyrexia

Name _____ Time

Wgt (kg) _____ Hours on treatment

DRUGS:

FLUIDS:

OBSERVE:
- Convulsions
- Passing urine
- Vomiting
- Drinking/sucking
- Eating
- Sitting
- Standing
- Walking

VITAL SIGNS:
- Respiratory rate
- Pulse rate
- Blood pressure (systolic)
- Blood glucose (mmol/L)
- Temperature (°C)
  - 40
  - 39
  - 38
  - 37
  - 36

COMA SCORE
- Best motor response
- Best verbal response
- Ability to watch
- TOTAL

- Parasites on blood film
- Haematocrit

**Figure 8.8** A flow chart developed for serial observations of children hospitalized with severe malaria at The Queen Elizabeth Central Hospital in Blantyre, Malawi.

**Table 8.2** *Recommended regimens for commonly used antimalarial drugs (see also Chapter 12, Tables 12.2, 12.3)*

| | Dosage | Caveats |
|---|---|---|
| **For oral use** | | |
| Chloroquine | 10 mg **base**/kg stat, followed by 10 mg **base**/kg at 24 h, 5 mg **base**/kg at 48 h | Take into consideration extent and degree of resistance |
| Sulfadoxine–pyrimethamine | 20 mg/kg sulfadoxine, 1 mg/kg pyrimethamine, single dose | Contraindicated in children sensitive to sulphonamides |
| Quinine sulphate | 10 mg **salt**/kg three times daily for 7 days | |
| Artesunate | 4 mg/kg daily for 3 days | Should be used with a second drug (e.g. mefloquine) to prevent recrudescence |
| Mefloquine | 15–25 mg/kg stat | Not recommended for children weighing less than 15 kg |
| **For parenteral use** | | |
| Quinine dihydrochloride (intravenous, intra-muscular [i.m.]) | Loading dose: 15–20 mg **salt**/kg over 2–4 h<br>Maintenance: 10 mg **salt**/kg over 2 h, every 8–12 h | Complete treatment with oral sulfadoxine/pyrimethamine or clindamycin when the patient is able to take medications by mouth |
| | | For intramuscular use, the drug should be diluted to a concentration of 60 mg/mL, and split between sites if the volume exceeds 5 mL |
| Quinidine gluconate | Loading dose: 20 mg **salt**/kg over 4 h<br>Maintenance: 10 mg **salt**/kg over 4 h, every 8–12 h | Administer with ECG monitoring |
| Artemisinins<br>  Artemether | Loading dose: 3.2 mg/kg i.m.<br>Maintenance: 1.6 mg/kg i.m. daily | Complete treatment with oral sulfadoxine/pyrimethamine, or clindamycin when the patient is able to swallow tablets |
|   Artesunate<br>    Intravenous<br>    Rectal suppository | Loading dose: 2.4 mg/kg<br>Maintenance: 1.2 mg/kg | |

and/or hypoglycaemia. It is important to check body temperature and blood glucose in children who are convulsing and to treat appropriately. If no such cause of convulsions can be found, seizures lasting longer than 5 minutes should be treated. Diazepam (0.4 mg/kg *per rectum*, 0.2 mg/kg intravenously) and paraldehyde (0.1 mL/kg intramuscular injection or *per rectum*) are both effective. Children receiving diazepam should be watched closely for signs of respiratory depression. Phenobarbitone is useful in children with repeated or continuous seizures, and can be given intravenously or as an intramuscular injection (15–20 mg/kg loading dose, 5–10 mg/kg daily). Phenytoin can

be used in these circumstances as well, but because electrocardiography monitoring is recommended, it is rarely practicable in most endemic areas. There is no evidence that anticonvulsants given routinely to all children with cerebral malaria will improve the prognosis, and some evidence suggests that this policy can be harmful (Crawley *et al.*, 2000).

## FEVER

Treating hyperpyrexia (temperature over 39 °C) in children with malaria may make the patient more comfortable and may decrease the risk of convulsions.

Paracetamol suppositories (30 mg/kg) are convenient and effective in those unable to take oral medicine; oral paracetamol (20 mg/kg) and ibuprofen are useful in children with uncomplicated malaria. Aspirin is effective, but should be avoided because of the association with Reye's syndrome. Tepid sponging and fanning, by enhancing evaporation from the skin surface, may, when used in conjunction with paracetamol, accelerate fever clearance times, but their effect on core temperature has not been determined.

## Detecting and correcting hypoglycaemia

Pretreatment and recurrent hypoglycaemia are common events in children with severe malaria; recognizing and correcting hypoglycaemia are important aspects of supportive care. There are theoretical objections to the administration of 50 per cent dextrose (1 mL/kg, diluted 1:3) in this setting (acidosis may worsen, rebound hypoglycaemia might ensue), but careful studies suggest that the practice is, in fact, safe. If blood glucose cannot be measured quickly, the patient should be assumed to be hypoglycaemic and treated accordingly. Intravenous fluids should contain dextrose in concentrations equal to or more than 5 per cent.

## Blood transfusions

Blood transfusions can be both life-saving and life-threatening in children with severe malarial anaemia. Because of the risks associated with transfusions in parts of the world where the capacity to screen for hepatitis B and HIV are limited, and where these two blood-borne infections are highly prevalent, most clinicians restrict transfusions. Generally, only anaemic children with severe acidosis, shock, high-output congestive heart failure, hyperparasitaemia and/or cerebral malaria are transfused. Most blood banks in malaria-endemic areas provide whole blood and, in general, a transfusion of 20 mL/kg will be sufficient. The risk of transfusion-associated pulmonary oedema is low and, in fact, most patients are sufficiently volume depleted that rapid transfusions are tolerated well (English et al., 1996).

Exchange transfusions have theoretical appeal (rapid removal of circulating parasites and correction of anaemia, minimal risk of volume overload), but have not been demonstrated to be superior to the standard approach judged by case fatality (Miller et al., 1989; Wilkinson et al., 1994). Because exchange transfusion requires several units of blood, there is an increased risk of transmission of infectious agents. The artemisinins are so fast acting and broad in their activity that even the possible benefit of more rapid removal of parasites by exchange transfusion may be minimal.

## Intravenous fluids

Intravenous fluid support is important for patients unable to take fluids by mouth. Children with severe malaria are sometimes severely hypovolaemic, but mild intravascular volume depletion is more common. Acidosis is a frequent concomitant, and usually resolves within 4–6 hours of starting intravenous fluids. Careful monitoring of infusion rates is recommended. Where intravenous fluid pumps are not available, a simple method using infusion chambers with removable labels indicating volumes and times can improve the delivery of intravenous fluids (Figure 8.9).

## Nursing care

Good nursing care is required for children with severe malaria. Simple measures, such as nursing a child on its side rather than supine or prone, or inserting a nasogastric tube, can decrease the risk of aspiration pneumonia. Children should be monitored regularly for vital signs, level of consciousness, hypoglycaemia, progressive anaemia, seizures and the complications of seizures.

### SERIAL ASSESSMENTS OF COMA

Repeated assessments of the level of consciousness are helpful. The Blantyre Coma Score (BCS; Table 8.3) is a useful measure, particularly in children with cerebral malaria who are over 8 months of age (Molyneux et al., 1989). Pressure is applied to a nailbed and the responses (both verbal and motor) are observed. If the patient withdraws, pressure is applied to the sternum and/or the supraorbital ridge to assess whether they are capable of localizing the painful stimulus. Finally, an attempt is made to see if

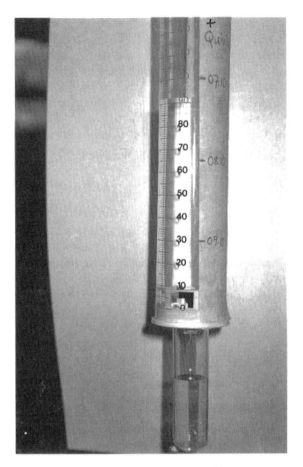

**Figure 8.9** *A drip chamber with a removable label devised to monitor rates of fluid administration in clinical situations in which infusion pumps are impracticable. (Queen Elizabeth Central Hospital, Blantyre, Malawi.)*

**Table 8.3** *Components of the Blantyre Coma Score*

| | |
|---|---|
| **Best motor response** | |
| None, or extension | 0 |
| Withdrawal | 1 |
| Localizing | 2 |
| **Best verbal reponse** | |
| None | 0 |
| Moan, inappropriate cry | 1 |
| Normal cry, speaking | 2 |
| **Eye movements** | |
| Does not follow a moving object | 0 |
| Does follow a moving object | 1 |
| Total | (0–5) |

tric tube, should be initiated between 36 and 48 hours after the start of treatment. Local porridge or a nutritive mixture (milk, sugar, eggs, oil) is usually sufficient, and most of those who survive their illness can be fed by mouth within 2–3 days of starting nasogastric tube feeds.

## OVERVIEW

Most children in sub-Saharan Africa experience at least one malarial infection each year. The character of the illness resulting from an infection is influenced by many factors, including passive and acquired immunity and the usage and efficacy of antimalarial drugs. The vast majority of illnesses are uncomplicated and can be managed with an effective oral antimalarial drug. For reasons that have yet to be elucidated, some children develop more severe disease. Although only a small proportion of the paediatric population becomes severely ill, and although only 15–50 per cent of those with severe disease die, *P. falciparum* causes more deaths in African children than any other single organism. The commonest presenting syndromes associated with substantial mortality are cerebral malaria, recurrent convulsions, metabolic acidosis, hypoglycaemia and anaemia. Children at the highest risk of mortality are those in deep coma (BCS = 0) or with acidosis severe enough to produce deep breathing. Severe anaemia affects more children than either cerebral malaria or acidosis, but if antimalarial drugs and, when necessary, blood transfusions are administered promptly, the case fatality rate is much lower than for the other complications. The age distribu-

the patient is able to follow a moving object. Fully conscious children have a BCS of 5.

Failure to localize a painful stimulus is usually accompanied by an inadequate cry and failure to watch. Most cerebral malaria patients therefore have a BCS of 2 or less. The coma score should improve following the initiation of effective therapy; any deterioration should prompt reassessment for treatable causes (worsening anaemia, hypoglycaemia, convulsions).

### FEEDING

Although most patients with severe malaria recover within 24–36 hours, a proportion remain unconscious for longer. Nutritional support, via a nasogas-

tions of these syndromes are different (see Figure 8.7): severe anaemia affects younger children than cerebral malaria, whereas acidosis overlaps both.

Rapid treatment with an appropriate antiparasitic drug is important in the treatment of severe disease, but attention to the clinical complications is also vital. No animal model mimics the human disease sufficiently, and no surrogate measures for 'survival' have emerged, so large, multicentre, mortality-based clinical trials are required in order to evaluate new drugs and adjunct treatments. Interventions worth considering are aggressive fluid resuscitation, measures to reduce raised intracranial pressure or to lower lactate concentration, antipyretics, anticonvulsants, assisted ventilation, anti-inflammatory drugs and drugs that could improve microcirculatory blood flow.

# REFERENCES

Allen SJ, O'Donnell A, Alexander NDE, et al. Severe malaria in children in Papua New Guinea. Q J Med 1996; **89**: 779–88.

Bloland PB, Lackritz EM, Kazembe PN, Were JB, Steketee R, Campbell CC. Beyond chloroquine: implications of drug resistance for evaluating malaria therapy efficacy and treatment policy in Africa. J Infect Dis 1993; **167**: 932–7.

Boele van Hensbroek MB, Palmer, A, Jaffar S, Schneider G, Kwiatkowski D. Residual neurologic sequelae after childhood malaria. J Pediatr 1997; **131**: 125–9.

Brewster DR, Kwiatkowski D, White NJ. Neurological sequelae of cerebral malaria in children. Lancet 1990; **336**: 1039–43.

Crawley J, Smith S, Krikham FJ, Muthinji P, Waruiru C, Marsh K. Seizures and status epilepticus in childhood cerebral malaria. Q J Med 1996; **89**: 591–7.

Crawley J, Waruiru C, Mithwani S, et al. Effect of phenobarbital on seizure frequency and mortality in childhood cerebral malaria: a randomised, controlled intervention study. Lancet 2000; **355**: 701–6.

English M, Waruiru C, Lightowler C, Murphy SA, Kirigha G, Marsh K. Hyponatremia and dehydration in severe malaria. Arch Dis Child 1996; **74**: 201–5.

English M, Waruiru C, Marsh K. Transfusion for respiratory distress in life-threatening childhood malaria. Am J Trop Med Hyg 1996; **55**: 525–30.

Gupta S, Hill AVS, Kwiatkowski D, Greenwood AM, Greenwood BM, Day K. Parasite virulence and disease patterns in Plasmodium falciparum malaria. Proc Natl Acad Sci USA 1994; **91**: 3715–19.

Hien TT, White NJ. Qinghaosu. Lancet 1993; **341**: 603–8.

Krishna S, Waller DW, ter Kuile F, et al. Lactic acidosis and hypoglycaemia in children with severe malaria: pathophysiological and prognostic significance. Trans R Soc Trop Med Hyg 1994; **88**: 67–73.

Lewallen S, Harding SP, Ajewole J, et al. A review of the spectrum of clinical ocular fundus findings in P. falciparum malaria in African children with a proposed classification and grading system. Trans R Soc Trop Med Hyg 1999; **93**: 619–22.

Marsh K, Forster D, Waruiru C, et al. Indicators of life-threatening malaria in African children. N Engl J Med 1995; **332**: 1399–404.

Miller KD, Greenberg AE, Campbell CC. Treatment of severe malaria in the United States with a continuous infusion of quinidine gluconate and exchange transfusion. N Engl J Med 1989; **321**: 65–70.

Molyneux ME, Taylor TE, Wirima JJ, Borgstein A. Clinical features and prognostic indicators in paediatric cerebral malaria: a study of 131 comatose Malawian children. Q J Med 1989; **71**: 441–59.

Newton CR, Kirkham FJ, Winstanley PA, et al. Intracranial pressure in African children with cerebral malaria. Lancet 1991; **337**: 573–6.

Newton CRJC, Crawley J, Sowunmi A, et al. Intracranial hypertension in Kenyan children with cerebral malaria. Arch Dis Child 1997; **76**: 219–26.

Newton CRJC, Krishna S. Severe falciparum malaria in children: current understanding of pathophysiology and supportive treatment. Pharmacol Ther 1998; **79**: 1–52.

Newton CRJC, Peshu N, Kendall B, et al. Brain swelling and ischaemia in Kenyans with cerebral malaria. Arch Dis Childh 1994; **70**: 281–7.

Newton CRJC, Warrell DA. Neurological manifestations of falciparum malaria. Ann Neurol 1998; **43**: 695–702.

O'Dempsey TJ, McArdle TF, Laurence BE, Lamont AC, Todd JE, Greenwood BM. Overlap in the clinical features of pneumonia and malaria in African children. Trans R Soc Trop Med Hyg 1993; **87**: 662–5.

Redd SC, Bloland PB, Kazembe PN, Patrick E, Tembenu R, Campbell CC. Usefulness of clinical case-definitions in guiding therapy for African children with malaria or pneumonia. Lancet 1992; **340**: 1140–3.

Snow RW, Omumbo JA, Lowe B, et al. Relation between severe malaria morbidity in children and level of Plasmodium falciparum transmission in Africa. Lancet 1997; **349**: 1650–4.

Taylor TE, Borgstein A, Molyneux ME. Acid–base status in paediatric *Plasmodium falciparum* malaria. *Q J Med* 1993; **86**: 99–109.

Taylor TE, Molyneux ME, Wirima JJ, Fletcher A, Morris K. Blood glucose levels in Malawian children before and during the administration of intravenous quinine for severe falciparum malaria. *N Engl J Med* 1988; **319**: 1040–7.

Trape J-F, Pison G, Preziosi M-P, *et al.* Impact of chloro-quine resistance on malaria mortality. *Life Sci* 1998; **321**: 689–97.

Waller D, Krishna S, Crawley J, *et al.* Clinical features of severe malaria in Gambian children, *Clin Infect Dis* 1995; **21**: 577–87.

Warrell DA. Cerebral malaria. In *Tropical neurology*. Shakir RA, Newman PK, Poser CM, eds. London, WB Saunders, 1996, 213–45.

White NJ, Miller KD, Marsh K, *et al.* Hypoglycaemia in African children with severe malaria. *Lancet* 1987; **I**: 64–6.

Wilkinson RJ, Brown JL, Pasvol G, Chiodini PL, Davidson RN. Severe falciparum malaria: predicting the effect of exchange transfusion. *Q J Med* 1994; **87**: 553–7.

# 9

# Clinical features of malaria in pregnancy

CAROLINE SHULMAN AND EDGAR DORMAN

## INTRODUCTION

The clinical features of falciparum malaria in pregnancy depend to a large extent on the immune status of the woman, which in turn is determined by her previous exposure to malaria (see Clinical features of falciparum malaria, overleaf).

In pregnant women with little or no pre-existing immunity, such as those from non-endemic areas, infection is associated with extremely high risks of both maternal and perinatal mortality. This is well documented in the malaria epidemic that occurred in Ceylon in 1934–35, where maternal mortality in women treated for malaria with quinine was 13 per cent. Pregnancy failure (fetal loss or neonatal mortality) was 67 per cent (Wickramasuriya, 1937).

In areas of moderate or high transmission (holoendemic or hyperendemic), including large parts of sub-Saharan Africa, adults usually have a high level of immunity to malaria. Infection is frequently asymptomatic and severe disease is uncommon. During pregnancy, this immunity to malaria is altered. Infection is still frequently asymptomatic, so may go unsuspected and undetected, but is associated with placental parasitization. Malaria in pregnancy is a common cause of severe maternal anaemia and low-birth-weight babies, these complications being more common in primigravidae than multigravidae.

Virtually all the work on malaria in pregnancy has involved *Plasmodium falciparum*. However, recent evidence from Thailand and India indicates that *P. vivax* is also associated with adverse pregnancy outcomes (Nosten *et al.*, 1999; Singh *et al.*, 1999). (This is discussed at the end of the chapter.) The details that follow refer to falciparum malaria.

## PATHOLOGY/PATHOGENESIS

What is peculiar to malaria in pregnancy is the sequestration of parasites in the placenta, where infection is often extremely heavy. Parasites are seen in maternal erythrocytes in the intervillous space in active/acute infection (see Plate 39). If there is longer-standing infection, haemozoin (malaria pigment) is seen in fibrin deposits in the placenta (see Plates 13a and b). Past infection is indicated by the presence of pigment without parasites (Bulmer *et al.*, 1993a,b). An important feature of the disease is that peripheral blood films may be negative despite heavy placental infection.

The reasons for the apparently reduced immune response during pregnancy and the increased susceptibility of primigravidae compared to multigravidae are poorly understood. There is an alteration in humoral and cell-mediated immunity in pregnancy, the latter being modulated to favour survival of the fetoplacental allograft. However, these changes are not thought to lead to significant immune impairment and do not explain the increased susceptibility of primigravidae compared to multigravidae.

The uterine environment (and, in particular, the placenta) appears to act as a privileged site for parasite replication. Evidence for a mechanism to explain parasite binding within the placenta has been obtained recently by Fried and Duffy in western Kenya (Fried and Duffy, 1996; Fried et al., 1998). Parasites isolated from pregnant women and from their placentae cytoadhered to chondroitin sulphate A (CSA). This ligand is present at a high concentration on the surface of the syncytiotrophoblast, which covers the placental villi, and is the equivalent of the endothelium in the maternal vascular compartment of the placenta. The parasites isolated from non-pregnant women and from men in the same geographical area do not express binding to CSA. This raises the possibility that a clone of parasites capable of binding to CSA is selected for during pregnancy. Incubation with sera from mutigravidae inhibits the binding of these parasites to CSA *in vitro*, providing a possible explanation for why multigravidae are less susceptible to malaria infection than primigravidae.

## CLINICAL FEATURES OF FALCIPARUM MALARIA IN PREGNANCY

Pregnant women with little or no previous immunity to malaria are two or three times more likely to develop severe disease as a result of malaria infection than are non-pregnant adults living in the same area (Luxemburger et al., 1997). In addition, if they develop severe disease, they are at a higher risk of dying than their non-pregnant counterparts. Severe disease in pregnant women has been associated with 20–30 per cent maternal mortality and a very high risk of miscarriage, premature delivery or neonatal death (Meek, 1988). Particular dangers of malaria in pregnancy in women with absent or low levels of immunity are hyperpyrexia, hypoglycaemia, severe haemolytic anaemia, cerebral malaria and pulmonary oedema (Looareesuwan et al., 1985). Women of all parities are affected and any of the other manifestations of severe malaria may occur (see Chapter 7).

In contrast, among women living in areas of moderate or high transmission who have been regularly

**Table 9.1** *Consequences of malaria in pregnancy in areas of different transmission*

|  | Low transmission: little or no immunity | Moderate or high transmission: pre-existing immunity |
| --- | --- | --- |
| *Mother* | | |
| Groups at risk | All parities | Mainly primigravidae |
| High fever | Yes | Often asymptomatic |
| Maternal death | Yes | Yes, secondary to severe anaemia |
| Cerebral malaria | Yes | Rare |
| Pulmonary oedema | Yes | Rare |
| Hypoglycaemia | Yes | Rare |
| Severe anaemia | Yes | Yes, may develop slowly |
| *Fetus* | | |
| Miscarriage | Yes | Uncommon |
| Stillbirth | Yes | Unknown |
| Low birth weight | Yes | Yes |
| Prematurity | Yes | Yes |
| Intrauterine growth restriction | ? | Yes |
| *Neonate* | | |
| Congenital malaria | Yes: may be severe | Yes: parasites usually clear spontaneously |

exposed to malaria since childhood, malaria infection in pregnancy is often asymptomatic. In these areas, the main maternal effect of malaria infection is anaemia, which is often severe. The main effect on the baby is low birth weight. It is rare for pregnant women from areas of moderate or high transmission to suffer from other manifestations of severe disease.

Table 9.1 summarizes the clinical features and consequences of malaria in pregnancy in low-transmission compared to moderate-transmission and high-transmission areas.

The pattern of malaria in pregnancy varies between the two extremes described above. Outlined below are features of malaria that are of particular relevance to pregnant women.

## Fever

High fever, which is common among non-immune women, can precipitate miscarriage or premature labour. Although women from areas of moderate or high transmission often remain afebrile and asymptomatic despite high levels of parasitaemia (Steketee et al., 1996c), they probably suffer from more episodes of clinical malarial illness than non-pregnant women of the same age (Diagne et al., 1997).

## Severe anaemia

The World Health Organization defines severe anaemia in pregnancy as a haemoglobin below 7 g/dL, and very severe anaemia in pregnancy as a haemoglobin below 5 g/dL. When very severe, anaemia is an important contributor to maternal and perinatal mortality and morbidity (Lawson and Stewart, 1967; Brabin, 1991; Harrison et al., 2000).

The severe anaemia secondary to malaria infection results from several mechanisms (see Chapter 10). Malaria causes acute haemolysis of infected and uninfected erythrocytes. This is the main mechanism by which malaria causes severe anaemia in non-immune women. By increasing haemolysis, malaria infection also increases the risk of folate deficiency. Pregnant women are particularly vulnerable as demand for folate is already increased. Severe anaemia secondary to malaria is often associated with splenomegaly and may result from hyperreac-

tive malaria splenomegaly. It may also be the result of dyserythropoiesis.

In areas of moderate or high transmission, the anaemia secondary to malaria often does not appear until after the peripheral parasitaemia has cleared. Peak peripheral parasitaemia has been found to occur at 13–16 weeks' gestation, whereas the peak incidence of severe anaemia occurs at 20–24 weeks' gestation (Brabin, 1983). As the parasitaemia and severe anaemia are not concurrent, malaria may be overlooked as the cause of the severe anaemia.

Malaria is often the main cause of severe anaemia in primigravidae (Gilles et al., 1969; Shulman et al., 1996). In areas of seasonal malaria transmission, the prevalence of severe anaemia in pregnancy has been shown to be highest in the rainy season (Bouvier et al., 1997). A trial in Kenya has shown that 39 per cent of severe anaemia in primigravidae could be prevented by antimalarials (Shulman et al., 1999). Other risk factors for anaemia are inadequate iron and folate intake; infection with hookworm and other intestinal parasites; vitamin $B_{12}$ deficiency; advanced human immunodeficiency virus (HIV) infection and haemoglobinopathies (Fleming, 1989). In women already anaemic from other causes, malaria infection can quickly result in progressive severe anaemia.

Women with severe anaemia that has come on acutely are likely to have marked symptoms, such as breathlessness, dizziness, palpitations and difficulty walking. In semi-immune women, however, the severe anaemia secondary to malaria often develops insidiously. For this reason, its diagnosis is frequently overlooked, especially where routine testing of haemoglobin during pregnancy is not practised.

Labour is a particularly hazardous time in severely anaemic women (Lawson and Stewart, 1967; Harrison et al., 2000). At the time of placental separation, constriction of the uteroplacental circulation diverts blood back into the general circulation and causes an overall rise in systemic vascular resistance. This puts women who are severely anaemic or fluid overloaded at high risk of developing heart failure with pulmonary oedema (see below and Figure 7.9). In addition, in women who are severely anaemic, even a normal blood loss at the time of delivery may be life-threatening.

Severe maternal anaemia is also associated with fetal hypoxaemia, low birth weight and perinatal mortality.

## Cerebral malaria

Cerebral malaria has a higher case fatality rate in pregnancy (50 per cent) than in non-pregnant women (20 per cent) (Looareesuwan *et al.*, 1985). Convulsions may occur secondary to cerebral malaria or hypoglycaemia. It is important to consider the diagnosis of eclampsia in any pregnant women with convulsions (see below).

## Hypoglycaemia

Hypoglycaemia is a recognized complication of severe malaria, especially in pregnant and recently delivered non-immune women (White *et al.*, 1983; Looareesuwan *et al.*, 1985).

One cause of hypoglycaemia in malaria is quinine-induced hyperinsulinaemia, which results in reduced hepatic gluconeogenesis and increased uptake of glucose by peripheral tissues. However, in pregnancy, hypoglycaemia is commonly found in women with severe malaria before they receive quinine (Looareesuwan *et al.*, 1985). Reasons for this include: metabolism of glucose by the parasite, increased host-tissue metabolism, depletion of carbohydrate stores by starvation and malnutrition and glucose malabsorbtion from reduced splanchnic blood flow. Hypoglycaemia is more refractory to treatment in pregnancy and the puerperium, with recurrent episodes being particularly common in the quinine-treated patient. It also occurs in pregnant women with otherwise uncomplicated malaria.

Hypoglycaemia in pregnancy may be asymptomatic, but usually presents as an alteration in conscious level or as abnormal behaviour, often with sweating and an increased respiratory rate or dyspnoea. In uncomplicated malaria, a classical presentation would be of someone recovering from falciparum malaria and then suddenly losing consciousness. It can be confused with cerebral malaria, or even pulmonary oedema. In women with cerebral malaria, hypoglycaemia is usually characterized by deterioration in the level of consciousness, or relapse into unconsciousness after regaining consciousness. It may also present with abnormal posturing (see Figure 7.4, p. 195) and grand-mal seizures. Other differential diagnoses are sepsis, meningitis and eclampsia (see below).

If not promptly treated, hypoglycaemia is associated with lactic acidosis and a high mortality.

Hypoglycaemia is also dangerous for the baby, causing fetal bradycardia and other signs of fetal distress.

## Pulmonary oedema

Pregnant or recently delivered non-immune women with malaria are at particular risk of pulmonary oedema (Figure 7.9, p. 199)( Warrell *et al.*, 1990; WHO, 2000). The condition carries a mortality of more than 70 per cent. It may be associated with positive fluid balance, but it also frequently occurs without fluid overload. In these cases, the mechanism is thought to involve leucocyte- and complement-mediated endothelial damage, resulting in leaky pulmonary capillaries as in adult respiratory distress syndrome (ARDS; see Figure 10.11, p. 246). It may be a presenting feature of severe disease in pregnancy, or may develop unexpectedly several days after admission or immediately after childbirth.

## Fetus/newborn

Symptomatic malaria in non-immune women is associated with a high risk of miscarriage, premature delivery and perinatal death. Hyperpyrexia stimulates uterine contractions, and hypoglycaemia and severe anaemia increase the risk of fetal distress and hypoxia.

Malaria infection is associated with low birth weight (birth weight of less than 2500 g), which in turn is one of the main risk factors for infant mortality (McCormick, 1985). This is seen in all parities of non-immune women, even when there is active detection through screening and prompt treatment of malaria (Nosten *et al.*, 1991).

In areas of moderate or high transmission, the association between placental malaria and a reduction in birth weight is most apparent in primigravidae, the effect decreasing as parity increases, though an increased risk in grand-multiparae has also been described (Morley *et al.*, 1964; Greenwood *et al.*, 1989). In primigravidae, the mean difference in birth weight in women with placental malaria compared to women without is approximately 170–200 g. In Malawi, it has been estimated that placental malaria accounts for 5–14 per cent of low birth weight in the population (Steketee *et al.*, 1996b). As with severe anaemia, seasonal patterns in the prevalence of low birth weight are also seen, coinciding with the rainy season (Bouvier *et al.*, 1997).

The mechanisms by which malaria causes low birth weight are not fully understood and are likely to be multifactorial. In women with acute symptomatic disease, low birth weight can result from premature delivery. In areas of moderate or high transmission, low birth weight seems mainly to be due to intrauterine growth restriction. Both reduced nutrient and oxygen transfer across the infected placenta as well as maternal anaemia may be contributory factors.

## Congenital malaria

Congenital infection results from malaria parasites crossing the placenta into the fetal circulation. The mechanism by which this occurs is not known, but may be due to damage to the syncytiotrophoblast occurring during active placental infection.

Severe congenital malaria infection has been described among infants of non-immune women where there has been heavy placental infection (Covell, 1950). It may result in stillbirth or perinatal death, with massive infection in the brain and spleen at post mortem (Wickramasuriya, 1937). Alternatively, congenital infection can present with fever, anaemia, jaundice or splenomegaly up to 6 weeks post-delivery. It may be rapidly fatal.

In the babies of women with high levels of immunity, congenital infection is usually asymptomatic. The prevalence of cord parasitaemia ranges between less than 1 per cent and 25 per cent in different geographical sites. Infection rates are higher in women who are HIV infected (Steketee *et al.*, 1996a). In the majority of asymptomatic cases of congenital infection, parasites are rapidly cleared from the infant's blood. This may be explained by passive protection of the fetus/baby by maternal antibodies crossing the placenta, active immunity developing from exposure to soluble malarial antigens *in utero* and the high proportion of fetal haemoglobin present in the newborn, which retards parasite growth.

## HIV and malaria

The prevalence and intensity of malaria infection in pregnancy are higher in women who are HIV positive. In areas of moderate or high malaria transmission, HIV infection appears to render multigravidae as susceptible to malaria as primigravidae (Steketee *et al.*, 1996a).

Both HIV infection and malaria are independent risk factors for low birth weight and maternal anaemia, so where the two conditions co-exist, the risks for mother and baby are likely to be very high. Maternal morbidity ratios at the University Teaching Hospital in Lusaka, Zambia, have increased eight-fold over the past two decades despite improved obstetric practices (Ahmed *et al.*, 1999). This is attributed to dramatic increases in malaria, acquired immune deficiency syndrome (AIDS)-associated tuberculosis and unspecified 'chronic respiratory illness'.

## MANAGEMENT

It is critical that any febrile pregnant woman from a malarious area is treated promptly with effective antimalarials. Non-immune pregnant women with malaria infection are more ill, more anaemic, more hypoglycaemic and deteriorate faster than nonpregnant women. Thus, they must be treated more aggressively and transfused earlier than nonpregnant women. Those with severe disease should be transferred to an intensive care facility, if available. In a non-malarious area, a travel history should be taken from all pregnant women with a fever.

In areas of moderate or high transmission, malaria in pregnancy is often asymptomatic. Peripheral films may be negative despite placental parasitization, so malaria in pregnancy cannot easily be diagnosed or screened for. The mainstay of management in areas of moderate or high transmission is prevention of infection. In addition, effective antimalarial treatment should be part of the management of any febrile or severely anaemic pregnant women.

## Differential diagnosis

There are a number of important obstetric and non-obstetric conditions that should be considered alongside severe malaria in the differential diagnosis (see Table 7.5, p. 203). The obstetric conditions that need to be considered are mentioned briefly below, but a fuller description of these conditions can be found in most standard obstetric textbooks.

### SEPSIS

In the pregnant or recently delivered woman who presents with fever and abdominal pain, intrauterine infection and urinary tract infection should be considered. Septic abortion, chorioamnionitis, puerperal sepsis and pyelonephritis are all potentially fatal conditions.

### THE CONVULSING PATIENT

In the comatose or convulsing patient, eclampsia and meningoencephalitis should be considered alongside cerebral malaria or hypoglycaemia. Fever may be a feature of eclampsia and hypertension and albuminuria may be associated with cerebral malaria, so complicating the clinical picture.

### THE ACUTELY BREATHLESS PATIENT

Severely anaemic patients may become acutely breathless as they decompensate and develop pulmonary oedema. Massive pulmonary embolism or amniotic fluid embolism may present with similar features. Both conditions have a very high case fatality rate.

### POST-PARTUM HAEMORRHAGE

The collapsed, pale patient who has just delivered may have had acute or chronic severe anaemia due to malaria prior to delivery. Blood loss that is well tolerated by a non-anaemic woman may be rapidly fatal in a severely anaemic woman.

## Investigations

Basic investigations include:

- blood smear for malaria parasites (although this may be negative or of low density despite heavy placental infection in women with uncomplicated malaria from areas of moderate or high transmission),
- haemoglobin or haematocrit,
- blood sugar, monitored regularly.

Further investigations to confirm the diagnosis and guide management may be necessary, including:

- lumbar puncture to exclude meningitis,
- blood cultures to exclude sepsis,
- urinalysis for protein (to exclude eclampsia),
- urine microscopy and culture to exclude urinary tract infection/pyelonephritis,

- HIV test,
- blood gases.

## Antimalarials

Details of safety, effectiveness and dosages of antimalarials for treatment and prophylaxis in pregnancy are given in Table 9.2. The most appropriate antimalarial therapy will depend on local antimalarial drug resistance, the severity of the malaria and the degree of pre-existing immunity. The drugs used will often depend on what is locally available. For symptomatic malaria, prompt treatment with an effective antimalarial regime is vital. Concerns about possible adverse drug effects will be outweighed by the danger of malaria to the mother and fetus. In the first trimester, quinine and chloroquine have been widely used and found to be safe. There is less experience with most other antimalarials in pregnancy, but data suggest it is reasonable to use sulfadoxine–pyrimethamine in the first trimester for symptomatic disease. In the second or third trimester, in addition to these, artemesinin derivatives or amodiaquine could be used. Mefloquine should be used only if no other effective drug is available (see Table 9.2).

On the Thai–Burmese border in South-east Asia, where multidrug resistance of *P. falciparum* is a major problem, the treatment of uncomplicated malaria is currently with supervised oral quinine sulphate for 7 days, ideally in combination with clindamycin. A recurrent infection is treated with artesunate for 7 days. In this area, severe malaria is treated with intramuscular artemether in preference to intravenous quinine because of its ease of administration and the lower risk of hypoglycaemia (F. Nosten, personal communication).

In areas where there is chloroquine sensitivity, uncomplicated malaria can be treated with chloroquine. Where there is chloroquine resistance but sensitivity to sulfadoxine–pyrimethamine, the latter can be used. Quinine should be used if there is sulfadoxine–pyrimethamine resistance or severe malaria.

## Fever control

Temperature should be monitored regularly, and hyperthermia controlled by tepid sponging, fanning and paracetamol. This is particularly important

**Table 9.2** *Use of antimalarials for treatment and prevention of malaria during pregnancy*

| | Safety | Effectiveness | Use for treatment | Use for prevention |
|---|---|---|---|---|
| Chloroquine | Extensively used in pregnancy. No evidence of adverse effects | Widespread resistance of *P. falciparum*. Effective mostly against *P. vivax*, though some evidence of resistance developing | *P. vivax* and in areas where *P. falciparum* is sensitive<br><br>**Dose**: 600 mg **base** (4 tablets) on day 1, 600 mg on day 2 then 300 mg on day 3 (or the equivalent of 10 mg/kg day 1, 10 mg/kg day 2, then 5 mg/kg day 3) | *P. falciparum* in areas where it is sensitive. Role in preventing *P. vivax* being evaluated<br><br>**Dose**: treatment dose followed by 300 mg weekly. Intermittent presumptive treatment being evaluated in West Africa |
| Amodiaquine | Not much used in pregnancy, but WHO state there is no evidence for it to be contraindicated in pregnancy for **treatment** (WHO, 1995) | More effective than chloroquine for the **treatment** of *P. falciparum* malaria in chloroquine-resistant areas in children and non-pregnant adults (Olliaro *et al.*, 1996). Less bitter and causes less itching than chloroquine. May develop cross-resistance with chloroquine | Potential, though not evaluated | Not recommended because of toxic hepatitis and agranulocytosis (Phillips-Howard and West, 1990); may be considered for intermittent treatment after further evaluation |
| Sulfadoxine–pyrimethamine | Not recommended in 1st trimester, except for treatment of clinical disease where benefits outweigh the risks. However, no evidence of teratogenicity from inadvertent use in the 1st trimester. In 3rd trimester, there is a theoretical, but unproven, risk of kernicterus. Risk of Stevens Johnson syndrome, mainly when used as weekly prophylaxis for travellers (Phillips-Howard and West, 1990) | High resistance in SE Asia, spreading in sub-Saharan Africa | 3 tablets orally stat. Each tablet: pyrimethamine 25 mg, sulfadoxine 500 mg | Not recommended for prophylaxis because of toxicity (Stevens Johnson syndrome). Two or three doses of 3 tablets orally stat. given at least 4 weeks apart as intermittent preventive treatment in 2nd and 3rd trimesters (Schultz *et al.*, 1994; Parise *et al.*, 1998; Shulman *et al.*, 1999). Each tablet: pyrimethamine 25 mg, sulfadoxine 500 mg |
| Proguanil | Extensively used in pregnancy. No evidence of adverse effects | Pharmacokinetics altered in pregnancy, resulting in lower concentrations of the active metabolite cycloguanil. Hence need for higher maintenance doses (Wangboonskul *et al.*, 1993) | No | Yes, but should be started after parasite clearance with another drug. Needs to be taken daily so concerns over compliance. 2 tablets of 100 mg each, once daily |

**Table 9.2** (*Continued*)

| | Safety | Effectiveness | Use for treatment | Use for prevention |
|---|---|---|---|---|
| Pyrimethamine | Teratogenic and embryotoxic in animal models but used extensively in pregnancy as weekly prophylactic with no evidence of adverse effects | Widespread resistance | No, not alone | No, not alone |
| Maloprim/Deltaprim: (pyrimethamine–dapsone) | No evidence of toxicity in pregnant women (Greenwood et al., 1989; Phillips-Howard and Wood, 1996). Dapsone is excreted in sufficient quantities in breast milk to cause dapsone toxicity. Exposed infants should be monitored for anaemia and methaemoglobinaemia. When used for prophylaxis in Europeans twice a week, it caused agranulocytosis in about 1:15 000 subjects. Used for many years in Zimbabwe for routine prophylaxis | Increasing resistance | Yes | Yes. Pyrimethamine 12.5 mg and dapsone 100 mg once every 2 weeks |
| Mefloquine | Inadvertent use during pregnancy not associated with increased rate of adverse pregnancy outcomes (abortions and congenital malformations) compared to chloroquine, proguanil or sulfadoxine–pyrimethamine prophylaxis (Phillips-Howard et al., 1998; Vanjauwere et al., 1998). In Malawi, mefloquine in the 2nd and 3rd trimesters was not associated with any more side-effects or adverse pregnancy outcomes (miscarriages or stillbirths) than chloroquine (Steketee et al., 1996d). However, in Thailand, women receiving mefloquine during pregnancy had a higher rate of stillbirths than those receiving quinine (Nosten et al., 1999). | Yes, though increasing resistance in SE Asia (McGready et al., 1998) | Well tolerated and effective in the second half of pregnancy | Used for weekly prophylaxis in SE Asia and in Malawi. **Dose**: 750 mg as a single dose followed by 250 mg weekly. Safety issues need to be resolved before its use for prophylaxis or intermittent preventive treatment can be generally recommended |

| Drug | | | | |
|---|---|---|---|---|
| | avoided during pregnancy if effective alternatives are available. Pregnancy should be avoided for 3 months after completing prophylaxis (WHO, 1995). However, inadvertent use during pregnancy should not be viewed as an indication to terminate a pregnancy | | | |
| Quinine | Therapeutic doses do not induce labour or fetal distress (Phillips-Howard and Wood, 1996). However, quinine can increase the risk of hypoglycaemia. Methods of preventing, monitoring and treating hypoglycaemia should accompany the treatment with quinine | Increasing resistance in SE Asia (McGready et al., 1998) | **Severe disease:** **Dose:** 20 mg **salt**/kg i.v. or i.m. within 4 h, followed at 8 h with 10 mg/kg 8-hourly; Change to oral medication of 10 mg/kg as soon as this can be tolerated. Treat for a total of 7 days Uncomplicated disease: 10 mg/kg three times a day for 7 days | No |
| Artemisinin derivatives | Pre-clinical trials do not suggest mutagenicity or teratogenicity, but there was fetal resorption in rodents. In Thailand, treatment of falciparum malaria in pregnancy is not associated with congenital abnormality or other adverse effects (McGready et al., 1998). Not recommended in the 1st trimester, but can be used in the treatment of multi-drug resistance in the 2nd and 3rd trimesters when no other effective treatment available (WHO, 1995) | Effective and widely used in China and Asia for **treatment** of multi-drug-resistant malaria | **Severe disease:** **Dose:** i.m. artemether: 3.2 mg/kg on day 1 followed by 1.6 mg/kg on day 2 and every 24 h until oral artesunate is tolerated. Give the equivalent of 12 mg/kg over 7 days Uncomplicated: artesunate 2 mg/kg daily for 7 days | No |
| Clindamycin | Used in combination with quinine for **treatment** of multi-drug-resistant *P. falciparum* malaria. Unlike tetracyclines, it has not been reported to cause adverse events in pregnancy, but does cross placenta and may accumulate in fetal liver (WHO, 1995) | Yes, based on studies in Africa and South America | Only in combination with quinine | Not evaluated |

**Potential new drug**: chlorproguanil/dapsone (Lapdap), a new combination for treatment and possible prophylaxis of resistant falciparum malaria (see Chapter 12). Experience in pregnancy is limited, so studies are needed to assess efficacy and safety for treatment and prevention (possibly as intermittent presumptive treatment) in pregnancy.
**Not recommended for use in pregnancy**: halofantrine, tetracycline, doxycycline and primaquine (WHO, 1995).

during pregnancy, as high fever is a risk factor for miscarriage and premature labour and can cause fetal distress. Aspirin and non-steroidal anti-inflammatory agents should not be given, as it may precipitate premature closure of the fetal ductus arteriosus.

# Coma and convulsions

General care of the unconscious pregnant patient should include nursing on the side (to avoid aortocaval compression and aspiration pneumonia), with regular turning and attention to airway and fluid balance. Antibiotics should be given in addition to antimalarials until meningoencephalitis has been ruled out by lumbar puncture. Convulsions should be managed with intravenous diazepam, phenytoin or phenobarbitone.

### DIAZEPAM

Diazepam should be given by slow intravenous injection in 5–10 mg boluses, up to a maximum of 20 mg. It may also be given rectally if intravenous access is not possible. Recurrent seizures should be treated with phenytoin. Beware of respiratory depression. If the pregnant woman has serious respiratory depression after treatment with benzodiazepines for convulsions, this can clearly be life-threatening as she will have an unprotected airway and will be at risk of aspiration. Flumazenil may be used to reverse diazepam toxicity at a dose of 200 μg intravenously, followed by 100 μg boluses according to response, up to 600 μg in total.

### PHENYTOIN

Phenytoin should be given as a loading dose of 15 mg/kg in 100 mL intravenous fluid over 30 minutes. This should be followed by maintenance therapy of 100 mg 6-hourly, as an intravenous infusion or orally.

### PHENOBARBITONE

Phenobarbitone should only be given if neither of the other drugs is available: 10 mg/kg should be given by slow intravenous injection over 15 minutes, followed by maintenance therapy of 60–180 mg/day, intravenously, intramuscularly or orally.

Anticonvulsants may be the cause of respiratory and neurological depression in the neonate, so if delivery occurs after the administration of anticonvulsants, resuscitation and support of the neonate must be available. There may be some hypotonia.

### HYPOGLYCAEMIA

Hypoglycaemia – blood sugar less than 2.2 mmol/L (40 mg/dL) – should be excluded in all cases of severe malaria, as it may be asymptomatic in pregnancy. The treatment of hypoglycaemia should be with 50 mL of 50 per cent glucose intravenously. The response to treatment is usually rapid, but the blood sugar must be monitored closely and treatment continued until the patient has fully recovered, as relapses are frequent. Slow intravenous infusion of 10 per cent glucose should be used for recurrent hypoglycaemia, but even this may not prevent recurrent profound hypoglycaemia.

# Severe anaemia

### ACUTE ONSET

Women with falciparum malaria may haemolyse very quickly, resulting in a rapid fall in haemoglobin. This is particularly common in women with lower levels of immunity, but can also occur in areas of moderate or high transmission (Gilles *et al.*, 1969).

The decision about whether to transfuse depends on haemoglobin concentration, parasitaemia, clinical condition, gestation and the availability of blood that has been screened for HIV and other infections. The severity of symptoms depends on the speed with which anaemia has developed. Transfusion should be considered in women at or above 34 weeks' gestation, who have a haemoglobin of less than 7 g/dL, as it is important that severe anaemia is corrected prior to delivery. It is very important that women are transfused before developing very severe anaemia, as a haemoglobin less than 4 g/dL is associated with imminent heart failure and acute pulmonary oedema and carries a high risk of mortality.

When transfusion is indicated, it should be given slowly using packed cells, and given with 20 mg frusemide intravenously. Women should be monitored with extreme vigilance. Transfusion should be avoided in the third stage of labour, due to the risks of overload associated with placental separation. Exchange transfusion has been used successfully to treat women with heart failure secondary to severe anaemia (Lawson and Stewart, 1967). Up to 2500 mL of packed cells can be transfused slowly, while simultaneously venesecting a similar volume through a large-bore cannula in the opposite arm. Very careful control must be exercised over the volumes transfused and withdrawn. A simple system of a syringe and three-way tap in series with the line on each side enables the operator to control the procedure in alternating aliquots.

## INSIDIOUS ONSET

One of the specific features of the severe anaemia in women from areas of moderate or high transmission is that it may be insidious in onset, developing over a number of weeks, often against a background of iron and folate deficiency. Anaemia that develops insiduously is better tolerated and compensated for than more rapid falls in haemoglobin.

These relatively asymptomatic women may be overlooked until they are very severely anaemic and beginning to decompensate. It is vital that in these settings anaemia is screened for and, once detected, that there is a high index of suspicion for malaria. Any pregnant woman from a malarious area who has severe anaemia should be treated with effective antimalarials, irrespective of whether she has peripheral parasitaemia or other signs of clinical disease. The level of haemoglobin at which transfusion is required may be lower in women whose anaemia has developed slowly than in those in whom acute rapid haemolysis has occurred. However, it is still vital that severe anaemia be corrected prior to delivery.

Rarely, women may continue to haemolyse despite treatment with antimalarials and blood transfusion/ haematinics. In Nigeria, Fleming found that high-dose prednisolone was effective in stopping the continuing haemolysis in some of these women. The prednisolone was often needed for a number of weeks, the dose gradually being reduced after the cessation of haemolysis (Fleming and Allan, 1969). Further studies are needed to clarify the role of steroids in the management of women with this potentially life-threatening condition.

## Pulmonary oedema

This is an acute medical emergency and may be rapidly fatal. Its prevention, by strict monitoring and calculation of fluid balance, should always be a key aim in the management of a pregnant woman with malaria. The management of pulmonary oedema should include intravenous frusemide and fluid restriction in the presence of fluid overload, oxygen and propping up the patient. Where available, tracheal intubation and positive pressure ventilation may greatly improve the chances of survival. Measures to expedite delivery should also be considered, as ventilation in these severely ill patients is much more difficult while the gravid uterus continues to impair diaphragmatic movement.

## Fetal monitoring

Monitoring of the fetus in a woman with symptomatic malaria (Figure 9.1) may detect signs of fetal distress, such as fetal bradycardia, tachycardia or late decelerations in heart rate in relation to uterine contraction (see Figure 9.2). The decision to intervene (with forceps, ventouse or caesarean section) must take into account the condition of the mother, whether labour has started and the gestation of the pregnancy.

## PREVENTION OF MALARIA

## Antenatal screening

In areas of low or unstable transmission, prompt treatment of women with clinical malaria with effective antimalarials forms the mainstay of management. However, regular screening and prompt treatment of women with parasitaemia may be an effective option. In Thailand, in an area of low, seasonal transmission where a high proportion of pregnant women are non-immune, weekly antenatal screening has resulted in a large reduction in maternal and perinatal morbidity and mortality (Nosten et al., 1991).

In areas of moderate or high transmission, examining for peripheral parasitaemia is not a sensitive way of screening for malaria infection. In a number of studies, only about half of the women with placental infection at delivery were found to have concurrent peripheral parasitaemia. Screening women and treating only those with positive blood

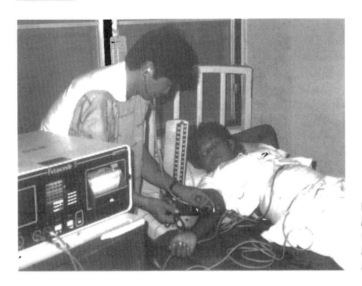

**Figure 9.1** *Monitoring of fetal heart rate, uterine contractions and blood pressure in a Thai woman with severe falciparum malaria in the third trimester of pregnancy. (Copyright DA Warrell.)*

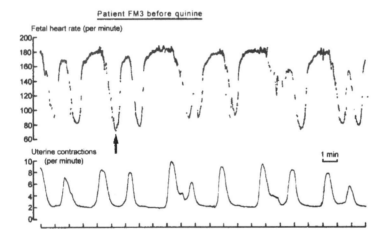

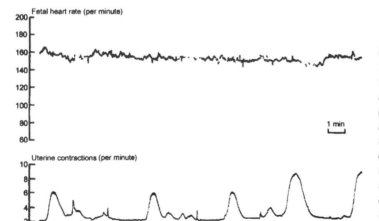

**Figure 9.2** *Cardiotocographic tracings in a 17-year-old primigravida, 35 weeks pregnant, who had been feverish for 3 days (falciparum malaria). The recordings were made before (top) and 3 hours after (bottom) starting quinine (10 mg salt/kg). Premature uterine contractions that were painless and late (type II) and deceleration in fetal heart rate in relation to the contractions are seen before treatment. After cooling the mother and starting antimalarial treatment, fetal tachycardia, late decelerations (a sign of fetal distress) and frequency of uterine contractions are diminished. (See Looareesuwan et al., 1985.)*

smears will therefore miss many women with placental infection and many women who have asymptomatic infection.

## Chemoprophylaxis or intermittent preventive treatment (Table 9.2)

In areas of moderate or high transmission, the prevention of malaria in pregnancy with effective antimalarial prophylaxis or intermittent preventive treatment has been shown to increase haemoglobin and birth weight.

Most countries in malaria-endemic areas of sub-Saharan Africa have had policies for the prevention of malaria in pregnancy. Historically, the mainstay of this prevention has been with chloroquine, but, with increasing levels of resistance, this is now inadequate in most places. In parts of West Africa, pyrimethamine has been used for many years for prophylaxis in pregnancy, but high levels of parasite resistance to single-agent pyrimethamine has rendered this approach ineffective. Proguanil is safe in pregnancy, but needs to be given daily, and must be preceded by effective parasite clearance. Fortnightly pyrimethamine–dapsone (Maloprim/Deltaprim) has been shown to be effective in increasing birth weight and reducing anaemia in primigravidae in The Gambia. In South-east Asia and in Malawi, weekly prophylaxis with mefloquine has been effectively used to prevent malaria in pregnancy (Nosten et al., 1994; Steketee et al., 1996d). Although the large study in Malawi found that mefloquine was not associated with an increased risk of stillbirths or miscarriages (Steketee et al., 1996d), a recent report has found an increased risk of stillbirths in women taking mefloquine compared with other antimalarials (Nosten et al., 1999). In the light of this contradictory evidence, mefloquine should be used in pregnancy only if no alternative is available.

### INTERMITTENT PREVENTIVE TREATMENT

Even if drug sensitivity is high, poor compliance may limit the effectiveness of prophylactic regimes. To try to overcome these problems, trials of intermittent preventive treatment with sulfadoxine–pyrimethamine have been undertaken. Full treatment doses are given to all women, irrespective of whether or not they have peripheral parasitaemia, at specified intervals during the second and third trimesters of pregnancy.

Sulfadoxine–pyrimethamine given two or three times during pregnancy has been shown to be effective in reducing placental parasitaemia, improving birth weight (Parise et al., 1998) and reducing severe maternal anaemia in primigravidae (Shulman et al., 1999) This is an operationally feasible regime that can be given when women come to antenatal clinic, as it does not rely on medication being taken regularly at home. HIV-positive women appear to respond less well to intermittent treatment than HIV-negative women, and may require more doses of treatment (Parise et al., 1998). Parasite resistance to sulfadoxine–pyrimethamine is increasing in many areas, and in Malawi where intermittent preventive treatment with sulfadoxine–pyrimethamine is national policy, there are indications that the strategy is no longer effective. Theoretically, there might be a risk of kernicterus in the fetus if sulphonamides were administered in late pregnancy, just before delivery. However, there has been no documented case of this complication.

The World Health Organization (WHO) currently recommends that intermittent preventive treatment with an effective, preferably single-dose, antimalarial drug should be made available to primigravidae and secundigravidae as an appropriate and effective means of reducing the consequences of malaria in pregnancy in highly endemic areas. Such intermittent preventive treatment should be started from the second trimester onwards and not be given more frequently than once each month.

## Mosquito bite prevention

### INSECTICIDE-TREATED BED-NETS

In some areas of moderate or high transmission, insecticide-treated bed-nets (ITNs), used without additional preventive measures, did not offer sufficient protection to pregnant women. In Kenya and Ghana, they had no impact on maternal anaemia or parasitaemia (Shulman et al., 1998; Browne et al., 2000). However, in Siaya/Bondo districts of western Kenya, ITNs proved very effective, reducing the incidence of maternal anaemia by 50 per cent, of low birth weight babies by 28 per cent, of combined low birth weight, stillbirths and intrauterine growth retardation by 25 per cent, and of anaemia in children in the first 2 years of life by 60 per cent (F. ter Kuile and P. Phillips-Howard, personal communication). In an area of low transmission in Thailand (Dolan *et al.*, 1993) and an area of highly seasonal transmission in The Gambia (D'Alessandro *et al.*, 1996), ITNs were shown to be associated with a reduction in maternal anaemia. Pregnant women should be a target group for ITNs *as an addition* to other preventive measures.

### REPELLENTS

There has been little work assessing the impact of repellents or other means of personal protection on pregnancy outcome. One study in Thailand has shown that repellents may have had a small effect on reducing the incidence of infection (R McGready, personal communication).

## HAEMATINICS AND MALARIA

Most developing countries have a policy of giving ferrous sulphate and folic acid to pregnant women routinely. These haematinics are important in the prevention and treatment of anaemia in pregnancy, as the requirement for them increases during pregnancy. There are a few issues relevant to malaria in pregnancy and haematinics that need to be considered.

## Supplementation with ferrous sulphate

Various studies in children have shown that iron supplementation is associated with a small increase in the risk of malaria infection. Little work has been conducted on this specifically in pregnant women. A study conducted in multigravidae did not show any increase in malaria with iron supplementation (Menendez *et al.*, 1994), but there has not been good evaluation of this in primigravidae. It is likely that, in a population with a high prevalence of iron deficiency, the risks of iron supplementation are small compared with the benefits, especially where women are receiving antimalarials in the form of chemoprophylaxis or intermittent treatment.

## Supplementation with folic acid

The haemolysis in malaria puts pregnant women at increased risk of folate deficiency and megaloblas-

tic anaemia (Fleming *et al.*, 1968), so they should be supplemented during pregnancy. However, there is a potential risk that folic acid may reduce the efficacy of antifolate antimalarials, such as sulfadoxine–pyrimethamine. With current knowledge, however, folate supplements should not be withheld from pregnant women who are taking sulfadoxine–pyrimethamine, though it may be beneficial to delay supplementation for 1 week following antimalarial treatment.

## VIVAX MALARIA AND PREGNANCY

It had been assumed that only falciparum malaria was associated with detrimental outcomes. In the Ceylon epidemic of 1934–35, *P. vivax* played a predominant part during the early stages of the epidemic, which affected one-third to one-half of the total population of the island (Gill, 1936).

Wickramasuriya (1937) reported that, out of 253 deliveries, 208 (82.2 per cent) were premature, and intrauterine fetal death occurred in 82 out of the 253 deliveries (32.4 per cent). It is reasonable to assume, therefore, that some of these fetal deaths and premature deliveries were due to *P. vivax*, although the author does not make this clear in his monograph. The relative prevalence in November to March was *P. vivax* 62.2 per cent, *P. falciparium* 36.7 per cent and *P. malariae* 1.1 per cent.

A prospective, controlled study in Chandigarh, India, showed that the severity of clinical illness was significantly higher in pregnant patients with *P. vivax* than in non-pregnant women with malarial infection and that there was no consistent difference between primigravidae and multigravidae (Sholapurkar *et al.*, 1988). The mean weight of babies born to mothers infected with *P. vivax* was found to be 390 g less than that of the control group (Nair and Nair, 1993).

Recently, it has been demonstrated in Thailand and India that infection with *P. vivax* is associated with lower haemoglobin levels and reduced birth weight (Nosten *et al.*, 1999; Singh *et al.*, 1999). However, the effects are less profound than with *P. falciparum*. These findings suggest that antimalarial prophylaxis for vivax malaria may be justified. Trials of chloroquine prophylaxis are currently underway in Thailand and Indonesia.

## ANTIMALARIAL TREATMENT FOR BREAST-FEEDING MOTHERS

Most antimalarial drugs are excreted in breast milk in low concentrations. Drugs that are believed to be safe in breast-feeding include chloroquine, proguanil, artemesinins and quinine. Amodiaquine and clindamycin also appear to be safe, although few data are available. Breast-feeding by mothers taking mefloquine is usually contraindicated, although the amount ingested is likely to be too small to produce adverse effects. Sulfadoxine–pyrimethamine is generally safe, although it should be avoided in mothers of preterm or very young infants, because of a theoretical risk of kernicterus in the newborn (see above). Maloprim is best avoided where possible (see Table 9.2). Tetracyline, doxycycline and halofantrine are contraindicated in both pregnancy and breast-feeding mothers.

## ACKNOWLEDGEMENTS

The authors are extremely grateful for the valuable input to this chapter received from Professor Bernard Brabin, Professor Brian Greenwood, Professor Sornchai Looareesuwan, Dr François Nosten, Dr Aafje Rietveld, Dr Alastair Robb and Dr Frances Sanderson.

## REFERENCES

Ahmed Y, Mwaba P, et al. A study of maternal mortality at the University Teaching Hospital, Lusaka, Zambia: the emergence of tuberculosis as a major non-obstetric cause of maternal death. Int J Tuberc Lung Dis 1999; 3: 675–80.

Bouvier P, Doumbo O, Breslow N, et al. Seasonality, malaria, and impact of prophylaxis in a West African village I. Effect of anemia in pregnancy. Am J Trop Med Hyg 1997a; 56: 378–83.

Bouvier P, Breslow N, Doumbo O, et al. Seasonality, malaria, and impact of prophylaxis in a West African village. II. Effect on birthweight. Am J Trop Med Hyg 1997b; 56: 384–89.

Brabin BJ. An analysis of malaria in pregnancy in Africa. Bull World Health Organization 1983; 61: 1005–16.

Brabin BJ. The risks and severity of malaria in pregnant women. TDR/FIELDMAL Appl Field Res Malaria Rep World Health Organ, 1991.

Browne ENL, Mande GH, Binka FN. The impact of insecticide-treated bednets on malaria and anaemia in pregnancy in Kassena-Nankara district, Ghana: a randomised controlled trial. Trop Med Int Hlth 2001; 6: 667–76.

Bulmer JN, Rasheed FN, Francis N, Morrison L, Greenwood BM. Placental malaria. I. Pathological classification. Histopathology 1993a; 22: 211–8.

Bulmer JN, Rasheed FN, Francis N, Morrison L, Greenwood BM. Placental malaria. II. A semi-quantitative investigation of the pathological features. Histopathology 1993b; 22: 219–25.

Covell G. Congenital malaria. Trop Dis Bull 1950; 47: 1147–67.

D'Alessandro U, Langerock P, Bennett S, Francis N, Cham K, Greenwood BM. The impact of a national impregnated bed net programme on the outcome of pregnancy in primigravidae in The Gambia. Trans R Soc Trop Med Hyg 1996; 90: 487–92.

Diagne N, Rogier C, Cisse B, Trape JF. Incidence of clinical malaria in pregnant women exposed to intense perennial transmission. Trans R Soc Trop Med Hyg 1997; 92: 166–70.

Dolan G, ter-Kuile FO, Jacoutot V, et al. Bed nets for the prevention of malaria and anaemia in pregnancy. Trans R Soc Trop Med Hyg 1993; 87: 620–6.

Edozien JC, Gilles HM, Udeozo IOK. Adult and cord-blood gamma globulin and immunity to malaria in Nigerians. Lancet 1962; 2: 951–4.

Fleming AF. Tropical obstetrics and gynaecology. 1. Anaemia in pregnancy in tropical Africa. Trans R Soc Trop Med Hyg 1989; 83: 441–8.

Fleming AF, Allan NC. Severe haemolytic anaemia in pregnancy in Nigerians treated with prednisolone. BMJ 1969; 4: 461–6.

Fleming AF, Hendrickse JP, Allan NC. The prevention of megaloblastic anaemia in pregnancy in Nigeria. J Obstet Gynaecol Br Commonw 1968; 75: 425–32.

Fried M, Duffy PE. Adherence of Plasmodium falciparum to chondroitin sulfate A in the human placenta. Science 1996; 272: 1502–4.

Fried M, Nosten F, Brockman A, Brabin B, Duffy P. Maternal antibodies block malaria. Nature 1998; 395: 851–2.

Gill CA. Some points in the epidemiology of malaria arising out of the study of the malaria epidemic in Ceylon in 1934–35. Trans R Soc Trop Med Hyg 1936; 29: 427–80.

Gilles HM, Lawson JB, Sibelas M, Voller A, Allan N. Malaria, anaemia and pregnancy. *Ann Trop Med Parasitol* 1969; **63**: 245–63.

Greenwood BM, Greenwood AM, Snow RW, Byass P, Bennett S, Hatib-N'Jie AB. The effects of malaria chemoprophylaxis given by traditional birth attendants on the course and outcome of pregnancy. *Trans R Soc Trop Med Hyg* 1989; **83**: 589–94.

Harrison KA. Malaria in pregnancy. In *Maternity care in developing countries*. Lawson JB, Harrison KH, Bergstrom S, eds. London, Royal College of Obstetricians and Gynaecologists, 2000.

Lawson JB, Stewart DB. Anaemia in pregnancy. In *Obstetrics and gynaecology in the tropics and developing countries*. Clayton LP, ed. London, Edward Arnold, 1967; 73–99.

Looareesuwan S, White NJ, Silamut K, Phillips RE, Warrell DA. Quinine and severe falciparum malaria in late pregnancy. *Lancet* 1985; **2**: 4–8.

Luxemburger C, Ricci F, Nosten F, Raimond D, Bathet S, White NJ. The epidemiology of severe malaria in an area of low transmission in Thailand. *Trans R Soc Trop Med Hyg* 1997; **91**: 256–62.

McCormick MC. The contribution of low birth weight to infant mortality and childhood mortality. *N Engl J Med* 1985; **312**: 82–90.

McGready R, Cho T, Cho JJ, *et al.* Artemisinin derivatives in the treatment of falciparum malaria in pregnancy. *Trans R Soc Trop Med Hyg* 1998; **92**: 430–3.

McGready R, Cho T, Hkirijaroen L, *et al.* Quinine and mefloquine in the treatment of multidrug-resistant Plasmodium falciparum malaria in pregnancy. *Ann Trop Med Parasitol* 1998; **92**: 643–53.

Meek SR. Epidemiology of malaria in displaced Khmers on the Thai–Kampuchean border. *Southeast Asian J Trop Med Public Health* 1988; **19**: 243–52.

Menendez C, Todd J, Alonso PL, *et al.* The effects of iron supplementation during pregnancy, given by traditional birth attendants, on the prevalence of anaemia and malaria. *Trans R Soc Trop Med Hyg* 1994; **88**: 590–3.

Morley D, Woodland M, Cuthbertson WFJ. Controlled trial of pyrimethamine in pregnant women in an African village. *BMJ* 1964; **1**: 667–8.

Nair LS, Nair AS. Effects of malaria infection in pregnancy. *Indian J Malariol* 1993; **30**: 207–14.

Nosten F, McGready R, Simpson J, *et al.* The effects of P. vivax in pregnancy. *Lancet* 1999; **354**: 546–9.

Nosten F, ter-Kuile F, Maelankiri L, *et al.* Mefloquine prophylaxis prevents malaria during pregnancy:

a double-blind, placebo-controlled study. *J Infect Dis* 1994; **169**: 595–603.

Nosten F, ter-Kuile F, Maelankirri L, Decludt B, White NJ. Malaria during pregnancy in an area of unstable endemicity. *Trans R Soc Trop Med Hyg* 1991; **85**: 424–9.

Nosten F, Vincenti M, Simpson J, *et al.* The effects of mefloquine treatment in pregnancy. *Clin Infect Dis* 1999; **28**: 808–15.

Olliaro P, Nevill C, LeBras J, *et al.* Systematic review of amodiaquine treatment in uncomplicated malaria. *Lancet* 1996; **348**: 1196–201.

Parise ME, Ayisi JG, Nahlen BL, *et al.* Efficacy of sulfadoxine–pyrimethamine for prevention of placental malaria in an area of Kenya with a high prevalence of malaria and human immunodeficiency virus infection. *Am J Trop Med Hyg* 1998; **59**: 813–22.

Phillips-Howard PA, Steffen R, Kerr L, *et al.* Safety of mefloquine and other antimalarial agents in the first trimester of pregnancy. *J Travel Med* 1998; **5**: 121–6.

Phillips-Howard PA, West L. Serious adverse reactions to pyrimethamine–sulphadoxine, pyrimethamine–dasone and to amodiaquine in Britain. *J R Soc Med* 1990; **83**: 82–5.

Phillips-Howard PA, Wood D. The safety of antimalarial drugs in pregnancy. *Drug Saf* 1996; **14**: 131–45.

Schultz LJ, Steketee RW, Macheso A, Kazembe P, Chitsulo L, Wirima JJ. The efficacy of antimalarial regimens containing sulfadoxine–pyrimethamine and/or chloroquine in preventing peripheral and placental *Plasmodium falciparum* infection among pregnant women in Malawi. *Am J Trop Med Hyg* 1994; **51**: 515–22.

Sholapurkar SL, Gupta AN, Mahajan RC. Clinical course of malaria in pregnancy – a prospective controlled study from India. *Trans R Soc Trop Med Hyg* 1988; **82**: 376–9.

Shulman CE, Dorman EK, Cutts F, *et al.* Intermittent sulphadoxine–pyrimethamine to prevent severe anaemia secondary to malaria in pregnancy: a randomised placebo-controlled trial. *Lancet* 1999; **353**: 632–6.

Shulman CE, Dorman EK, Talisuna AO, *et al.* A community randomized controlled trial of insecticide-treated bednets for the prevention of malaria and anaemia among primigravid women on the Kenyan coast. *Trop Med Int Health* 1998; **3**: 197–204.

Shulman CE, Graham WJ, Jilo H, *et al.* Malaria is an important cause of anaemia in primigravidae: evidence from a district hospital in coastal Kenya. *Trans R Soc Trop Med Hyg* 1996; **90**: 535–9.

Singh N, Shukla MM, Sharma VP. Epidemiology of malaria in pregnancy in central India. *Bull World Health Organization* 1999; **77**: 567–72.

Steketee RW, Wirima JJ, Bloland PB, *et al*. Impairment of a pregnant woman's acquired ability to limit Plasmodium falciparum by infection with human immunodeficiency virus type-1. *Am J Trop Med Hyg* 1996a; **55**(Suppl. 1): 42–9.

Steketee RW, Wirima JJ, Hightower AW, Slutsker L, Heymann DL, Breman JG. The effect of malaria and malaria prevention in pregnancy on offspring birthweight, prematurity, and intrauterine growth retardation in rural Malawi. *Am J Trop Med Hyg* 1996b; **55**: 33–41.

Steketee RW, Wirima JJ, Slutsker L, Breman JG, Heymann DL. Comparability of treatment groups and risk factors for parasitemia at the first antenatal clinic visit in a study of malaria treatment and prevention in pregnancy in rural Malawi. *Am J Trop Med Hyg* 1996c; **55**(Suppl. 1): 17–23.

Steketee RW, Wirima JJ, Slutsker L, Khoromana CO, Heymann DL, Breman JG. Malaria treatment and prevention in pregnancy: indications for use and adverse events associated with use of chloroquine or mefloquine. *Am J Trop Med Hyg* 1996d; **55**(Suppl. 1): 50–6.

Vanjauwere B, Maradit J, Kerr L. Post-marketing surveillance of prophylactic mefloquine (Larium) use in pregnancy. *Am J Trop Med Hyg* 1998; **58**: 17–21.

Wangboonskul J, White NJ, Nosten F, ter-Kuile F, Moody RR, Taylor RB. Single dose pharmacokinetics of proguanil and its metabolites in pregnancy. *Eur J Clin Pharmacol* 1993; **44**: 247–51.

Warrell D, Molyneux M, Beales P. Severe and complicated malaria. *Trans R Soc Trop Med Hyg* 1990; **84**(Suppl. 2): 43–4.

White NJ, Warrell DA, Chanthavanich P, *et al*. Severe hypoglycemia and hyperinsulinemia in falciparum malaria. *N Engl J Med* 1983; **309**: 61–6.

Wickramasuriya GAW. *Malaria and ankylostomiasis in the pregnant woman*. Oxford, Oxford University Press, 1937.

WHO. Expert Committee on Malaria. Technical Report Series 892. Geneva, World Health Organization, 2000.

WHO. *Management of uncomplicated malaria and the use of antimalarial drugs for the protection of travellers*. Report of an informal consultation. Geneva, World Health Organization, 1995.

# 10

# Pathology and pathophysiology of human malaria

DAVID A WARRELL, GARETH DH TURNER AND NICK FRANCIS

## INTRODUCTION

Human malaria is caused by infection with four species of the *Plasmodium* parasite: *P. falciparum, P. vivax, P. ovale* and *P. malariae*. Most severe and fatal illness is caused by *P. falciparum*, although *P. vivax* and *P. malariae* infections can also cause severe immunological consequences, affecting the spleen, liver and kidneys.

Following anopheline mosquito transmission, sporozoites injected by the mosquito into the bloodstream immediately invade the liver, where they undergo an initial pre-erythrocytic or exo-erythrocytic cycle. In the case of vivax and ovale infections, the development of some sporozoites is arrested in hepatocytes, resulting in latent or dormant forms (hypnozoites) from which the infection may relapse months or years later. The pre-erythrocytic stage of infection produces minimal histopathological changes (see Plate 14) and absolutely no detectable symptoms or functional disturbances in the host. Infection with erythrocytic stages via blood transfusion or parenteral accidents does not involve the liver; hypnozoites do not develop and there is no risk of relapse. Pathological processes in malaria are the result of the erythrocytic cycle. After developing in hepatocytes for 7–10 days, schizonts rupture, releasing merozoites which invade erythrocytes, where they develop through ring forms to trophozoites and finally to multisegmented schizonts. In the case of *P. falciparum*, this process results in the following changes to the infected erythrocyte: altered membrane transport mechanisms, decreased deformability and other mechanical and rheological changes, development (in some strains) of electron-dense protuberances or knobs beneath the surface membrane, expression of (strain-specific) variant surface neoantigens, development of cytoadherent and rosetting properties resulting in sequestration of erythrocytes containing later trophozoites and schizonts in deep vascular beds and digestion of haemoglobin to pigment.[1]

The secondary effects of these changes are related to the host's immunological response to parasite antigens and altered red cell surface membranes: stimulation of the reticuloendothelial system, changes in regional blood flow and vascular endothelium, systemic complications of altered biochemistry, anaemia, tissue and organ hypoxia and a marked systemic inflammatory response characterized by release of cytokines such as tumour necrosis factor-$\alpha$ (TNF$\alpha$) and interleukins (Day *et al.*, 1999).

The fever, febrile paroxysms, headache, a variety of aches and pains and prostration – the most familiar and consistent ('flu-like') symptoms of an acute malaria attack – are probably caused by cytokines released from macrophages at the time of schizont rupture (merogony). The malarial 'toxin' released at schizont rupture may be the lipid glycosyl phosphatidyl inositol (GPI) anchor of a parasite membrane protein – possibly merozoite surface protein 1 (MSP-1). Of the various cytokines, including interleukins (ILs) and interferons, released by activated macrophages, TNFα has been implicated as the cause of malarial fever. Earlier work in the precytokine era had detected the release of 'endogenous pyrogen' at the time of the febrile paroxysm (Cranston, 1966). An anti-TNFα monoclonal antibody produced dose-related suppression of fever in Gambian children with cerebral malaria (Kwiatkowski et al., 1993).

The role of the host's immune response in modifying the symptoms of disease is crucial (Bull et al., 1998). In endemic malarial regions, patients exposed to repeated infection rapidly develop resistance to the symptoms of disease, and some become resistant to infection. The role of host genetic polymorphisms is increasingly recognized as affecting both the susceptibility of the host and disease progression (see Chapter 11). The well-known association of sickle cell trait with protection from malaria is now one of many, as more information emerges from genetic approaches to analysing malarial disease (Kwiatkowski, 1999). There are also parasite virulence factors that may account for the wide variation in clinical symptoms, including the many facets of cytoadhesion and the initiation of host cytokine release. However, an important finding to emerge from more recent co-ordinated and comparative clinico-pathological studies of severe malaria is that there are definite clinical, pathophysiological and, presumably, physiological differences in severe malaria in populations differing in age, geographical location and genotype. Thus, the outcome of a malaria infection is not a single homogeneous disease, but reflects a number of different possible pathophysiological processes arising from the exposure of genetically diverse populations to parasite strains of variable virulence.

## THE CLINICAL SPECTRUM OF MALARIA

Infection with P. falciparum can cause disease patterns of various intensities, including mild, almost asymptomatic, disease, an acute but self-limiting febrile illness with constitutional symptoms such as myalgia, nausea, vomiting and diarrhoea, and severe life-threatening illness. Severe malaria is defined by the discovery of asexual blood-stage infection with P. falciparum, in association with a number of different clinical and laboratory abnormalities known to carry a bad prognosis (see Chapters 7–9 and Table 7.2) (WHO, 2000). These include severe anaemia, respiratory distress, cerebral malaria, jaundice, renal failure, shock, acidosis, metabolic and haemostatic abnormalities.

## PATHOLOGICAL AND PATHOPHYSIOLOGICAL CHANGES IN ORGANS AND TISSUES IN MALARIA

### Brain

The commonest severe complication of malaria is cerebral malaria, a diffuse encephalopathy associated with fitting and loss of consciousness, which can be rapidly fatal but is also potentially reversible.

Cerebral involvement is confined to P. falciparum infection. More than 95 per cent of adults and more than 85 per cent of children who recover from cerebral malaria show no persistent neurological sequelae, suggesting that much of the pathology must be transient and reversible. Interpretation of pathology should be carefully considered in relation to the clinical picture, which falls into four broad groups:

1. Patients fulfilling strict clinical criteria of cerebral malaria (see Chapters 7 and 8) but with no other features of severe disease. These patients usually make a full or partial recovery.
2. Patients fulfilling strict clinical criteria of cerebral malaria but with additional features of severe disease. The mechanism of coma may be different from that in 'isolated' or 'pure' cerebral malaria. Less than 70 per cent of these patients make a full or partial recovery.
3. Fatal cerebral malaria.
4. Malaria without clinical evidence of cerebral involvement.

Obviously, studies of post-mortem brain tissue confine our knowledge of the pathology to severe cases of cerebral malaria or those dying of other complications of severe malaria.

## MACROSCOPICAL APPEARANCE

The brains of some, but not all, cases of fatal cerebral malaria have been described as macroscopically swollen. Cerebral oedema is detected even less commonly during life, using such techniques as computed tomography (CT) and NMR scans. In two out of 10 unusually severe cases of cerebral malaria in Thailand, cerebral oedema developed as an agonal phenomenon. Evidence of cerebral or cerebellar herniation is extremely unusual. Engorgement of arachnoid blood vessels with erythrocytes containing mature pigmented parasites results in the classical leaden or plum-coloured brain (see Plate 15). Pigment deposition causes a grey cortex. The cut surface of the brain may exhibit numerous small, petechial haemorrhages, which can occur throughout the cortex and cerebellum, but often have a characteristic distribution within the subcortical white matter (see Plate 16). Infarction, necrosis and large haemorrhages are, however, rare. In fatal malaria without neurological symptoms, the brain usually shows no detectable macroscopic abnormalities.

## MICROSCOPICAL APPEARANCE

Common to most pathological descriptions is the presence of large numbers of parasitized red blood cells (PRBCs) undergoing schizogony, in the small capillaries and venules (see Plates 17 and 18; Figure 10.1) and, to a lesser extent, margination of infected erythrocytes in larger calibre vessels (see Plate 19).

Electron microscopic examination of sequestered parasites shows electron-dense knob proteins under the erythrocytic membrane, forming focal contacts between the PRBC and endothelial cell (Figure 10.2). In addition, intracytoplasmic breakdown of haemoglobin by the parasite causes accumulation of intra-erythrocytic pigment globules. Pigment deposition in the brain is often marked, with pigment granules bound to ghosted erythrocyte membranes, which remain adherent to endothelial cells following merogony, or phagocytosed within circulating monocytes or in meningeal/choroid plexus cells. Haemorrhages are common and can be of several types, including simple petechial or perivascular haemorrhages and more complex ring haemorrhages with their characteristic zoned architecture around a central necrotic vessel (see Plates 20 and 21). Parenchymal responses to haemorrhage include microglial nodules, astrocytic activation and focal collections of activated astroglial cells surrounding a resolving haemorrhage termed Dürck's granuloma (see Plate 22).

Although intravascular fibrin–platelet thrombi have been described, especially in African children, they are not common and some detailed studies have failed to detect them (Macpherson et al., 1985). It may be that the presence of significant fibrin–platelet thrombi in the brain or elsewhere is a manifestation of disseminated intravascular coagulation rather than a direct consequence of malarial infection. The reduced deformability of PRBCs together with their cytoadherence to endothelium and to uninfected cells (rosetting: Figure 10.3) leads to impairment of blood flow.

Cellular inflammatory responses can be marked, with intravascular collections of monocytes and lymphocytes, and perivascular activated macrophages

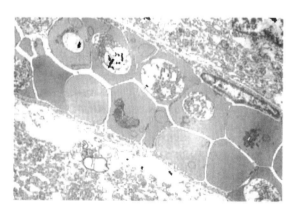

**Figure 10.1** *Cerebral malaria electron micrograph showing numerous parasitized erythrocytes packing cerebral vessels. (Copyright Nick Francis.)*

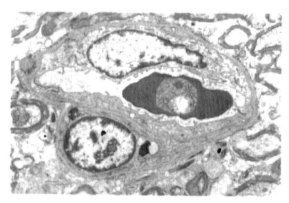

**Figure 10.2** *Cerebral malaria electron micrograph showing endothelial cell microvilli making contact with a parasitized erythrocyte via electron-dense strands (upper right). (Copyright Nick Francis.)*

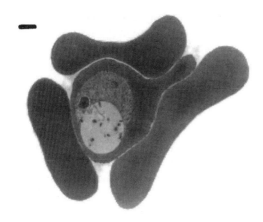

**Figure 10.3** *Rosetting* in vitro *(bar is 1 μm). (Copyright David Ferguson.)*

and pericytes. The degree of microscopic oedema in the brain varies, although some cases show marked perivascular, pericellular and parenchymal oedema. Focal areas of white matter rarefaction and necrosis can be seen.

Several large clinico-pathological correlations of cerebral malaria are currently underway in Thailand, Vietnam, Kenya and Malawi (Turner, 1997; Brown *et al.*, 2001). These studies have begun to provide evidence of pathological as well as of clinical differences among these populations (see Chapters 7 and 8). Pathologically, there appears to be a higher incidence of brain swelling in African children than in South-east Asian adults, with more intravascular monocytic cell infiltrates and fibrin–platelet thrombi at the centre of haemorrhages. Some of these differences may reflect variations in treatment, time to death and host genetic responses. A number of different mechanisms may contribute to the pathophysiology of cerebral malaria, all acting through a final common pathway of neuropathological changes to cause coma and, in some cases, death.

One direct consequence of sequestration is the local production of lactate and the systemic induction of IL-1 and TNFα by macrophages. Ultrastructurally, cerebral endothelial cells show the formation of microvillous cytoplasmic projections, some of which link to erythrocyte membrane knobs via thin, electron-dense strands (Macpherson *et al.*, 1985) (see Figure 10.2). The cause of these changes is not known, but they have been seen in experimental systems in association with free oxygen radical production.

Clinical evidence of cerebral herniation in African children with cerebral malaria (Newton *et al.*, 1997) (see Chapter 8) has prompted a search for grooving of the midbrain by the free edge of the notch of the tentorium cerebellae and damage to the cerebellar tonsils caused by their herniation through the foramen magnum. So far, very little evidence has emerged that herniation of the brain is an important terminal event in patients dying with cerebral malaria.

## PATHOPHYSIOLOGY OF CEREBRAL MALARIA

Several hypotheses have been proposed to explain the development of coma. The permeability hypothesis arose from studies of *P. knowlesi*-infected rhesus monkeys which suggested that a circulating malarial toxin, possibly a kinin, caused increased cerebral vascular permeability, leakage of plasma across the blood–brain barrier, cerebral oedema and resulting coma (WHO, 2000). However, there is now considerable evidence against the permeability hypothesis, at least in South-east Asian adults. A small increase in capillary permeability has been demonstrated from the measurement of the transcapillary escape rate of radiolabelled albumin and urinary microalbumin and by fluorescein angiography (Brown *et al.*, 1999, 2000). However, the passage of $^{125}$I-labelled human serum albumin across the blood–cerebrospinal fluid (CSF) barrier in comatose humans was 300 times less than in the rhesus monkey model and did not decrease during convalescence (Warrell *et al.*, 1986). Recent studies of blood–brain barrier permeability in South-east Asian adults and African children with cerebral malaria suggest a degree of dysfunction in both series, although this appears more marked in children. In comparison with other neurological diseases characterized by severe structural compromise to the blood–brain barrier, cerebral malaria involves less severe, and thus possibly reversible, changes. However, African children with cerebral malaria show a significantly higher level of blood–brain barrier permeability, as judged by CSF/serum albumin index, than non-cerebral cases (Brown *et al.*, 2001). The 'leakage' of plasma proteins into the perivascular space is difficult to demonstrate by immunohistochemistry, although immunohistochemical data indicate disruption of cerebral endothelial cell junctional proteins, which co-localizes with parasite sequestration. In addition, widespread perivascular monocyte activation occurs, which might increase the release of cytokines and other mediators, leading to a direct link between the presence of sequestered parasites within a vessel and neuroactive mediator release within the surrounding parenchyma.

Cerebral oedema is demonstrable in only a small minority of comatose adult patients, and the CSF opening pressure measured at lumbar puncture was normal in 80 per cent of patients, in a few of whom it was measured repeatedly during coma (Warrell et al., 1986). Finally, dexamethasone, the most potent anti-inflammatory drug in experimental bacterial meningitis, did not benefit adult patients with cerebral malaria (Warrell et al., 1982). However, the recent finding of elevated CSF opening pressures in African children with cerebral malaria indicates that, in this age group at least, intracranial pressure is usually elevated (Newton et al., 1997). This could be the result of raised intracranial blood volume, perhaps caused by massive sequestration of parasitized erythrocytes and vasodilatation caused by their products, or to cerebral oedema (Carr et al., 1998; Newton et al., 1998).

There is increasing evidence in support of the mechanical hypothesis, which postulates cytoadherence of parasitized erythrocytes to the endothelium of cerebral venules, resulting in the sequestration and tight packing of infected cells in these vessels. In severe malaria, the deformability of PRBCs and uninfected erythrocytes is reduced (Dondorp et al., 2000). Both abnormalities will tend to decrease blood flow and thus the supply of oxygen and other nutrients to the brain, causing coma, or stimulate the release of cytokines and activation of endothelial cells to generate nitric oxide, which can disturb neurotransmission (Maneerat et al., 2000).

Cerebral malaria is restricted to falciparum malaria, P. falciparum being the only species which sequesters in cerebral microvessels. Quantitative studies have shown a close association between the presence of sequestered PRBCs and the incidence of coma (Macpherson et al., 1985; Pongponratn et al., 1991; Silamut et al., 1999). The adhesion of PRBCs has been investigated in vitro, and is due to specific receptor-mediated events between parasite ligands such as PfEMP-1, expressed on the infected erythrocyte surface, and host endothelial adhesion molecules such as intracellular adhesion molecule 1 (ICAM-1), CD36 and thrombospondin (Table 10.1). Despite extensive research on the molecular mechanisms underlying sequestration, it remains unclear how this process is linked to the pathogenesis of cerebral malaria. Localization of PRBCs or host leucocytes within cerebral vessels could affect intraparenchymal brain function in a number of ways, including mechanical obstruction and resultant hypoxic–ischaemic damage, perturbation of the blood–brain barrier or metabolite competition, and by starving the brain of oxygen, glucose or other nutrients. Release of toxins might influence host cells, although no specific malaria toxin has yet been fully characterized. Damage to host endothelial cells by lymphocytes or platelets has been proposed. Some patients with cerebral malaria have raised intracranial pressures and brain swelling, which can be fatal. However, few patients develop fatal cerebral oedema, and cerebral blood flow can be normal (WHO, 2000). Adhesion to cerebral endothelial cells may have some effect on blood–brain barrier permeability, and evidence is accumulating that intraparenchymal inflammatory and immune response may play a role in translating the effects of sequestration into local neuronal dysfunction. These may include the local release of cytokines or neuroactive mediators and induction of intrinsic nitric oxide synthetase (iNOS) increasing nitric oxide production or changes in levels of other

**Table 10.1** *Cerebral malaria: cytoadherence and rosetting candidate receptors*

| Infected erythrocyte surface | Vascular endothelium | |
|---|---|---|
| PfEMP-1 | Thrombospondin | } all |
| Sequestration | CD36 | } parasites |
| Modified red blood cell band 3 | ICAM-1 (cerebral malaria) | |
| Rosetting | VCAM | |
| Pf332 | E-selectin (ELAM-1) | |
| (CRI-rosetting) | Chondroitin sulphate | } placenta |
| | Hyaluronic acid | |
| | CD31 (PECAM-1) | |
| | $\alpha_v \beta_3$ integrin | |

neurotransmitters (Taylor *et al.*, 1998). Nitric oxide production was inversely related to severity in both Tanzanian children and Vietnamese adults with severe malaria (Day *et al.*, 1991; Anstey *et al.*, 1996).

The molecular basis for cytoadherence is of great interest and potential importance because of the possibility of preventing or reversing this key pathogenic process by anti-disease vaccines, therapeutic antibodies or competitively antagonistic, soluble, synthetic peptide fragments. The large malarial protein PfEMP-1 shows appropriate properties and strain-specific diversity to be an important adhesin. Parasite-induced changes to the band 3 protein of the erythrocyte surface membrane may also allow binding to endothelial receptors. Candidate endothelial ligands are shown in Table 10.1. Clones of *P. falciparum* show a high rate of antigenic variation (perhaps 2 per cent per generation), allowing them to express, in successive generations, adhesins that bind with a repertoire of endothelial receptors, including the ones so far identified. Rosetting, the adhesion of non-parasitized to parasitized erythrocytes, is a property exhibited *in vitro* (see Figure 10.3) and *ex vivo* in the rat's mesoappendix by some strains of *P. falciparum* and some sequestering animal malarias (*P. chabaudi, P. fragile* and *P. coatneyi*). Rosetting is affected by heparin (including non-anticoagulant analogues), divalent cations, pH and antibodies directed against the malarial protein HRP-1. In Gambian children with cerebral malaria, all parasite isolates were able to form rosettes *in vitro* and the sera of these children lacked anti-rosetting antibodies.

Some predictions of the mechanical hypothesis have been tested in human patients. In Thai adults comatose with cerebral malaria, cerebral blood flow was reduced relative to arterial oxygen content, one of its principal physiological determinants (Warrell *et al.*, 1988). Cerebral oxygen consumption and cerebral arteriovenous oxygen content difference were decreased and cerebral venous $Po_2$ increased. Arterial lactate concentration and cerebral lactate production were significantly higher while the patients were comatose than when they had just recovered consciousness, and the CSF lactate concentration was elevated in patients with cerebral malaria and was significantly higher in fatal cases than in survivors. These results confirm a switch to anaerobic cerebral glycolysis in patients comatose with cerebral malaria.

The cytokine hypothesis is based on the observation that in African children with cerebral malaria, plasma concentrations of TNFα, IL-1, IL-6 and IL-8 correlate with disease severity, as judged by parasitaemia, hypoglycaemia, case fatality and the incidence of neurological sequelae. There may be a relative failure of IL-10 production, which would normally inhibit pro-inflammatory cytokine release (Ho and White, 1999). Cytokines released by macrophages under the influence of a malarial toxin (possibly GPI anchor) released at schizont rupture could be involved in enhancing cytoadherence by increasing the expression of endothelial receptors such as ICAM-1 and CD36, and can induce fever, hypoglycaemia, coagulopathy, dyserythropoiesis and leucocytosis. The most convincing evidence of a role for TNF was the finding in The Gambia that a genetic polymorphism of the TNFα promotor region conferred a seven-fold increased risk of either death or neurological deficit from severe malaria (McGuire *et al.*, 1994).

## Haematological changes

In the bone marrow there is sequestration of PRBCs (Figure 10.4) and pigmented macrophages and pigment deposition. Some marrow sinusoids are packed with and appear completely obstructed by PRBCs. Iron sequestration, erythrophagocytosis and dyserythropoiesis (see Plate 23) were found in the acute phase of falciparum malaria. Maturation defects were present in the marrow for at least 3 weeks after clearance of parasitaemia. Dyserythropoietic changes have also been found in the marrow of patients with vivax malaria, most of whom did not become anaemic. Increased numbers

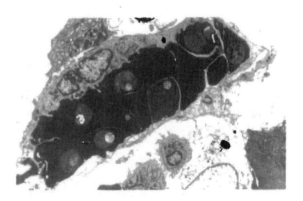

**Figure 10.4** *Bone marrow: sinusoid choked with parasitized erythrocytes. (Copyright Professor SN Wickramasinghe.)*

of large, abnormal-looking megakaryocytes have been found in the bone marrow, and the circulating platelets may also be enlarged, suggesting dyspoietic thrombopoiesis.

## PATHOPHYSIOLOGY

### Anaemia

Anaemia is an inevitable consequence of erythrocyte parasitization as all PRBCs are destroyed at merogony. However, other processes, such as dyserythropoiesis, enhanced splenic clearance and even blood loss, contribute to malaria anaemia. The survival of non-parasitized erythrocytes was found to be reduced for several weeks after clearance of parasitaemia in patients with falciparum and vivax malarias (WHO, 2000). In Gambian children, initial studies showed a correlation between severe anaemia and a positive direct antiglobulin (Coombs') test, implying immune haemolysis. Later studies failed to confirm this finding (WHO, 2000). Results of studies in Thai adults with falciparum malaria were conflicting. In an earlier investigation, there was no increase in IgG coating of erythrocytes and no corrleation between the number of IgG molecules per cell and the severity of anaemia (Lee et al., 1989; WHO, 2000). However, IgG-coated cells appeared to be cleared more rapidly by the spleen for a period of several weeks after the acute infection. Later, a strong correlation was found between anaemia and the clearance of erythrocytes coated with relatively low numbers of IgG molecules (Ho et al., 1990; WHO, 2000). The survival of radioisotope-labelled compatible donor erythrocytes was significantly shorter than that of the patient's own (autologous) erythrocytes, which were presumably survivors of the enhanced splenic clearance of ageing or subtly altered cells. Patients with splenomegaly showed markedly accelerated clearance of labelled, heat-damaged erythrocytes and a lower mean haematocrit than those without splenomegaly (WHO, 2000).

The membrane fluidity of PRBCs is much lower than that of uninfected cells, and this renders PRBCs less flexible, more liable to damage in the circulation, and more susceptible to splenic clearance. However, uninfected red cells also show alterations in their rheological characteristics during malaria, which also may render them more susceptible to damage or splenic clearance. In many parts of the tropics, repeated attacks of malaria eventually lead to profound anaemia, espe-cially if there is a background of chronic blood loss from hookworm infection, malnutrition, pregnancy and persisting relapsing or recrudescent parasitaemia.

### Thrombocytopenia

Thrombocytopenia is a common finding in falciparum and vivax malarias. Its degree, if not its presence, has some prognostic significance. Platelet survival is reduced to 2–4 days in severe falciparum malaria. Platelet-associated IgG and IgG coating of platelets have not been consistent findings (WHO, 2000). Enhanced splenic uptake or sequestration may contribute to thrombocytopenia and, in patients with DIC, platelets may be removed from the circulation at sites of fibrin deposition. Histopathological studies of South-east Asian adults indicate that fibrin–platelet thrombi are rarely found in cerebral blood vessels in patients dying with cerebral malaria, but in African children they are often seen at the centre of petechial and ring haemorrhages (Lou et al., 1997; WHO, 2000).

### Leucopenia and leucocytosis

Mild leucopenia has been described in uncomplicated malarias, but a neutrophil leucocytosis is an important abnormality in patients with severe falciparum malaria and is associated with a bad prognosis. TNFα may be responsible for this leucocytosis, which may be associated with a complicating Gram-negative rod or other bacteraemia. The proportion of circulating blood polymorphonuclear leucocytes that contain visible malarial pigment is of prognostic significance (see Chapter 7).

## Spleen and lymphoreticular system

Splenic enlargement is a feature of infection by all four species of human malaria parasites. In acute falciparum infections, the spleen is enlarged, soft or firm in consistency, varying from dark red to dark or slate grey in colour, depending on the duration of the infection and the amount of pigment present. Rapid enlargement of the spleen, with or without trauma, may lead to splenic rupture (see Plate 24). There is congestion with hyperplasia of the red and white pulp (see Plate 25). Large numbers of PRBCs are present, showing all stages of development. Splenic cords and sinuses are massively congested, with monocytes and macrophages containing pigment (see Plate 26), PRBCs and non-infected red cells. The red pulp is expanded by lymphocytes, immunoblasts and plasma cells and extramedullary haemopoiesis is common. Focal haemorrhage and infarction may also be seen. Numerous PRBCs are seen by electron microscopy. During migration through the splenic cords, littoral cells phagocytose pigment and can also extract the malaria parasite from PRBCs, a process known as 'pitting' (Figure 10.5). PRBCs adhere to macrophages via their surface knobs (Figure 10.6) and degenerating forms of parasites may be seen within some macrophages. These features are also seen in bone marrow sinusoids, together with morphological abnormalities of erythroblasts, phagocytosis of parasitized red cells and increased numbers of plasma cells and macrophages. In patients with repeated attacks of malaria, lymphoid compartments of the white pulp may show considerable depletion. The red pulp still shows reticuloendothelial hyperplasia and the fibrous trabeculae and capsule are thickened. The colour may vary with the amount of pigment and this may persist for a year or more after the last acute attack, although it will eventually be removed. The spleen may exceed 20 times its normal weight in tropical splenomegaly syndrome (hyperimmune malarial splenomegaly).

In vivax malaria, the enlargement of the spleen is more rapid, with marked lymphoid hyperplasia and an increased risk of rupture. It also shows active phagocytosis of infected red cells.

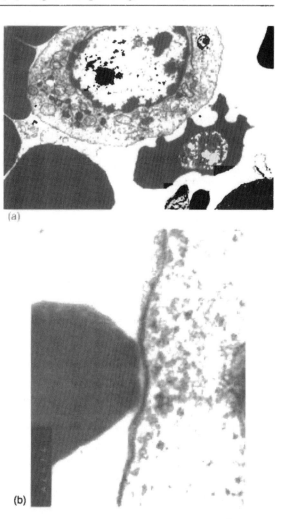

(a)

(b)

**Figure 10.6** *(a) Spleen electron micrograph showing adherence of infected red cell to splenic macrophage. (b) Higher power view of (a) showing cytoadherence via knobbed surface to macrophage. (Copyright Nick Francis.)*

## PATHOPHYSIOLOGY

The pathophysiology of the spleen's involvement in malaria is poorly understood, although it clearly plays a major role in clearance of the infection. Splenectomized patients frequently show hyperparasitaemia, high circulating levels of PRBCs with circulating mature trophozoites and schizonts, and modulation of the cytoadherence characteristics of circulating PRBCs. Immunohistochemical analysis of leucocyte and dendritic cell responses to malaria antigens in the spleen may increase our understanding of its important role in co-ordinating immune responses to malaria infection (Ho *et al.*, 1990; Urban *et al.*, 1999).

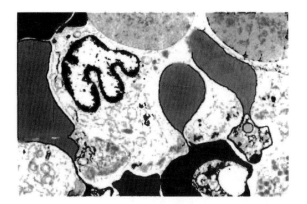

**Figure 10.5** *Spleen electron micrograph showing pitting of parasitized erythrocyte by splenic cord. (Copyright Nick Francis.)*

## LYMPH NODES

In acute falciparum infection, clinical lymph-adenopathy is uncommon, a distinguishing feature from other causes of fever. Histologically, there may be paracortical and medullary expansion and the infiltration of subcapsular sinuses by pigmented macrophages and relatively small numbers of PRBCs. The cellular proliferation is similar to that in the spleen. This may reflect a systemic response of the reticuloendothelial system to the massive intravascular antigen challenge associated with acute malaria infection.

# Kidney

### FALCIPARUM MALARIA

Renal involvement in severe falciparum malaria varies considerably in geographically distinct populations, being common in adult, South-east Asian and Indian populations, but rare in African children (Barsoum, 1998). More than one-third of non-immune adults with severe falciparum malaria will show biochemical evidence of renal dysfunction.

Several distinct patterns of renal dysfunction can be seen in falciparum malaria. Acute renal failure may develop, with associated anuria and acidosis, as part of a multisystem illness with associated haemodynamic shock ('algid' malaria) and jaundice. Haemodynamic measurements have shown that there is pre-renal failure, associated with the shock, and also a renal component (Day *et al.*, 2000b). The pathological picture is of acute tubular necrosis (Figure 10.7). PRBCs and host leucocytes, including pigment-laden macrophages, are seen within glomerular capillaries and interstitial vessels. The density of parasite sequestration (Figures 10.8 and 10.9) often appears less marked than in other organs from the same patient, although the number of lymphocytes is often more marked (see Plates 27 and 28). Fibrin thrombi can be seen in some glomerular capillaries (see Plate 28), and tubular red cell casts may be present.

In blackwater fever and in patients with inherited erythrocyte enzyme defects such as glucose-6-phosphate dehydrogenase (G6PD) deficiency who have been given oxidant drugs, large amounts of haemoglobin and other products of erythrocyte breakdown are cleared by the kidney following intravascular haemolysis. This may cause oliguric or anuric acute

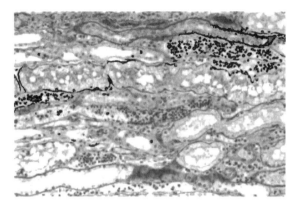

**Figure 10.7** *Kidney electron micrograph showing early, acute tubular necrosis with congestion of peritubular capillaries by large numbers of mononuclear inflammatory cells. (Copyright Nick Francis.)*

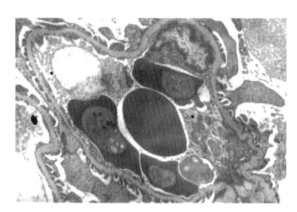

**Figure 10.8** *Kidney electron micrograph showing a capillary loop containing three parasitized erythrocytes (note pigment granules in the parasites) and a circulating mononuclear cell. (Copyright Nick Francis.)*

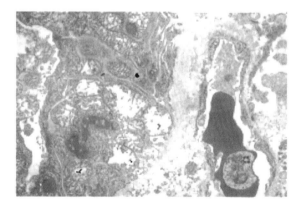

**Figure 10.9** *Kidney electron micrograph showing a parasitized erythrocyte in a peritubular capillary with apparent adherence to an endothelial cell. (Copyright Nick Francis.)*

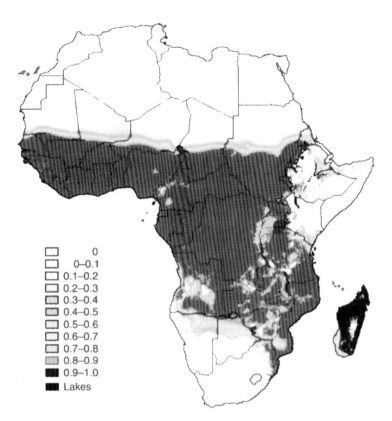

**Plate 1** *Climate model of distribution of stable P. falciparum transmission in Africa (Craig et al., 1999). Combined temperature and rainfall were used to define the vector and parasite viability for transmission within fixed seasonal windows of time. Fuzzy logic models were used to define the suitability for stable malaria transmission across Africa at a resolution of approximately 5 X 5 km. The model was structured to define distribution by setting the lower temperature cut-off at 18 °C and assuming a saturation of the temperature effect by 22 °C; similarly, rainfall values between 0 and 80 mm demarcate the range within which transmission is limited. Combined, these features must coincide on a month-to-month basis for five consecutive months and a frost-factor (minimum temperature of less than 5 °C) would eliminate transmission at any point in a contiguous period. In North Africa, high temperatures combined with a rapid onset of a short-duration rainfall allow for a limited transmission period of less than 3 months. The model provides fuzzy membership, or climate suitability values, ranging from 0 (unsuitable) to 1 (very suitable). See page 94.*

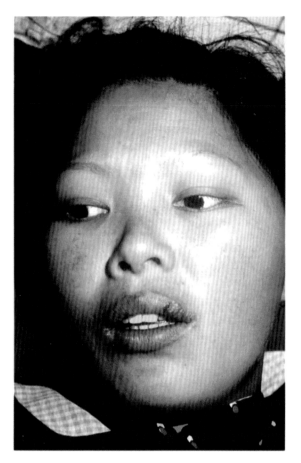

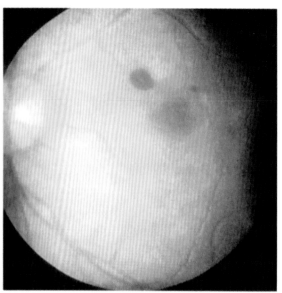

**Plate 3** *Retinal haemorrhages in a Thai man with cerebral malaria showing typical 'Roth's spot' pattern, with pale centres clustered around the macula. (Copyright DA Warrell.) See page 196.*

**Plate 2** *Herpes simplex ('cold sores') on the lips of a Vietnamese woman with acute falciparum malaria. (Copyright DA Warrell.) See page 192.*

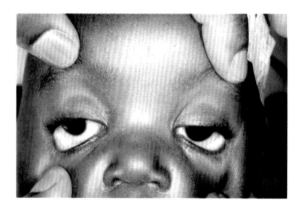

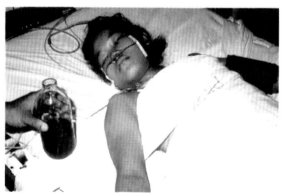

**Plate 4** *Profound anaemia (haemoglobin 1.2 g/dL) in a young Kenyan boy with heavy Plasmodium falciparum parasitaemia. (Copyright DA Warrell.) See page 197.*

**Plate 5** *Vietnamese girl with haemoglobinuria complicating severe falciparum malaria with coma and renal failure. (Copyright DA Warrell.) See page 198.*

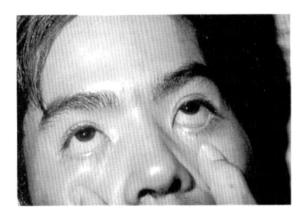

**Plate 6** *Deep jaundice in a Vietnamese man with severe falciparum malaria. (Copyright DA Warrell.) See page 198.*

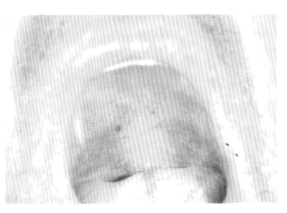

**Plate 7** *Palatal petechiae in a British patient with imported falciparum malaria complicated by severe thrombocytopenia. (Copyright DA Warrell.) See page 198.*

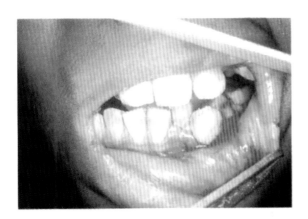

**Plate 8** *Bleeding from the gingival sulci in a Thai patient with cerebral malaria complicated by disseminated intravascular coagulation. (Copyright DA Warrell.) See page 198.*

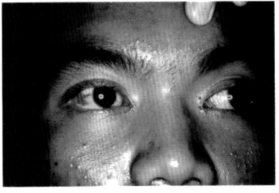

**Plate 9** *Subconjunctival haemorrhage in a jaundiced Thai man with severe falciparum malaria. (Copyright DA Warrell.) See page 198.*

(a) (b)

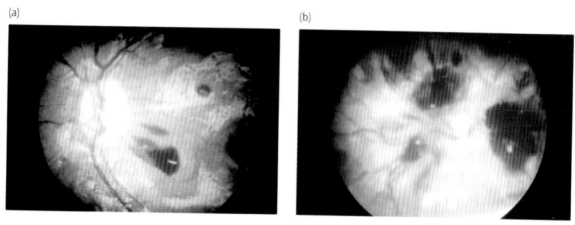

**Plate 10** *(a,b) Multiple retinal haemorrhages in Kenyan children with cerebral malaria. (Copyright K Marsh.) See page 209.*

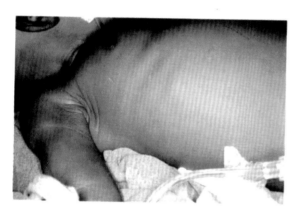

**Plate 11** *Chest retraction (recession of the intercostal spaces) in a Kenyan child with respiratory distress associated with metabolic acidosis in severe malaria. (Copyright DA Warrell.) See page 212.*

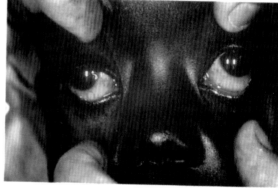

**Plate 12** *Jaundice, an unusual feature of severe malaria in African children. (Copyright DA Warrell.) See page 212.*

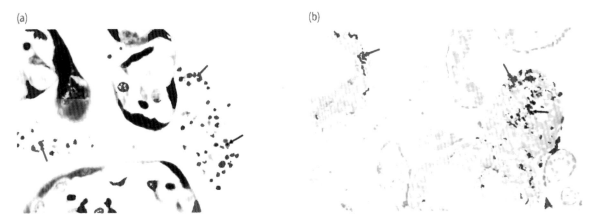

**Plate 13** *Histological slides from placentas of two women delivering in Kenya. (a) Active infection, with parasites in maternal erythrocytes in the intervillous space (Giemsa, ×1000). (b) Past infection, demonstrating haemozoin in perivillous fibrin deposits (H&E ×400). See page 219.*

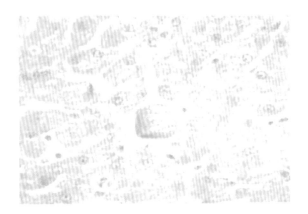

**Plate 14** *Central liver cell swollen with merozoite development in extra-erythrocytic phase (H&E). (Copyright Nick Francis.) See page 236.*

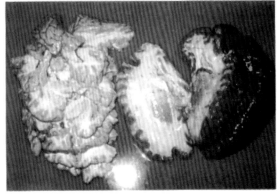

**Plate 15** *Characteristic macroscopic appearance of the brain in cerebral malaria (right), showing leaden/slatey or plum-coloured cortex and petechial haemorrhages in the white matter compared with a normal brain (left). (Copyright Dr U Hla Mon.) See page 238.*

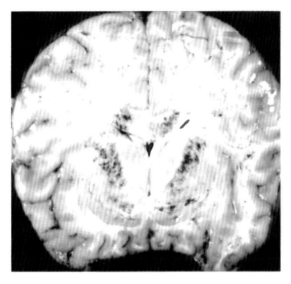

**Plate 16** *Macroscopic appearances of brain slice in cerebral malaria, showing multiple petechial haemorrhages concentrated within the subcortical white matter band, and the corpus callosum. (Copyright Dr Peter King, SAIMR, Johannesburg.) See page 238.*

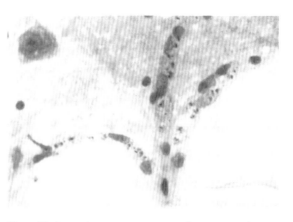

**Plate 17** *Smear from postmortem needle necropsy of brain in a victim of cerebral malaria, showing choking of small capillaries and venules with erythrocytes containing mature forms of the parasite with pigment. (Copyright Dr MJ Warrell.) See page 238.*

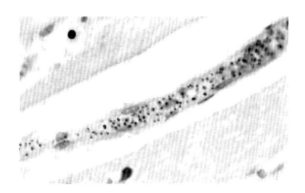

**Plate 18** *Cerebral microvascular sequestration in cerebral malaria; the vessels are packed with infected erythrocytes, recognized by pigment granules and parasite nuclei (×400, H&E). (Copyright DGH Turner.) See page 238.*

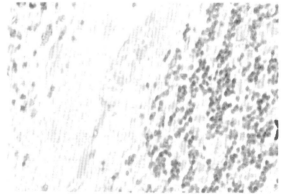

**Plate 19** *Section from cerebellum with parasitized red cells marginating in vessel (H&E). Note lack of oedema and lack of any inflammatory response. (Copyright Nick Francis.) See page 238.*

**Plate 20** *Brain showing ring haemorrhage (H&E): small central vessel contains parasitized erythrocytes with pigment. Extravasated erythrocytes are largely non-parasitized; a few contain pigment. (Copyright Nick Francis.) See page 238.*

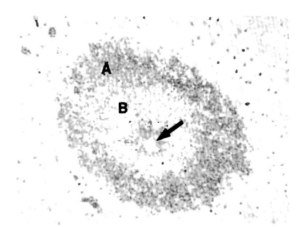

**Plate 21** *Cerebral malaria: characteristic zonal architecture of a ring haemorrhage in the brain. A central necrosed vessel (arrow) is seen surrounded by an inner ring of ischaemic change, gliosis and uninfected erythrocytes (B) and an outer ring of parasitized erythrocytes and host monocytic cells (A) (×400, H&E). (Copyright GDH Turner.) See page 238.*

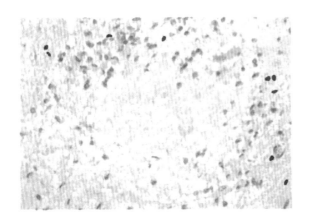

**Plate 22** *Dürck's granuloma (H&E): demyelinized central part with ring of migroglial cell proliferation. A small central vessel lumen is visible, and parasitized erythrocytes in marginal small vessels are also visible. (Copyright Nick Francis.) See page 238.*

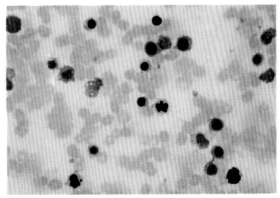

**Plate 23** *Dyserythropoietic changes in the bone marrow of a patient with severe falciparum malaria. Normoblasts show intercytoplasmic bridging and multinuclearity. (Copyright Dr Szu Hee Lee.) See page 241.*

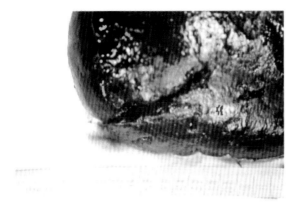

**Plate 24** *Ruptured spleen in a patient with falciparum malaria. (Copyright Professor J-E Touze.) See page 242.*

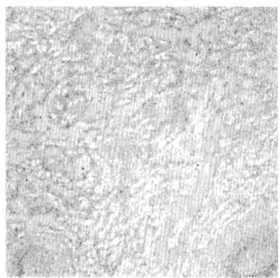

**Plate 25** *Low-powered view of the spleen from a case of fatal malaria, showing expansion of the sinusoids, reduction in white pulp lymphoid follicles and massive congestion of the red pulp with infected erythrocytes and monocytic cells (×250, H&E). (Copyright GDH Turner.) See page 242.*

**Plate 26** *Spleen (H&E): expanded red and white pulp. Red pulp shows increased white cells and macrophages plus diffuse pigment deposition. (Copyright Nick Francis.) See page 243.*

(a) 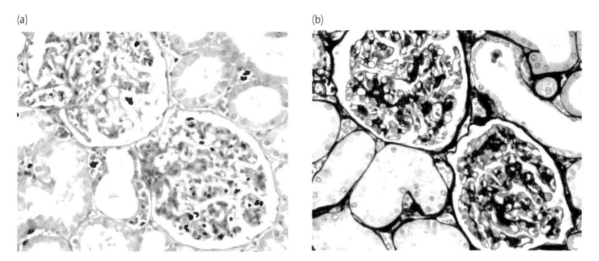 (b)

**Plate 27** *(a) Micrograph of a section of kidney from a Vietnamese adult who died with both cerebral malaria and renal failure. Parasitized erythrocytes can be seen in interstitial blood vessels and some glomerular capillary loops, as well as occasional pigmented monocytes. There is a mild increase in glomerular cellularity, but no crescent formation or obvious glomerulonephritis. No interstitial inflammatory infiltrate or severe tubular necrosis is seen (×400, H&E). (b) A micrograph of the same area as in (a) stained with silver stain to show no abnormality of the capillary basement membrane or evidence of membranous glomerulonephritis (Jones Hexamine Silver stain ×400). (Copyright GDH Turner.) See page 244.*

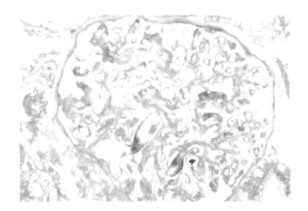

**Plate 28** *Kidney PTAH stain showing extensive capillary fibrin thrombi. (Copyright Nick Francis.) See page 244.*

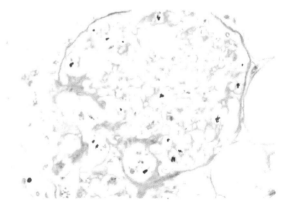

**Plate 29** *Kidney (PAS): hypercellular glomerulus with pig-ment-laden macrophages in capillary lumina. (Copyright Nick Francis.) See page 245.*

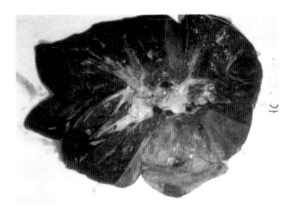

**Plate 30** *Haemorrhagic lung in a patient who died of severe falciparum malaria. (Copyright DA Warrell.) See page 245.*

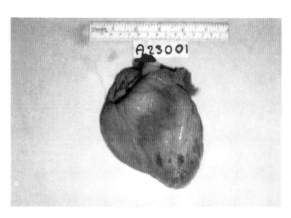

**Plate 31** *Epicardial petechial haemorrhages in a fatal case of algid malaria. (Copyright DA Warrell.) See page 246.*

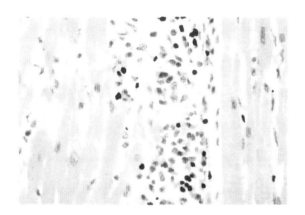

**Plate 32** *Heart (H&E): interstitial chronic inflammation between myocardial fibres and small vessels (upper centre) showing parasitized erythrocytes. (Copyright Nick Francis.) See page 246.*

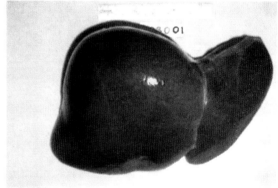

**Plate 33** *Characteristic enlarged black liver in severe falciparum malaria. (Copyright DA Warrell.) See page 246.*

(a)

(b)

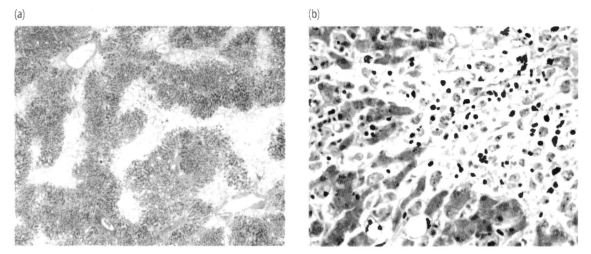

**Plates 34** *(a) Low-power micrograph showing histopathological features of the liver in a fatal case of severe malaria associated with shock and jaundice. The periportal zones are expanded and markedly congested (×250, H&E). (b) Higher power micrograph of the same section as in (a), showing mild portal tract inflammation and marked malaria pigment deposition in monocytes and Kupffer cells (×400, H&E). (Copyright GDH Turner.) See page 247.*

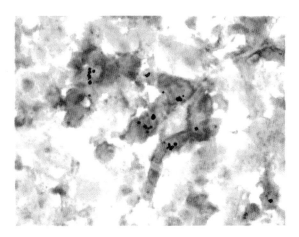

**Plate 36** *Liver showing portal and sinusoidal inflammation and marked pericentral necrosis (mid-right). (Copyright Nick Francis.) See page 247.*

**Plate 35** *Immunohistochemical staining of a liver section from a fatal malaria case showing anti-CD68 labelling of Kupffer cells with phagocytosed malaria pigment within the cytoplasm (×400, APAAP staining with haematoxylin counterstain). (Copyright GDH Turner.) See page 247.*

(a)

(b)

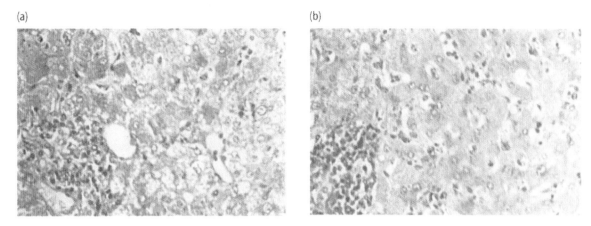

**Plate 37** *Liver from a fatal case of severe falciparum malaria showing periodic acid–Schiff stain for glycogen (a) before and (b) after digestion of glycogen with diastase. (Copyright Dr MS Dunnill.) See page 247.*

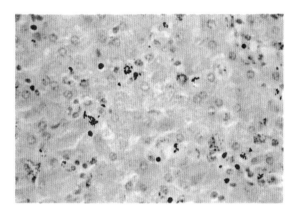

**Plate 38** *Liver (H&E) showing extensive pigment granule deposition in hepatic sinusoids, with parasitized erythrocytes discernible and minimal liver cell damage. (Copyright Nick Francis.) See page 247.*

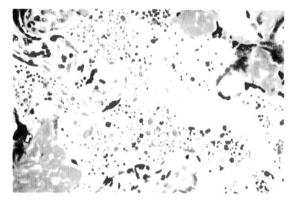

**Plate 39** *Placental villi packed with parasitized erythrocytes. (Copyright Sebastian Lucas.) See page 248.*

renal failure (Tran *et al.*, 1996). The pathophysiology of blackwater fever is discussed in Chapter 7.

In acute falciparum malaria, an acute, self-limiting mesangio-proliferative glomerulonephritis is common. It is usually associated with proteinuria, with or without microscopic haematuria. The glomeruli are hypercellular (see Plate 27a), with expansion of mesangial ground substance, focally thickened glomerular basement membranes, swollen glomeruli and focal adhesions to Bowman's capsule. There are granular, electron-dense deposits in the mesangium, paramesangium and subendothelial areas of the capillary wall, representing immune complex deposition (see Plate 29; Figure 10.10). IgM, IgG, β-1c globulin and *P. falciparum* antigens can be demonstrated in the deposits. The presence of circulating immune complexes with reduced serum C3 and C4 supports the view that this is an immune complex glomerulonephritis. It is rarely, if ever, of clinical significance.

## PATHOPHYSIOLOGY

The mechanism of renal dysfunction is uncertain, but, as mentioned above, in many of the patients there is a pre-renal factor, probably dehydration. In many, renal function is restored to normal by simple rehydration. In patients with hyperparasitaemia, jaundice or haemoglobinuria, renal impairment may persist despite rehydration. Studies of renal cortical blood flow by the [133]Xe clearance method, angiography and contrast urography have demonstrated reduced cortical perfusion during the acute stage of the disease, as in other forms of acute tubular necrosis (Day *et al.*, 2000b).

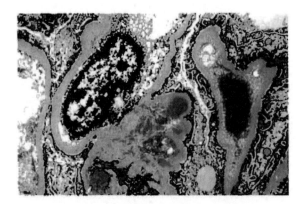

**Figure 10.10** *Kidney electron micrograph to illustrate mesangial and paramesangial electron-dense deposits (centre and bottom centre). The capillary loop to the right is plugged with fibrin thrombus. (Copyright Nick Francis.)*

## QUARTAN MALARIAL NEPHROSIS (MALARIAL NEPHROPATHY) (Barsoum, 1998)

*Plasmodium malariae* infection can cause a chronic, progressive, post-infectious glomerulonephritis, presenting as chronic nephrotic syndrome (Hendrickse *et al.*, 1979). This can cause end-stage renal failure despite active treatment. There is considerable evidence, including work in animal models, that this is an immune complex disease caused by the *in situ* formation of IgM–malaria antigen complexes in the glomerular basement membrane. There is a variety of microscopic patterns ranging from minimal change to membranous, the latter referred to as quartan malarial nephropathy because of its prominent membrane changes and lack of mesangial proliferation. Immunoglobulins (predominantly IgM), complement components, malarial antigens and electron-dense deposits have been found in the abnormal glomerular tufts.

# Lung

The older literature claimed that a variety of pneumonic, fibrotic and other syndromes were related specifically to malaria. Pneumonia is a familiar and frequently fatal complication of severe falciparum malaria and is usually attributable to aspiration or bacteraemic spread from another site of infection.

Respiratory complications of severe malaria are relatively frequent, although it is increasingly recognized that tachypnoa and abnormal breathing patterns are often related to respiratory acidosis and may reflect generalized metabolic abnormalities or intracranial events rather than primary lung disease (Crawley *et al.*, 1998).

Malaria infection can cause pulmonary oedema, seen as both free alveolar fluid and interstitial oedema. Macroscopically, the lung is dark, with scattered haemorrhages (see Plate 30). Numerous alveolar and septal haemorrhages may be present, together with large collections of leucocytes in alveolar vessels. The alveoli are congested with pigment-laden macrophages, plasma cells, neutrophils and PRBCs. Leucocytes are seen adherent to alveolar endothelial cells (Figure 10.11). Activated macrophages and lymphocytes are also present, and this picture may represent a stage in the development of an acute pulmonary syndrome which can clinically mimic 'shock lung'.

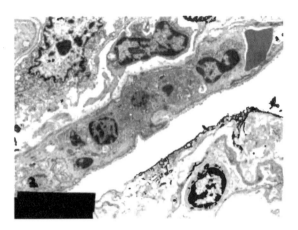

**Figure 10.11** *Lung electron micrograph showing adhesion of a leucocyte to pulmonary capillary endothelium. (Copyright GG MacPherson.)*

Laminated periodic acid–Schiff (PAS)-positive hyaline membranes may develop in more severe cases, representing a stage in the process of diffuse alveolar damage. This can progress to full-blown adult respiratory distress syndrome (ARDS), or be complicated by pneumonia. Pulmonary oedema (ARDS) has also been described in cases of proven vivax malaria (Figure 7.10, p. 199).

## PATHOPHYSIOLOGY

Acute pulmonary oedema, whether the result of iatrogenic fluid overload and associated with elevated pulmonary artery wedge pressures or of ARDS type with normal or low hydrostatic pressures in the pulmonary vascular bed, is a grave complication of severe falciparum malaria. It was a universal finding among Spitz's autopsy series of American soldiers in the Second World War (Spitz, 1946).

The pathogenesis of malarial pulmonary oedema is unclear. However, studies in animal models have indicated a role for cytokines, platelets and host lymphocyte responses in damage to microvascular endothelial cells in the lung, which may initiate the pathological processes similar to those seen in shock lung (Lucas *et al.*, 1997).

## Heart and cardiovascular system

Hypotensive shock, which has been termed 'algid malaria' or 'asthenic collapse', is a common terminal event in severe malaria in adults and children.

Previous pathological studies showed lipid depletion of the adrenal gland, which was thought to be due to secondary activation of the sympathetic nervous system during shock. Secondary haemorrhages or necrosis of the adrenal glands are rarely seen.

In patients dying of malaria, the heart shows little macroscopic abnormality. Petechial haemorrhages of the epicardial or endocardial surfaces may be found (see Plate 31), but the most striking findings are microscopical. There is congestion of the myocardial capillaries and of those of pericardial fat with PRBCs, pigment-laden macrophages, lymphocytes and plasma cells (see Plate 32). In a few cases, fatty changes of the myocardium and capillary fibrin thrombi with well-demarcated myocardial necrosis have been seen.

## PATHOPHYSIOLOGY

Shock is not attributed to effects on cardiac function of sequestered PRBCs. Myocardial function appears normal in severe falciparum malaria. Most patients have an elevated cardiac index attributable to cytokine-mediated vasodilatation, low systemic vascular resistance and low or normal pulmonary arterial wedge pressures. The mean arterial pressure is usually reduced. Profound hypotension or shock ('algid malaria') is unusual, except as a terminal phenomenon, and may be difficult to treat. In some cases it is explained by a complicating Gram-negative rod septicaemia. Cardiac arrhythmias are very uncommon (Bethell *et al.*, 1996).

## Liver and gastrointestinal system

### LIVER

Findings are similar in all forms of malaria, but tend to be more severe in *P. falciparum* infection. The major changes are in hepatic sinusoids and lining cells, but there is relatively little damage to hepatocytes and no specific malarial 'hepatitis'. The liver is enlarged as a result of sequestered blood cells and sinusoidal engorgement. Its colour varies from tan-pink to brown and eventually to black due to the deposition of malarial pigment (see Plate 33). In acute infection, the liver may be friable, becoming firm with repeated attacks. Lobular accentuation is attributable to pigment in the portal tracts.

The extra-erythrocytic or pre-erythrocytic phase of the life cycle may sometimes be detectable. Intrahepatocyte schizonts and merozoites can be seen, with displacement of the liver cell nucleus but without inflammatory changes (see Plate 14). In vivax malaria, small, non-dividing parasites 5–6 μm in diameter, which resemble the hypnozoites of experimental *P. cynomolgi* infection in rhesus monkeys, have been found in human liver biopsies and *in vitro* in cultured hepatocytes.

In early infection, there is sinusoidal dilatation and congestion, with Kupffer cell hyperplasia (initially in the periportal zone), PRBCs and fine pigment in red cells and Kupffer cells. There is phagocytosis of PRBCs and non-infected erythrocytes by Kupffer cells, endothelial cells and sinusoidal macrophages, which are increased in number and are probably recruited from the spleen (see Plates 34 and 35). Infective erythrocytes fill the sinusoids, causing reduced hepatic circulation and associated splanchnic constriction.

Small areas of centrilobular zone necrosis (see Plate 36) may be attributable to shock or disseminated intravascular coagulation rather than being specific effects of malaria, as has been claimed by Sherlock. There is often reduced hepatocyte glycogen, on PAS staining (see Plate 37) and ultrastructurally (Figure 10.12), which may explain in part the hypoglycaemia of acute hepatic dysfunction in malaria. Histological severity does not correlate well with abnormalities of liver function. Later in the disease, pigment becomes

clumped, macrophages are increased in the sinusoids (see Plate 38) and there is a chronic inflammatory infiltrate and pigment deposition in the portal tracts. Ultrastructurally, most of the PRBCs contain trophozoites, which may be knobbed or knobless and contain characteristic crystalline malarial pigment granules (Figure 10.13). Partially degenerate erythrocytes are also seen. Sites of attachment between knobbed PRBCs and phagocytic cells can be demonstrated. The hepatocytes, apart from containing lipofuscin and sometimes haemosiderin, show some fat droplet formation and swollen mitochondria, which may become depleted (Figure 10.14). There is also narrowing of the space of Disse, with loss of microvilli of the bile canaliculi, features which have been suggested as the basis for hepatic dysfunction and cholestasis. In patients with disseminated intravascular coagulation (DIC), fibrin may

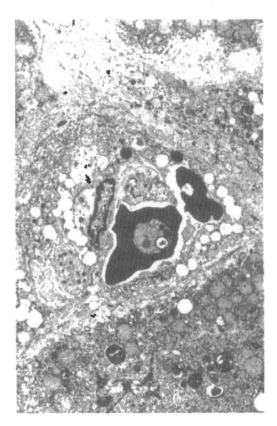

**Figure 10.13** *Liver electron micrograph showing erythrocytes in a sinusoid, with a trophozoite in one and a pigment granule in the other deformed red cell. (Copyright Nick Francis.)*

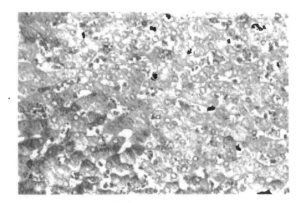

**Figure 10.12** *Liver (periodic acid–Schiff stain) showing extensive pigment in hepatic sinusoids with increased sinusoidal macrophages. Also shown is lack of glycogen in most of the field, with some residual glycogen in the lower left. (Copyright Nick Francis.)*

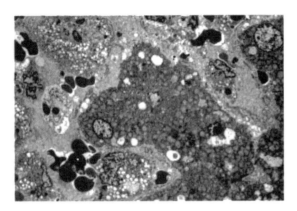

**Figure 10.14** *Liver electron micrograph showing liver sinusoids containing numerous parasitized erythrocytes, with swollen endothelial cells and fat droplet formation within hepatocytes. (Copyright Nick Francis.)*

be seen in sinusoids and, when there is associated anaemia, extramedullary haemopoiesis is found in the periportal area.

In *tropical splenomegaly syndrome*, there is a characteristically dense lymphocytic infiltrate of the sinusoids, which may resemble leukaemia, and Kupffer cell hyperplasia, with some pigment and variable portal tract chronic inflammation. Marked lobular or portal tract inflammation, hepatocyte destruction or chronic fibrosis is not seen. PRBCs are rarely detected.

**Pathophysiology**

In severe falciparum malaria, hepatic dysfunction is reflected by blood coagulation abnormalities, hypoalbuminaemia and reduced metabolic clearance of many substances, including alanine, lactate and antimalarial drugs. Hepatic blood flow is reduced during the acute phase of severe non-cerebral malaria, returning to normal during convalescence. One possible explanation for this finding would be sequestration or microcirculatory obstruction in the portal circulation. Portal vein constriction was found in rhesus monkeys infected with *P. knowlesi*. The use of the term 'malarial hepatitis' in jaundiced patients is rarely justified histopathologically.

**GASTROINTESTINAL TRACT**

Gastrointestinal symptoms, notably nausea, vomiting, abdominal pain and diarrhoea, are common in falciparum malaria. Sequestration and cytoadherence have been seen in small and large bowel, predominantly within the lamina propria capillaries, but also in larger submucosal vessels. In many severe cases, mucosal ulceration and haemorrhage may ensue and in some of these fibrin thrombi are found in small blood vessels (Dudgeon and Clark, 1917). Massive gastrointestinal haemorrhage may occur, especially if there are underlying haemostatic problems or inappropriate use of heparin.

**Pathophysiology**

Malabsorption of amino acids, sugars, fats, chloroquine and quinine have been described, although in practice drug absorption from the gut appears to be adequate in all but the most severely ill patients. In the acute phase of falciparum malaria, adult Thai patients showed greatly reduced absorption of sugars, which rely on mediated mechanisms and unmediated diffusion. Absorption returned to normal in convalescence. The pattern of reduced absorption was not characteristic of mucosal damage, but could have resulted from impaired splanchnic blood flow. Neither sugar absorption nor liver blood flow was reduced in uncomplicated falciparum malaria.

## Placenta

Malaria contracted during pregnancy can be relatively asymptomatic, but may cause pathology in the placenta and sometimes congenial transmission to the fetus. Maternal malaria is associated with decreased birth weight and premature delivery (see Chapter 9). The pathological findings in the placenta after birth vary (Bulmer *et al.*, 1993; Ismail *et al.*, 2000).

In active infection the placenta is black or slatey grey. The sinusoids are packed with PRBCs and increased numbers of pigment-laden macrophages (see Plates 13 and 39). Syncytiotrophoblastic necrosis and loss of microvilli, fibrinoid necrosis of the villi, proliferation of cytotrophoblastic cells and thickening of the trophoblastic basement membrane have been observed and may provide a basis for impaired fetal nutrition. In previous or resolved infection, variable amounts of pigment are seen in perivillous fibrinoid material and placental bed tissue (see Plate 13b). If the infection is recently resolved, pigment may be seen in syncytiotrophoblasts and circulating mononuclear cells or macrophages. Transmission of infection across an intact placenta to the fetus is considered uncommon, especially in immune and semi-immune mothers, but PRBCs are sometimes seen in fetal vessels in infected placentas (Matteelli *et al.*, 1997).

## PATHOPHYSIOLOGY

This is an area of active research because the placenta offers an accessible human tissue model of the comparative effects of parasite and leucocyte cytoadherence, host cytokine release and other pathophysiological factors in the causation of tissue damage during severe malaria. PRBC sequestration to trophoblastic cells appears to be mediated by matrix adhesion molecules such as chondroitin sulphate A and hyaluronic acid (Rogerson and Beeson, 1999; Beeson *et al.*, 2000). It may involve only certain clones of *P. falciparum* (Fried and Duffy, 1996). These receptors are different from those mediating cytoadherence in other organs of the body, and the development of maternal antibodies against parasite strains binding to these receptors appears to protect the mother against subsequent episodes of maternal malaria. The vulnerability of primigravidae to symptomatic malaria, even those brought up in malaria endemic areas, may be explained by lack of these antibodies. An animal model (*P. coatneyi* in *Macaca mulatta*) may help with the understanding of these issues (Davison *et al.*, 1998, 2000).

## Metabolic disturbances

### HYPOGLYCAEMIA

Hypoglycaemia is an increasingly recognized complication of falciparum malaria. The *Cinchona* alkaloids, quinine and quinidine, release insulin from pancreatic islet cells. This reduces hepatic gluconeogenesis and increases peripheral glucose uptake by tissues, resulting in hypoglycaemia. In this situation, inappropriately high plasma insulin concentrations will be associated with increased lactate and alanine and low ketone concentrations.

Glucose consumption may be increased in patients with malaria as a result of fever, infection and anaerobic glycolysis in the host tissues and by the parasite burden.

Glycogen reserves may be depleted, especially in children and pregnant women as a result of fasting and 'accelerated starvation'. Inhibition of hepatic gluconeogenesis by TNFα and other cytokines could be the cause of a common hypoglycaemic syndrome in African children with severe malaria, adult patients with severe disease and pregnant women who have elevated plasma lactate and alanine concentrations and in some cases moderately increased ketone bodies. Counter-regulatory hormone levels are usually very high. Similar disturbances have been found in other severe infections such as bacillary dysentery in children.

### ACIDOSIS

Acidosis is an important feature of severe adult and childhood falciparum malaria (English *et al.*, 1996; Day *et al.*, 2000a).

Recent studies suggest a multifactorial origin involving tissue hypoxia, liver dysfunction and impaired renal handling of bicarbonate. Many of these metabolic abnormalities may be due to widespread sequestration in a number of different organs, but the role of systemic cytokine release is also likely to be an important factor.

## ENDNOTE

1. Malarial pigment is a blackish-brown, acid haematin with characteristic birefringence with polarized light but without any positive staining characteristics with special staining techniques. Ultrastructurally, it can be identified by its rectangular crystalline structure and solubility in alkaline lead citrate, leaving electron-lucent clear spaces.

## REFERENCES

Anstey NM, Weinberg JB, Hassanali MY, *et al.* Nitric oxide in Tanzanian children with malaria: inverse relationship between malaria severity and nitric oxide production/nitric oxide synthase Type 2 expression. *J Exp Med* 1996; **184**: 557–67.

Barsoum RS. Malarial nephropathies. *Nephrol Dial Transplant* 1998; **13**(6): 1588–97.

Beeson JG, Rogerson SJ, Cooke BM, *et al.* Adhesion of *Plasmodium falciparum*-infected erythrocytes to hyaluronic acid in placental malaria. *Nat Med* 2000; **6**(1): 86–90.

Bethell DB, Phuong PT, Phuong CX, *et al*. Electrocardiographic monitoring in severe falciparum malaria. *Trans R Soc Trop Med Hyg* 1996; **90**(3): 266–9.

Brown HC, Chau TTH, Mai NTH, *et al*. Blood–brain barrier function in cerebral malaria and CNS infections in Vietnam. *Neurology* 2000; **55**(1): 104–11.

Brown H, Turner G, Rogerson S, *et al*. Cytokine expression in the brain in human cerebral malaria. *J Infect Dis* 1999; **180**(5): 1742–6.

Brown H *et al*. Evidence of blood–brain barrier dysfunction in human cerebral malaria. *Neuropathol Appl Neurobiol* 1999; **25**: 331–40.

Brown H, Rogerson S, Taylor T, *et al*. Blood–brain barrier function in cerebral malaria in Malawian children. *Am J Trop Med Hyg* 2001; **64**: 207–13.

Bull PC, Lowe BS, Kortok M, Molyneux CS, Newbold CI, Marsh K. Parasite antigens on the infected red cell surface are targets for naturally acquired immunity to malaria. *Nat Med* 1998; **4**(3): 358–60.

Bulmer JN, Rasheed FN, Francis N, Morrison L, Greenwood BM. Placental malaria. I. Pathological classification. *Histopathology* 1993; **22**(3): 211–18.

Carr RA, Molyneux ME, Mwenechanya JJ, *et al*. Macroscopic evidence of moderate brain swelling in pediatric cerebral malaria: an autopsy study. *Proc Am Soc Trop Med Hyg* 1998; **59**(Suppl.): 239.

Cranston WI. Temperature regulation. *Br Med J* 1966; **2**: 69–75.

Crawley J, English M, Waruiru C, Mwangi I, Marsh K. Abnormal respiratory patterns in childhood cerebral malaria. *Trans R Soc Trop Med Hyg* 1998; **92**(3): 305–8.

Davison BB, Cogswell FB, Baskin GB, *et al*. *Plasmodium coatneyi* in the Rhesus monkey (*Macaca mulatta*) as a model of malaria in pregnancy. *Am J Trop Med Hyg* 1998; **59**: 189–201.

Davison BB, Cogswell BB, Baskin GB, *et al*. Placental changes associated with fetal outcome in the *Plasmodium coatneyi*/Rhesus monkey model of malaria in pregnancy. *Am J Trop Med Hyg* 2000; **63**: 158–73.

Day NP, Hien TT, Schollaardt T, *et al*. The prognostic and pathophysiologic role of pro- and anti-inflammatory cytokines in severe malaria. *J Infect Dis* 1999; **180**(4): 1288–97.

Day NP, Phu NH, Mai NT, *et al*. The pathophysiologic and prognostic significance of acidosis in severe adult malaria. *Crit Care Med* 2000a; **28**(6): 1833–40.

Day NP, Phu NH, Mai NT, *et al*. Effects of dopamine and epinephrine infusions on renal hemodynamics in severe malaria and severe sepsis. *Crit Care Med* 2000b; **28**(5): 1353–62.

Dondorp AM, Kager PA, Vreeken J, White NJ. Abnormal blood flow and red blood cell deformability in severe malaria. *Parasitol Today* 2000; **16**(6): 228–32.

Dudgeon L, Clark C. A contribution to the microscopical histology of malaria. *Lancet* 1917; **ii**: 153–6.

English M, Waruiru C, Amukoye E, *et al*. Deep breathing in children with severe malaria: indicator of metabolic acidosis and poor outcome. *Am J Trop Med Hyg* 1996; **55**(5): 521–4.

Fried M, Duffy PE. Adherence of *Plasmodium falciparum* to chondroitin sulfate A in the human placenta. *Science* 1996; **272**(5267): 1502–4.

Hendrickse RG, Adeniyi A. Quartan malarial nephrotic syndrome in children. *Kidney Int* 1979; **16**(1): 64–74.

Ho M, White NJ. Molecular mechanisms of cytoadherence in malaria. *Am J Physiol* 1999; **276** (6 Pt 1): C1231–42.

Ho M *et al*. Splenic Fc receptor in host defence and anemia in acute *Plasmodium falciparum* malaria. *J Infect Dis* 1990; **161**: 555–61.

Ismail MR, Ordi J, Menendez C, *et al*. Placental pathology in malaria: a histological, immunohistochemical, and quantitative study. *Hum Pathol* 2000; **31**(1): 85–93.

Kwiatkowski D. The molecular genetic approach to malarial pathogenesis and immunity. *Parassitologia* 1999; **41**(1–3): 233–40.

Kwiatkowski D, Molyneux ME, Stephens S, *et al*. Anti-TNF therapy inhibits fever in cerebral malaria. *Quart J Med* 1993; **86**: 91–8.

Lee SH *et al*. Antibody dependent red cell removal during *P. falciparum* malaria: the clearance of red cells sensitized with IgG anti-D. *Br J Haematol* 1989; **73**: 396–402.

Lou J, Donati YR, Juillard P, *et al*. Platelets play an important role in TNF-induced microvascular endothelial cell pathology. *Am J Pathol* 1997; **151**(5): 1397–405.

Lucas R, Lou J, Morel DR, Ricou B, Suter PM, Grau GE. TNF receptors in the microvascular pathology of acute respiratory distress syndrome and cerebral malaria. *J Leukoc Biol* 1997; **61**(5): 551–8.

Macpherson G, Warrell M, White N, Looareesuwan S, Warrell D. Human cerebral malaria – a quantitative ultrastructural analysis of parasitized erythrocyte sequestration. *Am J Pathol* 1985; **119**: 385–401.

Maneerat Y, Viriyavejakul P, Punpoowong B, *et al*. Inducible nitric oxide synthase expression is increased in the brain in fatal cerebral malaria. *Histopathology* 2000; in press.

Matteelli A, Caligaris S, Castelli F, Carosi G. The placenta and malaria. *Ann Trop Med Parasitol* 1997; **91**(7): 803–10.

McGuire W, Hill AV, Allsopp CE, *et al*. Variation in the TNF-alpha promotor region associated with susceptibility to cerebral malaria. *Nature* 1994; **371**: 508–10.

Newton CR, Crawley J, Sowumni A, *et al*. Intracranial hypertension in Africans with cerebral malaria. *Arch Dis Child* 1997; **76**(3): 219–26.

Newton CR, Taylor TE, Whitten RO. Pathophysiology of fatal falciparum malaria in African children. *Am J Trop Med Hyg* 1998; **58**(5): 673–83.

Pongponratn E, Riganti M, Punpoowong B, Aikawa M. Microvascular sequestration of parasitized erythrocytes in human falciparum malaria. *Am J Trop Med Hyg* 1991; **44**: 168–75.

Rogerson SJ, Beeson JG. The placenta in malaria: mechanisms of infection, disease and foetal morbidity. *Ann Trop Med Parasitol* 1999; **93**(Suppl. 1): S35–42.

Sanni LA, Thomas SR, Tattam BN, *et al*. Dramatic changes in oxidative tryptophan metabolism along the kynurenine pathway in experimental cerebral and noncerebral malaria. *Am J Pathol* 1998; **152**(2): 611–19.

Silamut K, Phu NH, Whitty C, *et al*. A quantitative analysis of microvascular sequestration of malaria parasites in the human brain. *Am J Pathol* 1999; **155**: 395–410.

Spitz S. The pathology of acute falciparum malaria. *Milit Surg* 1946; **99**: 555–72.

Taylor AM, Day NP, Sinh DX, *et al*. Reactive nitrogen intermediates and outcome in severe adult malaria. *Trans R Soc Trop Med Hyg* 1998; **92**: 170–5.

Tran TH, Day NP, Ly VC, *et al*. Blackwater fever in southern Vietnam: a prospective descriptive study of 50 cases. *Clin Infect Dis* 1996; **23**(6): 1274–81.

Turner GDH. Cerebral malaria. *Brain Pathol* 1997; **7**: 569–82.

Urban BC, Ferguson DJ, Pain A, *et al*. *Plasmodium falciparum*-infected erythrocytes modulate the maturation of dendritic cells. *Nature* 1999; **400**(6739): 73–7.

Warrell DA, Looareesuwan S, Phillips RE, *et al*. Function of the blood–cerebrospinal fluid barrier in human cerebral malaria: rejection of the permeability hypothesis. *Am J Trop Med Hyg* 1986; **35**: 882–9.

Warrell DA, Looareesuwan S, Warrell MJ, *et al*. Dexamethasone proves deleterious in cerebral malaria. A double blind trial in 100 comatose patients. *N Engl J Med* 1982; **306**: 313–9.

Warrell DA, White NJ, Veall N, *et al*. Cerebral anaerobic glycolysis and reduced cerebral oxygen transport in human cerebral malaria. *Lancet* 1988; **ii**: 534–8.

WHO. Severe falciparum malaria. *Trans R Soc Trop Med Hyg* 2000; **94**(Suppl. 1): S1–S90.

# Immunology of malaria

KEVIN MARSH

Malaria is an important cause of morbidity, but not everyone infected with the malaria parasite becomes seriously ill or dies. In areas of stable endemicity, repeated exposure to the parasite leads to the acquisition of specific immunity, which restricts serious problems to young children; malaria in older subjects causes a relatively mild febrile illness. However, even in people exposed to malaria for the first time, there is a range of possible outcomes, from death at one extreme to the occasional subject who appears resistant to infection at the other. In this case, any resistance is non-specific; it does not depend on prior exposure to malaria and may be either acquired or innate. Of course, the situation is not necessarily clear-cut and in any one individual several factors may interact, for instance when innate genetic factors exert their effect on the acquisition of specific immunity. Much of this chapter is concerned with specific acquired immunity to malaria; how it might work, what goes wrong with it and the possibilities for manipulation by vaccination. However, we begin with a brief outline of important innate and acquired factors that lead to non-specific immunity.

## INNATE RESISTANCE TO MALARIA

The malaria parasite faces a succession of challenges within the host. It has to attach to, enter and thrive in, first, hepatocytes and then erythrocytes. Having overcome these hurdles, it has to leave the host to carry on the next part of its cycle in the mosquito. Along its way, the parasite is susceptible to a whole range of potential interruptions, including simple physical barriers, non-specific protective responses, alterations in the supply of essential nutrients and the operation of specific immune mechanisms. Many host genes will be involved in the control of the internal environment which faces the parasite, and the major disadvantages of being parasitized should favour the survival of those host gene polymorphisms that afford any degree of protection against the parasite. Finding out which human genes are important is difficult, although more is probably known about the selective effect of malaria on the human genome than any other infection. This is due not only to malaria having been such a potent selective force but also to the fact that the red cell, the most important host environment for the parasite, is relatively easy to characterize in terms of genetic differences. The effect of host genetics on other aspects of parasite success, such as interactions with the hepatocyte, the generation of immune responses and even the ability to form infective gametocytes, are less well understood.

## RED CELL POLYMORPHISMS AND MALARIA

Hundreds of genetic variations have been described that affect human red blood cells (Weatherall, 1987). The variants of most interest are those that have achieved polymorphic status, i.e. alternative versions of the same gene co-exist in a population at frequencies well above those that could be explained simply by the repeated occurrence of the mutation which produces the variant. At a time when the only well-recognized red cell polymorphisms were those giving rise to the thalassaemic states, JBS Haldane suggested that their geographical distribution was due to a selective effect of malaria on the heterozygote, i.e. the carriers of the genes enjoyed some advantage that balanced the disadvantage of the homozygotic states. This 'malaria hypothesis' was a key insight into the interaction of human genetics and infectious diseases.

The red cell polymorphisms for which there is now reasonable evidence to support a 'malaria hypothesis' include conditions affecting the structure of the β-globin chain of haemoglobin (HbS, HbC and HbE), rates of synthesis of globin chains, (α-thalassaemia and β-thalassaemia), the level of a key red cell enzyme, glucose-6-phosphate dehydrogenase (G6PD), and conditions affecting the red cell membrane and cytoskeleton (Duffy blood group negativity and hereditary ovalocytosis). There are also a number of less clear-cut cases affecting both membrane structure and other red cell enzymes for which either the degree of polymorphism is less or the possibility of protection is not yet clearly established; these will not be discussed.

In most cases, the strongest evidence for the malaria hypothesis is epidemiological, although there is clear-cut clinical evidence of protection for sickle cell trait (the carrier state for HbS) and, to a lesser extent, with β-thalassaemia and G6PD deficiency. Several potential mechanisms of protection have been shown

*in vitro*. They include interference with the complex events of red cell invasion and metabolic effects on the parasite, either by not providing the optimum intracellular environment or by increasing the susceptibility of the infected cell to oxidant damage. In many cases it is likely that several mechanisms operate together. There is emerging evidence for increased immunological clearance of infected variant cells, providing a potential 'unified theory' to underpin the malaria hypothesis.

## Haemoglobin S

The haemoglobin molecule is a tetramer; the normal haemoglobin of adults (HbA) comprising two α chains and two β chains. Haemoglobin S is formed when there is a particular amino acid substitution (valine for glutamic acid at position 6) in the β chain. The resulting abnormal chain can still combine with α chains, but the haemoglobin molecule formed has altered physicochemical characteristics. Normally there are two functional β genes, one inherited from each parent. Heterozygotes for HbS have one normal and one defective β gene (they are said to have sickle trait and are designated AS). Their red cells, which contain a mixture of HbA and HbS, function fairly normally in most situations. By contrast, red cells of homozygotes (designated SS) contain HbS, as both β globin genes are of the abnormal type. Their cells assume an abnormal shape (sickle) under conditions of low oxygen tension, which leads to both increased red cell lysis and obstruction of vascular flow as the abnormal cells lodge in small blood vessels. Except under circumstances with a high availability of medical care, the homozygous condition (sickle cell disease) is often fatal in childhood, indicating that there must be a very powerful advantage to the heterozygote in maintaining the gene at high frequencies.

Haemoglobin S is found at increased frequencies only in malarious areas. It reaches very high levels in parts of Africa where over 20 per cent of the population are heterozygotes. It occurs at lower frequencies in some Mediterranean populations, in the Middle East and in parts of India. The selective advantage is exercised predominantly in childhood. The overwhelming evidence is that this is due to a strong protection against the clinical effects of malaria, rather than an effect on susceptibility to malaria infection *per se*, which is not markedly less common in AS individuals (Bayoumi, 1987). A number of protective mechanisms have been suggested. Infected AS cells sickle more readily than uninfected cells, which may lead to increased reticulo-endothelial clearance. Parasite growth is inhibited in AS cells under conditions of low oxygen tension, possibly due to an alteration in red cell potassium levels. A number of studies have shown differences in immune responses to malaria in AS individuals and it is possible that altered reticuloendothelial clearance of infected cells leads to better natural immunization against subsequent malaria.

## Haemoglobin C

Haemoglobin C is formed by substitution of a lysine for glutamate at position 6 in the β chain. It is present at high frequencies in a localized part of West Africa, around Burkina Faso and Ghana. Cells from the homozygote CC are refractory to parasite growth in culture, possibly due to their resistance to bursting and releasing merozoites rather than to any deficit in the intracellular environment. However, AC cells support parasite growth normally. An interesting twist is added by the fact that, in West Africa, sickle cell gene frequencies are also very high and individuals carrying one S gene and one C gene (i.e. SC) are not uncommon and parasite growth is particularly poor in SC cells. Since it seems unlikely that HbC has been maintained by an advantage of AC heterozygotes, or that homozygote advantage has been the selective force, it is possible that the high frequencies are not even related to malaria. An interesting possibility is that it is SC individuals who have been at a particular advantage, protection against severe malaria more than balancing the reduced fertility of SC females.

## Haemoglobin E

Haemoglobin E is probably the commonest haemoglobin variant in the world. It is caused by a single mutation of glutamine to lysine at position 26 in the β chain and is common throughout South-east Asia. The mechanism of protection is not clear; there is evidence of reduced parasite growth in cells from both homozygotes and heterozygotes, possibly exacerbated under conditions of oxidant stress. In addition, both parasitized EE and AE erythrocytes are phagocytosed more readily than parasitized AA erythrocytes, raising the possibility that protection derives in part from an interaction with the host immune system.

## The thalassaemias

The thalassaemias are a heterogeneous group of conditions in which there is a reduced rate of production of one or more of the globin chains of haemoglobin. The β-thalassaemias usually result from single base changes or small deletions in the β globin genes. They occur widely in areas that are, or have been, malarious, being common in the Mediterranean basin, the Middle East and South-east Asia. They occur at lower frequencies in sub-Saharan Africa; this has been explained as the result of the β-thalassaemia genes being in competition with the strongly protective sickle cell gene. Although this makes sense, it is less clear why both β-thalassaemia and HbE genes co-exist at such high frequencies in parts of South-east Asia.

Humans have four α globin genes, a duplicated pair being inherited from each parent. The α-thalassaemias result from defects in one or more of these genes. The effects cover a wide spectrum: from asymptomatic individuals with one α gene affected, to the absence of all four functional genes, a condition which is incompatible with life and results in stillbirths with Hb Barts hydrops syndrome. Because the more minor forms are without obvious clinical consequences, the epidemiology of the α-thalassaemias has had to await the availability of molecular typing techniques. These techniques have shown that α-thalassaemia genes are widely distributed throughout every part of the world that has been endemic for malaria. Particularly high frequencies are reached in parts of South-east Asia and in Melanesia, where detailed epidemiological studies have provided strong evidence to support the malaria hypothesis (Flint et al., 1986).

As with the other red cell polymorphisms, the mechanisms by which the thalassaemias protect against malaria are not known with any certainty. There is reduced parasite growth in β-thalassaemia cells, particularly when exposed to oxidant stress. On the other hand, cells from individuals with single or double α gene deletions support parasite growth normally under all conditions. However, infected cells from both α-thalassaemia and β-thalassaemia subjects show enhanced antigen expression at the surface of the infected red cell, possibly leading to enhanced immune clearance. Recently, evidence has suggested that, far from being completely protected against malaria, children with α-thalassaemia may experience *more* attacks of mild malaria in early life, suggesting that longer-term protection may stem from better early immunization (Williams *et al.*, 1996).

## Glucose-6-phosphate dehydrogenase deficiency

G6PD is the first enzyme of the hexose monophosphate shunt and plays a critical role in the production of NADPH. There are numerous variants of the enzyme described, inheritance of some of which leads to deficiency of the enzyme. The gene for G6PD is on the X chromosome and severe deficiency is fully expressed only in male hemizygotes and rare female homozygotes. Under most circumstances, the malaria parasite is thought to use host pathways for NADPH production and it should be susceptible to changes in the level of the enzymes. Although variant genes leading to deficiency states have been found all over the world, they only reach polymorphic frequencies (with a few puzzling exceptions) in malaria-endemic regions, leading to the hypothesis that they, like genes for structural haemoglobin variants, have been selected for by malaria (Ruwende *et al.*, 1995). Epidemiological studies and *in vitro* studies of parasite growth in deficient cells have often produced equivocal results: it had previously been believed that only heterozygote females benefited from protection, something which was difficult to reconcile with the observation that parasite growth is retarded in G6PD-deficient cells. However, recent large case–control studies have shown clearly that hemizygote males are protected to the same degree from severe malaria.

## Innate resistance and the red cell membrane

As there are a number of human genetic polymorphisms affecting the structure and function of the red cell membrane, it might be expected that some of these will affect the parasite's ability to invade the red cell. The classical example is the Duffy blood group system and *P. vivax*. Red cells from Duffy-negative

individuals are completely resistant to *infection* with *P. vivax*, implying that this parasite uses the Duffy determinants during invasion. *P. vivax* is not endemic in West Africa, where the majority of people are Duffy negative, and is rare in other parts of Africa. This is usually interpreted as having come about by malaria selecting for humans who are negative; however, *P. vivax* causes little direct mortality and it would have to be argued either that there was considerable indirect mortality or that *P. vivax* has in the past been more virulent. Perhaps more likely is that Duffy negativity was already established in certain populations by other mechanisms and that the selection has been against the parasite invading these areas, rather than the other way round.

## Red cell cytoskeletal abnormalities

The only red cell cytoskeletal abnormality known to reach polymorphic frequencies is hereditary ovalocytosis. This is an autosomal dominant condition in which the red cells have an oval shape and a marked increase in membrane rigidity. The molecular basis of the condition appears to be modification of band 3, the major anion transporter of red cells. Ovalocytic red cells are highly resistant to invasion by both *P. vivax* and *P. falciparum* and this is reflected by lower parasite rates and densities in ovalocytic individuals. The gene frequency is high (up to 30 per cent) in many parts of South-east Asia through into Papua New Guinea. As the condition is not known to cause any ill-effects, it is a matter of speculation as to whether it is a balanced polymorphism or whether it is moving towards fixation, i.e. will become the 'normal' red cell type with the passage of time if a selective pressure from malaria is maintained in those populations.

## Other genetic polymorphisms and malaria

The relationship between malaria and the red cell has played a central role in the development of ideas on the selection of single genes by infective agents, but it seems certain that many other host genes will be important. Human leucocyte antigens (HLA) are a highly polymorphic family of proteins that play critical roles in the genesis of immune responses (see below). There is some evidence from studies in Sardinia of selection for particular HLA types in populations historically exposed to malaria when compared with populations of the same ancestral stock living at a higher altitude, where malaria has never been endemic. More recently, evidence has emerged for associations between a few HLA antigens common in African populations and protection from severe disease. An HLA class 1 antigen, HLA-BW53, and an HLA class 11 haplotype, DRBI*I302-DQB1*0501, have been associated with reduced susceptibility to severe disease (Hill *et al.*, 1991).

Increasingly, interest is focusing on host molecules thought to be involved in the pathogenesis of severe malaria, on the grounds that polymorphisms altering the function of these molecules would make them subject to either positive or negative selection, depending on the effect of the functional change on disease severity. Different polymorphisms affecting the promoter region of the gene coding for TNFα, which is believed to play an important role in severe malaria, have been shown to be associated with both protection and increased susceptibility (Knight *et al.*, 1999). Similarly, a polymorphism in intracellular adhesion molecule 1 (ICAM-1), one of the endothelial receptors for infected cell cytoadherence (see Chapter 10), is associated with an increased risk of cerebral malaria (Fernandez-Reyes *et al.*, 1997). Although more genetic polymorphisms have already been associated with malaria than with any other infectious disease, it seems likely that many more will be discovered over the next few years.

## ACQUIRED NON-SPECIFIC RESISTANCE TO MALARIA

Not all mechanisms of non-specific resistance to malaria are genetic. The relationship between nutritional status and malaria is contentious. It is often stated that it is unusual to see severe malaria in children with marasmus or kwashiorkor and there have been several reports of exacerbation of malaria when nutritional supplements have been introduced in times of famine. Deficiencies of several specific dietary components have been shown to have a protective effect against malaria in a variety of animal models, including iron, riboflavin and para-amino benzoic acid (PABA). Taken together, these observa-

tions are sometimes assumed to support the idea that undernutrition may be protective against malaria. This is difficult to reconcile with the undoubted importance of poor nutritional status as a determinant of overall childhood mortality in malaria-endemic areas. More recent studies show that even moderate undernutrition is, in fact, associated with increased severity of malaria and increased case fatality. Thus, it seems likely that, overall, poor nutritional status increases susceptibility to clinical malaria, but that *in extremis* an individual may become so starved that deficiency of specific nutrients may actually limit parasite growth.

It may seem strange to include drugs as an acquired resistance factor, but it should be recognized that community use of chloroquine in some areas is now so common that the drug, which has a long clearance time, can be detected in a large proportion of the population at any one time. Even with rapidly diminishing sensitivity to chloroquine, this is likely to have an effect on the epidemiology of malaria in these areas.

## ACQUIRED IMMUNITY TO MALARIA

In stable endemic areas, a heavy burden of morbidity and mortality falls on young children, but malaria is a relatively mild condition in adults (Baird, 1998). This is due to the acquisition of specific immunity. Children born to immune mothers appear themselves to be relatively immune to malaria for a period (Fried *et al.*, 1998). It is not rare to find low numbers of parasites in cord blood, but these do not usually give rise to overt infections (this contrasts with the situation in less stable areas, where clinically severe congenital malaria does occur). The child remains relatively protected for a period of around 3 months following birth. If transmission is heavy, the child may become parasitaemic during this period, and sometimes have fever, but rarely manifests any severe features of malaria. In short, very young infants behave rather like immune adults.

Following the period of relative protection, children become susceptible to the more severe clinical manifestations of malaria (see Chapters 7 and 8). However, it should be stressed that, even during the period of maximum susceptibility to severe disease, children spend the majority of their time parasitized but healthy. From around the fourth year of life, the severity of clinical attacks begins to decline, although parasite rates remain high (Gupta *et al.*, 1999). Death from malaria is rare after the fifth year and thereafter clinical attacks become less frequent and less severe until, in adulthood, significant disease is rare, although self-limiting attacks of fever and headache are common. Complete immunity to parasitization is probably never achieved and the cumulative parasite prevalence in adults is near 100 per cent. The above description is somewhat idealized and both the exact timing of events and the clinical manifestations of parasitization vary with the intensity of transmission (see Chapter 5); nonetheless, this sketch captures the essential epidemiological features of aquired immunity.

Once achieved, malaria immunity may not be stable and it is often reported that immune subjects who spend time outside an endemic area are prone to malaria on re-exposure. However, this is an area with far more anecdotes than hard facts and, although there is an increased susceptibility to minor symptoms, immunity to life-threatening disease probably persists for much longer. A second situation in which there is some apparent loss of immunity is pregnancy. This is manifest as an increased prevalence and increased density of parasitaemia which may lead to severe anaemia (see Chapter 9). At delivery, the placenta is often parasitized to a degree far beyond that expected from the peripheral parasitaemia. The fact that this phenomenon is particularly common in first pregnancies has led to the suggestion that it represents a failure of local immunity, and that such local immunity is acquired in subsequent pregnancies. It has recently been shown that parasites accumulating in the placenta do so by adhering to a specific receptor, chondroitin sulphate A, expressed on the syncytiotrophoblast, and that in subsequent pregnancies women develop specific antibodies which may block this interaction.

What general conclusions about the nature of immunity to malaria can be drawn from this epidemiological picture? First, it appears that a substantial degree of protection can be transferred from mother to child, implying an important role for humoral immune mechanisms. This is also supported by classical studies of the effects of immune globulin given to individuals with acute malaria. A second conclusion sometimes drawn is that, because children pass through a period when they commonly have high parasitaemia without serious disease, there must be a part of immunity which is not directly antiparasitic but is 'antitoxic', either by neutralizing toxic parasite products or by tempering the host's acute response to infection (see Chapter 10). Although such mechanisms may well be important, it needs to be recognized that, even when there is tolerance of parasites, there must at the same time be mechanisms acting to limit parasite multiplication, otherwise the child would die as its red cells were destroyed by the inexorable increase of parasites. The third and most important conclusion is that, if children who are immune to some parasites (i.e. able to live happily while parasitized) remain susceptible to disease, there must be a sense in which immunity is strain-specific. This is supported by many observations from experimental infections in humans and in a number of animal models of malaria. This leads to the idea that an individual must experience a repertoire of strains in order to build up substantial immunity. The fact that this commonly takes several years has led to the idea that the number of strains must be very large; however, two recent observations suggest that this may not necessarily be the case. First, non-immune adults moving into a malarious area become immune to malaria much more rapidly than children from the same population (Anders *et al.*, 1986). Second, even in African children, a considerable degree of immunity can be shown to be acquired after only one or two episodes of disease (Gupta *et al.*, 1999).

In order to explain these epidemiological observations, it will be necessary to examine the points in the malaria parasite's life cycle at which immune responses could act, and to identify the targets of these responses. However, first it is necessary to give a brief and somewhat simplified general overview of the elements of immune responses.

## Humoral and cell-mediated immunity

The immune system is made up of more or less specialized cells, which act collectively to protect the host against foreign organisms. The cells are produced in the bone marrow and subsequently move freely between the blood and sites such as the lymph nodes, spleen and liver. At the hub of the system are lymphocytes, which are responsible for the fundamental properties of specificity and memory and which are divided into subpopulations by the presence of surface markers (which have a reasonably close correspondence with function). The fundamental process of all

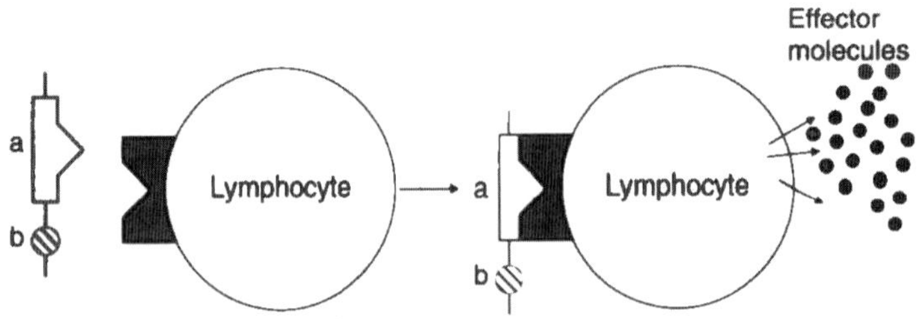

**Figure 11.1** *The essential feature of immune responses is the recognition of an epitope ('a') by a specific receptor on the surface of a lymphocyte and the consequent release of effector molecules by that lymphocyte.*

immune mechanisms is the same: lymphocytes recognize foreign material by way of specialized surface receptors. The recognition event leads to stimulation of the lymphocyte, resulting in the production of specialized effector molecules that either act directly on foreign organisms or recruit other effector cells do so (Figure 11.1).

It is traditional to consider the immune system as either humoral or cell-mediated. The central cell of the humoral arm is the B lymphocyte and the specialized effector molecules are the immunoglobulins or antibodies. T lymphocytes are the central cells of the cell-mediated arm of immunity and there is a range of effector molecules, including some that act to cause immediate damage in the area of release, those that enter the circulation and act at a distance, and those that recruit other, less specific cells (such as polymorphs and macrophages) to the site of action.

## Antibody-mediated immunity

Antibodies form a group of specialized proteins that have a shared basic structure of two pairs of polypeptide chains held together by interchain and intrachain disulphide bonds. This basic structure exists in either a monomeric form (of which there are four classes: IgG, IgA, IgD and IgE) or a pentameric form, IgM. Whatever the class, the essential feature of antibodies is the possession of a binding site capable of forming strong bonds in a highly specific way with parts (epitopes) of other molecules (antigens). In the case of infection with a large complex organism such as a malaria parasite, the host's immune system will be faced with hundreds of distinct antigenic molecules and even more potential epitopes. The first time that an individual is exposed to a particular antigen, the majority of antibody produced is IgM. In the absence of persisting antigen, the levels

of antibody decline rapidly. However, on re-exposure to the same antigen, the individual can now make a rapid secondary response in which large amounts of antibody of other classes are produced. This requires the presence not only of B cells but also of specific T cells, which are said to provide 'T-cell help' (Figure 11.2). When the B cell binds a piece of antigen by the epitope for which it has a specific receptor, it internalizes the antigen. Here, the antigenic molecule is broken down into pieces, which are re-exported to the surface of the B cell. It is these fragments (short peptides) that are recognized by specific receptors on T cells (i.e. these fragments are T-cell epitopes). Thus, it can be seen that the specificity of any T-cell clone to be able to deliver help to any given B-cell clone is determined by sequences in the same molecule that contains the B-cell epitope.

The best way to understand how cell-mediated, as opposed to humoral, immunity works is by analogy with the mechanism of T-cell help discussed above. The ability to process and export small pieces of molecules is not limited to B cells or specialist antigen-processing cells; indeed, almost all cells do it and it is probably a way of clearing intracellular debris. Cell-mediated immunity involves the recognition of such fragments (peptides) by T cells which, instead of delivering a help signal, deliver a damaging response, either the release of cytolytic substances (by cytotoxic lymphocytes or CTLs) or the release of cytokines, such as γ-interferon, which may have a local or more distant effect. Some cytokines act directly on foreign organisms, whereas others attract populations of non-specific effector cells into the area.

T-cell epitopes, whether for stimulating T-cell help to humoral immunity or when acting as the targets for cell-mediated T-cell attack, are not exported or recognized in their natural state, but rather in association with a class of specialized 'carrier' molecules, the HLA antigens. The actual determinant recognized

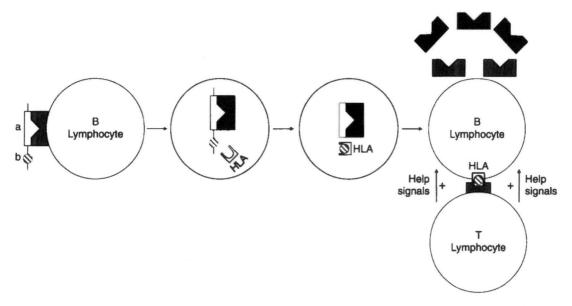

**Figure 11.2** *T-cell help to B cells. The antigenic molecule is recognized by a B cell through epitope 'a' and internalized. The molecule is broken down and epitope 'b' returned to the B-cell surface in specific conjunction with a human leucocyte antigen (HLA) molecule, the combination of which is recognized by a receptor on the surface of a T lymphocyte, stimulating it to deliver help signals for the B cell to produce antibody to epitope 'a'.*

by T-cell receptors is not the small piece of foreign material (peptide) alone, but the three-dimensional combination of HLA plus peptide. There are six important HLA genes and each one is present in the human population in numerous polymorphic forms. The particular combination of HLA molecules possessed by an individual has important effects in determining whether that individual can respond to a given antigen, and this is particularly important when only a limited set of antigens is presented, as will be the case with a malaria vaccine (see below) (Hill *et al.*, 1991).

## MECHANISMS OF ANTIMALARIAL IMMUNITY

Malarial parasites are complex organisms comprising thousands of different molecules, which in turn can be broken down into tens of thousands of epitopes capable of recognition by the immune system (Good and Doolan, 1999). Which of the many possible mechanisms in the repertoire of the immune system occur in response to malaria infections? Which ones are protective? What are the parasite

molecules responsible for inducing these responses and, therefore, which could be used to artificially induce protective responses? For many years, immunologists concentrated on the first two of these questions, using either animal models of malaria or observations in endemic areas. With the advent of *in vitro* culture of *P. falciparum* in 1976 (Trager and Jensen, 1997), it became possible to examine some of the mechanisms in more detail, but the biggest expansion in our knowledge has come with the explosion in biotechnology, particularly the production of monoclonal antibodies and gene cloning. Since the first malaria gene was cloned, there has been an ever-increasing number of genes characterized. This is a fast-moving field and any listing is bound to be outdated quickly; the best source of up-to-date information is the internet, where a search of 'malaria antigens' will identify several dedicated sites. Currently, an international effort to sequence the entire *P. falciparum* genome is well advanced and this will reveal thousands more genes, many of them potential targets of protective immune responses.

The identification of potential targets of immunity is closely linked to efforts to develop malaria vaccines, and in the sections below information from vaccine studies, animal models and studies in endemic areas is synthesized to provide a general overview of potential mechanisms and targets for protective immunity (Bull *et al.*, 1998).

## Pre-erythrocytic immunity

Following the bite of the female mosquito, sporozoites circulate in the bloodstream for a very brief period, some reaching the liver and entering hepatocytes, others being filtered out by a variety of nonspecific mechanisms. At this stage, the parasite would be susceptible to an antibody-mediated attack directed to components on the surface of the sporozoite. Such antibody could potentially exert its protective effect by any of a variety of mechanisms, including opsonization, complement-mediated lysis or neutralization (i.e. blocking the invasion of hepatocytes and thus aborting the infection). Once invasion of hepatocytes has taken place, the situation is different; now it would be difficult to envisage a role for antibody. On the other hand, hepatocytes have HLA molecules and could therefore present processed antigens derived from the parasite at their surface, leading to recognition and killing by either direct lysis or the range of soluble mediators discussed above.

There is no doubt that pre-erythrocytic immunity can be induced. Experimental immunization with live, irradiated sporozoites produces immunity to subsequent sporozoite challenge in a whole range of hosts, including mice, monkeys and humans (but such immunization gives no protection against infection initiated by blood stages, confirming the stage specificity of immunity). Initial interest focused on the possible roles of antibodies, particularly those directed at the major sporozoite surface protein (the circumsporozoite protein, CSP). The central part of the CSP comprises the same sequence of amino acids (NANP) repeated about 40 times and this seems to be an immunodominant epitope. Antibodies to this epitope protect animals against sporozoite challenge and block the invasion of hepatocytes in *in vitro* models. However, there is no convincing evidence that anti-sporozoite antibodies play an important role in naturally acquired immunity, and early vaccine studies in humans were disappointing. This does not preclude the possibility of engineering the response to be more effective, and more encouraging recent vaccine results are discussed below.

The problems encountered in the early development of sporozoite vaccines forced a re-appraisal of the potential mechanisms of pre-erythrocytic immunity. It is now clear that cell-mediated responses by T-cells recognizing processed antigens on the hepatocyte surface play the dominant role in most situations where immunity is induced by vaccination with sporozoites or sporozoite products. A number of mechanisms and cellular subsets may be involved, including direct cellular cytotoxicity and indirect effects of cytokine mediators. The role of γ-interfeon in inducing killing by local nitric oxide release seems to be particularly important. Several parasite molecules have been used to induce such protective responses, including two molecules from the sporozoite surface (CSP 1 and CSP 2, also known as thrombospondin-related adhesive protein, TRAP) as well as several liver-stage-specific antigens. As with humoral immunity to sporozoites, there is as yet little direct evidence that cell-mediated responses to the infected hepatocyte play a major role in naturally aquired immunity.

## Immunity to erythrocytic stages

At first glance, it looks as though the malaria parasite ought to be well protected once it leaves the liver and enters the erythrocytic cycle, because it spends most of its time inside the host erythrocyte. Only at schizont rupture is the parasite directly exposed to the host immune system, when, for a few seconds, daughter merozoites have to attach to and enter new red cells. Much attention has therefore been given to the merozoite as a potential target of host immune responses. Antibody-mediated protective responses directed against the surface of the merozoite could act either by blocking key steps in the invasion process or by rendering the merozoite susceptible to secondary effects such as phagocytosis or complement-mediated damage. Alternatively, an antibody-mediated response could be directed at non-surface molecules released transiently as part of the invasion process. In fact, there is experimental evidence for all these possibilities and, as with the sporozoite, the difficulty is in determining which, if any, are important. Two components of the merozoite surface coat seem to be particularly important. Vaccination with various parts of both merozoite surface protein 1 (MSP-1) and MSP-2 leads to protection in a number of animal models of malaria (Miller *et al.*, 1998). Interestingly, both proteins exist in two major allelic forms, though with many minor variations in sequence within these forms, and this could clearly fit with the idea that immunity is directed to a limited number of major strains. Although evidence is still limited, several field studies have suggested that antibody responses to parts of these molecules may play a role in protecting against clinical disease. Several parasite proteins produced in internal organelles of the merozoite, and playing a role in red cell invasion, are capable of inducing protective immune responses and are being considered for inclusion in potential vaccines.

Once inside the host red cell, the parasite appears well positioned to avoid host responses, but there are several potential chinks in its defences. Unlike other intracellular sites, there is not really the potential for direct T-cell-mediated responses to determinants presented at the host cell surface, as the erythrocyte has only low numbers of residual HLA molecules and no mechanism of producing, assembling or transporting new ones. However, the intracellular parasite might clearly be susceptible to soluble products of immune cells. In this case, some means of ensuring that parasites were exposed to high concentrations of the cytokines would be needed. A plausible scenario would be that initial parasite clearance by phagocytic cells in fixed parts of the reticuloendothelial system leads to the recruitment of antigen-specific lymphocytes and the production of cytokines. Parasites would then be damaged whenever they passed through this 'cytokine factory'. Such a scenario fits well with the known importance of the spleen in malarial immunity and the massive trafficking of immune cells to the spleen that is seen in experimental models.

Finally, the intracellular parasite is not nearly as unobtrusive as appears at first glance. As the parasite matures, it induces a series of morphological, functional and antigenic changes in the host red cell membrane. Some changes are a result of alteration of host constituents, perhaps by partial disruption of integral membrane proteins, but others result from the parasite inserting its own molecules into the host cell membrane. These 'neoantigens' are potentially important targets for immunity as they advertize the presence of a foreign organism within the cell. They also mediate the cytoadherence of infected cells to receptors on vascular endothelium, a function thought to be vital in the pathogenesis of malaria (see Chapter 10).

Recently, the molecular basis of these changes has begun to become clearer. A major parasite product expressed on the red cell surface is termed parasite erythrocyte membrane protein 1 (PfEMP-1) (Newbold *et al.*, 1997). This is coded for by a highly polymorphic family of genes (*Var* genes), of which each parasite genome contains around 50 different versions scattered amongst all of the 14 chromosomes. The parasite is capable of sequentially expressing different versions of this gene, a phenomenon known as antigenic variation. The host makes an antibody response to PfEMP-1, and field studies have shown that possession of antibodies to a particular version of PfEMP-1 protects against subsequent disease caused by parasites expressing that antigenic profile. Recently, the picture has become even more complicated by the discovery of a second family of antigenically variant parasite molecules, the Rifins, expressed at the infected red cell surface (Kyes *et al.*, 1999). At first glance, the enormous potential variation in molecules expressed at the surface of the infected red cell would seem to argue against any use in a vaccine. However, at the moment, not enough is known about possible conserved sequences within these highly variable molecules to preclude this possibility.

## Immunity to sexual stages

Host immune products ingested by the mosquitoes when taking a blood meal could potentially act on the parasite stages in the mosquito to interfere with transmission (Kaslow, 1997). Antibodies to the surface of gametocytes are found in humans naturally exposed to malaria, raising the question of whether anti-gametocyte immunity has a role in controlling transmission in endemic areas. In the case of *P. vivax*, the epidemiological picture in some areas is consistent with such a hypothesis; in the case of *P. falciparum*, there is not enough information to be sure, although it may be less likely as anti-gametocyte responses are a more prominent feature of non-immune individuals than of individuals living under constant transmission. There has been considerable interest in the possibility of using such responses in a vaccine against sexual stages. The feasibility of this approach has been shown by the experimental blocking of transmission by monoclonal antibodies against surface antigens of gametocytes, zygotes and ookinetes when fed to mosquitoes. This would offer no immediate advantage to the immunized person, and is sometimes referred to as an 'altruistic' vaccine. The uses of such a vaccine would depend on the level of transmission, but, in general, it is envisaged that they would be one part of a combined control strategy, for instance in limiting the transmission of parasites that escape immunity in individuals vaccinated against other stages.

## Parasite diversity

One way in which the molecular characterization of malaria parasites has thrown light on malarial immunity is the revelation of just how much diversity there is within a single species. The majority of malaria antigens examined show considerable polymorphism, ranging from single amino acid changes to very extensive deletions and recombinations. Of course, not all diversity is related to immune evasion, but much of it may be, especially in the light of evidence discussed earlier from experimental infections and the epidemiological picture, which suggest the importance of strain-specific responses. At the simplest level, a high level of polymorphism in critical epitopes may allow the parasite population to outflank the human immune response; thus, a single amino acid change in a T-cell epitope of the CSP may result in a given host being unable to mount a T-cell response, despite already having made good responses to very similar parasites. Other, more subtle, mechanisms may be important. Many malarial antigens have immunodominant sections made up of short motifs repeated several times. These often show subtle changes of length and sequence and there are considerable similarities between the repeats of different molecules. It has been suggested that such strongly immunogenic regions may act as decoy or smokescreen antigens and that small changes in otherwise similar sequences prevent the maturation of antibody responses to critical epitopes. A further evasion mechanism of great biological interest is clonal antigenic variation, whereby a single parasite has within its genome the capacity to express different versions of a particular antigen sequentially. As discussed above, this is the case for at least two families of malaria antigens expressed at the red cell membrane and presumably offers a way for the parasite to keep one step ahead of the host immune system. The importance of this high degree of diversity is two-fold: it makes it even more difficult to study naturally developing immunity and it presents potentially major problems for vaccine development.

## PROSPECTS FOR VACCINATION AGAINST MALARIA (see also CHAPTER 13)

The facts that humans do naturally develop effective immunity to malaria and that this can be induced in various animal models by a whole range of approaches to immunization support the idea that it is technically possible to develop a malaria vaccine. However, the problems are enormous and no vaccine of comparable complexity has been developed for use in humans. One of the issues that has to be dealt with is: what kind of vaccine is needed and for what purposes? Experimental and currently emerging vaccine trial data suggest that it may be feasible to block infection in the short term by vaccines directed against the pre-erythrocytic stages of the parasite. Such a vaccine would be ideal for short-term visitors to endemic areas. However, it seems unlikely that sterilizing immunity could be achieved in the long term in the face of continuing, repeated exposure. This is the situation faced by hundreds of millions of children in Africa. Here, the ideal is a vaccine that would prevent serious morbidity and mortality. Given the stage specificity of antimalarial immune responses, such a vaccine would have to be primarily directed at blood-stage parasites. Such vaccines are unlikely to be completely effective, but continuing low-level infection may not be a problem; indeed, it may be a good thing in providing continuing boosts to the immune response. Whatever the aims of vaccination, there is no obvious way in which biological material derived directly from parasites could be used, and realistic approaches to vaccine development had to await the advent of DNA technology. Initial approaches were based on the idea of identifying very specific subunits of the parasite, in the earliest case the repeating NANP motif, which appears to be the target of protective antibodies directed against the sporozoite surface. Early trials were disappointing, with only a few individuals showing any evidence of protection. More recently, studies have been carried out in volunteers using essentially the same part of the CSP molecule fused to part of the hepatitis B surface antigen (to provide better T-cell help) and newly developed powerful adjuvants. Vaccination induced good humoral and cell-mediated responses and led to protection in six of seven subjects immunized. Unfortunately, the protective effect was short-lived and attempts are currently being made to overcome this (Stoute *et al.*, 1997).

Given the complexity of the parasite and the diversity of host immune responses, most researchers now feel that the ideal vaccine will need to include a range of antigens, rather than single subunits. These could come from a single stage, or could include antigens from several stages in the life cycle. Several different approaches have already been taken along these lines. One vaccine, based on a synthetic fusion peptide representing four different antigens, produced encouraging results when used in South America and in a first trial in Africa. However, subsequent trials in Africa and South-east Asia have shown little or no protection (Alonso *et al.*, 1994; D'Alessandro *et al.*, 1995). Multi-epitope approaches currently under development include vaccines incorporating several different liver-stage antigens aimed at inducing cell-mediated responses and several different vaccines incorporating multiple T-cell and B-cell epitopes from liver, blood and sexual stages.

In addition to a proliferation of potential antigen combinations, there is also an increasing range of alternative modes of delivery. As well as simple synthetic peptides or fusion proteins, these include inserting the genes for vaccine antigens into modified bacteria or viruses such as vaccinia. Recently, the prospect of direct vaccination with DNA, rather than with protein products of DNA, has become a reality in a number of diseases, including malaria. Thus, at the time of writing, there are a whole range of alternative prototype vaccines at different stages of development and many can be expected to come to trial over the next few years. This in itself is a problem, as such trials are expensive and choosing which of many possible combinations to concentrate resources on is a major difficulty. Given the great technical difficulties involved in engineering a safe, effective, long-lasting immune response that can cope with the parasite's capacity for immune evasion, it may seem churlish to say that the development of a vaccine that works is only the first of many problems to overcome. Cost is an obvious problem: pneumococcal disease probably kills as many children as malaria and there is already a very effective vacccine that is currently precluded from use in Africa due to its expense. Large-scale international philanthropy may offer some hope here, but the logistics of delivery through failing health systems to the poorest populations in the world also present major problems and many children still die of diseases for which cheap vaccines exist. Despite these problems, there seems no doubt that an effective vaccine is the best hope of fundamentally changing the malaria situation in many parts of the world and, indeed, its development may turn out to be an essential spur to solve these problems for other vaccines.

## IMMUNOPATHOLOGY

As we have seen, infection with malaria induces a broad spectrum of immune responses. Only a small part of the total response is likely to be protective, and it might be expected that malaria would be associated with a wide range of immunopathology. Classical immunopathological reactions such as allergic responses or immune complex disease are rare. More important are effects on the regulation of the immune system. In malaria epidemic areas, normal individuals are 'hypergammaglobulinaemic'. Although the inhabitants of endemic areas are subjected to many infectious challenges, it does seem that hypergammaglobulinaemia is due predominantly to malaria, for when malaria is controlled levels fall remarkably. Part of the polyclonal antibody response includes the production of a wide range of autoantibodies (Daniel-Ribeiro *et al.*, 1991). These are found commonly following an acute attack of malaria and are also common in the population at large in an endemic area. The finding of autoantibodies does not have the significance that it would have in a non-endemic area; indeed, autoimmune diseases are generally rare in malaria-endemic areas. This appears to be an environmental effect, as the low prevalence is not maintained on migration away from endemic areas. There is intriguing evidence from experimental models that malaria may actually suppress the expression of autoimmune disease (Greenwood *et al.*, 1970).

## Immunopathology of acute malaria

It has often been suggested that immune responses play a role in the pathogenesis of disease. Circulating immune complexes (i.e. antigens, in this case from the parasite, bound tightly to antibody) are detectable in the majority of patients, levels rising over the 2 weeks following presentation (Adam et al., 1981). It has been reported that levels are higher in patients with cerebral malaria, but the significance of this is not clear. Immune complex deposition in the kidneys is probably common, but in P. falciparum it leads only to a subclinical glomerulonephritis, renal failure in acute malaria being predominantly a tubular, rather than a glomerular, problem. Immune complex renal disease is important in P. malariae infections (see below). Immune complexes may consume complement, and hypocomplementaemia is common during acute attacks of malaria, particularly low levels of C3 and C4 (Greenwood and Brueton, 1974). However, this is a transient depression, at least in African children, and normal levels are regained before the appearance of large amounts of immune complexes in the circulation.

Malaria induces a very marked rise in acute phase proteins, for example levels of C reactive protein and α-I-acid glycoprotein are well above those found in serious bacterial infections. The most compelling evidence for a role of immune mechanisms in pathogenesis is the relationship between the levels of various cytokines, particularly interleukin-1 (IL-1), IL-6 and tumour necrosis factor (TNFα), and the severity of disease. Thus, for example, there is a gradient in levels of TNFα, rising from non-severe disease through cerebral malaria, with the highest levels being found in the group who die (see Chapter 10).

Malaria is often said to be immunosuppressive and there is much experimental evidence for a whole range of mechanisms in animal models. When malaria is controlled, mortality from other causes usually falls too, suggesting that immunosuppression may be important in humans. However, there is surprisingly little direct evidence for an important clinical effect. Responses to some, but by no means all, vaccines are reduced in children when given during infection. There are conflicting views on whether malaria predisposes to other acute infections, for instance pneumonia, or whether the illnesses observed are in fact part of the clinical spectrum of malaria itself. There is an increased susceptibility to systemic infections with non-typhoid salmonella in children with malaria, and recent evidence suggests there may be a more general association with other invasive bacterial infections (Berkley et al., 1999).

## Plasmodium malariae nephropathy

The nephrotic syndrome (a condition in which the normally efficient filtering mechanisms of the kidneys are damaged, resulting in the loss of large amounts of protein in the urine) is common in many malaria-endemic areas. That this is due to P. malariae in a proportion of cases was established by a combination of epidemiological, experimental and clinical observations (Hendrickse et al., 1972). The syndrome is associated with a variety of histological pictures. In West African children, the findings are sufficiently distinct to allow the description of a specific 'quartan nephropathy'; in contrast, many different histological findings are described in patients in East Africa. It is an immune complex nephropathy, with deposits of both IgG and IgM in the basement membrane. In 50 per cent of cases, there is also complement deposition. When antibody is eluted from affected tissues, it has specificity for P. malariae antigens. The pathogenesis probably requires long-term infection. In a few reported cases where treatment was given as soon as the clinical features of nephropathy were noted, a complete cure was obtained. However, the general experience in African children is that, once established, the syndrome carries a very high mortality (around 80 per cent in 2 years) and progress is not modified by either antimalarial treatment or immunosuppressive drugs. It is striking that, although much more common, P. falciparum does not seem to give rise to this syndrome, despite commonly causing an asymptomatic glomerulonephritis.

## Anaemia

Some degree of anaemia is the rule in malarial infections and it is commonly of greater degree than can be accounted for by destruction of infected red cells. Several mechanisms may operate: during an acute attack of malaria, there is usually evidence of increased red cell destruction; at the other extreme, a proportion of patients show reduced red cell production, with a markedly dyserythropoietic bone marrow picture (Pasvoll and Weatherall, 1980; Weatherall et al., 1983). The question as to what extent immunopathological mechanisms play a role in the genesis of malarial anaemia is contentious. Uninfected host red cells commonly have increased levels of antibody bound to their surface after a malaria infection. This could occur by a number of mechanisms, including the production of anti-red cell autoantibodies, the binding of soluble malaria antigen to red cells and subsequent recognition by antimalarial antibodies or the binding of immune complexes. Increased levels of antibody on uninfected cells could lead to their more rapid clearance in the spleen and other sites. However, attempts to correlate the degree of antibody binding and anaemia have produced conflicting results, and in some communities antibodies on the red cells seem merely to act as a marker of recent malaria infection. Finally, evidence from experimental models suggests that immune mechanisms could play a role in the abnormal erythropoiesis of malaria through the effects of cytokines such as TNF; however, this remains to be established in human infections.

## Hyperactive malarial splenomegaly

Splenic enlargement is a characteristic feature of malaria infections and in endemic areas palpable splenomegaly is the norm rather than the exception during childhood. However, it is unusual for the spleen to remain palpable into adulthood. In all malaria-endemic areas, a certain number of subjects, often young adults, are found with marked splenic enlargement. In about half the cases there is no explanation found, and these cases are truly idiopathic, but others show a constellation of features that form a single, identifiable condition originally called tropical splenomegaly syndrome (TSS) and later renamed hyperreactive malarial splenomegaly (HMS). The three cardinal features are splenic enlargement, usually to between 6 and 15 cm, elevation of serum IgM to at least two standard deviations above the mean for that population (and often very much higher), and a positive response to antimalarial therapy. This often requires several months of prophylaxis before there is a regression in spleen size. The syndrome occurs only in malaria-endemic areas and disappears following malaria control. Unlike Burkitt's lymphoma (see below), there is not a close correlation with the degree of malaria endemicity or with any particular malaria species. In parts of South-east Asia and Papua New Guinea, the condition is extremely common, with over 50 per cent of the population fulfilling the criteria, i.e. it is almost the 'normal' response to malaria in those communities (Crane et al., 1972). In West Africa, HMS has a prevalence of around 1 in 1000. Several lines of evidence suggest that there is a strong genetic element to susceptibility. The basic deficit seems to be impaired suppressor T-cell function, leading to polyclonal B-cell expansion and massive overproduction of IgM. Recently, attention has been focused on the clinical and immunological similarities between HMS and the syndrome of splenic lymphoma with villous lymphocytes (SLVL), a B-cell monoclonal lymphoproliferative disorder (Bates et al., 1997). It has been proposed that HMS may evolve into a monoclonal disorder in a multistep process similar to that proposed for Burkitt's lymphoma (see below).

## Burkitt's lymphoma

Burkitt's lymphoma is the commonest childhood malignancy in Africa. It has a peak prevalence in 4–9 year-old children and presents as a rapidly growing tumour, usually in the jaw or abdomen. Although sporadic cases of lymphoma with the same features occur worldwide, it only reaches high prevalences (endemic Burkitt's lymphoma) in areas of high P. falciparum transmission. The evidence that this is due to an interaction between the Epstein–Barr virus (EBV, a herpes virus first discovered in Burkitt's tumour tissue) and malaria is very strong. The basic event appears to be a translocation of an oncogene from its normal position on chromosome 8 to one of several other positions in the genome. In Burkitt's lymphomas, the new position is always in the regions that regulate the expression of immunoglobin genes and it is assumed that this interferes with normal control over the oncogene, and the cell in which the event occurs (a B cell) goes on to divide in an uncontrolled way. The exact role of malaria is contentious, but it is clear that during malaria attacks normal immune surveillance of EBV-infected B cells is reduced, and it may be that the ensuing proliferation increases the chance of the required translocation taking place (Whittle et al., 1990).

## REFERENCES

Adam C, Geniteau M, Gougerot-Pocidalo M, et al. Cryoglobulins, circulating immune complexes, and complement activation in cerebral malaria. Infect Immun 1981; **31**: 530–5.

Alonso PL, Smith T, Schellenberg JR, *et al*. Randomised trial of efficacy of SPf66 vaccine against *Plasmodium falciparum* malaria in children in southern Tanzania. *Lancet* 1994; **344**: 1175–81.

Anders RF. Multiple cross-reactivities amongst antigens of *Plasmodium falciparum* impair the development of protective immunity against malaria. *Parasite Immunol* 1986; **8**: 529–39.

Baird JK. Age-dependent characteristics of protection v. susceptibility to *Plasmodium falciparum*. *Ann Trop Med Parasitol* 1998; **92**: 367–90.

Bates I, Bedu-Addo G, Rutherford TR, Bevan DH. Circulating villous lymphocytes – a link between hyperreactive malarial splenomegaly and splenic lymphoma. *Trans R Soc Trop Med Hyg* 1997; **91**: 171–4.

Bayoumi RA. The sickle-cell trait modifies the intensity and specificity of the immune response against *P. falciparum* malaria and leads to acquired protective immunity. *Med Hypoth* 1987; **22**: 287–98.

Berkley J, Mwarumba S, Bramham K, Lowe B, Marsh K. Bacteraemia complicating severe malaria in children. *Trans R Soc Trop Med Hyg* 1999; **93**: 283–6.

Bull PC, Lowe BS, Kortok M, Molyneux CS, Newbold CI, Marsh K. Parasite antigens on the infected red cell surface are targets for naturally acquired immunity to malaria. *Nat Med* 1998; **4**: 358–60.

Crane GG, Wells JV, Hudson P. Tropical splenomegaly syndrome in New Guinea. I. Natural history. *Trans R Soc Trop Med Hyg* 1972; **66**: 724–32.

D'Alessandro U, Leach A, Drakeley CJ, *et al*. Efficacy trial of malaria vaccine SPf66 in Gambian infants. *Lancet* 1995; **346**: 462–7.

Daniel-Ribeiro C, Ben Slama L, Gentilini M. Anti-nuclear and anti-smooth muscle antibodies in Caucasians, Africans and Asians with acute malaria. *J Clin Lab Immunol* 1991; **35**: 109–12.

Fernandez-Reyes D, Craig AG, Kyes SA, *et al*. A high frequency African coding polymorphism in the N-terminal domain of ICAM-1 predisposing to cerebral malaria in Kenya. *Hum Mol Genet* 1997; **6**: 1357–60.

Flint J, Hill AV, Bowden DK, *et al*. High frequencies of alpha-thalassaemia are the result of natural selection by malaria. *Nature* 1986; **321**: 744–50.

Fried M, Nosten F, Brockman A, Brabin BJ, Duffy PE. Maternal antibodies block malaria. *Nature* 1998; **395**: 851–2.

Good MF, Doolan DL. Immune effector mechanisms in malaria. *Curr Opin Immunol* 1999; **11**: 412–9.

Greenwood BM, Brueton MJ. Complement activation in children with acute malaria. *Clin Exp Immunol* 1974; **18**: 267–72.

Greenwood BM, Herrick EM, Voller A. Suppression of autoimmune disease in NZB and (NZB × NZW) F1 hybrid mice by infection with malaria. *Nature* 1970; **226**: 266–7.

Gupta S, Snow RW, Donnelly CA, Marsh K, Newbold C. Immunity to non-cerebral severe malaria is acquired after one or two infections. *Nat Med* 1999; **5**: 340–3.

Hendrickse RG, Adeniyi A, Edington GM, Glasgow EF, White RH, Houba V. Quartan malarial nephrotic syndrome. Collaborative clinicopathological study in Nigerian children. *Lancet* 1972; **1**: 1143–9.

Hill AV, Allsopp CE, Kwiatkowski D, *et al*. Common west African HLA antigens are associated with protection from severe malaria. *Nature* 1991; **352**: 595–600.

Kaslow DC. Transmission-blocking vaccines: uses and current status of development. *Int J Parasitol* 1997; **27**: 183–9.

Knight JC, Udalova I, Hivv AL, *et al*. A polymorphism that affects OCT-1 binding to the TNF promoter region is associated with severe malaria. *Nat Genet* 1999; **22**: 145–50.

Kyes SA, Rowe JA, Kriek N, Newbold CI. Rifins: a second family of clonally variant proteins expressed on the surface of red cells infected with *Plasmodium falciparum*. *Proc Nat Acad Sci USA* 1999; **96**: 9333–8.

Miller LH, Good MF, Kaslow DC. Vaccines against the blood stages of falciparum malaria. *Adv Exp Med Biol* 1998; **452**: 193–205.

Newbold CI, Craig AG, Kyes S, *et al*. PfEMP-1, polymorphism and pathogenesis. *Ann Trop Med Parasitol* 1997; **91**: 551–7.

Pasvol G, Weatherall DJ. The red cell and the malarial parasite. *Br J Haematol* 1980; **46**: 165–70.

Ruwende C, Khoo SC, Snow RW, *et al*. Natural selection of hemi- and heterozygotes for G6PD deficiency in Africa by resistance to severe malaria. *Nature* 1995; **376**: 246–9.

Stoute JA, Slaoui M, Heppner DG, *et al*. A preliminary evaluation of a recombinant circumsporozoite protein vaccine against *Plasmodium falciparum* malaria. RTSS Malaria Vaccine Evaluation Group. *N Engl J Med* 1997; **336**: 86–91.

Trager W, Jensen JB. Continuous culture of *Plasmodium falciparum*: its impact on malaria research. *Int J Parasitol* 1997; **27**: 989–1006.

Weatherall DJ, Abdalla S, Pippard MJ. The anaemia of *Plasmodium falciparum* malaria. *Ciba Found Symp* 1983; **94**: 74–97.

Weatherall DJ. Common genetic disorders of the red cell and the 'malaria hypothesis'. *Ann Trop Med Parasitol* 1987; **81**: 539–48.

Whittle HC, Brown J, Marsh K, Blackman M, Jobe O, Shenton F. The effects of *Plasmodium falciparum* malaria on immune control of B lymphocytes in Gambian children. *Clin Exp Immunol* 1990; **80**: 213–18.

Williams TN, Maitland K, Bennett S, *et al*. High incidence of malaria in alpha-thalassaemic children. *Nature* 1996; **383**: 522–5.

# Treatment and prevention of malaria

DAVID A WARRELL, WILLIAM M WATKINS AND PETER A WINSTANLEY

## CHEMOTHERAPY AND CHEMOPROPHYLAXIS

Antimalarial drugs have selective actions on the different phases of the parasite life cycle. Causal prophylactic drugs prevent the establishment of the parasite in the liver and blood schizontocidal drugs attack the parasite in the red blood cell, preventing or terminating the clinical attack.

Tissue schizontocides act on pre-erythrocytic forms in the liver. Gametocytocidal drugs destroy the sexual forms of the parasite in the blood. Some of these drugs are hypnozoitocidal: they will kill the dormant hypnozoites in the liver (responsible for relapses in *Plasmodium vivax* and *P. ovale*). Sporontocidal drugs inhibit the development of oocysts on the stomach wall of the mosquito that has fed on the human gametocyte carrier so that the mosquito cannot transmit the infection. The relationship between the phases of development and the action of the drug is shown diagrammatically in Figure 12.1 and, more simply, in Figure 12.2.

People who have, by repeated exposures to infection, acquired a degree of immunity can be cured or protected much more easily by drugs than those who

have not. Evidence obtained from the treatment or prevention of the partially immune groups cannot be applied to non-immunes or to other groups whose immunity may be less.

The ideal drug for antimalarial therapy would be effective in a single dose, so as to be practicable where supervision of protracted courses is impossible, and would be active on all stages of the parasite. Resistance of the malaria parasite, especially *P. falciparum*, to existing drugs is a serious problem in many parts of the world.

## THE SOURCE AND DEVELOPMENT OF CURRENT ANTIMALARIAL DRUGS

Almost all drugs are discovered and developed by the pharmaceutical industry at high financial risk. It costs about £150 million to take a compound to the marketplace, and the risk of losing the investment completely is often high. Thus, although industrial 'research and development' teams are often motivated by scientific and medical concerns, funds are usually provided with the expectation of profit, in which respect antimalarial drugs compete poorly with most

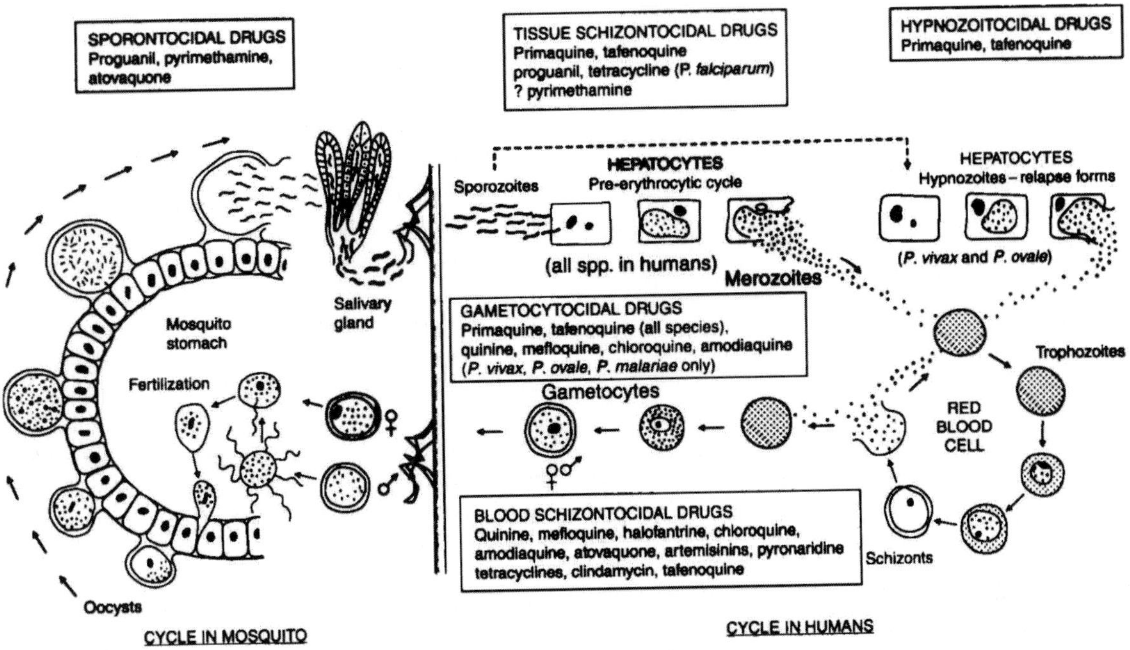

SPORONTOCIDAL DRUGS
Proguanil, pyrimethamine,
atovaquone

TISSUE SCHIZONTOCIDAL DRUGS
Primaquine, tafenoquine
proguanil, tetracycline (P. *falciparum*)
? pyrimethamine

HYPNOZOITOCIDAL DRUGS
Primaquine, tafenoquine

HEPATOCYTES
Pre-erythrocytic cycle

Sporozoites

(all spp. in humans) Merozoites

HEPATOCYTES
Hypnozoites – relapse forms

(*P. vivax* and *P. ovale*)

GAMETOCYTOCIDAL DRUGS
Primaquine, tafenoquine (all species),
quinine, mefloquine, chloroquine, amodiaquine
(*P. vivax, P. ovale, P. malariae* only)

Gametocytes

Mosquito
stomach

Salivary
gland

Fertilization

♀

♀♂ ♂

Trophozoites

RED
BLOOD
CELL

Schizonts

BLOOD SCHIZONTOCIDAL DRUGS
Quinine, mefloquine, halfantrine, chloroquine,
amodiaquine, atovaquone, artemisinins, pyronaridine
tetracyclines, clindamycin, tafenoquine

Oocysts

CYCLE IN MOSQUITO

CYCLE IN HUMANS

**Figure 12.1** *Action of antimalarial compounds at different stages of the development of the malaria parasite in* Anopheles *mosquitoes in the human host. (Redrawn after David Warhurst and David Payne.)*

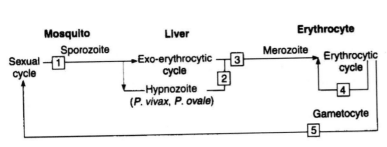

**Figure 12.2** *Stage specificity of antimalarial drugs: 1, sporontocidal (e.g. proguanil, pyrimethamine, atovaquone); 2, hypnozoitocidal (e.g. primaquine and tafenoquine); 3, tissue schizontocidal (primaquine, tafenoquine; P. falciparum only – proguanil, tetracyclines); 4, blood schizontocidal (most antimalarial drugs except primaquine); 5, gametocytocidal (e.g. primaquine, tafenoquine; P. vivax, P. ovale and P. malariae only – quinine, mefloquine, chloroquine, amodiaquine).*

other drug categories. As a result, many of our present compounds were discovered outside the pharmaceutical industry, often in academic settings. However, the development of these compounds to registration has always needed industrial skill and experience and adequate funding. Such commitment from pharmaceutical companies has usually resulted from a favourable balance between costs and the goodwill of national or international bodies. Unfortunately, the pace of antimalarial drug development has been too slow, and the drugs described in this chapter have not changed much in recent decades, even though antimalarial drug resistance is now a major threat to global health. Our need for industrial collaborations in antimalarial drug development has never been greater. It may be that awareness among the governments of the 'G8 nations' combined with a number of international initiatives will facilitate industrial involvement and lead to new drugs in coming years. However, for the present, we must continue to make the best use of the drugs we already have: it is in this area that carefully conducted research can provide new opportunities.

## USES OF ANTIMALARIAL DRUGS

Antimalarial drugs may be put to several uses, in each of which their efficacy may be determined by several factors including:

- The species of malaria parasite: for example, some species have a hypnozoite stage that is eradicated only by treatment with an 8-aminoquinoline (such as primaquine or tafenoquine).
- The parasite's sensitivity to the drug: *P. falciparum* has evolved multidrug resistance in many parts of the tropics, and some isolates of *P. vivax* have developed resistance to chloroquine.
- The host's degree of immunity to the parasite: some classes of drug are acceptable for the treatment of 'semi-immune' patients, but unacceptable for 'non-immunes'.
- Analysis of the benefits of treatment versus the risks of adverse effects: all drugs have adverse effects, and the physician must balance benefits against the possible risks.
- Drug cost: many antimalarial compounds are unaffordable by large groups of patients.
- Practicability of the treatment regimen: for both outpatient and inpatient treatment.

The main uses of antimalarial drugs are:

- Protective (prophylactic).
- Curative (therapeutic): the therapy of established infection, whether symptomatic or asymptomatic.
- Preventive of transmission: by preventing infection of mosquitoes either by effects on gametocytes in the host's blood or interruption of sporogony in the insect.

## CLINICAL PHARMACOLOGY OF THE MAIN ANTIMALARIAL DRUGS

The chemical structures of the drugs are shown in Figure 12.3 on pp. 272–3.

## Artemisinins

Artemisinin is the antimalarial principle isolated by Chinese scientists in 1972 from *Artemisia annua* (Klayman, 1985). High activity combined with low resistance makes artemisinin one of the most important drugs in antimalarial chemotherapy. Artemether, arteether and artesunate are derivatives in clinical use (Hien and White, 1993).

### MODE OF ACTION

Artemisinin is a sesquiterpene lactone, containing a labile peroxide bridge. The breakdown of this bridge generates free radicals that rapidly undergo alkylating reactions. Parasite membranes are particularly sensitive to this oxidative damage. Haemozoin catalyses the decomposition of the drug, which may explain why the malaria parasite is particularly sensitive to artemisinin and its derivative compounds; a chloroquine-resistant strain of *P. berghei* lacking haemozoin is resistant to artemisinin. Selectivity may also result from the high uptake and concentration of drug by the malaria parasite.

### PHARMACEUTICS

The poor solubility of artemisinin in both oil and water was the reason for developing derivative compounds. Dihydroartemisinin can be etherified or esterified to produce the more active compounds artemether, arteether or artesunate. Artemether, the methyl ether, is available as a solution in groundnut oil (1.0-mL ampoules containing 80 mg artemether) for intramuscular injection. Artesunate, the water-soluble and haemisuccinate ester, is administered intravenously or intramuscularly in solution as artesunic acid (60 mg per ampoule), or orally as 50 mg tablets. Artemisinin and artemether suppositories are available commercially.

### CLINICAL PHARMACOKINETICS

Extreme difficulties in analysis have hampered the pharmacokinetic study of the artemisinin compounds (White, 1985). Artemisinin and its derivatives are rapidly hydrolysed *in vivo* to dihydroartemisinin (DHA), the most potent of the artemisinins. Artemisinin and its derivatives are rapidly metabolized by the liver and have short elimination half-lives. Artemether absorption is slower, more variable and with lower biotransformation to DHA when administered by the intramuscular or intravenous routes in comparison to oral dosage.

### THERAPEUTIC USE

Artemisinins are used parenterally and by suppository for treating severe multiresistant falciparum malaria and orally for the treatment of uncomplicated multiresistant falciparum malaria (Nosten, 1994; The Artemether–quinine Meta-analysis Study Group, 2001). Because of their very rapid action, there is great interest in combining artemisinins with other antimalarial drugs (see 'Combination therapy', p. 285).

## ADVERSE EFFECTS

Artemether and arteether are neurotoxic in rats and dogs at doses higher than those used in the treatment of malaria in humans (Brewer *et al.*, 1993). However, few adverse effects have been reported in patients monitored during clinical trials of artemisinin or its derivatives. It is estimated that over 2 million malaria cases have been treated, with no reports of gross toxicity, suggesting that immediate and severe complications associated with this group of drugs are rare.

## ADVERSE DRUG INTERACTIONS

Artemisinin with mefloquine potentiates antimalarial activity. Artemisinin antagonizes the action of pyrimethamine–sulfadoxine (PSD) in the mouse model. This effect has not been explained and it is unknown whether significant antagonism occurs in the clinical use of artemisinin–PSD in humans.

# Atovaquone

## MODE OF ACTION

Atovaquone is structurally similar to ubiquinone (coenzyme Q), an electron carrier molecule in the mitochondria. It is thought to inhibit mitochondrial respiration by binding irreversibly to an 11 500-Da protein in the cytochrome $bc_1$ complex, causing inhibition of nucleic acid and adenosine triphosphate synthesis (Hudson, 1993). *In vitro*, atovaquone affects the maturation of trophozoites and gametocytes of *P. falciparum*. Synergistic combinations of atovaquone with proguanil and tetracycline are effective for infections with multidrug-resistant *P. falciparum* and also *P. ovale* and *P. malariae* (although it would not normally be used for infections with the latter species). In animal models, atovaquone inhibits ookinetes, oocysts and sporozoites of *P. berghei*. Resistance of *P. falciparum* to atovaquone is selected readily; whether resistance to

the combination atovaquone–proguanil will appear when this drug is widely used remains to be seen (see below).

## CLINICAL PHARMACOKINETICS

Ingested atovaquone is poorly and variably absorbed. Bioavailability is increased about four-fold by a fatty meal. The relationship between oral dose and peak drug concentration is not linear, possibly because absorption mechanisms become saturated. Selective tissue accumulation of the drug has not been found in animal models (Dollery, 1999). Plasma concentrations are several-fold higher than those in tissues and atovaquone is more than 99 per cent bound to plasma proteins. Almost all the drug is eliminated unchanged via the bile into the gut. There is enterohepatic circulation, resulting in a second 'peak' plasma concentration. Ninety-four per cent of an oral dose of atovaquone can be recovered unchanged in the faeces and less than 1 per cent from the urine (Roland *et al.*, 1994). No metabolites have been identified in humans. The elimination half-life is long (50–70 hours). Steady-state plasma concentrations are achieved in about 7 days.

## THERAPEUTIC USE

Atovaquone is used, only in combination with proguanil (as 'Malarone'), for the treatment and prophylaxis of multiresistant falciparum malaria.

## ADVERSE EFFECTS

Atovaquone is well tolerated. In acquired immune deficiency syndrome (AIDS) patients treated with atovaquone for opportunistic infections, the most common adverse effects have included:

- Rashes: maculopapular rash (in up to 40 per cent) and erythema multiforme.
- Gastrointestinal disturbances: abdominal pain, nausea, vomiting and diarrhoea.
- Fever: in up to 40 per cent.
- Central nervous system disturbances: headaches, dizziness and insomnia.

Atovaquone reduced fetal body weight in rabbits and so should not normally be given to pregnant women. It is excreted in the breast milk at concentrations around 30 per cent of those in the plasma.

*Arylaminoalcohols*

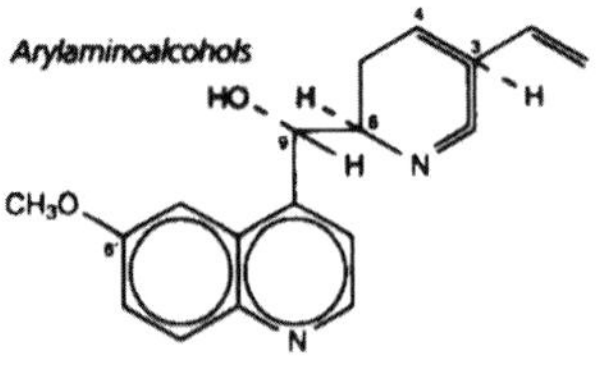

1. Quinine
(8S,9R)-6'-methoxycinchonan-9-ol

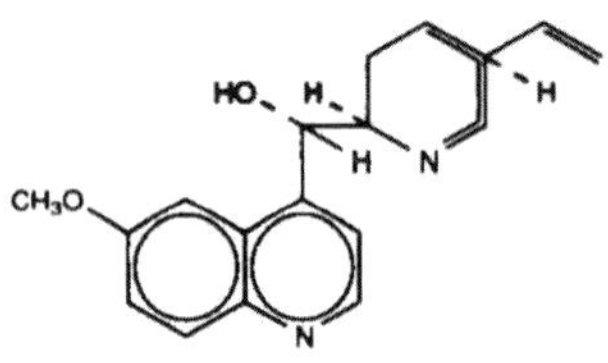

2. Quinidine
(8R,9S)-6'-methoxycinchonan-9-ol

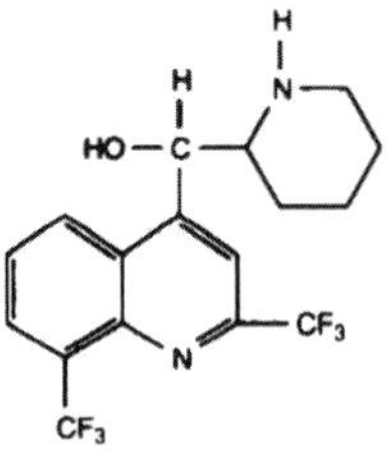

3. Mefloquine
α-(2-piperidyl)-2,8-bis(trifluoromethyl)-4-quinolinemethanol

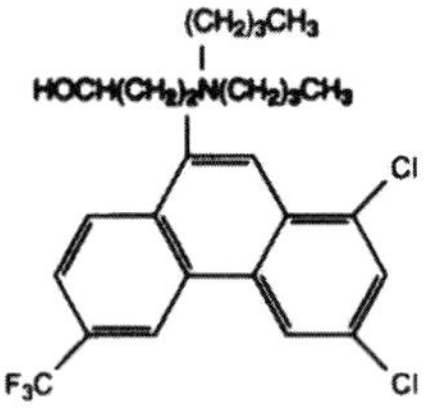

4. Halofantrine
1,3-dichloro-α-[2-(dibutylamino)-
ethyl]-6-(trifluoromethyl)-9-
phenantrenemethanol

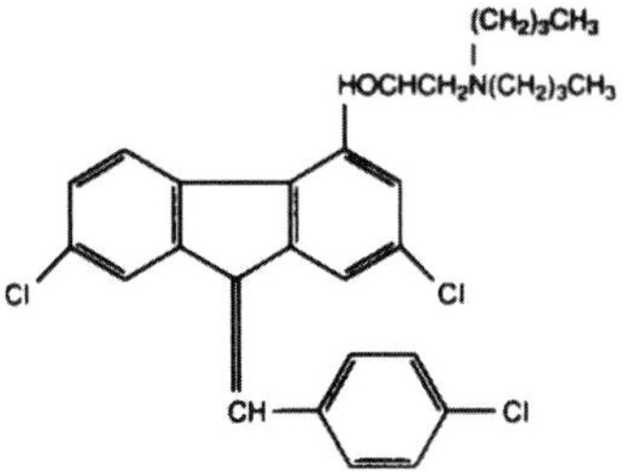

5. Lumefantrine (Benflumetol)
2-dibutylamino-1-[2,7-dichloro-9-(4-chloroen-
zylidene)-9H-fluoren-4-yl] ethanol

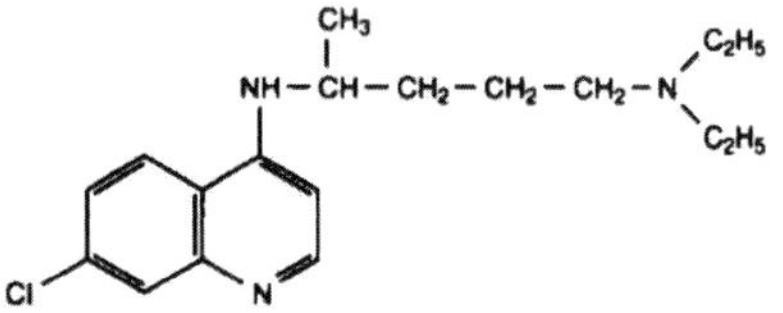

6. Chloroquine
7-chloro-4-(4'-diethyl-
amino-1'-methylbutyl-
amino)quinoline

*4-Aminoquinolines*

*Benzonaphthyridines*

*Sulphonamides*

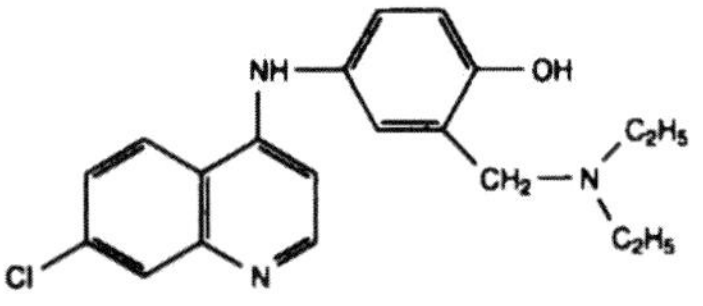

7. Amodiaquine
7-chloro-4-(3'-diethylamino-
methyl-4'-hydroxyanilino)-
quinoline

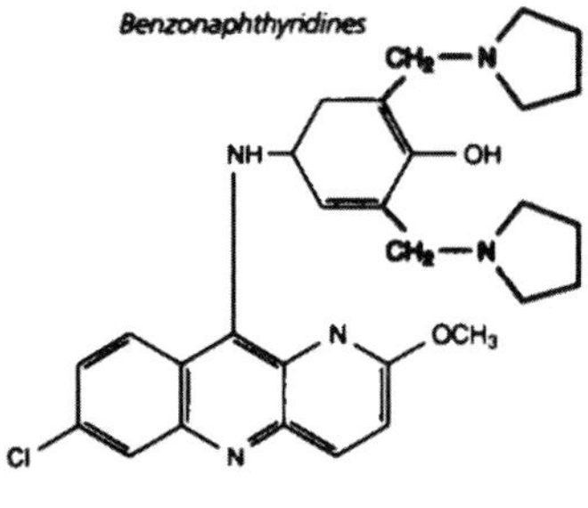

8 Pyronaridine(7351)
2-methoxy-6-chloro-9(3,5-
bis(1-pyrrolidinylmethyl)-
4-hydroxy]anilino-1-aza-
acridine

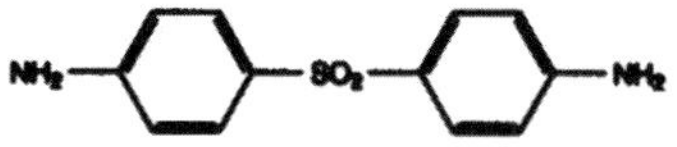

9. Dapsone
4,4'-diaminodiphenylsulfone

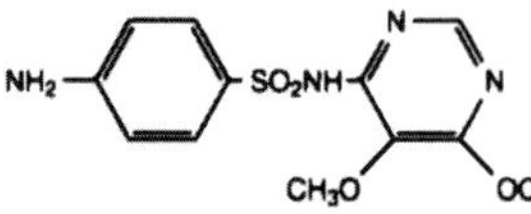

*Dihydrofolate reductase inhibitors*

*Biguanides*

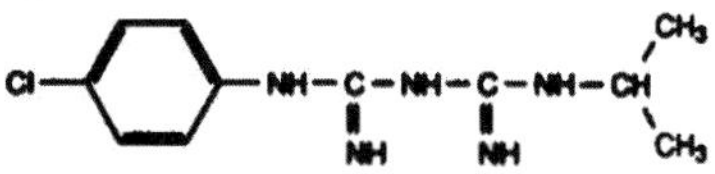

10. Sulfadoxine
N'-(5,6-dimethoxy-4-pyrimi-
dinyl)-sulfanilamide

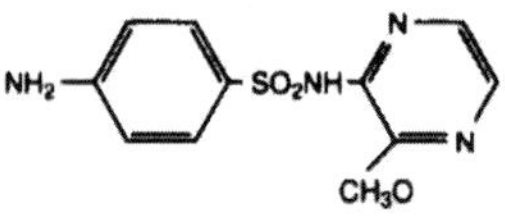

11. Sulfalene
N'-(3-methoxy-2-pyrazinyl)-
sulfanilamide

12. Proguanil
N'(p-chlorophenyl)-N$^\beta$-iso-
propyldiguanide

*8-Aminoquinolines*

*Diaminopyrimidines*

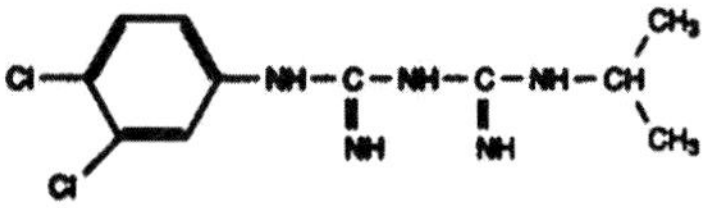

13. Chlorproguanil
N$^1$-(3,4-dichlorophenyl)-N$^\beta$-iso-
propyldiguanide

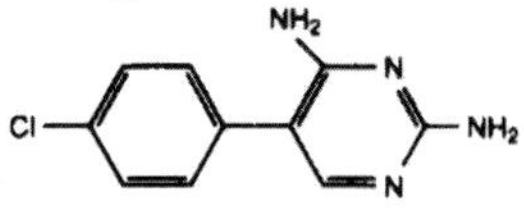

14. Pyrimethamine
2,4-diamino-5-p-chlorophenyl-6-
ethylpyrimidine

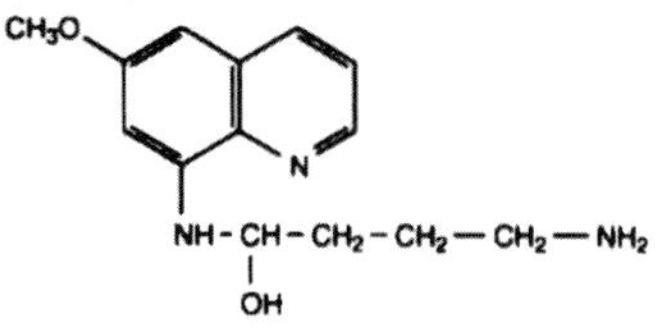

15. Primaquine
6-methoxy-8-(4'-amino-1'-
methylbutylamino)quinoline

**Figure 12.3** *Structures, chemical formulae and chemical names of principal antimalarial drugs.*

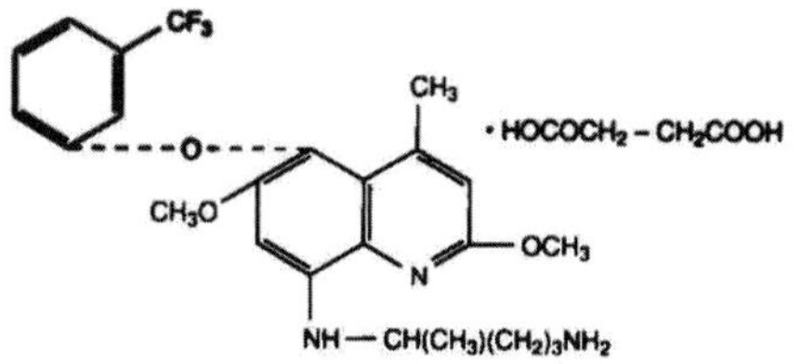

**16. Tafenoquine (WR 238,605)**
2,6-dimethoxy-4-methyl-5-
(3-trifluoromethyl)-phenoxy-8-
(4-amino-1-methylbutyl-
amino)quinoline

*Antibiotics*

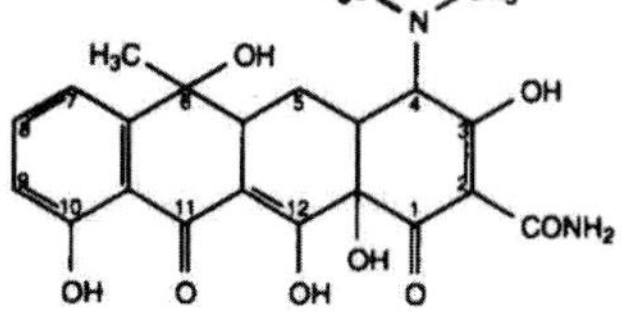

**17. Tetracycline**
4-dimethylamino-1,4,4a,5,5a,6,
11,12a-octahydro-3,6,10,12,12a-
pentahydroxy-6-methyl-1,11-di-
oxo-2-naphthacenecarboxamide

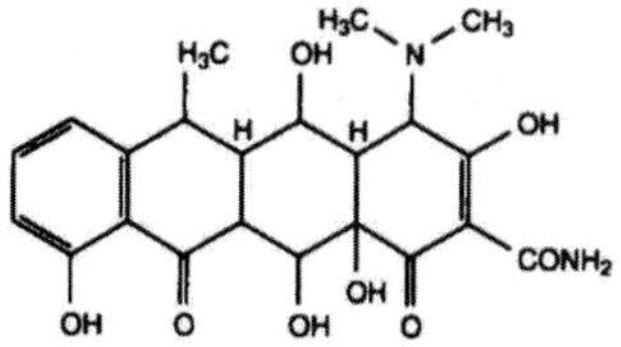

**18. Doxycycline**
4-dimethylamino-1,4,4a,5,5a,6,
11,12a-octahydro-3,5,10,12,12a-
pentahydroxy-6-methyl-1,11-di-
oxo-2-naphthecenecarboxamide

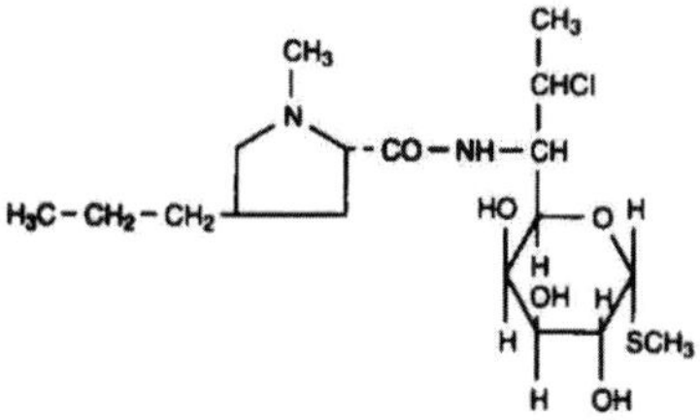

**19. Clindamycin**
methyl 7-chloro-6,7,8-tri-dioxy-6-
*trans*-(1-methyl-4-prophyl-L-2-
pyrrolidine-carboxamido)-1-
thio-L-*threo*-α-D-*galacto*-octo-
pyranoside or: 7-(5)-chloro-7-
desoxylinco-mycin)

*Sesquiterpene lactones*

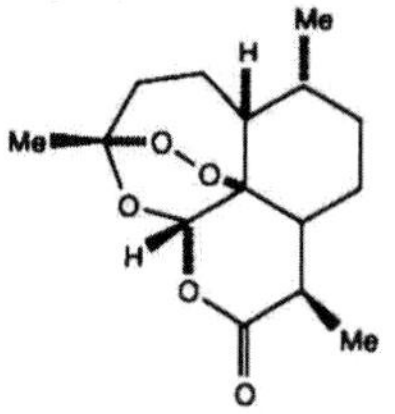

**20. Artemisinin**
(3R,5aS,6R,8aS,9R,12S,12aR)
octahydro-3,6,9-trimethyl-3,
12-epoxy-12H-pyrano[4,3-j]-
1,2-benzodioxepin-10(3H)-one

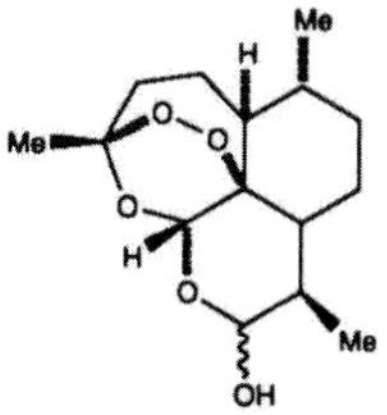

**21. Dihydroartemisinin**
3α, 12α-epoxy-3,4,5,5aα,6,7,8,
8aα,9,10,12β,12α-dodecahydro-
10β-hydroxy-3β,6α,9β-
trimethylpyrano[4,3-j][1,2]
benzodioxepin

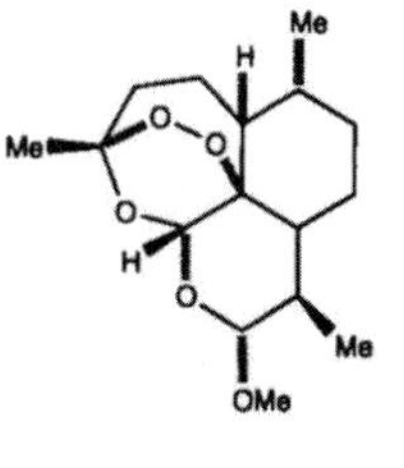

**22. 10β artemether (crystalline)**
3α,12α-epoxy-3,4,5,5aα,6,7,8,
8aα,9,10,12β,12α-dodecahydro-
10β-methoxy-3β,6α,9β-
trimethylpyrano[4,3-j][1,2]
benzodioxepin

10α artemether is an oil

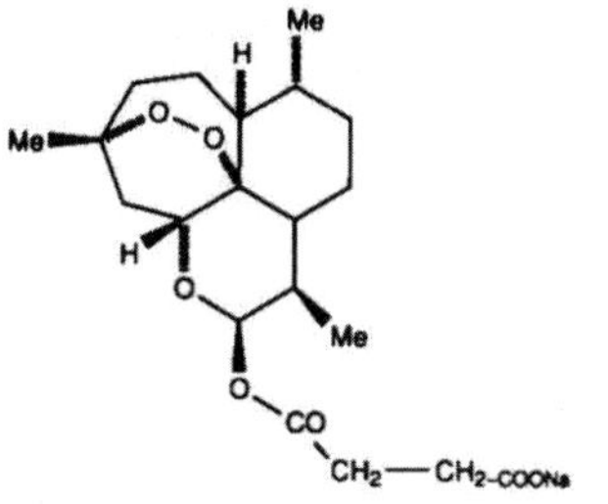

**23. Sodium artesunate**
3α,12α-epoxy-3,4,5,5aα,6,7,8,
8aα,9,10,12β,12α-dodecahydro-
3β,6α,9β-trimethylpyrano[4,3-j]
[1,2]benzodioxepin-10α-yl
sodium butanedioate

*Naphthoquinones*

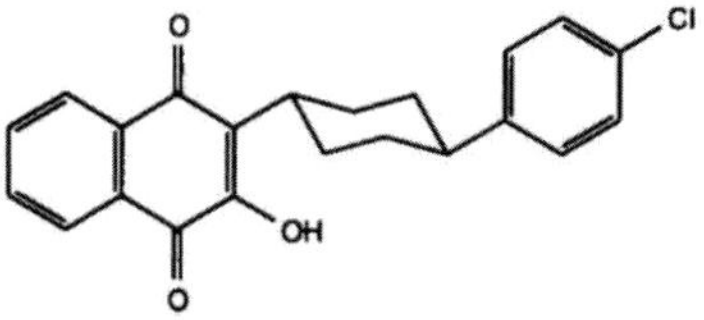

**24. Atovaquone (BW 566 C80)**
2-[*trans*-4-(4-chlorophenyl)
cyclohexyl]-3-hydroxy-1,
4 naphthoquinone

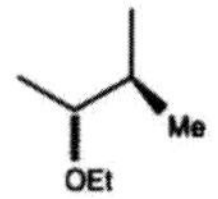

Arteether, as prepared by the
method recommended by
Brossi *et al.*, is composed of the
crystalline beta isomer only

3α,12α-epoxy-3,4,5,5aα,6,7,8,
8aα,9,10,12β,12α-dodecahydro-
10β-ethoxy-3β,6α,9β-
trimethylpyrano[4,3-j][1,2]
benzodioxepin

**Figure 12.3** (*Continued*)

## ADVERSE DRUG INTERACTIONS

Steady-state plasma atovaquone concentration is approximately halved and its half-life reduced if co-administered with rifampicin, whereas rifampicin concentrations may rise. Atovaquone causes a significant rise in steady-state concentrations of zidovudine and reduces didanosine (ddI) clearance.

## Benflumetol (lumefantrine)

### MODE OF ACTION

Benflumetol (lumefantrine) has structural similarities with quinine, mefloquine and especially halofantrine (Figure 12.3). Its mode of action is unknown, but it is thought to accumulate in the food vacuoles of parasites and bind to haemin, forming toxic complexes.

### CLINICAL PHARMACOKINETICS

When fasted, healthy, normal volunteers were given benflumetol–artemether by mouth, there was an initial lag time of 2 hours, followed by peak plasma concentrations about 8 hours after dosing. Benflumetol is eliminated slowly, with an apparent terminal half-life of 1–3 days in healthy volunteers and of 4–6 days in patients.

### THERAPEUTIC USE

Benflumetol is used only in combination with artemether (as Riamet or Co-artemether) for the treatment of uncomplicated multiresistant falciparum malaria (Hatz et al., 1998).

### ADVERSE EFFECTS

In combination with artemether, benflumetol appears to be well tolerated, but experience is limited. Unlike halofantrine, benflumetol does not cause prolongation of the electrocardiogram (ECG) QT interval.

## Chloroquine and amodiaquine

Despite the extensive spread of chloroquine-resistant strains of P. falciparum and the emergence of chloroquine-resistant P. vivax in New Guinea, chloroquine, which was first synthesized in 1934, is still by far the most widely used antimalarial drug worldwide. Chloroquine remains effective for P. vivax, P. ovale and P. malariae infections worldwide and for falciparum malaria in restricted areas such as Central America northwest of the Panama Canal, Haiti and the Dominican Republic (Hispaniola) and parts of the Middle East. Against sensitive strains, it is a rapidly effective blood schizonticide and is gametocytocidal against P. vivax, P. malariae and P. ovale.

### MODE OF ACTION

Chloroquine acts only against those stages of the malaria life cycle which actively digest haemoglobin within the erythrocyte (Peters, 1970). Ultrastructural studies suggest that the parasite's food vacuole is the target of chloroquine's activity. There is some evidence that chloroquine interferes with the parasite's mechanisms for detoxifying ferriprotoporphyrin IX and superoxide anions resulting from its digestion of haemoglobin so that the parasite is killed by accumulation of these toxic products (Rosenthal, 2001).

### Clinical pharmacokinetics

In healthy adults and patients with uncomplicated malaria, ingested chloroquine is rapidly absorbed. Peak plasma concentrations of around 250 μg/L are reached within 2 hours (White, 1985). Acute bioavailability is 70–75 per cent. After intramuscular or subcutaneous injection, absorption is very rapid, such that dangerously high peak plasma concentrations (500–3500 μg/L) may be reached within 5–20 minutes after a dose of 5 mg base/kg. Cases of children dying soon after intramuscular injection of chloroquine are probably explained by its rapid absorption and the resulting hypotension. This can be prevented by giving small, more frequent injections (for example, 3.5 mg base/kg 6-hourly or 2.5 mg base/kg 4-hourly) (White et al., 1988). In healthy volunteers, chloroquine is absorbed as rapidly from rectal suppositories as when ingested. Chloroquine is extensively bound to tissues, especially liver, connective tissue and pigmented tissues such as skin and retina. This explains its apparent enormous total volume of distribution. Chloroquine is concentrated in erythrocytes, granulocytes and platelets and 55 per cent is protein bound in plasma. Cerebrospinal fluid concentrations are very low (2.7 per cent of the whole blood concentration). About half of the absorbed chloroquine is cleared unchanged by the kidney. The rest is biotransformed in the liver to desethyl-chloroquine and bisdesethyl-chloroquine.

Although clearance is reduced in renal failure, it is not necessary to reduce the dose. Therapeutic blood concentrations persist for 6–10 days after a single dose, but the terminal elimination half-time is 1–2 months (Dollery, 1999).

## THERAPEUTIC USE

Oral chloroquine is used for the treatment and prophylaxis of vivax, ovale and malariae malarias and for uncomplicated chloroquine-sensitive falciparum malaria. Severe chloroquine-sensitive falciparum malaria can be treated with parenteral chloroquine.

## ADVERSE EFFECTS

Chloroquine is generally well tolerated but, when plasma concentrations exceed 250 µg/mL, unpleasant symptoms such as dizziness, headache, diplopia, disturbed visual accommodation, dysphagia, nausea and malaise may develop. These symptoms are most likely after intravenous infusion. Systolic hypotension and ECG abnormalities may occur during the initial distribution phase. In Africans, Haitians and dark-skinned Asians, pruritus of the palms, soles and scalp is a tiresome problem. Rare toxic effects include photoallergic dermatitis, aggravation of psoriasis, skin pigmentation, leucopenia, bleaching of the hair and aplastic anaemia. Chloroquine can exacerbate epilepsy.

### Acute toxicity

Overdose (ingestion of 20 mg base/kg or more at one time) produces symptoms within 30 minutes to 6 hours. These symptoms include nausea, headache, drowsiness, blurring of vision, malaise, vomiting, speech abnormalities, jaw contractions, hypokalaemia, thrombocytopenia, increased FDPs, coma, convulsions, hypotension, respiratory paralysis and cardiac arrest. Fatal cardiac arrest may occur as soon as 1 hour after ingestion. ECG changes include sinus tachycardia, bradycardia, prolonged QT interval, ectopic beats, ventricular tachycardia and fibrillation, idioventricular rhythm, torsade de pointes and asystole. Blood concentrations of more than 7 µmol/L, and certainly of more than 25 µmol/L, were fatal before the introduction of the modern treatment of chloroquine overdose. This consists of diazepam, adrenaline and mechanical ventilation (Riou et al., 1988). Diazepam competes with chloroquine for binding at benzodiazepine receptors in the heart muscle and adrenaline counteracts the effects of chloroquine on the myocardium and vasculature.

### Chronic toxicity

Continuous weekly antimalarial prophylaxis with chloroquine (cumulative dose >100 g) and especially the higher anti-inflammatory doses used in collagen vascular diseases may cause an irreversible retinopathy and also skeletal and cardiac myopathy.

Chloroquine prophylaxis depresses the immune response to rabies and tetanus vaccine.

## AMODIAQUINE

Chloroquine-resistant strains of P. falciparum may remain sensitive to amodiaquine. The drug is rapidly and extensively converted to a pharmacologically active metabolite, desethyl-amodiaquine. Another metabolite, a quinoneimine, is probably responsible for toxic hepatitis and potentially lethal agranulocytosis, which occurred in 1 in 2000 of those taking amodiaquine prophylactically. As a result, amodiaquine is no longer recommended for prophylaxis, but it may have limited use as an alternative to chloroquine.

# Clindamycin

## MODE OF ACTION

This semisynthetic lincosamide antibiotic was derived from lincomycin by halogenation in the 7-position, to which is attributed its antimalarial activity. In bacteria, it acts by binding to the 50S subunit of the bacterial ribosome, as with macrolides, inhibiting the early stage of protein synthesis. In parasites of the phylum Apicomplexa, including Plasmodium, Toxoplasma and Eimeria, clindamycin may inhibit protein synthesis in a plastid organelle (apicoplast). Clindamycin has a slow-action blood schizontocidal activity against P. falciparum, including isolates resistant to 4-aminoquinolines and dihydrofolate reductase (DHFR) inhibitors, but it should never be used alone. In sequence with quinine and possibly chloroquine, it has proved effective against multiresistant P. falciparum in South America, Africa and South-east Asia. This combination is particularly useful in pregnant women and young children, in whom quinine–tetracycline combinations are contraindicated. Unfortunately, clindamycin is too expensive for most developing countries.

## CLINICAL PHARMACOKINETICS

Ninety per cent of an ingested dose of clindamycin is absorbed, producing peak blood levels within 45 minutes. The drug is widely distributed, but does not penetrate the cerebrospinal fluid. It crosses the placenta and is excreted in breast milk. Its half-life is 1.5–3.5 (average 2.38) hours. It is metabolized in the liver and mainly excreted in the bile. About 10 per cent of the dose is excreted in urine as active drug or metabolites and about 4 per cent in the faeces and the rest as inactive metabolites.

## ADVERSE EFFECTS

Clindamycin produces gastrointestinal symptoms, notably diarrhoea, in 2–20 per cent of patients. *Clostridium difficile* toxin pseudomembranous colitis is a particular problem, commoner in women and in elderly patients. Rashes develop in 10 per cent of recipients. Toxicity of the quinine–clindamycin combination is reduced if the drugs are given sequentially rather than together.

# Halofantrine

Halofantrine is a phenanthrene methanol, identified by the US Army during the Second World War, but not developed until the 1980s, and not commercially available until the early 1990s (Cosgriff *et al.*, 1982).

## MODE OF ACTION

The mechanism of action of halofantrine seems to be similar to that of quinine and mefloquine, involving lysosomal trapping of the drug, followed by binding to haemin and prevention of haemin polymerization to relatively inert malarial pigment. Halofantrine exhibits high activity *in vitro* against chloroquine-resistant strains of *P. falciparum*, although cross-resistance to chloroquine and rapid acquisition of halofantrine resistance have been reported in the *P. berghei* mouse model. Early studies in humans confirmed efficacy of the drug against multidrug-resistant falciparum malaria in artificial infections and in the field (Watkins *et al.*, 1988).

## CLINICAL PHARMACOKINETICS

The absorption of halofantrine following oral administration is incomplete and variable, with non-linear absorption kinetics above the 500-mg single dose range – possibly a function of the poor solubility of the drug (Broom, 1990). Peak plasma concentrations occur after about 6 hours, and the apparent terminal half-life is 1–2 days. Peak concentrations of the major metabolite, N-desbutylhalofantrine, occur at about 12 hours after ingestion, and the metabolite has an apparent terminal elimination half-life of 3–5 days. The absorption of halofantrine can be markedly enhanced by high-protein, high-lipid content food (Milton *et al.*, 1989). In some populations, and in malaria patients, the time to reach peak concentrations, elimination times and the extent of absorption may be significantly different from the values above (Veenendall *et al.*, 1991). The extent of halofantrine absorption may be related to the severity of malaria (Watkins *et al.*, 1995).

## THERAPEUTIC USE

Mandatory electrocardiography to exclude susceptibility to halofantrine cardiotoxicity before treatment has greatly limited the usefulness of this drug.

## ADVERSE EFFECTS

The most important adverse effect is the increase is the ECG QT interval, apparent at the recommended dosage as well as at the higher doses that have been used in research. The risk of cardiotoxicity may be increased by facilitated absorption, when halofantrine is administered with a fatty meal, and is increased in patients previously treated with mefloquine. The package insert carries a warning that halofantrine should not be given to patients who might have a long QT interval (either as a familial condition or associated with other treatments, such as mefloquine), and that halofantrine should not be taken with food or by people deficient in thiamine, which is an additional risk factor for cardiac arrhythmia.

## MEFLOQUINE (LARIAM)

### Mode of action

Mefloquine forms complexes with haemin (ferriprotoporphyrin IX) in cultured *P. falciparum*. Blocking haemin release with a protease inhibitor antagonizes its antimalarial activity. This suggests that, like 4-aminoquinolines and quinine, mefloquine works by interaction with haemin and its polymer (Mungthin *et al.*, 1998).

Mefloquine acts against the asexual stages of all species of human malaria parasite. The drug has no useful activity against the exo-erythrocytic stages of *P. vivax* or *P. ovale*. It does not kill gametocytes of *P. falciparum*. Clinical resistance is common in South-east Asia (notably on the borders of Thailand with Burma and Cambodia and elsewhere).

## CLINICAL PHARMACOKINETICS

Oral bioavailability is about 80 per cent in fasting volunteers. An oral dose of 250 mg yields a peak concentration of about 300 μg/L after between 6 and 24 hours (Karbwang and White, 1990). It is highly lipid-soluble and extensively distributed, especially in lung, liver and lymphoid tissue. Cerebrospinal fluid concentrations are low. More than 95 per cent is bound to plasma proteins. About half of a mefloquine dose undergoes hepatic transformation to metabolites that lack antimalarial activity. About 9 per cent of the drug is eliminated unchanged in the urine. Unchanged drug and metabolites are eliminated mainly via the bile in the faeces; there is evidence of enterohepatic circulation. The elimination half-life is very long, ranging from 15 to 33 days; steady state is reached after 8 weeks of weekly dosing.

## THERAPEUTIC USE

Mefloquine is used for the prophylaxis and treatment of uncomplicated multiresistant falciparum malaria. In combination with artesunate, it has proved effective against uncomplicated falciparum malaria in areas, such as the Thai–Burmese border, where there is a high level of resistance to mefloquine alone.

## ADVERSE EFFECTS

Dose-related adverse reactions are common, usually mild and most frequently gastrointestinal. 'Serious' central nervous system events, including seizures, are estimated to occur in about 1 in 10 000 prophylactic users, which is about the same reported rate as for chloroquine. The estimated frequency of non-serious central nervous system events (including headache, dizziness, insomnia and depression) varies between 1.8 per cent and 7.6 per cent (and is generally higher in females than in males). These proportions are similar to those for chloroquine, but about five-fold higher than those reported by patients taking no prophylaxis.

Mefloquine and chloroquine–proguanil have been compared for the frequency, severity and type of adverse reaction. In a retrospective questionnaire-based study, 1214 adults taking mefloquine and 1181 taking chloroquine plus proguanil were surveyed (Phillips-Howard and TerKuile, 1995). Forty per cent of both groups reported adverse events, but neuro-psychiatric adverse events were significantly more common in travellers taking mefloquine (333/1214, compared with 189/1181 in the chloroquine–proguanil group); others present similar findings. In contrast, in a prospective, randomized, double-blind trial in soldiers, there was no difference in the incidence of central nervous system toxicity between mefloquine users and those taking chloroquine–proguanil; results of this latter study are in keeping with earlier findings in both military personnel and private travellers. A recent double-blind, randomized, placebo-controlled trial studied the frequency of adverse effects to mefloquine in volunteers. Mefloquine was associated with mild diarrhoea, ECG QT prolongation and a mean drop in plasma glucose of 0.5 mmol/L, but there was no excess of central nervous system adverse events and 'symbol digit modality' testing was unaffected by mefloquine.

Rarely, mefloquine has been associated with serious idiosyncratic adverse reactions, including exfoliative dermatitis, toxic epidermal necrolysis, cutaneous vasculitis and aplastic anaemia. The use of mefloquine during pregnancy increases the risk of stillbirth and the British National Formulary advises that pregnancy should be excluded before the drug is taken.

## ADVERSE DRUG INTERACTIONS

- Anti-arrhythmic drugs: risk of additive cardiac effects with amiodarone and quinidine.
- Anticonvulsants: mefloquine lowers seizure threshold.
- Antipsychotics: increased risk of ventricular arrhythmias.

# Primaquine and tafenoquine

Primaquine, an 8-aminoquinoline, was synthesized in the 1940s. Since 1950, it has been the drug of choice for the radical cure of *P. vivax* and *P. ovale* infections.

## MODE OF ACTION

The site of action is thought to be in the mitochondria, possibly by competitive inhibition of dihydro-orotate dehydrogenase involved in pyrimidine synthesis. Primaquine is active against exo-erythrocytic schizonts (causal prophylaxis) and is gametocytocidal for all species of human malaria parasite and hypnozoitocidal for *P. vivax* and *P. ovale*. The Chesson strain of *P. vivax* from New Guinea is relatively resistant to primaquine.

## CLINICAL PHARMACOKINETICS

Ingested primaquine has 72–76 per cent bioavailability, producing peak plasma concentrations within 2 or 3 hours. There is little tissue binding. Primaquine is rapidly metabolized in the liver; the main metabolite is carboxyprimaquine. The half-life is 5–6 hours.

## THERAPEUTIC USE

Primaquine is used for the radical cure of vivax and ovale malarias, as a community transmission-blocking (gametocytocidal) drug against *P. falciparum* and, to a very limited extent, for the prophylaxis of falciparum malaria.

## ADVERSE EFFECTS

Primaquine is well tolerated in normal therapeutic doses. However, in patients with inherited deficiencies of erythrocyte enzymes, notably glucose-6-phosphate dehydrogenase (G6PD), it may cause acute intravascular haemolysis and methaemoglobinaemia. This is most severe in people with Mediterranean and Asian variants of G6PD deficiency and is relatively mild in those with African variants. Gastrointestinal disturbances are also described.

## TAFENOQUINE (WR238605, ETAQUINE)

Tafenoquine is an 8-aminoquinoline drug developed by the US Army Program (Peters, 1999). It is a 5-phenoxy derivative of primaquine with a longer elimination half-life (14 days compared to 6 hours) and, in animal models, is seven times more active than primaquine as a hypnozoitocide, 14 times more active as a causal prophylactic and 100 times more active as a blood schizontocide. It is better tolerated than primaquine, but can cause haemolysis in people with G6PD deficiency. Tafenoquine has great potential as a causal prophylactic drug against *P. falciparum*, for the radical cure of *P. vivax*, as a gametocytocidal and possibly blood schizontocidal drug for *P. falciparum*.

# Proguanil and chlorproguanil

## MODE OF ACTION

The biguanides proguanil and chlorproguanil are metabolized *in vivo* to the triazine compounds cycloguanil and chlorcycloguanil, respectively, which are structurally similar to the diamino-pyrimidine pyrimethamine. Triazines are known as type 2 antifolate drugs because they specifically inhibit parasite DHFR, an enzyme that regenerates folate cofactors, which are essential for 2-carbon transfer reactions and the synthesis of parasite nucleic acids (Canfield *et al.*, 1995). Both triazines are competitive inhibitors of DHFR. Because they inhibit all growing stages of the malaria parasite, both proguanil and chlorproguanil have been used as causal prophylactics, and are effective in preventing the growth of sporogonic stages in the mosquito. Like pyrimethamine, triazines synergize with type 1 antifolate drugs (sulphonamides and sulphones). The biguanide pro-drugs, but not triazine metabolites, have a secondary site of action, independent of their effect on the parasite folate pathway (Kaneko *et al.*, 1999). Proguanil, but not cycloguanil, is synergistic in combination with atovaquone, a drug that inhibits parasite mitochondrial electron transport (see above). Proguanil–atovaquone synergy *in vitro* is independent of the extent of proguanil metabolism (see below).

## CLINICAL PHARMACOKINETICS

Following ingestion, peak plasma concentrations of proguanil are reached in 2–4 hours. The elimination half-life varies between 12 and 23 hours. For malaria prophylaxis, proguanil is administered daily and steady state is achieved within 3 days; therefore, the drug should be commenced a week before exposure to malaria. Cycloguanil usually reaches peak concentration within 4–9 hours of the proguanil dose. Proguanil is about 75 per cent bound to plasma proteins. The extent of proguanil metabolism varies considerably among individuals and populations (Helsby *et al.*, 1990). Metabolism is catalysed by enzymes of the cytochrome P450 group (CYP 2C19 and CYP 3A4), which are subject to genetic polymorphism. 'Poor metabolizers' of proguanil sustain low or undetectable concentrations of cycloguanil, which may jeopardize prophylactic efficacy, although it is possible that the prophylactic efficacy of proguanil is unrelated to metabolism status (Watkins *et al.*, 1990).

## PHARMACEUTICS

Proguanil is available as proguanil hydrochloride tablets B.P. 100 mg. The adult dose is 200 mg daily for the prevention and suppression of malaria. There is no paediatric formulation; for young children, tablets crushed and mixed with jam or honey are usually practicable. Chlorproguanil was marketed as Lapudrine, a once-weekly chemoprophylactic agent, because it was thought that the elimination of the biguanide and triazine metabolite was significantly slower than that of proguanil. However, the two drugs have similar pharmacokinetic properties, and weekly chlorproguanil does not provide adequate protection (Watkins *et al.*, 1987). Chlorproguanil in combination with dapsone may, however, have an important role in the treatment of falciparum malaria, especially in Africa (see below).

## THERAPEUTIC USE

Proguanil is used most commonly in combination with chloroquine for the prophylaxis of mildly chloroquine-resistant falciparum malaria and also in a fixed combination with atovaquone (as Malarone) (Canfield *et al.*, 1995).

## ADVERSE EFFECTS

Mild to moderate gastric intolerance and nausea can occur, which may subside as use continues. Mouth ulceration is common and may be severe (Drysdale *et al.*, 1990). Hair loss is reported. Megaloblastic anaemia and pancytopenia have been reported in patients with chronic renal failure.

## DRUG INTERACTIONS

Proguanil may affect the dose of anticoagulants needed for those on long-term treatment, and it is best to re-stabilize the anticoagulant dose in the presence of proguanil.

# Pyrimethamine

## MODE OF ACTION

Pyrimethamine, like the triazine metabolites of proguanil and chlorproguanil, is an 'antimetabolite'.

Activity arises from the selective, competitive inhibition of parasite, rather than host, enzymes; in this case the target enzyme is DHFR (Peterson *et al.*, 1990). Spontaneous mutations in the parasite gene encoding DHFR structure can have a pronounced effect on pyrimethamine action, by altering the configuration of the target enzyme and thus changing the drug–target binding characteristics. DHFR mutations that give rise to pyrimethamine resistance are very common in all parts of the world. Pyrimethamine is only used in synergic combination with a sulphonamide or sulphone, in regions where the parasite remains sensitive, mainly in Africa. However, the prevalence of mutations in DHFR and in dihydropteroate synthase (DHPS), which control parasite chemosensitivity to these combinations, is now increasing rapidly in Africa.

## CLINICAL PHARMACOKINETICS

Pyrimethamine is well absorbed after oral or parenteral administration in patients with malaria, reaching synergistic plasma concentrations within 1 hour. It is about 94 per cent bound to plasma proteins. Elimination half-lives in children with malaria average 81 hours and 124 hours after oral and intramuscular injection, respectively (Winstanley *et al.*, 1992). The long elimination phase of pyrimethamine, administered together with sulfadoxine, has been related to the selection of pyrimethamine-resistant parasites in Africa.

## PHARMACEUTICS

Pyrimethamine is available only as formulations with either a sulphonamide (sulfadoxine, sulfalene) or, for chemoprophylaxis, with dapsone (Maloprim®, Glaxo-Wellcome). PSD treatment for malaria is a single dose (three tablets for an adult; equivalent to 1.25 mg/kg pyrimethamine and 25 mg/kg sulfadoxine). Many manufacturers now produce tablets containing pyrimethamine 25 mg plus sulfadoxine 500 mg. Pyrimethamine–sulfalene has equivalent efficacy, and tablets are available. A solution containing pyrimethamine 10 mg/mL plus sulfadoxine 200 mg/mL is available for intramuscular injection (Hoffman LaRoche).

## THERAPEUTIC USE

Pyrimethamine in combination with dapsone (as Maloprim or Deltaprim) has been used for the prophylaxis of mildly chloroquine-resistant falciparum malaria (Dollery, 1991). Pyrimethamine in combination with sulfadoxine (as Fansidar) or with sulfalene (as Metakelfin) is used for the treatment of uncomplicated chloroquine-resistant falciparum malaria. Fansidar is also used in combination with short-course quinine in the treatment of uncomplicated multiresistant falciparum malaria and in two doses during pregnancy for the intermittent presumptive treatment of chloroquine-resistant falciparum malaria in Africa.

### ADVERSE EFFECTS

Acute poisoning in children is seen readily with doses greater than 25 mg (one tablet of PSD or Maloprim) and fatalities have been reported with doses exceeding 375 mg. Pyrimethamine causes concentration-dependent suppression of the marrow and may produce temporary pancytopenia or granulocytosis. Severe idiosyncratic reactions to pyrimethamine are uncommon.

### DRUG INTERACTIONS

The inhibition of host DHFR by pyrimethamine is mild, but it may produce an additive effect to that resulting from other drugs such as co-trimoxazole, trimethoprim and methotrexate.

## Pyronaridine

Drug-resistant malaria is making treatments redundant at a faster rate than new drugs can be developed. One consequence of this process is the renewed interest in older drugs, which were displaced by more acceptable compounds such as chloroquine. Pyronaridine is a promising acridine-based drug, synthesized in Shanghai in 1970. In China, it is used in both oral and parenteral forms for the treatment of chloroquine-resistant *P. falciparum* malaria, and is being developed further under the auspices of the World Health Organization (WHO) (Chang *et al.*, 1992).

### MODE OF ACTION

Pyronaridine is an azacrine-type Mannich base with structural similarities to both mepacrine and amodiaquine. Effects on haemoglobin degradation, haem polymerization and topoisomerase-2 activity have been suggested, but the precise mode of action remains unknown. There are conflicting reports on

cross-resistance between chloroquine and pyronaridine: studies in China and on isolates from Africa show no correlation, in contrast to studies on isolates from Thailand and Somalia (Elueze *et al.*, 1996). For parasites from a range of geographical locations, there is a positive correlation between chloroquine and pyronaridine chemosensitivity *in vitro* at the IC50 (50% inhibitory concentration), but not the IC90 (90% inhibitory concentration) level.

### PHARMACEUTICS

The Chinese formulation for oral use, an enteric-coated tablet, contains pyronaridine base 100 mg as the phosphate. There is evidence that these tablets are not fully bioavailable. Work is in progress on a capsule formulation with improved bioavailability.

### THERAPEUTIC USE

Pyronaridine is used for the treatment of uncomplicated chloroquine-resistant falciparum malaria.

### ADVERSE EFFECTS

Adverse effects seem to be mild, consisting mainly of headache, nausea and abdominal discomfort.

## Quinidine

Quinidine, the dextrorotatory diastereomer of quinine, is used as an anti-arrhythmic agent by cardiologists and so may be available in hospitals when parenteral quinine is not (see below).

## Quinine

In the seventeenth century, it was found that the bark of the fever tree (*Cinchona*; 'Peruvian bark', 'Jesuit's powder') cured 'agues'. Not until the nineteenth century was this activity against malaria attributed to the *Cinchona* alkaloids, of which quinine and, to a much lesser extent, quinidine are still in use today. Against *P. falciparum*, quinidine is more active than quinine *in vitro* and *in vivo*, but is more toxic.

### MODE OF ACTION

Like chloroquine, quinine interferes with parasite metabolism of haemin, a toxic product of haemoglobin digestion. It is possible that quinine opposes the polymerization of haemin into inert crystals of malarial pigment (haemozoin).

## CLINICAL PHARMACOKINETICS

Ingested quinine is largely absorbed and there is little first-pass metabolism. After intramuscular injection, the absorption half-time seems to vary with the drug concentration in the injectate, ranging from about 10 to 40 minutes. Areas under the concentration–time curve and maximum plasma concentrations are similar following the intramuscular and intravenous administration of quinine.

Quinine is extensively bound to plasma proteins, principally to the acute phase-reactant $\alpha_1$-acid glycoprotein, but also to albumin. In healthy subjects, about 80 per cent of the total plasma quinine concentration is bound, but in patients with malaria, $\alpha_1$-acid glycoprotein concentrations rise, and around 90 per cent is bound; this may explain the apparently lower toxicity of high quinine concentrations in patients with malaria. The binding of quinine to $\alpha_1$-acid glycoprotein is affected by pH *in vitro*. Quinine does not accumulate in erythrocytes, but concentrations in infected cells are higher than those in uninfected cells.

Quinine undergoes extensive hepatic biotransformation, first to 3-hydroxyquinine and 2-hydroxyquinine and then to a series of more polar water-soluble metabolites. Less than 20 per cent of the drug is excreted unchanged in urine, and the impact of renal failure on the disposition of quinine does not appear to be great. Dose reductions are not recommended in severe malaria complicated by either hepatic or renal impairment. In adults with uncomplicated malaria, the elimination half-time of quinine (16 hours) is longer than in health (11 hours), and is even longer in adults with cerebral malaria (18 hours). Quinine is eliminated in breast milk, the plasma:milk ratio being about 0.3:1. Women on standard quinine doses are unlikely to excrete enough drug to cause toxicity in the nursing infant. Quinine crosses the placenta, the cord blood:maternal blood concentration coefficient being about 0.3.

## PHARMACEUTICS

Quinine is available in oral and parenteral forms, and should be stored out of direct light. Unfortun-

**Table 12.1** *Salt–base equivalents of common quinoline antimalarial drugs*

| Antimalarial drug | Salt (mg) | Base (mg) |
|---|---|---|
| Amodiaquine sulphate | 130 | 100 |
| Chloroquine sulphate | 136 | 100 |
| Chloroquine phosphate | 161 | 100 |
| Chloroquine hydrochloride | 123 | 100 |
| Halofantrine hydrochloride | 107 | 100 |
| Mefloquine hydrochloride | 110 | 100 |
| Primaquine phosphate | 18 | 10 |
| Quinidine gluconate | 145 | 100 |
| Quinidine sulphate | 108 | 100 |
| Quinine bisulphate | 137 | 100 |
| Quinine dihydrochloride | 105 | 100 |
| Quinine hydrochloride | 105 | 100 |
| Quinine sulphate | 103 | 100 |

ately, medication is labelled with the mass of drug expressed as the salt, rather than as the base (the active drug); because the base content of the salts varies, confusion may result (Table 12.1). Parenteral quinine (as the dihydrochloride BP) is available as solutions of various strengths in distilled water:

- 500 mg of the salt (413 mg base) in 1 mL
- 600 mg of the salt (496 mg base) in 2 mL
- 1000 mg of the salt (826 mg base) in 2 mL.

## THERAPEUTIC USE

Quinine (and, in the USA, quinidine) is a drug of choice for the parenteral treatment of severe, and the oral treatment of uncomplicated, chloroquine-resistant falciparum malaria.

## ADVERSE EFFECTS

### Symptomatic adverse effects
'Cinchonism', comprising tinnitus, deafness, headache, nausea and visual disturbance, affects the majority of conscious patients with therapeutic levels and does not warrant dose reduction.

### Potentially life-threatening effects
- Hypersensitivity reactions are uncommon; they include rashes, thrombocytopenia with potentially fatal bleeding, leucopenia, disseminated intravascular coagulation, haemolytic–uraemic syndrome, bronchospasm and pancytopenia.

- Quinine stimulates the release of insulin from the pancreatic islets, determined in part by the rate of intravenous infusion. Because malaria itself can cause hypoglycaemia, blood glucose must be carefully monitored.

### Acute overdosage

- Toxicity from quinine can be seen with doses as low as 2 g of the anhydrous free base in adults; the fatal dose ranges from 8 to 15 g.
- Visual impairment is common and may be unilateral or bilateral, total or partial, permanent or temporary.
- Serious cardiovascular compromise is less common than oculotoxicity and is usually seen with higher drug concentrations. Arrhythmias include serious bradyarrhythmias, ventricular tachycardia (including torsade de pointes) and ventricular fibrillation.
- Hypotension may be caused by the negative inotropic effect of the drug and peripheral vasodilatation.
- At high concentration, quinine can cause coma and seizures.
- Activated charcoal has been shown to increase the clearance of quinine. Stellate ganglion block confers no benefit.

### Pregnancy

Quinine in standard doses has no deleterious effects in pregnancy. Pregnant women with falciparum malaria should be given the standard quinine regimen. High-dose quinine has been used as an abortifacient.

### ADVERSE DRUG INTERACTIONS

- Digitalis glycosides: quinine markedly reduces renal clearance.
- Flecainide: quinine reduces clearance.
- Warfarin: quinine may inhibit hepatic metabolism.
- Cimetidine: inhibits the hepatic metabolism of quinine.
- Hypoglycaemic drugs: diabetic control may be compromised by quinine-induced insulin secretion.
- Mefloquine: quinine and mefloquine are molecularly similar; they may exhibit additive toxicity.

### SULPHONAMIDES AND SULPHONES

Sulphonamides and sulphones are often referred to, collectively, as 'sulpha drugs'. First developed as antibacterial agents in the 1930s, this group includes sulphonamides (e.g. sulfadoxine) and sulphones (e.g. dapsone). The sulpha drugs are effective against *P. falciparum*, but relatively inactive against *P. vivax*.

### MODE OF ACTION

Sulpha drugs are structural analogues of p-aminobenzoic acid, and competitively inhibit DHPS – an early stage in *de novo* folate biosynthesis (Watkins *et al.*, 1984). In theory, sulpha drugs have selective activity against the malaria parasite because the host does not possess an endogenous pathway, and all folate cofactors are acquired from ingested food. On this basis, the sulpha drugs should be very potent antimalarial drugs, but in reality their activity is weak. One explanantion for this anomaly is that the parasite appears to utilize preformed folates under certain conditions. Sulpha drugs inhibit parasite DHPS at concentrations in the range 6–90 $\mu$molar, but inhibit the intact parasite *in vitro* at much lower cofcentrations (30–500 nmolar). This discrepancy may be due to active drug concentration by the parasite.

### CLINICAL PHARMACOKINETICS

Of the many thousands of sulpha drugs that have been synthesized and tested for use in medicine, only the sulphonamides sulfadoxine and sulfalene and the sulphone dapsone have been widely used in malaria chemotherapy. Sulfadoxine and sulfalene are long-acting drugs; they are rapidly and completely absorbed, reaching synergistic concentrations within 1 hour of dosing. The elimination half-life of sulfadoxine is between 100 and 200 hours (about 120 hours following oral or parenteral dosage in African children with malaria), that for sulfalene is significantly shorter – about 65 hours (Winstanley *et al.*, 1992). Both drugs are highly bound to plasma proteins and undergo limited metabolism (5 per cent to the acetyl derivative and 2–3 per cent to the glucuronide). Dapsone is rapidly absorbed, reaching peak plasma concentration in 3–6 hours. It is 75 per cent bound to plasma proteins and eliminated quickly in comparison with sulfadoxine, with a mean half-life of about 26 hours. There may be significant, race-linked differences in dapsone metabolism (Cook *et al.*, 1986).

## THERAPEUTIC USE

Sulphonamides in combination with pyrimethamine (for example as Fansidar) are used for the treatment of chloroquine-resistant falciparum malaria. Dapsone in combination with pyrimethamine (for example as Maloprim) is used for the prophylaxis of mildly chloroquine-resistant falciparum malaria. There are plans to use dapsone in combination with chlorproguanil (as LapDap) for the treatment of chloroquine-resistant falciparum malaria.

## ADVERSE EFFECTS

Severe allergic reactions to sulpha drugs are rare, but severe and life-threatening, and the drugs should be used with caution (Miller *et al.*, 1986). The main use of sulpha-containing regimens is for the treatment of non-severe or outpatient malaria in Africa, and there are no adequate data on the rate of adverse reactions in this context. The reported rates of severe adverse reaction to sulfadoxine–pyrimethamine prophylaxis vary between 1 in 5000–8000 and 1 in 150 000.

## Tetracyclines

The antimalarial activity of tetracyclines was first recognized in 1949. Like clindamycin, they are thought to affect protein synthesis in the plastid organelle (apicoplast). Slow activity against pre-erythrocytic and erythrocytic schizonts of *P. falciparum*, including chloroquine-resistant strains, has been demonstrated. Doxycycline alone is effective as prophylaxis against *P. falciparum*, but tetracyclines should never be used alone for treatment, only in combination with, for example with quinine.

### CLINICAL PHARMACOKINETICS

The absorption of ingested tetracyclines ranges from 30 to 80 per cent and is reduced by food, milk and antacids. Tetracyclines are widely distributed in tissues, notably to bone and the dentine and enamel of developing teeth. They cross the placenta and are excreted in milk. The half-life of doxycycline is 16 hours. Elimination is in the faeces and urine. Tetracyclines, with the exception of doxycycline, are contraindicated in severe renal failure.

## THERAPEUTIC USE

Tetracyclines are used in combination with quinine in the treatment of severe and uncomplicated multi-resistant falciparum malaria. Doxycycline is used for the prophylaxis of multiresistant falciparum malaria.

## ADVERSE EFFECTS

Tetracyclines are contraindicated in pregnant women and in children less than 8 years of age because of the risk of interference with the development of bone and teeth and the discoloration of teeth. High doses of tetracycline can damage the liver and kidney, especially if the drug is expired. Common side-effects of tetracyclines are gastrointestinal symptoms, notably diarrhoea, *Candida* vaginitis or stomatitis, light-sensitive rashes and itching of the skin, even in unexposed areas.

# PRACTICAL ANTIMALARIAL CHEMOTHERAPY

## Prescribing quinoline antimalarial drugs

The various salts of quinoline compounds (*Cinchona* alkaloids and related compounds such as mefloquine and halofantrine, 4-aminoquinolines and 8-aminoquinolines) contain greatly differing amounts of base (see Table 12.1). If the prescription fails to specify salt or base, or which particular salt is intended, serious problems of overdosing or underdosing can arise. Whenever possible, the dose of base should be prescribed. This is generally accepted for chloroquine, amodiaquine and primaquine, but, in the case of quinine, quinidine, mefloquine and halofantrine, doses of salts are usually quoted.

## Antimalarial chemotherapy: general considerations

### THE CRISIS IN AFRICA

Although malaria is a serious public health problem throughout the tropical regions of the world, its impact is greatest in Africa. In 1995, it was estimated that, among populations exposed to stable endemic malaria in sub-Saharan Africa, there were at least 207.5 million clinical attacks of malaria, leading to about 1 million deaths from the direct consequences of *P. falciparum* infection. These figures for Africa represent some 85 per cent of the global burden of malaria morbidity and mortality. This situation is not improving. Over the past 30 years, overall infant mortality rates in sub-Saharan African have generally changed little and there is evidence that malaria-associated mortality is increasing as a direct consequence of antimalarial drug resistance – primarily chloroquine resistance (Figure 12.4) (Trape *et al.*, 1998). This depressing scenario is not improved by the knowledge that, although cost-effective interventions are available, they tend to be unaffordable in the economically poor countries of sub-Saharan Africa. For Africa, the urgent need is to find new, effective and affordable drugs for the treatment of outpatient (non-severe) malaria.

## DIAGNOSIS

Ideally, the species of malaria parasite, the parasite density and the geographical origin of the infection should be known. In patients with features of severe malaria, a mixed infection including *P. falciparum* should be assumed even if only parasites of one of the other malaria species are identified in the blood smear. A therapeutic trial is justified in patients who were exposed to infection and develop severe symptoms, even if the blood smear is consistently negative.

## DETAILS OF THE PATIENT

The choice of treatment will depend on the age and genetic origin of the patients, their presumed immune status and, in the case of women, whether they are pregnant or lactating. The dose must be calculated from the patient's weight whenever possible.

## CLINICAL CONDITION

Clinical condition is of great importance. Patients with severe falciparum malaria and those who are vomiting will require parenteral treatment, at least during the initial phase of management.

## PRIOR TREATMENT

Prior treatment is extremely common, particularly in developing countries where drugs such as chloroquine are sold across the counter for the treatment of fevers and suspected malaria. Malaria that breaks through prophylaxis (for example with chloroquine) or which recrudesces or relapses after a recent course of chemotherapy is most likely to be caused by a parasite resistant to that drug. Even though the prophylactic drug has not prevented infection, it may have altered the morphology of the parasites and reduced their numbers, making diagnosis more difficult. *Patients being investigated for malaria should stop taking their malaria prophylaxis.* People who have taken an antimalarial drug within the previous 24–36 hours may develop toxic blood

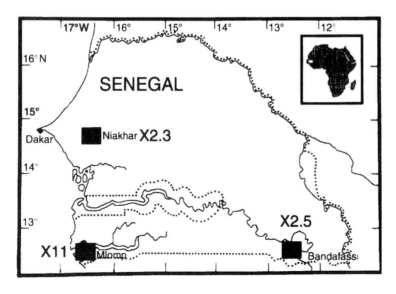

**Figure 12.4** *Increases in malarial mortality in children aged 0–4 years in three areas of Senegal: 1992–95 compared to 1985–91 (after Trape et al., 1998).*

levels if the same drug is given again or there may be adverse drug interactions if a different drug is given.

## OBJECTIVES OF CHEMOTHERAPY

These will differ between mild and severe infections and in different geographical and epidemiological situations. In the treatment of uncomplicated infections in endemic areas, the main objective is to produce symptomatic improvement to limit morbidity; radical cure may be an unrealistic objective where early reinfection is almost certain. In severe malaria, which can kill the patient within a few days, parasiticidal plasma concentrations of the antimalarial drug must be achieved as quickly and safely as possible and sustained for long enough to ensure rapid clearance of parasitaemia. Single-dose regimens to ensure compliance, the prevention of recrudescences and the killing of gametocytes, which may be important considerations in the treatment of uncomplicated malaria in endemic regions, are of little importance in the treatment of severe disease. Symptoms that are troublesome to the fully conscious patient with uncomplicated malaria and may reduce compliance, such as cinchonism or pruritus, are acceptable in the treatment of life-threatening disease and should not limit dosage.

## COMBINATION THERAPY

### Rationale

Recently, there has been renewed interest in the idea of using antimalarial drugs in combination. There is an obvious parallel with developments in the chemotherapy of tuberculosis (TB) and cancer, for which monotherapy resulted in the rapid development of drug resistance. The theory is based on the concept that drug resistance in infecting organisms arises from the selection of mutations in functional genes as a direct consequence of exposure of microbe populations to the drug. Where two drugs with different mechanisms of action are used together, the chance of a double mutation arising, and being selected, is far lower than the chance of selection of the individual mutations. This theory assumes that resistance to all antimalarial drugs is essentially mutation-dependent, but that it is not necessary to define the precise mutations involved. In TB and cancer chemotherapy this concept is paramount, and characterizes all treatments. In malaria chemotherapy, the threat of resistance was appreciated almost 100 years ago and the concept of combination

therapy promoted, notably by Wallace Peters, but, for various reasons, this has so far not been successfully implemented.

On the Thai–Burmese border, parasite resistance to mefloquine 25 mg/kg was 50 per cent in 1994. At this point, treatment was changed to mefloquine 25 mg/kg plus artesunate 4 mg/kg. Over the intervening period to 2000, mefloquine resistance has continued to increase in areas of Thailand where mefloquine monotherapy has been used. Conversely, while the cure rate of the mefloquine plus artesunate regimen has remained over 95 per cent, parasite chemosensitivity to mefloquine has increased rather than decreased. Artesunate is a rapidly acting blood schizontocide, reducing parasite density *in vivo* faster than any other antimalarial drug. Further, it has a pronounced inhibitory effect on gametocytes, which mefloquine alone does not, and so transmission is reduced. One effect of this double action has been to lower the *P. falciparum* case load in this area, as well as maintaining or improving therapeutic efficacy. The combination of mefloquine with an artemisinin is now national policy in Thailand, Vietnam and Cambodia. Studies in South-east Asia and Africa have demonstrated that in combinations of drugs with artemisinins (ACT) with mefloquine or sulfadoxine–pyrimethamine, 3 days of artemisinin are needed to improve cure rates of the partner drug alone.

An important aspect of combination therapy is the mutual simultaneous protection offered to each of the partner drugs. Ideally, no parasite is ever exposed to one drug in the absence of the other. Thus, resistance to each drug is delayed. Further, combination therapy allows the dose of individual drugs to be reduced. Artesunate alone must be given daily for 5 days to clear the infection, whereas, in the presence of mefloquine, a 3-day regimen is sufficient.

The largest clinical trials ever planned are now in progress to assess 'proof of concept' of combination therapy in Africa, South America and the Pacific. These trials are studying combinations of artesunate with amodiaquine, chloroquine, sulfadoxine–pyrimethamine and mefloquine and will be completed in 2001.

Combinations of drugs that do not contain artemisinins are also in use. In Africa, chloroquine has been used increasingly with sulfadoxine–pyrimethamine, in the face of spreading resistance to chloroquine. Chloroquine–sulfadoxine–pyrimethamine has the advantage of the rapid parasiticidal and antipyretic actions of chloroquine, with the additional inhibitory activity of the antifolate. There is strong clinical support for this development, where the doubling of drug costs is affordable. In areas of East and Central Africa, chloroquine efficacy is low, and sulfadoxine–pyrimethamine efficacy is decreasing quickly. This makes it difficult to change from chloroquine to sulfadoxine–pyrimethamine monotherapy, given the operational constraints, especially the time required for the implementation of a new treatment. Consequently, some National Malaria Control agencies are considering a change from chloroquine monotherapy to chloroquine–sulfadoxine–pyrimethamine combination therapy. However, where there is already some resistance to both partner drugs, chloroquine–sulfadoxine pyrimethamine must be regarded as merely an interim solution rather than a radical change. There is an urgent need for field data demonstrating a significant difference in efficacy between chloroquine or amodiaquine and their sulfadoxine–pyrimethamine combinations.

In ACT employing two drugs, A (artesunate) and B (any drug with a different mechanism of action), it is important that precise data are available on parasite chemosensitivity to the individual components. Where resistance to B is complete, A–B treatments do not constitute ACT, but rather artesunate monotherapy. This is a dangerous situation, because the artesunate component is not protected. Further, because artesunate monotherapy requires an extended dosage regimen, infections will not be cleared with the shorter artesunate regimens used in ACT. This will increase the selective pressure for resistance operating on the artemisinin component.

This emphasizes an important and basic concept: that combination therapy should not be used as a device to extend the useful therapeutic life of a *failing drug.*

The cost of therapy is another critical issue in malarial chemotherapy, especially in Africa. While the commercial cost of artemisinins is generally decreasing as the market expands, the additional cost of ACT remains a barrier to wide acceptance.

## Drugs used in combination therapy

In fixed-ratio combination therapy, the two drugs are formulated in a single tablet. In non-fixed-ratio combination therapy, separate formulations of the two drugs are administered at the same time.

*Benflumetol plus artemether (Riamet or Co-artemether)* Co-artemether is an interesting application of benflumetol (lumefantrine) that was synthesized in China, where all the original research was conducted, and latterly developed by Novartis (see above).

This combination has been registered while continuing field testing (phase 4) attempts to improve the cumbersome dosage regimen.

Potential problems include the poor absorption of the benflumetol component which, like halofantrine, is not fully absorbed unless accompanied by a fatty meal; the potential for rapid emergence and selection of benflumetol resistance; the mismatch of pharmacokinetics leaving benflumetol unprotected after elimination of artesunate; and the cost.

Potential advantages are the high efficiency of this ACT, which may be available to endemic countries at an affordable price.

*Amodiaquine plus artesunate* This ACT is being studied in both East and West Africa.

Potential advantages are that a 3-day regimen is appropriate for both components, so a fixed-ratio formulation is practicable and, throughout Africa, amodiaquine is significantly more effective than chloroquine or even sulfadoxine–pyrimethamine.

Potential disadvantages include the development and spread of amodiaquine resistance and the potential toxicity of repeated doses of amodiaquine.

*Sulfadoxine–pyrimethamine plus artesunate* This is an important concept for Africa, where sulfadoxine–pyrimethamine is beginning to fail in areas of chloroquine-resistant falciparum malaria. It is hoped that sulfadoxine–pyrimethamine ACT will reduce the rate of emergence of sulfadoxine–pyrimethamine resistance, and so prolong the useful therapeutic life of sulfadoxine–pyrimethamine, which is currently the last of the available, affordable treatments for uncomplicated malaria in this continent.

In the Gambia, the efficacy of single-dose sulfadoxine–pyrimethamine has been compared with sulfadoxine–pyrimethamine plus one dose of artesunate 4 mg/kg, and sulfadoxine–pyrimethamine plus three daily doses of artesunate 4 mg/kg. The addition of a single dose of artesunate had little effect on cure rate, but gametocyte carriage was significantly reduced. Sulfadoxine–pyrimethamine plus three doses of artesunate reduced gametocyte carriage even more.

Is it already too late to implement sulfadoxine–pyrimethamine ACT in Africa? Sulfadoxine–pyrimethamine resistance is strongly associated with mutations in parasite *dhfr* (see below). Although three mutations in *dhfr* are now prevalent in many parts of Africa, a fourth *dhfr* mutation, providing complete sulfadoxine–pyrimethamine resistance, has been reported only as a possible genotype at very low frequency. Models predict that sulfadoxine–pyrimethamine ACT will still delay the rate of selection of the quadruple mutation, if the triple combination is deployed widely before this genotype becomes prevalent. Infections with triple mutant *dhfr* parasites, with borderline susceptibility to sulfadoxine–pyrimethamine mono-therapy, might still become common, requiring treatment with sulfadoxine–pyrimethamine ACT. It is debatable whether, in this situation, the high cost of sulfadoxine–pyrimethamine ACT is justified, or whether a different combination, with greater activity in the partner drug, should be considered. Candidate ACTs would be amodiaquine ACT or benflumetol plus artemether.

### Experimental or theoretical artemisinin combination therapies

*Pyronaridine plus artesunate*  A major theoretical disadvantage of pyronaridine (see above) is the rate at which resistance develops in the mouse model. There are problems in drug absorption following oral dosage, and in constructing a suitable dosage regimen. The price of pyronaridine alone is expected to be comparatively high and the ACT formulation will be even more expensive. However, a regimen consisting of a maximum of three daily doses would be practicable.

*Chlorproguanil–dapsone with artesunate*  Chlorproguanil–dapsone (Lapdap) is being developed as an affordable and effective treatment for uncomplicated falciparum malaria, especially in Africa. An ACT formulation is also being developed.

### RISK–BENEFIT ANALYSIS

The choice of drugs for therapy and prophylaxis should depend on a proper assessment of the balance between the therapeutic needs and urgency in a particular case and on the risks of toxicity. In the case of pregnant or lactating women, the risks to the fetus or infant must also be taken into account.

### COST

Most malarious countries are relatively poor economically and so the choice of treatment will usually be determined by cost. In some estimates made by WHO using European prices, the costs of a course of treatment relative to that of chloroquine ($= 1$) were as follows: halofantrine 66.4, mefloquine 24.0, quinine 18.4, amodiaquine 1.75, Fansidar 1.6. Prices will vary a great deal in different countries and brand name antimalarials are considerably more expensive than their internationally traded generic equivalents.

Dosage recommendations for the principal antimalarial drugs are given in Tables 12.2 and 12.3.

## Treatment of uncomplicated malaria (see Table 12.2)

### CHLOROQUINE

Chloroquine remains the treatment of choice for *P. vivax*, *P. ovale*, *P. malariae*, monkey malarias and uncomplicated falciparum malaria in those few geographical areas where this drug can still be relied upon to achieve a satisfactory clinical response. Even in areas of long-established and high-level chloroquine resistance such as Vietnam, chloroquine is still the most widely used treatment for uncomplicated falciparum malaria and still produces a clinical response, albeit with RI or RII resistance in a majority of patients [RI implies delayed recrudescence (after 7 days), and RII early recrudescence (before 7 days) of parasitaemia after its initial disappearance in response to chemotherapy (Gilles and Warrell, 1993)]. Chloroquine is cheap, safe and, in the usual 3-day course, well tolerated, but, despite the clinical improvement attributable to its anti-inflammatory action, its failure to eliminate parasitaemia and the subsequent recrudescences may eventually lead to the development of profound anaemia. In many parts of the malaria-endemic area, a decision must soon be made to replace chloroquine as the first-line treatment for falciparum malaria with a more expensive, more toxic and less well-tolerated drug. The switch to pyrimethamine–sulphonamide combinations has been made in many countries and, unfortunately, resistance usually develops within a few years. Combinations such as Fansidar

**Table 12.2** *Antimalarial chemotherapy for adults and children who can swallow tablets*

| Chloroquine-resistant *P. falciparum* or origin of species unknown | Chloroquine-sensitive *P. falciparum* or *P. vivax, P. ovale, P. malariae* or monkey malarias |
|---|---|
| 1 *Mefloquine*<br>Adults: 15–25 mg **base**/kg[a] given as 2 doses 6–8 h apart<br><br>Children: 25 mg **base**/kg given as 2 doses 6–8 h apart | 1 *Chloroquine*[b]<br>Adults: 600 mg **base** on the 1st and 2nd days; 300 mg on the 3rd day<br>Children: approximately 10 mg **base**/kg on the 1st and 2nd days; 5 mg **base**/kg on the 3rd day |
| **or**<br><br>2 *Proguanil with atovaquone* (Malarone)<br>Adults: 4 tablets (each containing 100 mg proguanil and 250 mg atovaquone) once daily for 3 days<br>Children: 11–20 kg, 1 tablet; 21–30 kg, 2 tablets; 31–40 kg, 3 tablets, **all** once daily for 3 days | For radical cure of vivax/ovale add:<br>2 *Primaquine*<br>Adults (except pregnant and lactating women and G6PD-deficient patients): 15 mg **base**/day on days 4–17 *or* 45 mg/week for 8 weeks[c]<br>Children: 0.25 mg/kg per day on days 4–17 *or* 0.75 mg/kg per week for 8 weeks[c] |
| **or**<br>3 *Artemether with lumefantrine* (Riamet)<br>Adults: 4 tablets (each containing 20 mg artemether and 120 mg lumefantrine) twice daily for 3 days<br>Children: <15 kg, 1 tablet; 15–<25 kg, 2 tablets; 25–<35 kg, 3 tablets, **all** twice daily for 3 days | |
| **or**<br>4 *Quinine*<br>Adults: 600 mg **salt** 3 times daily for 7 days[d]<br>Children: approximately 10 mg **salt**/kg 3 times daily for 7 days | |
| **or**<br>5 *Chlorproguanil with dapsone* (Lapdap)<br>Adults and children: chlorproguanil 2.0 mg/kg with dapsone 2.5 mg/kg once daily for 3 days | |
| **or**<br>6 *Sulphonamide–pyrimethamine*[e]<br>Sulfadoxine (500 mg per tablet) or sulfalene (500 mg) plus pyrimethamine (25 mg)<br>Adults: 3 tablets as single dose<br>Children: < 5 years, 1/2 tablet; < 9 years, 1 tablet; < 15 years, 2 tablets, **all** as single doses | |

For **salt–base** equivalents see Table 12.1.
[a]Depending on geographical area and presumed immunity.
[b]For chloroquine-resistant *P. vivax*, repeat the course.
[c]For Chesson-type strains (SE Asia, W Pacific), use double dose or double duration up to a total dose of 6 mg **base**/kg in daily doses of 15–22.5 mg in adults.
[d]In areas where 7 days of quinine is not curative (e.g. Thailand), **add** tetracycline 250 mg 4 times each day or doxycycline 100 mg daily for 7 days except for children under 8 years and pregnant women **or add** clindamycin 10 mg/kg twice daily for 3–7 days.
[e]Sulfadoxine + pyrimethamine (Fansidar); sulfalene + pyrimethamine (Metakelfin). Contraindicated if patient has known sulphonamide hypersensitivity.

and 'Metakelfin' have the great advantage of being single-dose treatments that are usually well tolerated, except in people in with hypersensitivity to sulphonamide.

## CHLORPROGUANIL–DAPSONE (Lapdap)

This synergistic antifolate drug combination is not yet commercially available. It is being developed (as a

**Table 12.3** *Antimalarial chemotherapy in adults or children with severe malaria\* or in those who cannot swallow tablets*

| Chloroquine-resistant *P. falciparum* or origin unknown | Chloroquine-sensitive *P. falciparum*[a] or *P. vivax*, *P. ovale*, *P. malariae* or monkey malarias |
|---|---|
| 1 *Quinine*<br>Adults: 20 mg **salt**/kg (loading dose)[b] diluted in 10 mL/kg isotonic fluid by i.v. infusion over 4 h then, 8 h after the start of the loading dose, 10 mg **salt**/kg over 4 h, every 8 h until patients can swallow[c,d]<br><br>Children: 20 mg **salt**/kg (loading dose)[b] diluted in 10 mL/kg isotonic fluid by i.v. infusion over 2 h then, 12 h after the start of the loading dose, 10 mg **salt**/kg over 2 h, 12-hourly until patients can swallow[c,d] The 7-day course should be completed with quinine tablets approximately 10 mg **salt**/kg (maximum 600 mg) 8–12 hourly[c,d] | 1 *Chloroquine*[e]<br>25 mg **base**/kg diluted in isotonic fluid by continuous i.v. infusion over 30 h (or 5 mg **base**/kg over 6 h every 6 h) |
| **or**<br>2 *Quinine* (in intensive care unit) 7 mg **salt**/kg (loading dose)[b] i.v. by infusion pump over 30 min followed immediately by 10 mg **salt**/kg (maintenance dose) diluted in 10 mL/kg isotonic fluid by i.v. infusion over 4 h, repeated 8-hourly until patient can swallow etc.[c,d] | **or**<br>2 *Quinine*<br>(see left-hand column, above) |
| **or**<br>3 *Artesunate*[f]<br>2.4 mg/kg (loading dose) i.v. on the first day followed by 1.2 mg/kg daily for a minimum of 3 days until the patient can take oral therapy or another effective antimalarial | |
| **or**<br>4 *Artemether*<br>3.2 mg/kg (loading dose) i.m. on the first day, followed by 1.6 mg/kg daily for a minimum of 3 days until the patient can take oral treatment or another effective anti-malarial. In children, the use of a 1-mL tuberculin syringe is advisable because the injection volumes will be small | |
| **or**<br>5 *Quinidine* (in intensive care unit)<br>15 mg **base**/kg (loading dose)[b] i.v. by infusion over 4 h then, 8 h after the start of the loading dose, give 7.5 mg **base**/kg over 4 h every 8 h, until the patient can swallow,[c] then quinine tablets to complete 7 days treatment[d] **or** give a single dose of 25 mg/kg sulfadoxine and 1.25 mg/kg pyrimethamine | |
| **If it is not possible to give drugs by intravenous infusion**<br>1 *Quinine*<br>20 mg **salt**/kg diluted to 60–100 mg/mL (loading dose)[b] i.m. (anterolateral thigh, divided half into each leg), then 10 mg **salt**/kg 8-hourly until patient can swallow etc.[c,d] | 1 *Chloroquine*[e]<br>Total dose 25 mg **base**/kg given either (a) i.m. or s.c. 2.5 mg **base**/kg 4-hourly; or (b) i.m. or s.c. 3.5 mg **base**/kg 6-hourly |
| | **or**<br>2 *Quinine*<br>i.m. (see left-hand column, above) |

**Table 12.3** (*Continued*)

| Chloroquine-resistant *P. falciparum* or origin unknown | Chloroquine-sensitive *P. falciparum*[a] or *P. vivax*, *P. ovale, P. malariae* or monkey malarias |
|---|---|
| **If it is not possible to give drugs by injection (i.m./i.v.) or infusion** | |
| 1 *Suppositories of artemisinin*[g] <br> 40 mg/kg loading dose as suppositories intrarectally, followed by 20 mg/kg at 4, 24, 48 and 72 h followed by an oral antimalarial drug[h] <br> *Suppositories of artesunate*[g] <br> One 200 mg suppository intrarectally at 0, 4, 8, 12, 24, 36, 48 and 60 h followed by an oral antimalarial drug[h,i] | 1 *Chloroquine* <br> 10 mg **base**/kg of body weight as tablets/syrup by mouth or nasogastric tube, *then* refer the patient to a higher level of health care for parenteral treatment **or** continue 5 mg **base**/kg at 5, 24 and 48 h later[h] |
| **or** | **or** |
| 2 *Tablets of artemisinin* (artesunate, artemether, artemether with lumefantrine), quinine, mefloquine or other appropriate antimalarials[h] | 2 *Suppositories of artemisinin or artesunate, oral quinine, mefloquine or sulfadoxine/pyrimethamine* (see left-hand column)[h] |

For **salt/base** equivalents see Table 7.1 (p. 192).
*For definition, see Table 7.2 (p. 193).
[a]Currently restricted to Haiti, Dominican Republic, Central America and parts of the Middle East.
[b]Loading dose must not be used if patient received quinine, quinidine or halofantrine within preceding 24 h.
[c]In patients requiring more than 48 h of parenteral therapy, reduce the dose to 5.7 mg **salt**/kg 8-hourly or 3.75 mg quinidine **base**/kg 8-hourly.
[d]In areas where 7 days of quinine is not curative (e.g. Thailand), **add** tetracycline 250 mg four times each day or doxycycline 100 mg daily for 7 days, except for children under 8 years and pregnant women, **or add** clindamycin 10 mg/kg twice daily for 3–7 days.
[e]Parenteral chloroquine should be used with great caution in young children.
[f]Artesunic acid 60 mg is dissolved in 0.6 mL of 5% sodium bicarbonate diluted to 3–5 mL with 5% (w/v) dextrose and given immediately by intravenous ('push') bolus injection.
[g]Artemisinin and artesunate suppositories are registered for use in a few countries. If suppository formulations are not available, tablets of artemisinins should be given orally, if possible, or crushed and given by nasogastric tube.
[h]Transfer patient to hospital as soon as possible after initiating chemotherapy.
[i]In Vietnam, 4 mg/kg of artesunate in suppository form (China) intrarectally as a loading dose, followed by 2 mg/kg at 4, 12, 48 and 72 h followed by an oral antimalarial drug, proved as effective as artemisinin suppositories.

fixed-ratio tablet), primarily for the treatment of semi-immune patients in tropical Africa, where there is an urgent need for an inexpensive alternative to pyrimethamine combinations. Daily Lapdap for 3 days (chlorproguanil 2.0 mg/kg and dapsone 2.5 mg/kg daily) is an effective treatment for uncomplicated falciparum malaria in semi-immune patients and seems to be well tolerated. There is evidence that pyrimethamine–sulfadoxine treatment of parasite strains with *dhfr* mutations at positions 108, 51 and 59 often results in clinical failure; in contrast, the risk of clinical failure seems lower with Lapdap (Mutabingwa *et al.*, 2001). It is also possible that Lapdap exerts a smaller degree of 'selection pressure for resistance' than pyrimethamine–sulfadoxine. There is no experience of the use of Lapdap to treat non-immune patients, and the drug is not recommended for this group. In line with the strong arguments for 'combination therapy', work has started to manufacture a chloroproguanil–dapsone–artesunate triple combination tablet.

## QUININE

Quinine is an effective replacement for chloroquine and is a drug of choice for non-immune patients in most areas where multidrug-resistant strains of *P. falciparum* are prevalent. However, it has the disadvantages that it must be taken three times a day for 7 days, tastes bitter and produces unpleasant symptoms at normal therapeutic dose (cinchonism– see above). This creates severe problems with compliance. In some countries, a short course (3–5 days) of quinine followed by a single dose of pyrimethamine–sulphonamide or a short course of clindamycin is effective

In those parts of South-east Asia where parasite sensitivity to quinine is declining and where few alternatives are available, cure rates are improved if the drug is combined with tetracycline: 250 mg is usually given four times daily for 7 days. Tetracycline is contraindicated in children and pregnant women, but combinations of quinine with clindamycin have been used successfully, with treatment courses as short as 3 days.

## MEFLOQUINE

Mefloquine, given as a single dose of 15–25 mg base/kg or in divided doses 6–8 hours apart to reduce the risk of vomiting, was initially highly effective against multiresistant strains of falciparum malaria throughout the world. However, in some areas, notably in the border regions of Thailand, mefloquine resistance has developed rapidly and a combination of melfoquine with artesunate is currently used. A proportion of patients (varying from 5 to 50 per cent in different studies) suffer unpleasant gastrointestinal symptoms (nausea, vomiting, colicky abdominal pain and diarrhoea) and dizziness after taking mefloquine, and a few develop more severe symptoms (see above).

## HALOFANTRINE

Halofantrine causes dose-related prolongation of the ECG QTc interval and may induce fatal arrhythmias in susceptible individuals, making it too dangerous to administer under most circumstances.

## PROGUANIL HYDROCHLORIDE WITH ATOVAQUONE (MALARONE)

This new combination treatment contains 100 mg of proguanil and 250 mg of atovaquone in each tablet. In an adult dose of four tablets once daily for 3 days, it has proved highly effective against uncomplicated multidrug-resistant falciparum malaria in Thailand and elsewhere. However, there are concerns about whether the combination with proguanil will be effective in preventing the development of resistance, which happened so rapidly (within the space of a single infection) when atovaquone was used alone.

## ARTEMETHER WITH LUMEFANTRINE (BENFLUMETOL) (RIAMET, CO-ARTEMETHER)

This recently marketed combination drug contains 20 mg of artemether and 120 mg of lumefantrine in each tablet. The six-dose regimen (adult dose four tablets twice a day for 3 days) proved effective in multi drug-resistant falciparum malaria in northwestern Thailand and Africa. Cure rates were almost as good as with artesunate–mefloquine in Thailand and Fansidar in Africa. Artemether–lumefantrine was better tolerated than regimens containing mefloquine and there was no evidence of neurotoxicity or cardiotoxicity.

## TOLERABILITY OF INGESTED ANTIMALARIAL DRUGS

Most antimalarial drugs taste very bitter and must be given with a generous drink of milk (but not with tetracyclines!), fruit juice or other flavoured fluid. Feverish patients who are ill with acute malaria may vomit the tablets, creating concern about whether the dose should be repeated. The risk of vomiting can often be reduced by insisting that the patient lies down quietly for a while and is cooled by fanning and sponging with tepid water and by taking an antipyretic such as paracetamol (acetaminofen). They may then be able to tolerate the antimalarial tablets.

The oral administration of antimalarial drugs to infants and children with malaria is particularly difficult. Some antimalarial drugs are available as syrups or flavoured suspensions, or tablets can be crushed and attempts made to disguise their bitter flavour with honey, jam or chocolate.

It is surprising that more effort has not been put into the development of suppository formulations of antimalarial drugs. Artemisinin and artesunate suppositories have been used with great success, even in patients with cerebral and other severe forms of falciparum malaria. Patients who vomit persistently will require treatment by injection, nasogastric tube or (where available) suppository. If these patients have no other features of severe malaria, they may soon be able to continue treatment by mouth.

## ANCILLARY TREATMENT OF UNCOMPLICATED MALARIA

Rehydration is important, especially in hot climates where febrile patients may become dehydrated rapidly and children and pregnant women, whose tolerance of fasting is limited, may become hypoglycaemic. Mothers should be encouraged, through community education programmes, to give children with acute fevers oral rehydration solutions containing extra glucose, as in the home treatment of gastroenteritis.

Fever should be reduced by traditional methods such as removing the clothes, tepid sponging of a large area of skin and vigorous fanning. Paracetamol (acetaminofen) is the safest antipyretic drug; it can be given by mouth or suppository. Crushed tablets can be administered via a nasogastric tube. The few properly designed studies have failed to demonstrate more rapid fever clearance with paracetamol and this antipyretic is certainly no more effective than mechanical methods in relieving fever. However, the analgesic (against headache and musculoskeletal pains, which may be severe), anti-inflammatory and anti-emetic effects of paracetamol are beneficial and its use is recommended in patients undergoing treatment with antimalarial drugs and in conjunction with mechanical methods when the temperature rises above 39 °C. One study in children with uncomplicated falciparum malaria showed that parasitaemia was prolonged by paracetamol, but there was no evidence that this was harmful (Brandts *et al.*, 1997). Aspirin is contraindicated in children because of its assocation with Reye's syndrome and in patients of all ages because of its tendency to cause gastric bleeding. Injectable antipyretics such as metamizole sodium (Dipyrone) are widely used in developing countries, but the risk of agranulocytosis makes them unacceptable.

Patients with uncomplicated malaria are often found to be anaemic. The causes are often multiple and complicated, including the effect of repeated attacks of malaria, intestinal helminthic infections (especially hookworm), inheritable erythrocyte abnormalities, malnutrition and sometimes the haemolytic effect of oxidant antimalarial drugs. Treatment may be required with haematinics such as iron and folic acid, anthelminthics and, if safely screened blood is available, with blood transfusion.

## Treatment of severe falciparum malaria (Table 12.4)

### BASIC PRINCIPLES

- Treatment should be started immediately the diagnosis is proved or even suspected.

- A drug regimen should be chosen that is appropriate for the known local pattern of drug resistance.
- Dosage should be calculated according to the patient's body weight, rather than estimated.
- The antimalarial drug should be given parenterally wherever possible. Oral dosing (or administration via nasogastric tubes) is best avoided because the patient may be vomiting, there may be gastric stasis and drug absorption cannot be relied upon. Studies are in progress on the use of artesunate and artemisinin suppositories at peripheral levels of the health service, where parenteral administration may be impossible.
- A loading dose of quinine or quinidine should be given unless the patient has received parenteral quinine/quinidine or oral halofantrine within the previous 24 hours.
- Therapeutic response should be monitored frequently by:

   (i)   repeated clinical assessment
   (ii)  examination of blood films
   (iii) measurement of blood glucose, temperature, pulse and blood pressure.

- Drugs should be given orally as soon as patients are able to swallow and retain tablets.

### CLINICAL USE OF ANTIMALARIAL DRUGS (see Table 12.3)

Quinine has been the first-choice antimalarial drug for severe malaria since resistance to chloroquine became widespread. However, powerful clinical trials published between 1996 and 1998 have shown that intramuscular artemether is as effective as quinine and possibly more effective in South-east Asian adults (The Artemether–quinine Meta-analysis Study Group, 2001).

**Table 12.4** *Principles of management of severe falciparum malaria*

1. Suspect and attempt to confirm diagnosis
2. Make rapid clinical assessment, take blood etc. for laboratory investigations, check blood sugar and weigh the patient
3. Start appropriate parenteral antimalarial chemotherapy (or artemisinins by suppository)
4. Transfer to highest available level of medical care
5. Treat convulsions (cerebral malaria)
6. Detect complications such as hyperpyrexia and hypoglycaemia by monitoring and treat them
7. Correct fluid, electrolyte and acid–base imbalance
8. Nurse the patient appropriately (e.g. comatose patients on their side, clear airway, turn frequently)
9. Avoid harmful ancillary treatments such as corticosteroids, heparin etc.

## Quinine

Severe falciparum malaria in adults and children is treated with parenteral quinine until oral drugs can be taken. Severe malaria has a grave prognosis if treatment is delayed or inadequate, and quinine may be the only reliable drug available. The only contraindication to the use of quinine is reliable evidence of serious quinine allergy. Haemolysis, pregnancy, jaundice and renal failure are not contraindications.

Quinine has a narrow therapeutic range, and doses should always be adjusted for body weight (see Table 12.3); even unconscious patients should be weighed wherever possible. A loading dose should be given to achieve therapeutic concentrations more rapidly. There is some evidence from clinical trials of the clinical benefit of a loading dose, but the practice is based largely upon sound pharmacokinetic data and empirical medical practice. Contraindications to the use of a loading dose are:

- treatment with quinine or quinidine in the previous 24 hours
- treatment with halofantrine in the previous 24 hours.

Appropriate and safe dosage of quinine is least certain in very fat, very thin and elderly patients.

If patients develop severe malaria following mefloquine treatment, a full dose of quinine should be given. There is no evidence that mefloquine and quinine in combination are cardiotoxic. However, if a therapeutic dose of mefloquine has been taken in the 12 hours before starting treatment for severe malaria with quinine, ECG monitoring is advisable.

Quinine must never be given as a bolus intravenous injection; the risk of serious adverse reactions, including shock and arrhythmias, is high. The preferred means of administration is by slow, constant-rate infusion of the drug diluted in crystalloid solution (normal saline, 5 per cent dextrose, dextrose–saline or Ringer's solution). Delivery is best undertaken using either an infusion pump or a burette. Neither may be available, in which case the drug may be added to intravenous fluid in the bag. This may be difficult in young children because of the need for caution with fluid volumes.

If intravenous administration is impossible, quinine may be given intramuscularly; the doses are identical to those used intravenously. Coagulopathy is a relative contraindication to this route, but quinine is absorbed reliably, even in the sickest patients. The dose should be diluted (up to 1:5 v:v) with water for injections, as undiluted quinine dihydrochloride 300 mg/mL has a pH of 2 and is very painful. The loading dose should be divided between two or more sites. The skin of the anterolateral thigh should be cleaned with disinfectant and the injections should be given deep using a 1.5-inch (3.8-cm) long 21-gauge needle (in adults). These injections are painful if the patient is conscious. Severe tetanus has been associated with the use of intramuscular quinine and so meticulous cleaning of the skin is essential.

Maintenance quinine doses are usually given every 8 hours, but in African children 12-hourly maintenance is effective. In South-east Asia, quinine (combined with either tetracycline or clindamycin) is given for 7 days; shorter courses are associated with recrudescences. Courses are generally shorter in semi-immune African patients (5 days being standard in many countries), and combination with antibiotics or sulphonamide–pyrimethamine is not usual.

To prevent the accumulation of quinine, the maintenance dose should be reduced to one half after 48 hours of parenteral treatment, unless the patient is fit enough to switch to oral treatment. If it is possible to monitor plasma quinine/quinidine concentrations, the maintenance dose should be reduced if, at any stage, plasma concentrations exceed 15 mg/L (45 $\mu$mol/L).

Frequent blood glucose measurements are mandatory for patients on parenteral quinine because of the risk of drug-induced hypoglycaemia. The preferred frequency of measurement varies between cases and clinical judgement should be used. If possible, blood slides should be examined 6-hourly and a quantitative parasite count done (see Chapter 3). Parasite counts often remain unchanged, and may rise, during the first 18–24 hours of treatment with quinine; this is not reliable evidence for drug failure. After 24 hours of treatment, counts usually fall in a log-normal manner and asexual parasitaemia should disappear within 5 days (gametocytes may persist, but they are non-pathogenic and of no clinical, although of some public health, relevance). A rising, or unchanging, parasite count after 24 hours of quinine treatment may indicate drug resistance; this is particularly likely in infections acquired in South-east Asia.

In the USA, parenteral quinidine gluconate is currently regarded as the drug of choice for the treatment of severe *P. falciparum* malaria. The Centers for Disease Control Drug Service stopped supplying parenteral quinine dihydrochloride in 1991. Quinidine gluconate injection is often stocked by hospitals in the USA and continental Europe (but rarely in Britain) for the treatment of cardiac arrhythmias, and it can be used if there is likely to be any delay in obtaining parenteral quinine.

## Artemisinins

A meta-analysis has been carried out on the results of randomized comparisons of artemether with quinine in nearly 2000 patients suffering from cerebral and other severe forms of malaria in Africa, South-east Asia and Papua New Guinea (The Artemether–quinine Meta-analysis Study Group, 2001). Overall, there were no statistically significant differences between the two treatment groups in case fatality (artemether 14 per cent versus quinine 17 per cent, $p = 0.08$), coma recovery in patients with cerebral malaria, fever clearance times or the development of neurological sequelae. However, combined 'adverse outcome' (death or sequelae) was significantly less common in the artemether group ($p = 0.02$) and treatment with artemether was associated with a significantly faster parasite clearance ($p < 0.001$). Subgroup analyses by age and region suggested that, in adults and in Asian patients, artemether was significantly more effective than quinine in reducing mortality, perhaps explained partly by the greater prevalence of quinine resistance in Asia. These studies, the most powerful ever attempted in the history of antimalarial chemotherapy, indicated that artemether was a safe and effective alternative to quinine for the treatment of severe falciparum malaria in adults and children.

*Artemisinins for intramuscular injection* There is most clinical experience with the oil-based formulation of artemether that is now widely used throughout South-east Asia. Arteether is also being developed. Absorption may be seriously reduced in severely ill and especially shocked patients, as was observed during the early use of this drug in China. Water-soluble artesunate has the theoretical advantage of being less neurotoxic in animal models than oil-based formulations, but has the disadvantage of being unstable once reconstituted with bicarbonate. It is rapidly absorbed after intramuscular administration.

Artemether is usually dispensed in 1-mL ampoules containing 80 mg artemether in peanut oil. Artesunate is dispensed as dry artesunic acid powder, which is dissolved in 0.6 mL of 5 per cent sodium bicarbonate immediately before dilution in 3–5 mL of 5 per cent dextrose solution for intramuscular or intravenous injection.

An initial loading dose of both drugs is recommended, followed by once-daily administration of the maintenance dose for at least 3 days or until an oral formulation of an artemisinin or another antimalarial drug can be taken by mouth.

*Artemisinins for intravenous injection* Currently, only artesunate is available for intravenous administration, but there is no parenteral formulation produced to good manufacturing standards. Formulations of artenilic acid and dihydroartemisinin are also being developed for intravenous administration. A loading dose of artesunate, reconstituted as described above, is given by intravenous 'push' (bolus) injection followed by a maintenance dose given at 12 and 24 hours and then daily to complete 7 days of treatment.

In principle, artemisinin derivatives should never be used alone in the treatment of malaria to protect them against development of resistance.

*Artemisinins for rectal administration* Suppositories of artemisinin and artesunate have proved effective in adults and children with cerebral and other forms of severe malaria in China and South-east Asian countries. Although plasma concentration profiles are more erratic than with intravenous administration, inadequate absorption is unusual. This is a particularly promising route of administration for use at the most peripheral level of the health service. If malaria is suspected or confirmed in a patient with an acute fever who is unable to swallow tablets, these suppositories may prevent the evolution to severe disease. However, immediate use of artemisinin/artesunate suppositories should not discourage transfer to a hospital, when this is feasible.

If parenteral or rectal administration is not possible, patients with severe malaria should be encouraged to take oral drugs, particularly oral formulations of the rapid-acting artesunate and artemether.

Close surveillance of many thousands of patients treated with artemisinin derivatives has failed to reveal evidence of neurotoxicity or other serious effects. These drugs are usually very well tolerated. No deleterious effects have been detected in pregnant women or their babies.

### Sulfadoxine–pyrimethamine

A formulation containing 500 mg sulfadoxine and 25 mg pyrimethamine in a 2.5-mL ampoule has proved effective in a single dose for children and adults in parts of Africa, Thailand and Brazil. For severe malaria, it should be used only when effective alternatives are not available or cannot be given safely or when single-dose treatment is of particular advantage.

### Chloroquine

In geographical areas where *P. falciparum* remains fully sensitive to chloroquine, this drug is more rapidly effective than quinine. However, chloroquine should not be used unless the origin of the infection is known beyond doubt to be from Central America north-west of the Panama Canal or the islands of Hispaniola (Haiti and the Dominican Republic). The dangers of chloroquine's rapid absorption and distribution after parenteral administration should be borne in mind. Safe regimens involve continuous intravenous infusion over 30 hours or 6-hourly intramuscular or subcutaneous injections of the low dose of 3.5 mg base/kg.

## ANCILLARY TREATMENT OF SEVERE FALCIPARUM MALARIA (see Table 12.4)

## Hyperpyrexia

Ideally, core (rectal) temperature should be monitored continuously and should not be allowed to rise above 39 °C as such temperatures are associated with clinical deterioration, febrile convulsions in children and fetal distress in pregnant women. Methods of lowering the body temperature are described above. In the intensive care unit, the temperature of inspired gases, intravenous fluids, peritoneal dialysate and haemofiltrate can be reduced to aid cooling.

## Cerebral malaria

### CARE OF THE COMATOSE PATIENT

Unconscious patients should be nursed on their sides as vomiting is common and aspiration pneumonia is a common mode of death. A nasogastric tube should be passed and the stomach contents sucked out at frequent intervals to reduce the risk of aspiration. Patients should be turned regularly, at intervals of not more than 2 hours, and pressure areas carefully protected (Figure 12.5). The airway should be maintained by positioning of the head and jaw and, if necessary, with a rigid oral airway or even a cuffed endotracheal tube. Vital signs, level of consciousness (Glasgow Coma Scale – see Tables 7.4 and 8.3) and occurrence of convulsions should be recorded frequently.

### ANTICONVULSANTS

In adults, a single intramuscular dose of phenobarbital sodium (3.5 mg/kg) reduced the incidence of seizures four-fold without improving mortality, but, in African children, use of the much higher dose of 20 mg/kg was associated with a halving of the incidence of seizures but a doubling of case fatality, presumably due to respiratory depression (Crawley *et al.*, 2000). This intervention is not recommended. Generalized convulsions occur in about 20 per cent of adults with cerebral malaria. They are potentially harmful, leading to sustained neurological deterioration or aspiration pneumonia. Seizures must be treated promptly with a benzodiazepine drug such as diazepam (adult dose 10 mg by slow intravenous injection), chlormethiazole or lorazepam. There is a danger of inducing severe respiratory depression. Convulsions should always raise the possibility of hyperthermia or hypoglycaemia.

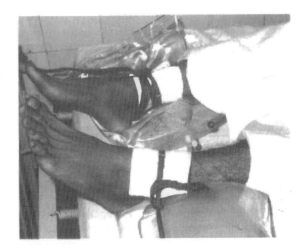

**Figure 12.5** *Protection of pressure areas: a clever makeshift device to protect a comatose patient's heels from pressure sores in use in a Vietnamese hospital. (Copyright DA Warrell.)*

## BRAIN SWELLING AND CEREBRAL HERNIATION

Although brain swelling is not thought to be part of the primary pathology of adult cerebral malaria, it may develop during prolonged intensive care or terminally. Deepening coma and signs of cerebral herniation are indications for computed tomography (CT)or magnetic resonance imaging (MRI) scanning or a trial of treatment to lower intracranial pressure, such as with the intravenous infusion of mannitol (1.0–1.5 g/kg of 10–20 per cent solution over 30 minutes) or mechanical hyperventilation to reduce the arterial $P_{CO_2}$ below 4.0 kPa.

## USE OF CORTICOSTEROIDS IN CEREBRAL MALARIA

Corticosteroids, especially dexamethasone, were widely used in the treatment of cerebral malaria until the early 1980s and there has been great interest in the use of this ancillary treatment to prevent complications, especially deafness, and to reduce case fatality in bacterial meningitis. However, two double-blind trials of dexamethasone (2 mg/kg and 11 mg/kg intravenously over 48 hours), involving mainly adult patients with severe cerebral malaria in South-east Asia, showed no reduction in mortality but prolongation of coma and an increased incidence of infection and gastrointestinal bleeding. However, the evidence of inflammatory processes in African childhood cerebral malaria and the observation of raised intracranial pressure and brain swelling suggest a possible therapeutic role for dexamethasone in this particular group of patients (Warrell, 1999).

Low-molecular-weight dextrans, osmotic agents, heparin, adrenaline, cyclosporin A, prostacyclin, pentoxifylline, hyperimmune globulin, iron chelators (desferrioxamine) and monoclonal anti-TNF (tumour necrosis factor) antibodies have also been advocated for the treatment of cerebral malaria, but without adequate evidence and in some cases despite severe side-effects.

## SEVERE ANAEMIA

Where blood, competently screened for human immunodeficiency virus (HIV), HTLV-1 (human T-cell leukaemia/lymphoma virus type 1) (where geographically relevant), hepatitis viruses and other important pathogens, is available, transfusion with packed cells (90 per cent of plasma removed) or whole blood should be considered when the haematocrit falls towards 20 per cent. Exchange transfusion is a safe way of correcting the anaemia without precipitating pulmonary oedema in those who are fluid overloaded or have been chronically and severely anaemic. The volume of transfused blood must be entered in the fluid balance chart. Diuretics such as frusemide can be given intravenously in a dose of 1–2 mg/kg to promote diuresis during the transfusion. Even the survival of compatible donor blood may be greatly reduced in patients during the acute and convalescent phases of falciparum malaria. This is not caused by quinine-mediated haemolysis.

Where screening of transfused blood is inadequate and infections such as HIV are prevalent, the criteria for blood transfusion have become much more strict. Under these conditions, plasma expanders (colloids) and oxygen should be used and clinical features such as shock, cardiac failure, hypoxia and extreme lethargy, rather than an arbitrary haematocrit value, should be used as an indication for transfusion. However, a haematocrit of 15 per cent in a normally hydrated child or adult is probably an absolute indication for blood transfusion. High parasitaemia (a presage of massive haemolysis), active or predicted bleeding (for example in a woman about to give birth) and other severe complications are also powerful indications for transfusion.

## HYPOGLYCAEMIA

Hypoglycaemia must be excluded in all patients with severe malaria. Frequent monitoring of the blood glucose is necessary, especially for patients with severe or deteriorating symptoms. A therapeutic trial of 50 per cent dextrose (1 mL/kg by intravenous bolus injection) should be given if hypoglycaemia is proved or suspected. This should be followed by a continuous infusion of 10 per cent dextrose. In adults, hypoglycaemia may develop or recur despite continuous intravenous infusions of 5 per cent or even 10 per cent dextrose. When the use of repeated doses of hypertonic dextrose for the treatment of quinine/quinidine-induced hyperinsulinaemic hypoglycaemia is contraindicated (for example in patients with electrolyte disturbances or incipient fluid overload), the synthetic somatostatin analogue octreotide (Sandostatin) can be used as a single subcutaneous dose of 50 μg or a continuous intravenous infusion of 50 μg/hour (adult dose). Glucagon (adult dose 1 mg subcutaneously) must be given as well, for somatostatin blocks glucagon release. Hypoglcyaemia is easily corrected in patients receiving peritoneal dialysis or haemodialysis or haemofiltration.

*Metabolic acidosis*  Lactic acidosis is best treated by correcting hypovolaemia and improving oxygenation. Sodium bicarbonate may be given if the arterial pH falls below 7.0, but the value of this treatment remains controversial. Dichloroacetate, which activates the pyruvate dehydrogenase complex of many tissues, especially in skeletal muscle, by inhibiting the kinase responsible for its phosphorylation and inactivation, can reduce circulating lactate levels, but its efficacy in human malaria has not been established.

## DISSEMINATED INTRAVASCULAR COAGULATION

If there is evidence of coagulopathy (spontaneous bleeding, oozing venepuncture sites, incoagulable blood, prolonged prothrombin time or International Normalized Ratio, INR), vitamin K in an adult dose of 10 mg should be given by slow intravenous injection. Fresh-frozen plasma or preferably cryoprecipitates should be given and platelet transfusion considered if the platelet count is less than $25 \times 10^9$/L or the bleeding time prolonged.

## DISTURBANCES OF FLUID AND ELECTROLYTE BALANCE

Especially in tropical climates, patients with severe malaria may be salt and water depleted as a result of fever, diarrhoea, vomiting, high insensible losses and poor intake. Others, particularly those in renal failure, may be fluid overloaded because of excessive intravenous replacement. Hypovolaemia will lead to hypotension, shock, acute tubular necrosis and lactic acidosis, and circulatory overload may precipitate pulmonary oedema. Fluid therapy should be controlled by measurements of jugular or central venous pressure, which should be maintained between 0 cm and 5 cm (Figure 12.6). Mild hyponatraemia (plasma sodium concentration 120–130 mmol/L) is common in severe malaria and is probably explained by salt depletion. More severe hyponatraemia may be caused by inappropriate antidiuretic hormone secretion. Hypoalbuminaemia is common and may result in low plasma calcium concentrations. Hypophosphataemia is a feature of severe malaria and may be exacerbated by intravenous glucose therapy.

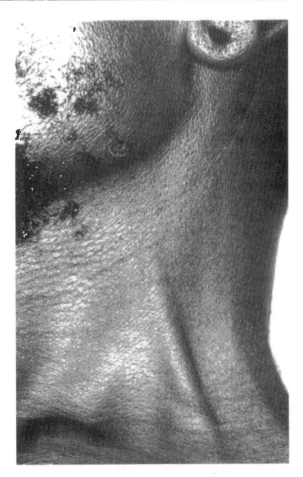

**Figure 12.6** *Observation of the jugular venous pulsation, in this case grossly elevated. (Copyright DA Warrell.)*

## RENAL FAILURE

Renal dysfunction is seen in about one-third of adult patients with severe falciparum malaria, but is uncommon in children. Serum creatinine or urea concentration and urine output should be carefully monitored. Most of these patients respond to a cautious fluid challenge of 20 mL/kg of 0.9 per cent saline intravenously over 60 minutes by increasing their urine output. In patients who have not been treated with diuretics, a urine specific gravity > 1.015 or a urinary sodium concentration < 20 mmol/L suggests dehydration. Patients who do not respond to the fluid challenge can be given an intravenous dose of loop diuretic (furosamide or bumetanide) and, if this fails, an intravenous infusion of dopamine (2.5–5 μg/kg per minute). Indications for dialysis (see Figure 12.7) or haemofiltration include

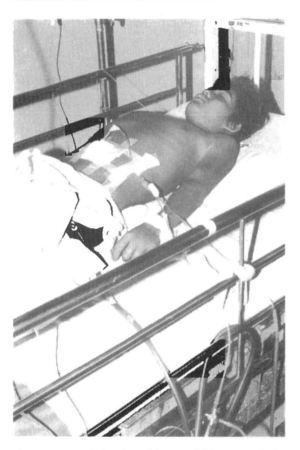

**Figure 12.7** *A Thai patient with severe falciparum malaria in acute renal failure receiving peritoneal dialysis. (Reproduced by courtesy of Dr RE Phillips.)*

hyperkalaemia, uraemia, metabolic acidosis and pulmonary oedema.

The treatment of massive intravascular haemolysis (blackwater fever etc.) involves correction of uraemia with dialysis and avoidance of fluid overload during blood transfusion, which is invariably necessary to maintain life. Quinine should be given in usual doses as the risk of untreated falciparum malaria outweighs the risk of quinine-related haemolysis in malaria.

### PULMONARY OEDEMA

This results from increased pulmonary capillary permeability (resembling adult respiratory distress syndrome, ARDS) or, less commonly, from fluid overload. Where facilities allow, the use of positive pressure ventilation with PEEP/CPAP (positive end-expiratory pressure/continuous positive airway pressure) to maintain adequate oxygenation and of haemofiltration to correct fluid overload can be life-saving. Elsewhere, fluid overload must be prevented by maintaining the central venous pressure between 0 and +5 cmH$_2$O, by nursing the patient propped up at 45° and by strict control of fluid intake. If pulmonary oedema develops, oxygen should be given by the most effective method available, a rapid-acting diuretic such as furosamide given by intravenous injection and, if all else fails, the patient should be venesected (see above).

### SEPTICAEMIC SHOCK ('ALGID MALARIA')

A secondary bacterial infection should always be suspected and blood, urine etc. should be sent for culture. Broad-spectrum antimicrobial treatment with an aminoglycoside such as gentamicin (for 48 hours only) with ceftazidime or cefuroxime and metronidazole should be started immediately. A less expensive combination would be gentamicin (for 48 hours only) with benzyl penicillin or cephalothin. Other causes of hypotensive shock in patients with malaria include hypovolaemia from dehydration or massive blood loss (e.g. ruptured spleen or gastrointestinal haemorrhage) and pulmonary oedema.

Treatment is the same as for septic shock: the correction of hypovolaemia and the use of increasing doses of dopamine (initially 2 μg/kg per minute) infused into a large central vein. Associated lactic acidosis and respiratory and renal problems are common.

### SECONDARY BACTERIAL PNEUMONIA

Aspiration or hypostatic pneumonia is a common complication and cause of death in severe falciparum malaria. Antimicrobial treatment consists of combinations of piperacillin or ceftazidime with gentamicin (for 48 hours only) and metronidazole or, if this cannot be afforded, benzyl penicillin or clindamycin or cephalothin.

### HYPERPARASITAEMIA

In non-immune patients, mortality increases with parasitaemia, exceeding 50 per cent at parasitaemias above 500 000/μL. It has been argued that exchange transfusion might reduce the parasitaemia more rapidly than chemotherapy alone and might also remove harmful metabolites, toxins, cytokines and other mediators and restore normal red cell mass, platelets, clotting factors, albumin and other depleted substances. These advantages must be balanced against the dangers of the procedure, including electrolyte disturbances (e.g. hypocalcaemia), cardiovascular complications and infection. The use of exchange transfusion has been reported in more than 150 patients. Some showed clinical improvement during or shortly after the procedure and most of the patients in the published reports survived, undoubtedly due in part to reporting bias. Manual exchange transfusion (alternating venesection and transfusion) and automated erythrocytopheresis (red cell exchange) have been used. There have been a few reports of ARDS developing during the procedure. Improved efficacy of exchange transfusion over optimal chemotherapy alone has not been proved and the rapid parasite clearance achieved by artemisinins may erode the putative advantage of this procedure. There is no consensus about the indications for exchange transfusion and, in most malarious parts of the world, it is impracticable because of the lack of adequate volumes of safe blood. However, where facilities allow, this procedure should be considered in non-immune patients who are severely ill, who have deteriorated despite optimal chemotherapy and who have parasitaemias in excess of about 10 per cent.

### RUPTURED SPLEEN

This potentially fatal complication of vivax and falciparum malaria must be suspected in patients who complain of abdominal pain (especially left upper quadrant), left shoulder tip pain and who become hypotensive and shocked. Free blood in the peritoneal cavity and a torn splenic capsule may be detected by ultrasound or combination therapy and confirmed by needle aspiration of the peritoneal cavity, laparoscopy or laparotomy. A trial of conservative management is increasingly favoured so that the spleen, with its important immunological functions, can be preserved. This involves blood transfusion, close observation in an intensive care unit and rapid access to surgical help should there be any sudden deterioration.

## RESISTANCE TO ANTIMALARIAL DRUGS

Antimalarial drug resistance is defined as 'the ability of a parasite to survive in the presence of concentrations of drug that normally destroy parasites of the same species or prevent their multiplication'. Drug resistance in malaria is a measure of the ability of the parasite to respond, through innate genetic diversity, to adverse conditions. Resistant genotypes with the ability to escape drug action survive chemotherapy at the expense of more sensitive organisms. All drugs represent a compromise between specificity and patient safety. The eventual emergence of parasite resistance is therefore the fate of all current treatments. The skill of malaria chemotherapy, as in other infectious diseases, is to use drugs in such a way that this selection process is minimized, extending the 'useful therapeutic life' (UTL) of the drug for as long as is practicable (Wernsdorfer, 1994; Plowe and Wellems, 1995; Peters, 1998).

## Mechanisms of parasite resistance

### CHLOROQUINE (AND OTHER 4-AMINOQUINOLINES)

The geographical extent of chloroquine-resistant falciparum malaria is almost coincident with that of the disease itself. Although isolated pockets exist where chloroquine-resistant fulciparum malaria is still rare, even in tropical Africa, resistance has been reported from all WHO regions except Central America and the Island of Hispaniola in the Caribbean. Continued drug use leads to a progressive increase in the degree of resistance, although in many cases treatment still reduces parasitaemia sufficiently to give clinical improvement (RI or RII response, in the old terminology, rather than RIII; see section on the *in vivo* test below). One of the most fascinating and unanswered questions about chloroquine-resistant fulciparum malaria is why resistance has not progressed to completion in areas where this drug has been used heavily for many years. The popularity of chloroquine for self-treatment, despite its diminished efficacy, explains why this drug is still the most commonly used antimalarial in Africa.

Chloroquine accumulates appreciably in the acid environment of the parasite food vacuole, where it interferes with the polymerization of toxic haem produced by the digestion of haemoglobin. In sensitive parasites, this leads to parasite death by haem poisoning. Chloroquine-resistant fulciparum malaria parasites accumulate less drug than sensitive parasites. This fact has generated two mechanistic hypotheses: the resistant parasite can either enhance the efflux of drug from the infected erythrocyte (Krogstad *et al.*, 1987), or reduce the initial uptake of drug itself. The latter hypothesis is at present the stronger, because it fits more closely with the known kinetics of drug movement into and out of the infected red cell. The finding that chloroquine resistance can be reversed by verapamil, an inhibitor of P glycoprotein-mediated drug transport (Martin *et al.*, 1987), focused attention on the transport homologues *pfmdr1* and *pfmdr2*, although initial attempts to link these genes with resistance were either inconclusive or negative. Reed *et al.* (2000) have recently conducted an elegant allelic exchange experiment with *pfmdr1* mutants, which confirms that mutations in *pfmdr1* are partially responsible for chloroquine resistance and a component of the verapamil effect, and also that these mutations increase parasite sensitivity to mefloquine and halofantrine. These data bring into question the conclusions drawn by Wellems and his colleagues following their classical genetic cross (Wellems *et al.*, 1991). They believed that chloroquine resistance was monogenic and linked with a 400-kb segment of *P. falciparum* chromosome 7. Within the original region, a 36-kb segment contained two genes, *cg1* and *cg2*, which were strongly associated with chloroquine-resistant falciparum malaria isolates from Asia and Africa, but not with sensitive parasites from the same regions. This suggested that African chloroquine-resistant falciparum malaria had originated in Indochina, and that it had a separate origin in South America. However, one Sudanese clone with chloroquine-resistant falciparum malaria polymorphisms and microsatellite markers was clearly chloroquine-sensitive *in vitro*, suggesting that another, complementary gene was involved in the resistance mechanism. The cg2 protein is localized in vesicle-like structures in the parasitopherous vacuole, not the plasma membrane, and does not have a structure typical of a membrane transporter protein; cg2 is not, therefore, simply controlling the entry of chloroquine into the parasite. The slow emergence of chloroquine resistance, in comparison with the rapid selection of resistance to the antifolate drugs, implies a multigenic mechanism. Interestingly, recent information would suggest that a gene positioned close to *cg2* is the major chloroquine-resistance locus, rather than *cg2* itself, although studies that have looked at the contribution of both *cg2* and *pfmdr1* genes, rather than a single gene, provide better correlation with parasite resist-

ance. The mechanism of chloroquine resistance is now being quickly unravelled, but the full picture is yet to emerge.

The only 4-aminoquinoline in clinical use, other than chloroquine, is amodiaquine. It is rapidly and completely metabolized to desethyl-amodiaquine (DESAQ), which is equally active against the parasite. For these reasons, Churchill has suggested that amodiaquine should be considered a pro-drug for DESAQ. In many locations in Africa, amodiaquine is more effective than chloroquine for treating malaria, suggesting a possible difference in resistance mechanisms. However, it is now apparent that differences in efficacy between 4-aminoquinoline drugs and their metabolites largely reflect differences in liposolubility; the degree of cross-resistance correlates well with the octanol:water partition coefficient. Amodiaquine and chloroquine share the same resistance mechanism and, although the degree of cross-resistance to amodiaquine is relatively small, the degree of cross-resistance to DESAQ (the active moiety *in vivo*) is complete. Whether the greater efficacy of amodiaquine has significant operational usefulness is still an open question, given the dangers of severe toxic reactions associated with frequent dosage.

## QUININE, MEFLOQUINE AND HALOFANTRINE

Although the P glycoprotein-mediated transporter genes appear not to be associated with chloroquine resistance, amplification of the *pfmdr1* gene has been associated with resistance to mefloquine, halofantrine and quinine in *P. falciparum*. In yeast, transformation of the *pfmdr1* gene confers resistance to mefloquine, halofantrine, quinine and the 9-aminoacridine drug mepacrine. The *pfmdr* genes, located on chromosome 5, code for a homologue of the mammalian P glycoprotein, termed Pgh1, which is present on the surface of the digestive vacuole of the parasite. The transfection study by Reed *et al.* (2000) confirmed a role for *pfmdr1* mutations in quinoline-methanol resistance. However, a simple explanation of amino-alcohol resistance, on the basis of a plasma membrane efflux pump, is not adequate in all cases, because resistance to amino-alcohols can be acquired by *P. falciparum in vitro* without any amplification of *pfmdr1*, increased expression of the Pgh1 protein or altered gene sequence. There are also theoretical difficulties in equating the increased chloroquine sensitivity that accompanies mefloquine and halofantrine resistance with a single protein model.

## ANTIFOLATE DRUGS

Resistance to the antifolate antimalarial drugs, as single entities, arose soon after their introduction into clinical use. Resistance to pyrimethamine in the *P. yoelii* and *P. chabaudi* models could be developed in a single step, and resistance of *P. vivax* to proguanil in Malaya increased several hundred-fold in 2 years (Peters, 1987). However, synergic antifolate combinations were more enduring. PSD proved an effective treatment for chloroquine-resistant falciparum malaria, including pyrimethamine-resistant infections. Similarly, pyrimethamine–dapsone (Maloprim), has proved a more effective chemoprophylactic agent than pyrimethamine alone.

Pyrimethamine and sulfadoxine both have long elimination half-lives. In the past, this was considered useful because these drugs could be administered in single dose for treatment and could be given once weekly for prophylaxis. However, long residence time in the body equates with a strong selective pressure for resistance, as new infections are exposed to eventual sub-inhibitory drug concentrations (Watkins and Mosobo, 1993). This was certainly one, and perhaps a major, reason for the short life span (approximately 5 years) of PSD in South-east Asia, and may presage a similarly short life in Africa, where PSD is now widely used. This is a particular cause for concern because PSD is the last of the affordable treatments available for large-scale use in Africa.

The mechanism of resistance to pyrimethamine and its analogues was shown to involve parasite DHFR with reduced drug affinity in 1970, although the pattern of cross-resistance between inhibitors was 'remarkably inconsistent' (Peters, 1970). With the advent of *in vitro* parasite chemosensitivity tests in the mid-1970s, it became possible to compare the activity of different DHFR inhibitors against laboratory strains of *P. falciparum*, and to examine cross-resistance in greater depth. One particular observation was the high *in vitro* activity that the biguanide metabolites cycloguanil and chlorcycloguanil retained against parasites which were pyrimethamine resistant, raising the possibility of drug-specific resistance mechanisms. Differential drug activity also offered an explanation for the effectiveness of chlorproguanil as a prophylactic drug in areas where pyrimethamine was completely ineffective.

Laboratory studies have shown that differential resistance results from specific mutations in the DHFR gene (Bzik *et al.*, 1987; Peterson *et al.*, 1988, 1990; Zolg *et al.*, 1989). The amino acid serine at codon 108 (Ser-108) is linked to sensitivity to both pyrimethamine and cycloguanil. A Ser-108 to Asn-108 mutation, the first mutation to appear in the field, confers resistance to pyrimethamine, but only slightly reduces sensitivity to cycloguanil. Subsequent mutations of Asn-51 to Ile-51, Cys-59 to Arg-59 enhance resistance, and Ile-164 to Leu-164 provides high-level resistance against both drugs. Analysis of the genotype and chemosensitivity profiles of *P. falciparum* field isolates has shown that Thr-108, which provides triazine-specific resistance, is uncommon (Nzila-Mounda *et al.*, submitted), suggesting that replacement of pyrimethamine by a biguanide inhibitor in synergic combinations may be advantageous.

Mutations in parasite DHPS correlate with *in vitro* sulphonamide chemosensitivity. Parasite lines exhibiting high-level resistance were found to carry either a double mutation, altering both Ser-436 and Ala-613, or a single mutation affecting Ala-581, and a fourth mutation at codon 437, which, although adjacent to the apparently crucial residue 436, showed no obvious correlation with resistance. A tight linkage was observed between DHPS mutations and sulfadoxine resistance in genetic cross experiments. Sulfadoxine susceptibility in most parasites is, however, strongly influenced by exogenous folate, suggesting that, *in vivo*, sulfadoxine susceptibility might be largely independent of DHPS status. In field studies, DHFR mutations at positions 51, 59 and 108 are widely correlated with PSD use and resistance, although this pattern is less clear for the DHPS mutations. The DHFR-164 mutation has not yet been reported in any of the African isolates, but is present in samples from South-east Asia and South America. The combinations of mutations that govern PSD resistance have yet to be defined precisely. However, DHFR mutations appear to be an essential requirement for PSD resistance, because parasites from cases of PSD resistance carry the triple mutant allele of DHFR with or without DHPS mutant alleles (Nzila *et al.*, in press).

## ATOVAQUONE

Atovaquone binds to the $bc_1$ complex of coenzyme Q (CoQ) in the malaria parasite with higher affinity than to the equivalent site in mammalian mitochondria.

However, *cyt b* gene sequence diversity is common in parasitic protozoa, including *P. falciparum*, and this is a potential mechanism for the resistance of *Plasmodium* cytochrome b to CoQ inhibitors. In phase II clinical studies of atovaquone monotherapy in Thailand, the cure rate to day 28 was 67 per cent, a significant rate of treatment failure, and the IC50 of recrudescent parasites was often 'markedly increased' from the IC50 of pretreatment isolates (Canfield *et al.*, 1995). In subsequent studies, atovaquone and the biguanide antimalarial proguanil were shown to be synergistic, and the combination, marketed as Malarone, was much more effective than atovaquone monotherapy against *P. falciparum* and against *P. ovale* and *P. malariae*. However, the possibility of early resistance development to the atovaquone–proguanil combination remains a valid concern, in view of the ease with which atovaquone-resistant *P. falciparum* can be selected by treatment. It has been argued that Malarone should be combined with a third drug, which has a different mechanism of action – the principle of 'combination therapy' (White *et al.*, 1999).

Recently, the molecular basis of atovaquone resistance has been reported (Cheng *et al.*, 1999). A unique single nucleotide mutation was found in the *cyt b* gene of parasites from a recrudescent parasitaemia following treatment. The fact that a different *cyt b* mutation could be induced by drug pressure *in vitro* demonstrates the potential genetic diversity at the target site. Both mutations were associated with reduced susceptibility to atovaquone, and related to putative atovaquone binding sites by molecular modelling.

# Geographical distribution of antimalarial resistance

## ASSESSING THE EFFICACY OF ANTIMALARIAL TREATMENT

### In vitro tests

Although 'in vitro tests' are still used to assess changes in parasite chemosensitivity in a locality over a period of time, the technology has not contributed much to malaria control. The reasons for this are complex. The tests themselves are robust, reproducible and provide reliable data, but they have not been employed widely throughout malarious regions, and use continues to decline. In part, this may be because the tests are complicated, time-consuming, and prone to failure. They are demanding in terms of the skills of handling parasitized blood and of maintaining controlled conditions for the 24 or 48 hours of culture. They also require a small volume of venous blood, which may be difficult to acquire under field conditions. The blood sample has to be cooled and transported to the field laboratory and the test set up within a limited time period in order to maximize test success rate.

As the molecular basis of drug resistance is identified for each antimalarial treatment drug, it is to be expected that *in vitro* tests will be replaced by molecular marker tests (Kublin *et al.*, 1998). Polymerase chain reaction (PCR) technology is far less demanding for the worker in the field, although just as demanding in the laboratory stage. The volume of blood required is minute; it can be collected on a filter paper strip, dried and packed into an envelope. The parasite DNA and RNA are completely stable, if dry, at tropical temperatures, so the samples can be transferred to the laboratory without the need for cooling – a considerable advantage. The test can be carried out at the convenience of the laboratory, because the test material is stable DNA, rather than fragile, viable parasites. This is a major advantage.

Some details of *in vitro* tests were provided in the previous edition of *Essential malariology* (Gilles and Warrell, 1993).

### In vivo tests

In the past, WHO *in vivo* tests were employed to assess response to treatment over 7 days (standard field test) or over 28 days (extended field test) (Gilles and Warrell, 1993). These tests were clinical, in the sense that patients were treated and clinically managed, but the entry requirements were imprecise: patients had to be infected with *P. falciparum*, but not necessarily to be suffering a clinical attack of malaria. Because asymptomatic patients are easier to find and to recruit than symptomatic patients, these tests were often a measure of parasitological response to treatment. The parasitological response is a useful assessment of drug action in the patient, and can reveal additional information on side-effects, patient compliance etc. However, for malaria control, especially in high-transmission settings, what is really needed is a measure of the efficacy of the drug as treatment for clinical malaria.

White (1992) suggested the necessary provisions of such a test. All patients, initially, are suffering from non-severe clinical malaria. Follow-up should differentiate between symptomatic and asymptomatic recrudescent infections, and the haemoglobin concentration should be used as an indicator of therapeutic response, because ineffective treatment is associated with a delayed recovery from anaemia. Patients previously treated for malaria should not be excluded from the test if the drug concerned is a 'genuine reflection' of drug-use patterns of the test population. The sample size for the test should depend upon the anticipated level of drug resistance, and therapeutic assessments should be stratified by patient age, to take account of the effect of malaria immunity.

Such a test is now available (WHO, 1996), and has become the standard WHO test method for monitoring therapeutic efficacy in treating children with uncomplicated malaria in areas of intense transmission. Recruitment into the test is dependent upon an initial clinical examination, parasite count, haemoglobin estimation and the use of a detailed list of inclusion criteria. Treatment starts on day 0. The clinical examination, including the axillary temperature, is repeated on days 1, 2, 3, 7 and 14. The blood-slide examination is repeated on days 3, 7 and 14, and haemoglobin on day 14. Therapeutic response is classified as an 'adequate clinical response' (ACR), or one of two failures: 'early treatment failure' (ETF) or 'late treatment failure' (LTF). An ACR is achieved if the patient is parasite-free and fever-free on day 14 and has not previously been classed as ETF or LTF. An ACR is still recorded if the patient has either parasitaemia or a fever, but not both, on day 14. ETF is defined by failure of the treatment to reduce both the parasite count and the fever within 3 days, under four precise sets of conditions. Similarly, LTF is defined by the return of parasitaemia with fever between days 4 and 14. The test method includes provision for quality control of test drugs and microscopy, for the recording of test results (usefully, on a single record page), for determining sample size and for adaptation to a 7-day or a 28-day test. The test is a major advance on its predecessors. Clinical response to treatment is the prime test outcome. The 14-day period is a sensible compromise between the time needed to 'trap' recrudescent infections and the practical and economic difficulties of maintaining teams in the field for prolonged periods. For drugs with very long elimination half-lives, e.g. mefloquine, for which a 14-day test is too short, the test can easily be extended.

## ANTIMALARIAL PROPHYLAXIS

Infection by any of the human malaria species produces symptoms which, in non-immune subjects, are at least temporarily debilitating and, in the case of *P. falciparum*, are potentially fatal. Every effort should therefore be made to prevent malaria.

## Avoidance of infection

None-immune people and other high-risk groups such as pregnant women, infants and young children, and people who are splenectomized or immunosuppressed should, if possible, avoid entering the malarious zone. Infection via blood transfusion should be prevented by screening donors or transfused blood (by microscopy, DNA probes or PCR methods) or by treating donors, transfused blood or recipients with antimalarial drugs. Malarial cross-infection in hospitals, by contamination of catheters and intravenous fluids, must be prevented. Most, but not all, of the anopheline vectors of malaria bite in or near human dwellings during the hours of darkness (see Chapter 4). The risk of infective mosquito bites can therefore be reduced by insect-proofing sleeping quarters or by sleeping under mosquito nets, preferably those that have been impregnated with an insecticide such as permethrin ($0.2 \text{ g/m}^2$ of material every 6 months). Bedrooms should be sprayed with a knock-down insecticide to kill any mosquitoes that may have entered the room during the day. Mosquitoes may also be killed or repelled by vapourizing synthetic pyrethroids on electrical heating devices (such as No Bite and Buzz Off; Bioallethrin 4.2 per cent w/w) or by burning mosquito coils. Ten to 35 per cent N,N-diethyl-3-methylbenzamide (DEET) is an effective repellent of mosquitoes, flies, midges, ticks, leeches etc. when applied to skin and clothing. Very rarely, skin application results in allergy, dermatitis and neurotoxicity in children (behavioural changes, ataxia, encephalopathy, seizures or coma) and adults (confusion, irritability and insomnia). Light-coloured protective clothing with long sleeves and trousers should be worn out of doors after sunset. Permethrin, or contact insecticide, can be applied to clothes and to other fabrics (curtains, tent walls, osquito nets) but not to skin.

Indigenous communities in many parts of the tropics have been protected by insecticide-impregnated bed-nets, screens or curtains, which can reduce the prevalence of parasitaemia and, among Gambian children, reduced malarial mortality.

# Chemoprophylaxis

The widespread use of antimalarial drugs for prophylaxis with the inevitably poor compliance and resulting underdosing has provided the selection pressure for the emergence of resistance to DHFRs, 4-aminoquinolines, pyrimethamine–sulphonamide/sulphone combinations and, most recently, to mefloquine. Over the last 40 years, the development of resistance to pyrimethamine, proguanil and chloroquine in particular has greatly complicated the choice of prophylactic drugs and the criteria for their use. These three drugs were remarkably safe, except for the cumulative retinal toxicity of chloroquine, whereas newer compounds, forced into use as a result of the declining efficacy of the original chemoprophylactic agents, have proved toxic. Amodiaquine causes agranulocytosis and hepatitis, pyrimethamine–sulphonamide combinations cause Stevens–Johnson syndrome and toxic epidermal necrolysis, doxycycline causes photosensitization and mefloquine causes gastrointestinal symptoms and sometimes neurotoxicity.

## PEOPLE REQUIRING PROPHYLAXIS

Those at most risk of contracting debilitating or life-threatening malaria are:

- Indigenous populations in malarious areas before they have acquired protective immunity (i.e. infants and children up to the age of about 5 years), pregnant women (especially during their first pregnancy), people who have been away from the endemic area for several years and those with certain types of immunosuppression.
- Non-immune immigrant workers, military personnel, game wardens and members of other task forces working in malarious areas.
- The increasing number of non-immune travellers and expatriates visiting or residing in malarious areas.

# Prophylactic drugs

More detailed descriptions of these drugs are given above.

Causal prophylactics prevent the infection from becoming established; most prophylactic drugs prevent the erythrocytic cycle by their blood schizontocidal activity. Recommended regimens of chemoprophylactic drugs and the choice of chemoprophylaxis and standby treatment for non-immune travellers in different geographical areas are given in Tables 12.5–12.7.

## BIGUANIDES

Biguanides such as proguanil are causal prophylactics for P. falciparum, P. vivax and P. ovale as they kill the pre-erythrocytic tissue (liver) stages of these parasites. They are also slow-acting blood schizontocides. They do not kill hypnozoites of the relapsing malarias. They have been used for prophylaxis, either alone or, more recently, in combination since the 1940s. Resistance developed rapidly in P. falciparum and has also been reported with P. vivax, but biguanides may remain active against the pre-erythrocytic stages of resistant parasites. Proguanil has most often been used in combination with chloroquine. The daily dose of proguanil has been increased from 100 mg to 200 mg, based on observations made by Bruce-Chwatt in Nigeria many years ago. He found that increasing the dose from one to two tablets daily significantly reduced the breakthroughs of malaria among oil company employees. Proguanil is also combined in a fixed-dosage tablet with atovaquone (Malarone, GlaxoSmithKline) and with chloroquine (Savarine, AstraZeneca). The increased recognition of side-effects of proguanil in recent years (reversible hair loss, mouth ulcers, scaling of the palms and soles, indigestion and diarrhoea) may result partly from the higher dose now used and its combination with chloroquine. Warfarin is potentiated by proguanil and in patients with severe renal failure there may be accumulation of the drug, causing megaloblastic anaemia and pancytopenia.

**The proguanil–chloroquine combination is acceptably safe, but is no longer a sufficiently effective prophylactic regime against P. falciparum in South-east Asia, Papua New Guinea, sub-Saharan Africa and the Amazon Basin.**

## PYRIMETHAMINE

Pyrimethamine is a causal prophylactic for P. falciparum and for some strains of P. vivax, but resistance is now so widespread that it is used only in combination with dapsone (as Maloprim or Deltaprim) or with

**Table 12.5** *Recommended chemoprophylactic regimens for non-immune travellers to malarious areas*

| Regimen | Dose for adult | Dose for child[a] (per kg body weight) |
|---|---|---|
| 1 Chloroquine | 300 mg **base** (2 tablets) once every week | 5 mg **base**/kg |
| 2 Proguanil | 200 mg (2 tablets) once every day | 3 mg/kg |
| 3 Proguanil + chloroquine (weekly) (doses above) | | |
| 4 Maloprim | 12.5 mg pyrimethamine + 100 mg dapsone (1 tablet) once every week | 0.2 mg/kg[b] + 1.5 mg/kg |
| 5 Maloprim (weekly) + chloroquine (weekly) (doses above) | | |
| 6 Mefloquine | 250 mg **base** (1 tablet) once every week | 5 mg **base**/kg[c] |
| 7 Doxycycline | 100 mg (1 tablet/capsule) once every day | (3 mg/kg)[d] |
| 8 Malarone | 100 mg proguanil + 250 mg atovaquone (1 tablet) once every day | Proguanil 2 mg/kg + atovaquone 6 mg/kg |

[a]See Table 12.6.
[b]Not recommended for children less than 6 weeks old.
[c]Not recommended for children less than 1 year old.
[d]Contraindicated in children less than 8 years old.
In all cases, continue for 4 weeks after leaving the malarious area, *except* Malarone: continue for 7 days.

chloroquine (as Daraclor). Deltaprim is used widely in Zimbabwe for prophylaxis for plantation workers and their families. Over many years of use, it has proved effective and no toxicity has been reported, even in pregnant women and children. Maloprim proved safe and effective in young children in The Gambia and, in combination with chloroquine (to cover vivax malaria), it was effective in the West Pacific area.

Pyrimethamine has been blamed for cases of nodular eosinophilic pneumonia in patients taking Maloprim and Daraclor. Dapsone given every day in higher doses (50–100 mg) for the treatment of leprosy and other skin diseases has caused haemolysis, methaemoglobinaemia, Heinz body formation, leucopenia, agranulocytosis and pseudoleukaemia. When used in a single adult dose of 100 mg/week in combination with pyrimethamine

**Table 12.6** *Antimalarial prophylaxis: doses for children*

| Age | Chloroquine 150-mg (base) tablet 5 mg base/kg weekly | Proguanil 100-mg tablet 3 mg/kg daily | Mefloquine 250-mg tablet 5 mg/kg weekly | Maloprim Pyrimethamine 12.5 mg Dapsone 100 mg |
|---|---|---|---|---|
| 0–5 weeks | 0.25 tablet | 0.25 tablet | Not recommended | Not recommended/ applicable |
| 6–52 weeks | 0.5 tablet | 0.5 tablet | | |
| 1 year | 0.75 tablet | 0.75 tablet | | |
| 2–5 years | 1 tablet | 1 tablet | 0.25 tablet | |
| 6–8 years | 1.5 tablet | 1.5 tablet | 0.5 tablet | 0.5 tablet |
| 9–11 years | | | 0.75 tablet | |
| ≥12 years | 2 tablets | 2 tablets | 1 tablet | 1 tablet |

**Doxycycline** 100-mg tablet/capsule:
  <12 years contraindicated
  12–14 years 0.75 tablet
  >14 years 1 tablet/capsule.

**Table 12.7** *Choice of chemoprophylaxis and standby treatment for non-immune travellers to malarious areas[a]*

| Geographical area | Prophylactic regimen[b] | Standby treatment |
|---|---|---|
| A  Armenia, Azerbaijan, Tajikistan (S border), Turkey (Adona, Side, SE Anatolia, March–November), Egypt (El Faiyoum, June–October), Iraq (rural N, May–November), Syria (N border, May–October), Mauritius (rural) | C/P | C |
| B  Afghanistan (< 2000 m, May–November), Iran (March–November), Oman, Saudi Arabia (except N, E and central provinces, Asir, W border cities), Yemen, United Arab Emirates (rural N) | C + P | F/M/Q |
| C  Sub-Saharan Africa including São Tomé, Principe, Madagascar and Comoro Islands | M/D/Malarone | F/M/Q |
| E  Mexico (rural), Central America, Haiti, Dominican Republic, Paraguay (rural, October–May), Argentina (NW only) | C/P | C |
| F  South America (except in E above and G and L below) | C + P/Malarone | M/Q/Malarone |
| G  Brazil (Amazonas, Mato Grosso, Maranhão), Colombia (< 800 m), French Guiana, Guyana (interior), Surinam (not Paramaribo and coast), Bolivia and Venezuela (Amazon regions only) | M/D/Malarone | M/Q/Malarone |
| H  South-east Asia including some areas of rural China, Sabah (except in I and L below) | M/D | M/Q |
| I  Thailand, borders with Cambodia and Burma (Myanmar) (except L below), western Cambodia | D/Malarone | Q/R |
| J  South Asia (Indian subcontinent, Bangladesh – not Dhaka, Sri Lanka – not Colombo, Nepal Terai – not Kathmandu, Bhutan, Indonesia except K and L below) | C + P | F/M/Q |
| K  West Pacific (Irian Jaya/Papua New Guinea and adjacent islands, Solomon Islands, Vanuatu) | M/Maloprim + C | M/Q |
| L  North Africa and Middle East (except in A above); South-east Asia – tourist areas and cities of Peninsular (W) Malaysia, Bali, Thailand, China, Sarawak, Hong Kong, Macao, Philippines, Brunei, Singapore, Maldives; South America – Uruguay | None | None |

[a]Revised November 2001.
[b]Prophylactic regimens see Tables 12.5 and 12.6.
C = chloroquine; D = doxycycline; F = Fansidar/Metakelfin; M = mefloquine; P = proguanil; Q = quinine; R = Riamet (benflumetol plus artemether).
Based on Bradley and Bannister (2001).

12.5 mg/week as Maloprim, serious toxicity is very uncommon, but mild haemolysis and methaemoglobinaemia are seen in children and in patients with erythrocyte enzyme defects (see above). The incidence of agranulocytosis is about 1 in 10 000 prescriptions at this dose, but may be as high as 1 in 2000 if the dose is doubled. Haematological monitoring is recommended for people taking Maloprim prophylaxis.

## CHLOROQUINE

Chloroquine is an effective suppressive prophylactic against chloroquine-sensitive strains of *P. falciparum* and other malarias, but does not prevent relapses of vivax or ovale malaria. For use on its own, chloroquine is now only suitable for areas where only vivax malaria occurs (for example Turkey) or for the few remaining areas where *P. falciparum* is sensitive to chloroquine. Combination of chloroquine with proguanil is described above. Chloroquine should be added to pyrimethamine–sulphone combinations in areas where vivax malaria is a problem.

Cumulative, irreversible retinal toxicity from chloroquine is seen after a life-time dose of 50–100 g base (i.e. after 3–6 years of taking 300 mg of base per week). Because chloroquine prophylaxis cannot prevent the establishment of hypnozoites in the liver and, therefore, relapses of vivax and ovale malaria, people who have been exposed to these infections for more than about 6 months should be given a course of primaquine for radical cure once they leave the endemic area.

## DOXYCYCLINE

Doxycycline has proved 87–98 per cent effective for prophylaxis against vivax and resistant falciparum malaria in Thailand and 93 per cent effective in Kenya. However, among US troops in Somalia, it proved five times less effective than mefloquine. Toxicity associated with prolonged use is uncertain, but recognized problems include photosensitization, gastrointestinal symptoms such as nausea, oesophagitis and diarrhoea (reduced by taking the capsules with a meal) and monilial vaginitis. Doxycycline and other tetracyclines should not be used in pregnant women or in children less than 8 years of age.

## AZITHROMYCIN

Azithromycin, an azalide antibiotic related to the macrolides, proved effective prophylaxis against falciparum malaria in Kenya in a dose of 250 mg/day. Side-effects were similar to those associated with doxycycline prophylaxis, but, unlike doxycycline, azithromycin could be used in children less than 8 years old and in pregnant women. However, this drug is expensive: in Britain, azithromycin prophylaxis would cost more than 13 times the cost of an equivalent course of proguanil and chloroquine.

## MEFLOQUINE

Early reports probably exaggerated the toxicity of mefloquine because comparative groups of subjects taking other antimalarial drugs were not included. There is also racial variation in the incidence of side-effects and women seem to be more vulnerable than men. Mefloquine will probably produce dizziness or gastrointestinal symptoms in about 5–10 per cent of people. The true incidence of neuropsychiatric complications is not yet known, but at prophylactic doses it is likely to be less than 1 per cent. It is now clear that other antimalarial drugs such as chloroquine can also cause psychosis and exacerbate epilepsy. Breakthroughs will occur unless the drug is taken every week in the recommended adult dose of 250 mg. The

rapid increase in resistance to mefloquine resulting from its uncontrolled use as a prophylactic now makes it unsuitable and ineffective for prophylaxis in border areas of Thailand and Cambodia. Despite the uncommon neurological side-effects, mefloquine prophylaxis has not caused problems in people such as airline pilots, drivers and soldiers, whose work requires fine co-ordination and spatial discrimination. Mefloquine is not recommended for prophylactic use in travellers known to be hypersensitive to the drug and in pregnant women. Dosage is practically impossible in children weighing less than 15 kg (less than 2 years old) because the 250-mg tablet cannot be divided into less than quarters. There is no convincing evidence to contraindicate mefloquine in people using beta blockers, calcium channel blockers or other drugs that may affect cardiac conduction.

## ATOVAQUONE WITH PROGUANIL (MALARONE)

Atovaquone with proguanil (Malarone) has proved effective in preventing vivax and multiresistant falciparum malaria infections in adults and children. Both components are causal prophylactic agents and therefore, after leaving a malarious area, treatment only needs to be continued for 7 days, rather than the 4 weeks required in the case of prophylaxis with (suppressive) blood sporontocides. Malarone is well tolerated (see above). One disadvantage is the high cost of the treatment. In Britain, the cost of Malarone is more than seven times the cost of an equivalent course of proguanil and chloroquine.

## PRIMAQUINE

Primaquine, in a dose of 30 mg/day, proved 94 per cent effective against falciparum malaria in Colombia, 95 per cent effective in Indonesia and 85 per cent effective in Kenya. Efficacy may be less against vivax malaria. The major disadvantage of this drug is that it cannot be used in people with inherited erythrocyte enzyme deficiencies such as G6PD deficiency and is not suitable for use in pregnant women or mothers who are breast-feeding.

## PORPHYRIAS AND ANTIMALARIAL DRUGS

People with acute intermittent and variegate porphyrias and hereditary coproporphyrinuria should never be given Maloprim, Fansidar, doxycycline, sulphonamides or sulphones as these will precipitate attacks. It is uncertain whether chloroquine and pyrimethamine are porphyrinogenic, but quinine and primaquine are safe and can be used to treat attacks of malaria.

## DRUGS NOT RECOMMENDED FOR PROPHYLAXIS

The following antimalarial drugs are not recommended for chemoprophylaxis: mepacrine, artemisinins, quinine, pyrimethamine–sulphonamide combinations (Fansidar, Metakelfin), amodiaquine and halofantrine.

## Principles of chemoprophylaxis

### NON-IMMUNE TRAVELLERS

Before prescribing chemoprophylaxis, a risk–benefit analysis should be carried out according to the algorithm (Figure 12.8). The risk of malaria infection, as

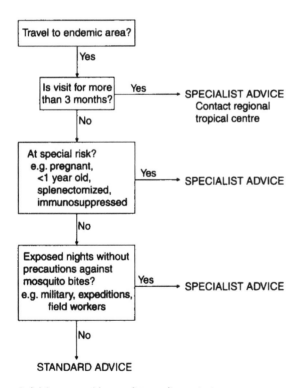

1. Advice on avoidance of mosquito contact
2. Warn traveller any fever may be malaria
3. Drug prophylaxis

**Figure 12.8** *A simple algorithm for malaria prophylaxis (adapted from Peto and Gilks, 1986).*

assessed by knowledge of the duration of foreign travel, itinerary and activities in the malarious area, and therefore the potential benefit of prophylaxis, is balanced against the risk of toxicity of the prophylactic drug. The following points should always be borne in mind:

- Although malaria may be widespread in a particular country, there may be a negligible risk of infection in the popular tourist sites. For example, although Thailand is a malarious country, the most popular tourist sites – Bangkok, Pattaya, Phuket, Chiang Rai, Chiangmai and Ko Samui – are malaria-free.
- No chemoprophylactic drug is totally effective, even when compliance is perfect, and all have some toxic effects. However, taking a chemoprophylactic drug may reduce the risk of severe and fatal malaria while not preventing infection.
- People who have been to a malarious area should see a doctor and mention the possibility of malaria if they become febrile or ill within a year of leaving the transmission zone.
- Malaria may be acquired during stopovers or while the aircraft waits at an airport in a malarious country ('runway malaria'), even though the country where the flight originated is malaria-free. Rarely, people living near an international airport in a temperate country may be bitten by an infected, imported mosquito ('airport malaria') and infection may result from routes other than mosquito bites.
- An alternative or supplement to chemoprophylaxis is 'standby treatment' (sometimes referred to as 'presumptive treatment'), to be taken if the traveller becomes feverish and unwell in a place remote from medical care and diagnostic facilities (Table 12.7). Rapid treatment with such 'standby drugs' or 'drugs in the pocket' may be preferable to chemoprophylaxis for those at increased risk of toxic reactions, such as pregnant women, young children and people with drug allergies.
- The cost of prophylaxis may be an important factor. In Britain, the costs of prophylactic regimens relative to chloroquine (adult dose 300 mg base/week) are as follows: chloroquine phosphate (=1), Maloprim 1, proguanil (200 mg/day) 11, mefloquine (250 mg/week) 19, doxycycline (100 mg/day) 20, Malarone (250 mg/day) 140, azithromycin (250 mg/day) 164.

- When to start taking prophylactic drugs:

  (i) Chloroquine, because of its slow elimination from the body, is accumulated. Higher blood levels may afford better protection and so it makes sense pharmacologically to start weekly chloroquine 1–2 weeks before entering the malarious area or to start chloroquine prophylaxis with a loading dose of 5 mg base/kg per day on two consecutive days and to continue with a weekly dose of 5 mg base/kg.

  (ii) Relatively toxic drugs such as Maloprim and mefloquine should be started 3–4 weeks before departure to allow time for side-effects to become apparent, in which case another drug can be substituted. In the case of Maloprim, haematological screening for haemolysis, methaemolgobinaemia and pancytopenia may be helpful. If primaquine is to be used, the recipient should be screened for G6PD deficiency first. The test may be negative if there has been recent haemolysis. Suppressive schizontocidal prophylactic drugs should have reached effective blood concentrations by the time that merozoites first enter the bloodstream 6–14 days after first exposure to infection.

- When to stop chemoprophylactic drugs: drugs (except Malarone) must be continued for 4 weeks after leaving the malarious area so that schizontocidal concentrations of the drug are present in the blood when merozoites emerge from the liver after a maximum prepatent period. Prophylactic drugs – with the exception of biguanides, atovaquone, primaquine and possibly pyrimethamine – have no effect on pre-erythrocytic (hepatic) forms.

- Apart from primaquine, the prophylactic drugs listed above cannot be relied upon to prevent the development of hypnozoites of *P. vivax* and *P. ovale* in the liver. After substantial exposure to these infections (for example 6 months), it is therefore worthwhile to give a radical cure with primaquine.

## CHEMOPROPHYLAXIS FOR INDIGENOUS POPULATIONS

There is reassuring evidence that, in children under the age of 5 years who are growing up in malarious areas, continuous prophylaxis does not suppress the acquisition of immunity. Some degree of immunity will increase the efficacy of chemoprophylactic regimens. Chemoprophylaxis of the two groups most obviously at risk of severe malaria – young children and pregnant women – remains controversial because of the increasing difficulty in choosing acceptably safe chemoprophylactic drugs and because poor compliance further reduces their efficacy. Other strategies in these groups are to improve the speed of diagnosis and treatment in peripheral paediatric and antenatal clinics and to institute anti-mosquito measures such as the use of impregnated bed-nets. However, it is clear from studies in The Gambia and elsewhere that many African children die of malaria without access to medical care and that even enthusiastic antenatal clinic surveillance cannot prevent the damaging effects of acute malaria in pregnancy.

Intermittent preventive treatment of pregnant women in Africa with one or two doses of Fansidar during the course of the pregnancy has reduced the incidence of placental infection and low birth weight and has had no toxic effects on the fetus or neonate.

## CHEMOPROPHYLAXIS FOR LONG-TERM, NON-IMMUNE EXPATRIATE RESIDENTS IN THE MALARIOUS AREA

Depending on the particular circumstances, long-term chemoprophylaxis with drugs of relatively low toxicity (and probably of only moderate efficacy) and/or early treatment of febrile illnesses with stand-by drugs may be recommended. The cumulative toxicity of chloroquine must not be forgotten. Ophthalmological checks are recommended within between 3 and 6 years of starting continuous chloroquine prophylaxis; after 6 years, an alternative chemoprophylactic drug should be prescribed.

## RECOMMENDED CHEMOPROPHYLAXIS

Recommendations are quickly overtaken by developments in the emergence and geographical distribution of drug-resistant parasites, in the recognition of new toxic effects of drugs, by changes in drug supply and in the global epidemiology of malaria. The recommendations given in Table 12.7 are therefore tentative and based on information available in November 2001.

# REFERENCES

Andersen SL, Oloo AJ, Gordon DM, *et al*. Successful double-blinded, randomised, placebo-controlled field trial of azithromycin and doxycycline as prophylaxis for malaria in western Kenya. *Clin Infect Dis* 1998; **26**: 146–50.

Artemether–quinine Meta-analysis Study Group. A meta-analysis using individual patient data of trials comparing artemether with quinine in the treatment of severe falciparum malaria. *Trans R Soc Trop Med Hyg* 2001; **95**: 1–14.

Beerahee M. Clinical pharmacology of atovaquone and proguanil hydrochloride. *J Travel Med* 1996; **6**(Suppl. 1): S13–17.

Bradley DJ, Bannister B. Guidelines for malaria prevention in travellers from the United Kingdom. *Comn Dis Publ Hlth* (PHLS, Colindale, London) 2001, **4**(2): 84–101.

Brandts CH, Ndjavé M, Graninger W, Kremsner PG. Effect of paracetamol on parasite clearance time in *Plasmodium falciparum* malaria. *Lancet* 1997; **350**: 704–9.

Brewer TG, Grate SJ, Peggins JO. Fatal neurotoxicity in animals due to arteether and artemether. *Am J Trop Med Hyg* 1994; **51**: 251–9.

Broom C. Human pharmacokinetics of halofantrine hydrochloride. Proceedings of the British Pharmacological Society Meeting, 12–14 September 1990, pp. 15–20.

Brueckner RP, Lasseter KC, Lin ET, *et al*. First-time-in-humans. Safety and pharmacokientics of WR238605, a new antimalarial. *Am J Trop Med Hyg* 1998; **58**: 645–9.

Bzik DJ, Li WB, Horii T, Inselberg J. Molecular cloning and sequence analysis of the *Plasmodium falciparum* dihydrofolate reductase-thymidylate synthase gene. *Proc Natl Acad Sci USA* 1987; **84**: 8360–4.

Canfield CJ, Pudney M, Gutteridge WE. Interactions of atovaquone and other antimalarial drugs against *Plasmodium falciparum* in vitro. *Exp Parasitol* 1995; **80**: 373–81.

Chang C, Lin-Hua T, Jantanavivat C. Studies on the new antimalarial compound: pyronaridine. *Trans R Soc Trop Med Hyg* 1992; **86**: 7–10.

Cheng Q, Korsinczky M, Chen N, Kotecka B, Rieckmann K. Mutations in *Plasmodium falciparum* cytochrome B that are associated with atovaquone resistance are located in a putative drug-binding site. Proceedings of the 48th Annual Meeting of the American Society of Tropical Medicine and Hygiene. *Am J Trop Med Hyg* 1999; **61**(3): 340.

Cook IF, Cochrane JP, Edstein MD. Race-linked differences in serum concentrations of dapsone, monoacetyldapsone and pyrimethamine during malaria chemoprophylaxis. *Trans R Soc Trop Med Hyg* 1986; **80**: 897–901.

Cosgriff TM, Boudreau EF, Pamplin CL, *et al*. Evaluation of the antimalarial activity of the phenanthrenemethanol halofantrine (WR 171669). *Am J Trop Med Hyg* 1982; **31**: 1075–9.

Crawley J, Waruiru C, Mithwani S, *et al*. Effect of phenobarbital on seizure frequency and mortality in childhood cerebral malaria: a randomised, controlled intervention study. *Lancet* 2000; **355**: 701–6.

Dollery C. (ed.). *Therapeutic drugs*. Edinburgh, Churchill-Livingstone, 1991, 314–17.

Dollery C. (ed.). *Therapeutic drugs*. Edinburgh, Churchill-Livingstone, 1999, A233–6.

Drysdale SF, Phillips-Howard PA, Behrens RH. Proguanil, chloroquine and mouth ulcers. *Lancet* 1990; **1**: 164.

Elueze EI, Croft SL, Warhurst DC. Activity of pyronaridine and mepacrine against twelve strains of *Plasmodium falciparum* in vitro. *J Antimicrob Chemother* 1996; **37**: 511–18.

Fichera ME, Roos DS. A plastic organelle as a drug target in Apicomplexan parasites. *Nature* 1997; **390**: 407–9.

Fradin MS. Mosquitoes and mosquito repellants: a clinician's guide. *Ann Intern Med* 1998; **128**: 931–40.

Fryauff DJ, Baird JK, Basri H, *et al*. Randomised, placebocontrolled trial of primaquine for prophylaxis of falciparum and vivax malaria. *Lancet* 1995; **346**: 1190–3.

Fryauff DJ, Church LW, Richards AL, *et al*. Lymphocyte response to tetanus toxoid among Indonesian men immunized with tetanus-diphtheria during extended chloroquine or primaquine prophylaxis. *J Infect Dis* 1997; **176**: 1644–8.

Gilles HM, Warrell DA. (eds). *Bruce-Chwatt's essential malariology*, 3rd edition. London, Edward Arnold, 1993.

Hatz C, Abdullah S, Mull R, *et al*. Efficacy and safety of CGP56697 (artemether and benflumetol) compared with chloroquine to treat acute falciparum malaria in Tanzanian children aged 1–5 years. *Trop Med Int Health* 1998; **3**: 498–504.

Helsby N, Ward SA, Edwards R, *et al*. The pharmacokinetics and activation of proguanil in man: consequences of variability in drug metabolism. *Br J Clin Pharmacol* 1990; **30**: 593–8.

Hien TT, Phu NH, Mai NTH *et al*. An open randomised comparison of intravenous and intramuscular artesunate in severe falciparum malaria. *Trans R Soc Trop Med Hyg* 1992; **84**: 584–5.

Hien TT, White NJ. Qinghasu. *Lancet* 1993; **341**: 603–8.

Hudson AT. Atovaquone – a novel broad-spectrum antiinfective drug. *Parasitol Today* 1993; **9**(2): 66–8.

Kaneko A, Bergqvist Y, Takechi M, *et al.* Intrinsic efficacy of proguanil against falciparum and vivax malaria independent of the metabolite cycloguanil. *J Infect Dis* 1999; **179**: 974–9.

Karbwang J, White NJ. Clinical pharmacokinetics of mefloquine. *Clin Pharmacokinet* 1990; **19**(4): 264–79.

Klayman DL. Qinghaosu (artemisinin): an antimalarial drug from China. *Science* 1985; **228**: 1049–55.

Krogstad DJ, Gluzman IY, Kyle DE, *et al.* Efflux of chloroquine from *Plasmodium falciparum*: mechanism of chloroquine resistance. *Science* 1987; **238**: 1283–5.

Kublin JG, Witzig RS, Shankar AH, *et al.* Molecular assays for surveillance of antifolate-resistant malaria. *Lancet* 1998; **351**: 1629–30.

Kuschner RA, Heppner DG, Andersen SL, *et al.* Azithromycin prophylaxis against a chloroquine-resistant strain of *Plasmodium falciparum*. *Lancet* 1994; **343**: 1396–7.

Lell B, Faucher J-F, Missinou MA, *et al.* Malaria chemoprophylaxis with tafenoquine: a randomised study. *Lancet* 2000; **355**: 2041–5.

Lobel HO, Kozarsky PE. Update on prevention of malaria for travelers. *JAMA* 1997; **278**: 1767–71.

Martin SK, Oduola AM, Milhous WK. Reversal of chloroquine resistance in *Plasmodium falciparum* by verapamil. *Science* 1987; **235**: 899–901.

Miller K, Lobel H, Satriale R, *et al.* Severe cutaneous reactions among American travellers using pyrimethamine–sulfadoxine for malaria prophylaxis. *Am J Trop Med Hyg* 1986; **35**: 451–8.

Milton KA, Edwards G, Ward SA, *et al.* Pharmacokinetics of halofantrine in man: effects of food and dose size. *Br J Clin Pharmacol* 1989; **28**: 71–7.

Mungthin M, Bray PG, Ridley RG, Ward SA. Central role of hemoglobin degradation in mechanisms of action of 4-aminoquinolines, quinoline methanols, and phenanthrene methanols. *Antimicrob Agents Chemother* 1998; **42**(11): 2973–7.

Murphy SA, Mberu E, Muhia D, *et al.* The disposition of intramuscular artemether in children with cerebral malaria; a preliminary study. *Trans R Soc Trop Med Hyg* 1997; **91**: 331–4.

Mutabingwa T, Nzila A, Mberu E, *et al.* Chlorproguanil–dapsone for treatment of drug-resistant falciparum malaria in Tanzania. *Lancet* 2001; **358**: 1218–23.

Nosten F. Artemisinin: large community studies. *Trans R Soc Trop Med Hyg* 1994; **88**(Suppl. 1): 45–6.

Nzila-Mounda A, Mberu EK, Sibley CH, Plowe CV, Winstanley PA, Watkins WM. Kenyan *Plasmodium falciparum* field isolates: correlation between pyrimethamine and chlorcycloguanil activity *in vitro* and point mutations in dihydrofolate reductase. *Antimicrob Agents Chemother* [submitted]

Nzila AM, Mberu EK, Sulo J, *et al.* Towards an understanding of the mechanism of pyrimethamine/sulfadoxine resistance in *Plasmodium falciparum*: the genotyping of dihydrofolate reductase and dihydropteroate synthase of Kenyan parasites. *Antimicrob Agents Chemother* (in press)

Ohrt C, Richie TL, Widjaja H, *et al.* Mefloquine compared with doxycycline for the prophylaxis of malaria in Indonesian soldiers. *Ann Intern Med* 1997; **126**: 963–72.

Peters W. *Chemotherapy and drug resistance in malaria*. London, Academic Press, 1970.

Peters W. *Chemotherapy and drug resistance in malaria*, 2nd edition. London, Academic Press, 1987.

Peters W. Drug resistance in malaria parasites of animals and man. *Adv Parasitol* 1998; **41**: 1–62.

Peters W. (1999) The evolution of tafenoquine – antimalarial for a new millennium? *J R Soc Med* 1999; **92**: 345–52.

Peterson DS, Milhous WK, Wellems TW. Molecular basis of differential resistance to cycloguanil and pyrimethamine in *Plasmodium falciparum* malaria. *Proc Natl Acad Sci USA* 1990; **87**: 3018–22.

Peterson DS, Walliker D, Wellems TE. Evidence that a point mutation in dihydrofolate reductase–thymidylate synthase confers resistance to pyrimethamine in falciparum malaria. *Proc Natl Acad Sci USA* 1988; **85**: 9114–19.

Peto TEA, Gilks CF. Strategies for the prevention of malaria in travellers: comparison of drug regimens by means of risk–benefit analysis. *Lancet* 1986; **i**: 1256–61.

Phillips-Howard P, TerKuile FO. CNS adverse events associated with antimalarial agents: fact or fiction? *Drug Saf* 1995; **12**: 370–83.

Plowe CV, Wellems TE. Molecular approaches to the spreading problem of drug resistant malaria. *Adv Exp Med Biol* 1995; **390**: 197–209.

Pukrittayakamee S, Chantra A, Vanijanonta S, *et al.* Therapeutic responses to quinine and clindamycin in multidrug-resistant falciparum malaria. *Antimicrob Agents Chemother* 2000; **44**: 2395–8.

Reed MB, Saliba K, Caruna SR, Kirk K, Cowman AF. Pgh1 modulates sensitivity and resistance to multiple antimalarials in *Plasmodium falciparum*. *Nature* 2000; **403**: 906–9.

Riou B, Barriott P, Rimailho A, *et al.* Treatment of severe chloroquine poisoning. *N Engl J Med* 1988; **318**: 1–6.

Roland PE, Mercer AJ, Weatherley BC, *et al*. Examination of some factors responsible for a food-induced increase in absorption of atovaquone. *Br J Clin Pharmacol* 1994; **37**(1): 13–20.

Rosenthal PJ (ed.). Antimalarial chemotherapy. Mechanisms of action, resistance, and new directions in drug discovery. Totowa, Humana Press, 2001.

Shanks GD, Kremsner PG, Sukwa TY, *et al*. Atovaquone and proguanil hydrochloride for prophylaxis of malaria. *J Travel Med* 1999; **6**(Suppl. 1): S21–7.

Soto J, Toledo J, Rodriquez M, *et al*. Primaquine prophylaxis against malaria in non-immune Colombian soldiers, efficacy and toxicity. A randomised, double-blind, placebo-controlled trial. *Ann Intern Med* 1998; **129**: 241–4.

Supanaranond W, Suputtamongkol Y, Davies TME, *et al*. Lack of a significant adverse cardiovascular effect of combined quinine and mefloquine therapy for uncomplicated malaria. *Trans R Soc Trop Med Hyg* 1977; **91**: 694–6.

Taylor DN, Wasi C, Bernard K. Chloroquine prophylaxis associated with a poor antibody response to human diploid cell rabies vaccine. *Lancet* 1984; **I**: 1405.

Trape JF, Pison G, Preziosi MP, *et al*. Impact of chloroquine resistance on malaria mortality. *Comp Rendus Acad Sci Paris* Series III, 1998; **321**: 689–97.

Veenendall JR, Parkinson AD, Kere N, *et al*. Pharmacokinetics of halofantrine and n-desbutylhalofantrine in patients with falciparum malaria following a multiple dose regimen of halofantrine. *Eur J Clin Pharmacol* 1991; **41**: 161–4.

Warrell DA. Management of severe malaria. *Parassitologia* 1999; **41**: 287–94.

Watkins WM, Brandling-Bennett AD, Oloo AJ, *et al*. Inadequacy of chlorproguanil 20 mg per week as chemoprophylaxis for falciparum malaria in Kenya. *Lancet* 1987; **1**: 125–8.

Watkins WM, Mberu EK, Nevill C, *et al*. Variability in the metabolism of proguanil to the active metabolite cycloguanil in healthy Kenyan subjects. *Trans R Soc Trop Med Hyg* 1990; **84**: 492–5.

Watkins WM, Mosobo M. (1993) Treatment of *Plasmodium falciparum* infections with pyrimethamine–sulfadoxine: selective pressure for resistance is a function of long elimination half life. *Trans R Soc Trop Med Hyg* 1993; **87**: 75–8.

Watkins WM, Oloo JA, Lury JD, *et al*. Efficacy of multiple-dose halofantrine in treatment of chloroquine-resistant falciparum malaria in children in Kenya. *Lancet* 1988; **2**: 247–50.

Watkins WM, Sixsmith DG, Chulay JD, *et al*. Antagonism of sulfadoxine and pyrimethamine antimalarial activity *in vitro* by p-aminobenzoic acid, p-aminobenzoylglutamic acid and folic acid. *Mol Biochem Parasitol* 1984; **14**: 55–61.

Watkins WM, Winstanley PA, Mberu EK, *et al*. Halofantrine pharmacokinetics in Kenyan children with non-severe and severe malaria. *Br J Clin Pharmacol* 1995; **39**: 283–7.

Weiss WR, Oloo AJ, Johnson A, *et al*. Daily primaquine is effective for prophylaxis against falciparum malaria in Kenya: comparison with mefloquine, doxycycline, and chloroquine plus proguanil. *J Infect Dis* 1999; **171**: 1569–75.

Wellems TE, Walker-Jonah A, Panton LJ. Genetic mapping of the chloroquine-resistance locus on *Plasmodium falciparum* chromosome 7. *Proc Natl Acad Sci USA* 1991; **88**: 3382–6.

Wernsdorfer WH. Epidemiology of drug resistance in malaria. *Acta Trop* 1994; **56**: 143–56.

White NJ. Clinical pharmacokinetics of antimalarial drugs. *Clin Pharmacokinet* 1985; **10**: 187–215.

White NJ. Antimalarial drug resistance: the pace quickens. *J Antimicrob Chemother* 1992; **30**: 571–85.

White NJ. The treatment of malaria. *N Engl J Med* 1996; **335**: 800–6.

White NJ, Miller KD, Churchill FC, *et al*. Chloroquine treatment of severe malaria in children; pharmacokinetics, toxicity and new dosage recommendations. *N Engl J Med* 1988; **319**: 1493–500.

White NJ, Nosten F, Looareesuwan S, *et al*. Averting a malaria disaster. *Lancet* 1999; **353**: 1965–7.

Winstanley PA, Watkins WM, Newton CRJC, *et al*. The disposition of oral and intramuscular pyrimethamine–sulfadoxine in Kenyan children with high parasitaemia but clinically non-severe falciparum malaria. *Br J Clin Pharmacol* 1992; **33**: 143–8.

Winstanley PA. Chemotherapy for falciparum malaria: the armoury, the problems and the prospects. *Parasitol Today* 2000; **16**: 146–53.

WHO. *Assessment of therapeutic efficacy of antimalarial drugs for umcomplicated falciparum malaria in areas with intense transmission*. WHO/MAL/96.1077. Geneva, World Health Organization, 1996.

World Health Organization. Severe falciparum malaria. *Trans R Soc Trop Med Hyg* 2000; **94**(suppl.): 1–90.

Zolg JW, Plitt JR, Chen G-X, Palmer S. Point mutations in the dihydrofolate reductase–thymidylate synthase gene as the molecular basis for pyrimethamine resistance in *Plasmodium falciparum*. *Mol Biochem Parasitol* 1989; **36**: 253–62.

# 13

# Malaria vaccines

STEPHEN L HOFFMAN AND JUDITH E EPSTEIN

## TARGET POPULATIONS FOR A MALARIA VACCINE

Many malariologists believe that different types of malaria vaccines may be necessary for different populations. Whether or not this turns out to be the case, we find it useful to think about the extremes of requirements for a malaria vaccine. One requirement is to reduce the incidence of severe malaria and malaria-associated mortality in infants and children with heavy exposure to *Plasmodium falciparum*, such as those living in sub-Saharan Africa (type 1 vaccine) (Table 13.1). At the other extreme is the requirement to prevent all clinical manifestations of malaria in individuals from areas with no exposure who travel to regions where malaria is endemic, primarily malaria caused by *P. falciparum* and *P. vivax* (type 2 vaccine). This 'extremes' approach to malaria vaccine development does not take into account specifically populations affected by malaria who fall between these extremes, particularly individuals in endemic regions at high risk of *P. vivax* infections. As type 1 and type 2 vaccines are developed, they will need to be assessed in many different types of populations.

For the type 1 vaccine designed to reduce mortality among children in sub-Saharan Africa, the problem is not as clear as one might think. In areas with extremely intense transmission, such as northern Ghana, it is primarily infants who are dying of malaria, with severe anaemia a major cause of death. In areas with less intense transmission, such as The Gambia, it appears to be 2–5-year-olds who are most at risk of dying, with cerebral malaria as the major cause of death. It is possible that different vaccines will be required for infants who would die of severe anaemia and for older children who would die of cerebral malaria (see Chapter 8).

The epidemiology of malaria must be understood in any given area in order to adequately design vaccine trials to try to reduce mortality. If most deaths from malaria are in 6–12-month-old infants, it would be foolish to do a vaccine trial in 2–4-year-olds. Likewise, if most deaths are in 2–4-year-olds, data on vaccine efficacy will be acquired most rapidly if we vaccinate 1–2-year-olds, not newborn infants. Furthermore, if certain groups in the population almost never die of malaria because of the genes that they have inherited, it makes no sense to include them in a vaccine trial aimed at determining whether a vaccine reduces mortality.

**Table 13.1** *Models for malaria vaccine development*

| Vaccine | Goal | Primary target population | Model | Primary mechanisms | Antigenic targets |
| --- | --- | --- | --- | --- | --- |
| Type 1 vaccine | Reduce the incidence of severe malaria and malaria-associated mortality | Infants and children living in areas with significant exposure to *P. falciparum* | Naturally acquired immunity: No deaths or severe disease after 10 years of age Decreased incidence, prevalence and density of infection with age | Antibodies (CD4+ T cells) | Parasite proteins expressed on the surface of merozoites and infected erythrocytes (B-cell epitopes) |
| Type 2 vaccine | Prevent all clinical manifestations of malaria | Travellers to malaria endemic areas with little or no immunity to *Plasmodium* species parasites | Irradiated-sporozoite immunization: Greater than 95% protection Protection not strain-specific Protection lasts for at least 10 months | CD8+ T cells (antibodies, CD4+ T cells) | Parasite proteins expressed by irradiated sporozoites in liver cells (T-cell epitopes) Sporozoite surface proteins (B-cell epitopes) |

For the type 2 vaccine designed to prevent all clinical manifestations of malaria in non-immune travellers to malaria-endemic areas, the target populations are also not as clear-cut as they might initially seem. One generally thinks that the major recipients of such a vaccine would be travellers from North America, Europe, Japan, Australia and other malaria-free areas of the world. However, there are hundreds of millions of people living in non-malarious areas who travel to malarious areas of their own country. For example, it is not infrequent for someone born in western Kenya, where transmission is high, to attend university in Nairobi, where there is no malaria transmission, and then get a job, get married, raise a family and settle in Nairobi. The children of these Nairobi residents are non-immune to malaria. When they visit their families in western Kenya on holidays, they are at high risk of contracting malaria and rapidly developing severe disease. There is very little mention in the malaria literature of the increasing numbers of non-immunes living in countries with endemic malaria who must receive short-term protection against malaria by a vaccine. Because of their susceptibility to rapidly developing severe disease, because they will not have the repeated exposure that could lead to boosting of vaccine-induced immunity, and because they are only visitors, we think that their parents would want them to have a vaccine with the same protective profile as a vaccine required by travellers from North America or Europe.

There is a third type of vaccine being developed, a transmission-blocking vaccine. This is not designed to protect the immunized individual, but the entire community, by reducing transmission intensity. We believe that such a vaccine will eventually be combined with the type 1 and/or type 2 vaccines described above. The target populations for such a vaccine are not yet clearly defined. Such a vaccine would unquestionably be of great value, perhaps even on its own, on islands with malaria, and in areas with only modest transmission. It might also be useful during prolonged epidemics. It is not clear how useful such a vaccine will be in areas like sub-Saharan Africa, where transmission is intense.

## WHY IS THERE NO MALARIA VACCINE?

Despite decades of effort, the goal of an effective malaria vaccine has remained unrealized. Infection with *P. falciparum* presents the human host with a formidable, protean foe. When *P. falciparum* sporozoites are inoculated into humans by *Anopheles* sp. mosquitoes, they circulate extracellularly in the bloodstream for less than 30 minutes before entering the liver. Within the hepatocyte, a uninucleate sporozoite develops into a schizont with more than $10^4$ uninucleate merozoites. These merozoites rupture from the hepatocyte and each can invade an erythrocyte, initiating the cycle of intra-erythrocytic stage development, rupture and re-invasion that leads to a 10–20-fold increase in the numbers of parasites in the bloodstream every 48 hours. These asexual erythrocytic stage parasites are responsible for the clinical manifestations and pathology of malaria.

There are a number of reasons for the failure to develop an effective vaccine (Figure 13.1):

- *P. falciparum* has a multistage life cycle, with stage-specific expression of proteins. Thus, even if a vaccine elicits high levels of antisporozoite antibodies, those antibodies will generally not recognize the blood-stage of the parasite's life cycle.
- *P. falciparum* has a large genome of 25–30 megabases on 14 chromosomes and an estimated 5000–6000 genes, for many of which allelic or antigenic variation has been demonstrated. A single individual can be infected simultaneously with at least eight different strains of *P. falciparum* (Felger et al., 1999) and a parasite protein expressed on the surface of erythrocytes (PfEMP-1) is encoded by 50–100 different genes, each with some variation in its sequence (Baruch et al., 1995). The parasite probably expresses only one at a time, thereby escaping from antibodies that recognize the first sequence. PfEMP-1 is thought to mediate cytoadherence of infected erythrocytes to endothelial cells in the microcircuation during maturation of the parasite, thereby preventing removal of the infected erythrocyte in the spleen during this vulnerable phase of its life cycle. Cytoadherence is thought to be responsible for the microcirculatory obstruction so important to the pathogenesis of severe disease (Brown and Rogerson, 1996). Thus, antigenic variation is critical to the parasite, and extremely unfavourable for the host.
- The complexity of the immune response to infection adds to the difficulty of developing a vaccine. Human host genetics, transmission dynamics of the parasite and, probably, even the age of the host contribute to this complexity. Although it is clear that sickle-cell trait protects against severe

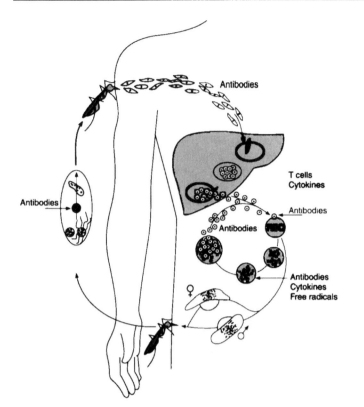

Reasons for difficulties in developing malaria vaccines include:

1. Multistage life cycle with stage-specific expression of proteins.

2. Large genome: 25–30 mega-bases, 5000–6000 genes, 14 chromosomes.

3. Allelic/antigenic variation.

4. Complex, genetically variable, human immune response.

5. Parasite adaptations to avoid immune response.

**Figure 13.1** *Life cycle of* Plasmodium falciparum, *primary protective immune responses expected at each stage of the life cycle, and reasons for difficulties in developing malaria vaccine.*

disease, and that other genetic traits may influence outcome, our understanding of the relationship of host genetics and the response to infection is very limited. The elucidation of the sequence of the human genome and the development of scientific tools to use these data should lead to a much better understanding of the role of host factors in determining the severity of disease associated with infection. The human immune response is also dependent on transmission dynamics. In areas where transmission of *P. falciparum* is most intense, infants are at highest risk of developing severe and fatal malaria, whereas, in areas with less intense transmission, older children have a higher incidence of severe and fatal disease than do infants (see Chapters 5, 8 and 11). The age of the individual may also play a role in determining the immune response. A number of reports have suggested that, among non-immune children and non-immune adults, adults are actually more susceptible than children to developing severe disease after their first

infection (Baird *et al.*, 1998). However, adults acquire immunity faster than children.

## HUMAN MODELS FOR TYPE 1 AND TYPE 2 VACCINES

Existing human models indicate the possibility of developing type 1 and type 2 vaccines (Table 13.1). For a type 1 vaccine to prevent death and severe disease, naturally acquired immunity is the model. If someone survives past a certain age in the areas where malaria is transmitted, they will become re-infected and clinically ill, but they will not develop severe disease or die (Figure 13.2). For a type 2 vaccine to prevent all manifestations of malaria, immunization with radiation-attenuated sporozoites is the model (Figure 13.3). Exposure of humans to bites by more than 1000 irradiated mosquitoes carrying *P. falci-parum* sporozoites in their salivary glands over 4–6

(a)

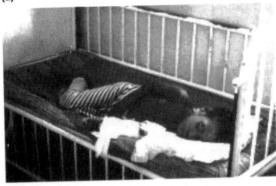

(b)

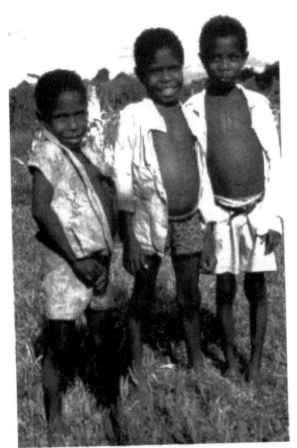

**Figure 13.2** *Naturally acquired immunity. (a) A child in Indonesia with cerebral malaria. (b) Children in Kenya (where up to 98 per cent of the population may have parasitaemia at any time) with recurrent* P. falciparum *infection. Children in Kenya who survive past 5–10 years of age have a very low risk of suffering severe malaria.*

months protects virtually all recipients against exposure to five infected mosquitoes 2 weeks after the last dose of irradiated sporozoites (Clyde *et al.*, 1973; Rieckmann *et al.*, 1974; Herrington *et al.*, 1991; Egan *et al.*, 1993). Thus, there is no genetic restriction of protection. The protection lasts for at least 10 months and is not strain-specific. Individuals immunized with parasites from Africa and challenged with parasites from South America are protected.

Attempts have been made to identify the mechanisms and targets of protective immunity in the human model systems, and then to develop a vaccine delivery system that induces the required immune responses against these targets. In the case of naturally acquired immunity and the irradiated sporozoite vaccine, the protective immunity in the model is elicited by exposure to the whole parasite. The aim is to take the parasite apart and create a vaccine composed of key components of the parasite – a 'subunit' vaccine. There are very few vaccines that have been developed this way, and none against an infectious agent as complex as *P. falciparum* or *P. vivax*.

Naturally acquired immunity provides an obvious model for a type 1 vaccine to prevent death and severe disease in infants and children living in heavily endemic regions. In areas with annual, stable transmission, neither severe malaria nor malaria-associated deaths are frequent after the age of 7–10 years. In areas with the most intense transmission, the transition to this immunity against severe malaria occurs even earlier, perhaps during the second to third year of life. Even adults become infected and develop symptoms attributed to malaria, but the incidence of new infection and the density of

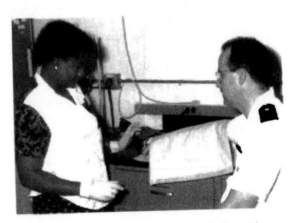

**Figure 13.3** *A volunteer receiving immunization with irradiated sporozoites.*

parasitaemias decrease with age. Antibodies against parasite proteins expressed on the surface of infected erythrocytes and merozoites and in apical organelles are thought to play a central role in this naturally acquired disease modulating immunity (Figure 13.4) (Hoffman *et al.*, 1996). However, biologically active molecules, including cytokines, nitric oxide and free oxygen intermediates, released from either CD4+ T cells after an antigen-specific interaction or from reticuloendothelial or other cells after non-specific activation, may also contribute to this immunity. The pathogenesis of the disease may be mediated by these same host-derived biologically active molecules, perhaps elicited by putative toxins released from the infected erythrocytes. Antibodies against these toxins may contribute to naturally acquired immunity. It seems likely that immune responses against sporozoites or infected hepatoctyes that limit the numbers of parasites that emerge from the liver into the bloodstream will also play an important role.

How rapidly does naturally acquired immunity develop? In *Aotus* monkeys, which are not a natural host for *P. falciparum*, the first exposure to infected erythrocytes of the FVO strain of *P. falciparum* is almost always fatal. However, most survive a second challenge, and all that do so will survive a third (Jones *et al.*, 2000). When patients with neurosyphilis were treated by infection with *P. falciparum*, a similar pattern was reported. A recent report suggested that, in areas with intense transmission of *P. falciparum*, immunity to fatal disease may develop after only one or two exposures to *P. falciparum* (Gupta *et al.*, 1999). However, this may vary with the transmission dynamics and epidemiology of the disease and requires further study.

The model for the type 2 vaccine, to prevent all clinical manfestations of malaria in non-immune hosts, is immunization with radiation-attenuated sporozoites. This would be an ideal vaccine for travellers, but it has been impracticable to immunize hundreds of thousands of people by the bites of thousands of infected mosquitoes. Considerable efforts have been made over the last 30 years to understand irradiated sporozoite-induced protection, and to develop a subunit vaccine that duplicates this excellent immunity. We believe that the primary protective immune mechanism in the irradiated sporozoite model involves CD8+ T-cell recognition of parasite-infected hepatocytes (Schofield *et al.*, 1987; Weiss *et al.*, 1988; Hoffman *et al.*, 1996; Doolan and Hoffman, 2000), although antibodies and CD4+ T cells may also play a role. The targets of the CD8+ T cells (and CD4+ T cells) are parasite proteins expressed by irradiated sporozoites within hepatocytes. Sporozoite surface proteins are the target of inhibitory antibodies.

The aim of a pre-erythrocytic stage vaccine is to prevent sporozoites from entering or developing within hepatoctyes. The irradiated sporozoite vaccine does not elicit immune responses against the major merozoite surface proteins. However, a pre-erythrocytic stage vaccine could be designed to elicit antibodies that recognized proteins on the surface of merozoites released from hepatocytes, and thereby eliminate parasites that have survived antisporozoite, and anti-liver stage blockade. Parasites that invade erythrocytes and begin the process of development will cause disease. A pre-erythrocytic stage vaccine that protected as well as irradiated sporozoite immunization and prevented all clinical manifestations of malaria would eliminate severe malarial disease and mortality while it was effective.

However, whether a pre-erythrocytic stage vaccine on its own would reduce mortality in children in Africa is unknown. If such a vaccine were perfect, it would certainly prevent disease and death, because no parasites would escape from the liver into the bloodstream. If it were less than perfect, substantial anti-asexual erythrocytic stage immunity would be needed. In fact, most of the intended recipients, including infants, are likely to possess some degree of anti-asexual stage immunity.

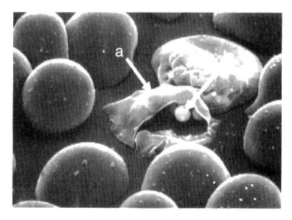

**Figure 13.4** *Antibodies against parasite proteins expressed on the surface of infected erythrocytes (a) and merozoites (b) are thought to play a significant role in naturally acquired disease modulating immunity. (Scanning electron micrograph of infected erythrocytes.)*

A difficult question is: what would happen if such a vaccine was perfect or almost perfect for a year or more, and then rapidly became ineffective? Would overall malaria morbidity and mortality worsen because recipients would not have developed anti-erythrocytic stage immunity (Snow *et al.*, 1997)? Fortunately, preliminary reports from long-term studies of insecticide-impregnated bed-nets do not suggest any delayed increase in morbidity or mortality. Because one could even characterize insecticide-impregnated bed-nets as being analogous to imperfect ('leaky') pre-erythrocytic stage vaccines, this suggests to us that a pre-erythrocytic stage vaccine has the possibility of being effective in reducing morbidity and mortality in young children.

We feel it is important to point out that naturally acquired immunity is not a model for a vaccine to prevent all clinical manifestations of malaria in travellers, because it does not prevent the development of blood-stage parasitaemia. The data included in Figure 13.5 were generated in 1986 in Saradidi in western Kenya (Hoffman *et al.*, 1987). Almost identical data have been generated recently in a study in Navrongo in northern Ghana. When adults who have lived their entire lives in areas of intense malaria transmission are radically cured of malaria, virtually all of them become re-infected within 4–6 months.

## THE CASE FOR A TRANSMISSION-BLOCKING VACCINE

During the past two decades, there has much interest in developing a vaccine that induces antibodies to attack the sexual stage of the parasite (gametocytes, gametes, zygotes, ookinetes), either in the human host or within the mosquito (Kaslow, 1996). If administered alone, such a vaccine would not provide any direct benefit to the recipient but could reduce transmission in the community ('altruistic vaccine'). Such immunity could also be extremely helpful in 'protecting' a type 1 or type 2 vaccine. For example, if the parasite developed a mutation within an epitope that allowed it to escape from potent vaccine-elicited immune responses, immunity against the sexual stage would reduce the chance that the mutant would be transmitted to other individuals.

Transmission-blocking vaccines could play a role on their own as part of a multifaceted strategy directed at the elimination of parasites from low-transmission areas, especially islands. Such vaccines will be important components of multistage type 1 vaccines designed to reduce severe disease and mortality in areas of intense transmission of *P. falciparum*, both by their direct anti-transmission effects and by their capacity to reduce the emergence of parasites resistant to vaccine-induced immunity against the pre-erythrocytic and asexual erythrocytic stages of the life cycle.

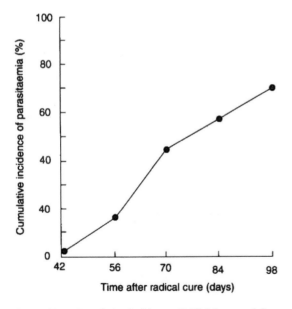

**Figure 13.5** *Cumulative incidence of* P. falciparum *infections from day 42 through day 98 in 83 Kenyan adult males treated with three tablets of Fansidar on day 0 and 100 mg of doxycycline twice a day on days 1–7. (From Hoffman* et al., *1987.)*

## CURRENT APPROACHES TO MALARIA VACCINE DEVELOPMENT

Currently, three general approaches to malaria vaccine development are being pursued:

- The most work has been done and progress achieved in attempts to maximize the magnitude and quality of immune responses to a single or a few key antigens, such as the circumsporozoite protein (CSP) and merozoite surface protein 1 (MSP-1), by immunizing with synthetic peptides or recombinant proteins in an adjuvant. These vaccines are being designed primarily to induce antibody and CD4+ T-cell responses, but there is also interest in eliciting CD8+ T-cell responses.

- The second approach is to induce good or optimum immune responses against all of the approximately 15–20 identified potential target proteins by immunizing with DNA vaccines and boosting with DNA vaccines, recombinant viruses or bacteria, or recombinant proteins in adjuvant. The goal is to elicit CD8+, antibody and CD4+ T-cell responses.

- The third approach is to try to duplicate the whole-organism immunity induced by immunization with radiation-attenuated sporozoites and natural exposure to malaria. Success in this area will be dependent on the sequencing of the *P. falciparum* genome and developing methods for exploiting this genomic sequence data. It remains to be established how such vaccines will be constructed.

## Current status of clinical trials

**Maximizing the magnitude and quality of immune responses to a few key antigens (recombinant proteins and synthetic peptides in adjuvant).**

### PRE-ERYTHROCYTIC STAGES

A number of clinical trials with pre-erythrocytic stage *P. falciparum* vaccines have already been completed and numerous others are planned or in progress. The Walter Reed Army Institute of Research (WRAIR) and GlaxoSmithKline Biologicals (GSK) have done extensive work on a CSP recombinant vaccine, RTS,S/AS02 (Stoute *et al.*, 1997, 1998). The vaccine is formulated with an oil-in-water emulsion plus the immunostimulants monophosphoryl lipid A (MPL) and the saponin derivative QS21. It consistently protects 40–50 per cent of volunteers experimentally challenged 2–3 weeks after their last immunization (Kester *et al.*, 2001). When five protected volunteers were rechallenged 6 months after the last immunization, only one of the five was protected (Stoute *et al.*, 1998). The first field trials with this vaccine have been conducted in The Gambia by the Medical Research Council. Vaccine efficacy (end-point defined as 'time to first infection') was 71 per cent (95 per cent CI =

46–85 per cent) during the first 9 weeks of surveillance but subsequently declined to 0 per cent (95 per cent CI = −52 to 34 per cent) in the last 6 weeks (Bojang *et al.*, 2001). The first trial of RTS,S/AS02 in a paediatric population (6–11-year-olds) began in The Gambia in May 2001. Efforts to improve the vaccine include use of better adjuvants and combination with other pre-erythrocytic and erythrocytic stage antigens.

A synthetic multiple antigen peptide (MAP) malaria vaccine developed at New York University, containing minimal *P. falciparum* CSP repeat epitopes, elicited high levels of parasite-specific antibodies and CD4+ T cells in volunteers of specific human leucocyte antigen (HLA) genotypes (Nardin *et al.*, 2000). More recently, this group, in collaboration with the University of Geneva, has demonstrated the immunogenicity of a synthetic triepitope polyoxime malaria vaccine containing B-cell epitopes and a universal T-cell epitope of PfCSP. In an open-labelled phase I study, volunteers of diverse HLA types developed anti-repeat antibodies and T cells specific for the universal T-cell epitope (Nardin *et al.*, 2001).

A carboxy terminal synthetic peptide from the PfCSP has been developed by the University of Lausanne. Based on a phase I trial demonstrating induction of CSP-specific antibodies as well as CD4+ and CD8+ T-cell responses (Lopez *et al.*, 2001), the European Malaria Vaccine Initiative (EMVI), in collaboration with researchers in Nijmegen, The Netherlands, plans to bring this vaccine into phase IIa testing at the end of 2001. Clinical trials with several *P. falciparum* liver-stage antigen 3 (PfLSA-3) constructs, including an LSA-3 long synthetic peptide, are planned to take place in Nijmegen in early 2002.

### ASEXUAL ERYTHROCYTIC STAGES

A number of human trials are planned or in progress of erythrocytic stage *P. falciparum* vaccines. The most work has been done with SPf66, which was developed at the Institute of Immunology in Bogota, Colombia. SPf66 is a polymer containing an 11 amino acid sequence from the N′-terminus of PfMSP1, the four amino acid repeat of PfCSP, and two other short amino acid sequences thought to be from *P. falciparum*, but not yet proved to be so. Initial trials in Colombia (Valero *et al.*, 1996) and Tanzania (Alonso,

1998) demonstrated moderate efficacy in adults and children aged 1–5 years of age. More recently, trials in The Gambia (6–12-month-olds) (d'Alessandro *et al.*, 1995), Thailand (2–15-year-olds) (Nosten *et al.*, 1996), Tanzania (infants) (Acosta *et al.*, 1999) and Brazil (7–70-year-olds) (Urdaneta *et al.*, 1998) have shown no significant efficacy.

In Australia and Papua New Guinea, trials have been conducted with vaccines containing purified recombinant proteins based on three blood-stage *P. falciparum* proteins (a fragment of MSP-1, MSP-2 and a portion of RESA [ring-infected erythrocyte surface antigen]) formulated in the adjuvant Montanide ISA 720, demonstrating induction of both T-cell and antibody responses (Saul *et al.*, 1999; Lawrence *et al.*, 2000). A field trial in 5–9-year-olds has shown promising results. The first phase I trial with the apical membrane antigen-1 (AMA-1) was initiated by this group. Another group, the National Institutes of Allergy and Infectious Diseases (NIAID) Malaria Vaccine Development Unit (MVDU), is hoping to start phase I clinical trials with PfAMA-1 recombinant vaccine in 2002.

A phase I dose-escalation trial of a purified recombinant PfMSP-1 has been conducted by WRAIR, with phase IIa testing continuing. The EMVI, together with investigators at the Institut Pasteur in Paris and the University of Lausanne, has initiated a phase I trial in Lausanne with an MSP-3 synthetic peptide,

with phase IIa testing tentatively planned for early in 2002. EMVI, in collaboration with Statens Serum Institut in Denmark, started a clinical trial in the Netherlands in September 2001 with a glutamate-rich protein (GLURP) synthetic peptide vaccine.

### SEXUAL STAGES

The NIAID MVDU is currently developing candidate transmission-blocking vaccines based on sexual stage antigens of *P. falciparum* and *P. vivax*, Pfs25 and Pvs25. Phase I clinical trials are expected to begin in 2002.

### Induction of immune responses to multiple antigens from different stages (DNA vaccines and prime-boost strategies).

### PRE-ERYTHROCYTIC STAGES

At the Naval Medical Research Center (NMRC), we have conducted two phase I safety and immunogenicity clinical trials of a PfCSP DNA vaccine. In both studies, the vaccine appeared to be safe and well tolerated and most of the volunteers developed antigen-specific, genetically restricted CD8+ cytotoxic lymphocytes (Wang *et al.*, 1998, 2001). In the second trial, comparing needle and needle-free Biojector® jet injection (Figure 13.6), antigen-specific CD8+

(a)

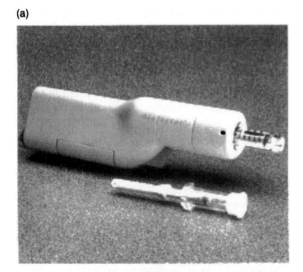

(b)

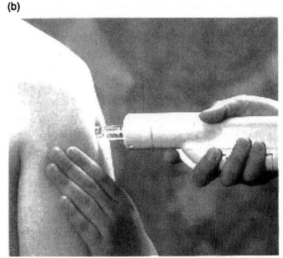

**Figure 13.6** (a) Needleless, single-use jet injection device, Biojector® 2000 used by Naval Medical Research Center to deliver PfCSP DNA vaccine. Biojector® uses compressed carbon dioxide as a safe power source. (b) Immunization using the device.

T-cell-dependent interferon-gamma (IFN-γ) responses were detected in all 14 volunteers, with the Biojector® intramuscular route appearing to be most immunogenic. In August 2000, we initiated a trial of a five-plasmid pre-erythrocytic stage DNA vaccine that includes genes encoding five proteins expressed by irradiated sporozoites in hepatocytes with a plasmid encoding human granulocyte–macrophage colony-stimulating factor (GM-CSF). This project, called MuStDO 5.1 (Multi-Stage Malaria DNA-based Vaccine Operation – 5 gene, iteration 1), is a collaboration among NMRC, Vical Inc., the United States Agency for International Development (USAID) and the Institut Pasteur in Paris.

At Oxford University, phase I/IIa trials were recently conducted with a *P. falciparum* pre-erythrocytic stage vaccine expressing multiple malaria CD8+ T-cell epitopes and the entire SSP2/TRAP antigen. Recipients received the priming doses of a DNA vaccine, delivered either by intramuscular needle or by Powderject gene gun, and booster doses of a recombinant attenuated vaccinia virus(MVA) expressing the same ME-TRAP insert delivered intradermally. This group has begun to test the DNA prime-MVA boost strategy in a field trial in The Gambia.

## COMBINED PRE-ERYTHROCYTIC AND ERYTHROCYTIC STAGE VACCINES

As mentioned above, the NMRC (in collaboration with multiple partners, including USAID, the Noguchi Memorial Institute of Medical Research in Accra, Ghana, and the Navrongo Health Research Center in Navrongo, Ghana) has been moving forward with a vaccine programme known as the Multi-Stage Malaria DNA Vaccine Operation (MuStDO). The cloning of the genes has taken place and the construction of plasmids will be done at NMRC, Monash University (Melbourne, Australia), and Entremed Inc. (Maryland, USA), with manufacturing at Vical Inc. (California, USA). The programme is based on the concept that an effective malaria vaccine will require a two-tiered immune response, the first tier attacking pre-erythrocytic stage parasites, and the second blood-stage parasites that break through the pre-erythrocytic defence. Thus, the final product would be a vaccine that incorporates both the type 1 and type 2 vaccines. The pre-erythrocytic component of the vaccine will be designed to induce antibodies that bind to the sporozoite surface before hepatocyte invasion

and, most importantly, CD8+ and CD4+ T cells that recognize parasite-derived peptides complexed with class I and class II HLA molecules, respectively, on the surface of infected hepatocytes. The hypothesis is that the pre-erythrocytic stage component will drastically reduce the number of parasites emerging from the liver. The erythrocytic component of the vaccine will be designed to prime the immune system to antigens from parasite proteins expressed on infected erythrocytes. These immune responses should limit replication of the parasite, thereby preventing severe disease and death in those experiencing breakthrough parasitaemia.

We are focusing on DNA vaccines as our core technology for this effort, because of their demonstrated ability to preferentially induce CD8+ T-cell and Th1-type immune responses, which has been difficult with the more traditional vaccines, and because of their simplicity of design and the ease with which they can be modified. As described above, the first trial of a five-gene pre-erythrocytic stage DNA vaccine, known as MuStDO 5.1, is in progress. This is an open-labelled, phase I/IIa trial of a vaccine incorporating five Pf pre-erythrocytic stage antigens (CSP, SSP2, Exp-1, LSA-1, LSA-3) along with escalating doses of the human GM-CSF plasmid, all administered by needle-free Biojector® injection. Depending upon the results of this trial, subsequent multivalent vaccines may supplement the five pre-erythrocytic stage antigens with four or more erythrocytic stage antigens. Eventually, the testing of DNA vaccines in healthy non-immune adults in the USA will be followed by testing in semi-immune adults in the region of Accra, Ghana, in collaboration with the Noguchi Institute of Medical Research, and finally in younger children and infants in highly endemic regions of northern Ghana in collaboration with the Navrongo Health Research Centre. The DNA plasmids used in future trials will differ from those used in the current MuStDO 5.1 trial in that *P. falciparum* gene inserts have been changed to synthetic genes with codon usage more similar to *Homo sapiens* than to *P. falciparum* (Kumar S, unpublished data).

However, DNA vaccines on their own do not induce an optimal immune response. Prime boost is dramatically more immunogenic and protective than DNA vaccination alone. Trials will soon be underway evaluating priming with DNA plasmids followed by boosting with the poxvirus construct encoding the same antigen and/or the homologous recombinant proteins.

## DUPLICATE WHOLE-ORGANISM-ELICITED IMMUNITY (UTILIZE MALARIA GENOME PROJECT)

This approach is based on the idea of duplicating immunity induced by exposure to the whole parasite (irradiated sporozoites or natural exposure). We have described an approach based on immune responses to one, two or three of the proteins encoded by the estimated 6000 genes in the *P. falciparum* genome, generally by a combination of recombinant protein or synthetic peptide and adjuvant. A second approach involves DNA-based immunization against 15 proteins, most of the known targets of protective immunity. Human models include immunization with the whole organism, either by natural exposure or by exposure to radiation-attenuated sporozoites. The strength of the immunity induced in these situations may be dependent on immune responses to hundreds or thousands of parasite proteins. The entire *P. falciparum* genome is being sequenced and the results of 6 per cent of the genome have been published (Gardner *et al.*, 1998; Bowman *et al.*, 1999). The complete sequence is expected by early 2002. Thousands of new proteins identified in this way will be assessed by applied genomics for potential inclusion in vaccines (Hoffman *et al.*, 1998; Carucci *et al.*, 2000; Hoffman, 2000). The integration of microbial and human genomics with molecular and cell biology, immunology and epidemiology in this century may provide many of the answers to the questions we have been struggling with for so long.

## The challenge of designing and executing field trials of malaria vaccines: research requirements

It will be critical to consider which outcome variables to measure in field trials of malaria vaccines, and which populations to study. A primary goal is to reduce mortality and severe disease. There is a potential problem that a vaccine may be discarded as a result of initial studies because the proper outcome variable(s) was not measured. It will be difficult to use severe disease and death as the primary outcome variables in initial studies, because of the very large sample sizes required. It is important to identify groups at highest risk so that sample sizes can be reduced. Some groups are working on identifying

surrogates of severe disease and death: parasitological, haematological, biochemical or clinical manifestations that are predictive of severe outcome.

Several other areas of field research could provide data to help vaccine development. The most important is the identification of target groups for vaccines in different areas (see above) and the exclusion of groups, like those with sickle-cell trait, who are at decreased risk and do not need to be immunized. It is important to determine if there are measurable outcome variables that have a high predictive value for severe disease and malaria-associated mortality. The impact of bed-nets and other interventions on epidemiology and the age-specific attributable reduction in mortality must be assessed. Better assays are needed for predicting protective immunity, involving more detailed characterization of the proteins and epitopes on these proteins involved in protective immunity. Epidemiological data will be more important in malaria vaccine development and the design of field trials than will acquisition of immunological data or the mapping of epitopes.

## PROSPECTS FOR MALARIA VACCINES

The human models (irradiated sporozoite and naturally acquired immunity) indicate that the development of a malaria vaccine is feasible. Genomics, proteomics, molecular biology, molecular immunology, vaccinology, population genetics, population biology and quantitative epidemiology have created great expectations for the development, licensing and deployment of effective malaria vaccines. It will be a formidable task to determine which antigens/epitopes from which stages of the life cycle are required for sustainable protection, how to measure immune responses that predict protection, which vaccine delivery systems are optimal, who and when in life to immunize, and what is the true impact of a malaria vaccine. However, we believe that the next 10–25 years will see the development of effective malaria vaccines, and that these will be used to control the effects of the disease worldwide and, when combined with other interventions, will be able to eradicate malaria from many areas.

The importance and difficulty of this task must not be underestimated. In 1962, malaria was an

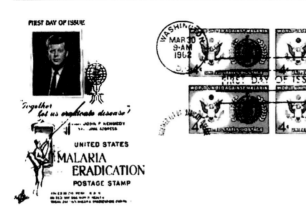

**Figure 13.7** 'Malaria Eradication Stamp', released in the USA in 1962.

important enough problem for the USA, along with many other countries, to release stamps commemorating attempts to eradicate malaria (Figure 13.7). That was at about the same time that President Kennedy vowed to put a man on the moon. The first man walked on the moon in 1969, but we are still far from eradicating malaria. We believe that the development of malaria vaccines will be crucial to realizing the dream of malaria eradication.

## REFERENCES

Acosta CJ, Galindo CM, Schellenberg D, *et al.* Evaluation of the SPf66 vaccine for malaria control when delivered through the EPI scheme in Tanzania. *Trop Med Int Health* 1999; **5**: 368–76.

Baird JK, Masbar S, Basri H, Tirtokusuomo S, Subianto B, Hoffman SL. Age-dependent susceptibility to severe disease with primary exposure to *Plasmodium falciparum. J Infect Dis* 1998; **178**: 592–5.

Baruch DI, Pasloke BL, Singh HB, *et al.* Cloning the *P. falciparum* gene encoding PfEMP1, a malarial variant antigen and adherence receptor on the surface of parasitized human erythrocytes. *Cell* 1995; **82**: 77–87.

Bojang K, Milligan PJM, Pinder M, *et al.* Randomized, double-blind controlled trial of efficacy of RTS,S/AS02 malaria vaccine against *Plasmodium falciparum* infection in semi-immune adult men in The Gambia. *The Lancet,* 2001, in press.

Bojang KA, Obaro SK, D'Alessandro U, *et al.* An efficacy trial of the malaria vaccine SPf66 in Gambian infants – second year of follow-up. *Vaccine* 1998; **16**(1): 62–7.

Bowman S, Lawson D, Basham D, *et al.* The complete nucleotide sequence of chromosome 3 of *Plasmodium falciparum. Nature* 1999; **400**: 532–8.

Brown GV, Rogerson SJ. Preventing cytoadherence of infected erythrocytes to endothelial cells and non-infected erythrocytes. In *Malaria vaccine development.* Hoffman SL, ed. Washington DC, ASM Press, 1996; 145–66.

Carucci DJ, Hoffman SL. The Malaria Genome Project: from sequence to functional. *Nat Med* Special Focus: Malaria; 2000; 6–8.

Clyde DF, Most H, McCarthy VC, Vanderberg JP. Immunization of man against sporozoite-induced falciparum malaria. *Am J Med Sci* 1973; **266**: 169–77.

D'Alessandro U, Leach A, Drakeley CJ, *et al.* Efficacy trial of malaria vaccine SPf66 in Gambian infants. *Lancet* 1995; **346**(8973): 462–7.

Doolan D, Hoffman SL. The complexity of protective immunity against liver-stage malaria. *J Immunol* 2000; **165**(3): 1453–62.

Egan JE, Hoffman SL, Haynes JD, *et al.* Humoral immune responses in volunteers immunized with irradiated *Plasmodium falciparum* sporozoites. *Am J Trop Med Hyg* 1993; **49**: 166–73.

Felger I, Irion A, Steiger S, Beck H-P. Epidemiology of multiple *Plasmodium falciparum* infections: 2. Genotypes of merozoite surface protein 2 of *Plasmodium falciparum* in Tanzania. *Trans R Soc Trop Med Hyg* 1999; **93**(Suppl. 1): S1/3–S1/9.

Galindo CM, Acosta CJ, Schellenberg D, *et al.* Humoral immune responses during a malaria vaccine trial in Tanzanian infants. *Parasite Immunol* 2000; **22**(9): 437–43.

Gardner MJ, Tettelin H, Carucci DJ, *et al.* Chromosome 2 sequence of the human malaria parasite *Plasmodium falciparum*. [Published erratum appears in *Science* 1998; **282**(5395): 1827.] *Science* 1998; **282**: 1126–32.

Gupta S, Snow RW, Donnelly CA, Marsh K, Newbold C. Immunity to non-cerebral severe malaria is acquired after one or two infections. *Nat Med* 1999; **5**: 340–3.

Herrington DA, Davis J, Nardin E, *et al*. Successful immunization of humans with irradiated sporozoites: humoral and cellular responses of the protected individuals. *Am J Trop Med Hyg* 1991; **45**: 539–47.

Hoffman SL. Infectious disease. Research (genomics) is crucial to attacking malaria. *Science* 2000; **290**: 1509.

Hoffman SL, Franke ED, Hollingdale MR, Druihle P. Attacking the infected hepatocyte. In *Malaria vaccine development*. Hoffman SL, ed. Washington DC, ASM Press, 1996, 15–34.

Hoffman SL, Oster CN, Plowe CV, *et al*. Naturally acquired antibodies to sporozoites do not prevent malaria: vaccine development implications. *Science* 1987; **237**: 639–42.

Hoffman SL, Rogers WO, Carucci DJ, Venter JC. From genomics to vaccines: malaria as a model system. *Nat Med* 1998; **4**: 1351–3.

Jones TR, Obaldia III N, Gramzinski RA, Hoffman SL. Repeated infection of *Aotus* monkeys with *Plasmodium falciparum* induces protection against subsequent challenge with homologous and heterologous strains of parasite. *Am J Trop Med Hyg* 2000; **62**: 675–80.

Kaslow DC. Transmission-blocking vaccines. *Malaria vaccine development*. Hoffman SL, ed. Washington DC, ASM Press, 1996; 181–228.

Kester KE, McKinney DA, Tornieporth N, *et al*. Efficacy of recombinant circumsporozoite protein vaccine regimens against experimental *Plasmodium falciparum* malaria. *J Infect Dis* 2001; **183**: 640–7.

Lawrence GW, Cheng Q, Reed C, *et al*. Effect of vaccination with 3 recombinant asexual-stage malaria antigens on initial growth rates of *Plasmodium falciparum* in non-immune volunteers. *Vaccine* 2000; **18**: 1925–31.

Lopez JA, Weilenmen C, Audran R, *et al*. A synthetic malaria vaccine elicits a potent CD8+ and CD4+ T lymphocyte immune response in humans. Implications for vaccine strategies. *Eur J Immunol* 2001; **31**: 1989–98.

Nardin EH, Calvo-Calle JM, Oliveira GA, *et al*. A totally synthetic polyoxime malaria vaccine containing *Plasmodium falciparum* B cell and universal T cell epitopes elicits immune responses in volunteers of diverse HLA types. *J Immunol* 2001; **166**(1): 481–9.

Nardin EH, Oliveira GA, Calvo-Calle JM, *et al*. Synthetic malaria peptide vaccine elicits high levels of anti-

bodies in vaccinees of defined HLA genotypes. *J Infect Dis* 2000; **182**(5): 1486–96.

Nosten F, Luxemburger C, Kyle DE, *et al*. Randomised double-blind placebo-controlled trial of SPf66 malaria vaccine in children in northwestern Thailand. *Lancet* 1996; **348**(9029): 701–7.

Rieckmann KH, Carson PE, Beaudoin RL, Cassells JS, Sell KW. Sporozoite induced immunity in man against an Ethiopian strain of *Plasmodium falciparum*. *Trans R Soc Trop Med Hyg* 1974; **68**: 258–9.

Saul A, Lawrence G, Smillie A, *et al*. Human phase I vaccine trials of 3 recombinant asexual stage malaria antigens with Montanide ISA720 adjuvant. *Vaccine* 1999; **17**(23–4): 3145–59.

Schofield LJ, Villaquiran J, Ferreira A, Schellekens RS, Nussenzweig RS, Nussenzweig V. Gamma-interferon, CD8+ T cells and antibodies required for immunity to malaria sporozoites. *Nature* 1987; **330**: 664–6.

Snow RW, Omumbo JA, Lowe B, *et al*. Relation between severe malaria morbidity in children and level of *Plasmodium falciparum* transmission in Africa. *Lancet* 1997; **349**: 1650–4.

Stoute JA, Kester KE, Krzych U, *et al*. Long-term efficacy and immune responses following immunization with the RTS,S malaria vaccine. *J Infect Dis* 1998; **178**: 1139–44.

Stoute JA, Slaoui M, Heppner DG, *et al*. A preliminary evaluation of a recombinant circumsporozoite protein vaccine against *Plasmodium falciparum* malaria. *N Engl J Med* 1997; **336**: 86–91.

Urdaneta M, Prata A, Struchiner CJ, Tosta CE, Tauil P, Boulos M. Evaluation of SPf66 malaria vaccine efficacy in Brazil. *Am J Trop Med Hyg* 1998; **58**(3): 378–85.

Valero MV, Amador R, Aponte JJ, *et al*. Evaluation of SPf66 malaria vaccine during a 22-month follow-up field trial in the Pacific coast of Colombia. *Vaccine* 1996; **14**(15): 1466–70.

Wang R, Doolan DL, Le TP, *et al*. Induction of antigen-specific cytotoxic T lymphocytes in humans by a malaria DNA vaccine. *Science* 1998; **282**: 476–80.

Wang R, Epstein J, Baraceros F, *et al*. Induction of CD4+ T cell-dependent CD8+ type 1 responses in humans by a malaria DNA vaccine. *Proc Natl Acad Sci USA* 2001; **98**: 10 817–22.

Weiss WR, Sedegah M, Beaudoin RL, Miller LH, Good MF. CD8+ T cells (cytotoxic/suppressors) are required for protection in mice immunized with malaria sporozoites. *Proc Natl Acad Sci USA* 1988; **85**: 573–6.

# Appendix: Characteristics of some major *Anopheles* vectors of human malaria[1]

MIKE W SERVICE

## 1. MALARIA VECTORS OF AFRICA SOUTH OF THE SAHARA

### *Anopheles gambiae* complex

This complex consists of seven very similar species, separated by banding patterns of their polytene chromosomes. They differ in certain aspects of their biology, behaviour, vector status and distribution.

#### ANOPHELES GAMBIAE

It is widespread in nearly all African countries south of the Sahara and is probably the world's most efficient malaria vector. Larvae occur mainly in temporary habitats such as pools, puddles, hoof prints, borrow pits, but also in rice fields. The adult bites humans both indoors and outdoors; in some areas, it also feeds on domestic animals. Adults rest predominantly indoors after feeding, but may rest outdoors.

Mainly after Service (2000).

#### ANOPHELES ARABIENSIS

It is also widespread in most African countries, but often prefers drier savannah areas. Larval habitats are the same as those of *A. gambiae*. Adults bite humans and animals, indoors and outdoors, and afterwards rest indoors or outdoors. This species usually has a greater tendency than *A. gambiae* to bite animals and rest outdoors. It is an important malaria vector, but not as efficient as *A. gambiae*.

#### ANOPHELES MELAS

A salt-water breeding species of the *gambiae* complex, it occurs along the coast of West Africa to Angola. It is very common in lagoons and mangrove swamps and does not breed in fresh water. Adults behave very similarly to *A. gambiae*. It is a malaria vector in many coastal areas.

#### ANOPHELES MERUS

The East African equivalent to *A. melas*, it breeds in salt-water lagoons and swamps along the coast of East

Africa. Occasionally, it is found in inland habitats such as in Tanzania, South Africa and Zimbabwe. The biting behaviour of adults is similar to that of *A. gambiae*, but it is often more exophilic. It is a vector in certain coastal areas.

### ANOPHELES QUADRIANNULATUS

It occurs in Ethiopia, Tanzania, Zimbabwe, Mozambique and southern Africa. It is not a malaria vector as it feeds mainly on cattle.

### ANOPHELES QUADRIANNULATUS SPECIES B

It is a newly described species that is very similar to *A. quadriannulatus*, but differs chromosomally. It is only known from Ethiopia. It is not a malaria vector.

### ANOPHELES BWAMBAE

It is known only from mineral springs in the Semliki forest of Uganda. It is a rare species and is not considered an important malaria vector, although it can transmit malaria within a very restricted area.

## Anopheles funestus

Widespread in Africa south of the Sahara, it is the most important vector after *A. gambiae* and *A. arabiensis*. Larvae occur in more or less permanent waters, especially with vegetation, such as swamps, marshes, edges of streams, rivers and ditches. It prefers shaded habitats. The adult bites humans predominantly, but also domestic animals. It feeds both indoors and outdoors, and after feeding rests mainly indoors.

## Other Anopheles

*Anopheles nili, A. moucheti, A. hargreavesi, A. hancocki* and *A. pharoensis* may also be malaria vectors of minor importance in certain localities.

## 2. MALARIA VECTORS OF EUROPE, NORTH AFRICA AND THE MIDDLE EAST

## Anopheles atroparvus

One of 11 species in the *A. maculipennis* complex, it is found in Europe, mainly in the coastal areas of the Netherlands, northern Germany, France, Portugal and in central Europe and north of the Caspian Sea, extending eastwards to Russia and Mongolia. Larvae are found in fresh or brackish marshes, lagoons and rice fields. The adult bites humans and domestic animals both inside and outside. During the winter, females enter partial hibernation, sheltering in houses and animal sheds, periodically emerging to bite people and livestock. There has been no malaria transmission since eradication in endemic areas, but potential capacity is present.

## Anopheles labranchiae

One of 11 species in the *A. maculipennis* complex, it is found in Italy, Sicily, Corsica, Sardinia to Morocco, Algeria and Tunisia, but is now a vector only in North Africa. It prefers brackish waters in coastal marshes, fresh waters of rice fields, marshes and edges of grassy streams and ditches, and prefers sunlight. The adult bites humans and also domestic animals indoors and outdoors, and rests mainly in houses or animal shelters after feeding. It overwinters as hibernating adults.

## Anopheles pharoensis

It is found in Egypt, Sudan, Saudi Arabia, Yemen and most of Africa south of the Sahara. It is a vector of importance in Egypt. It prefers marshes, swamps, rice fields and ponds, especially those with abundant grassy or floating vegetation. The adult bites humans and animals indoors and outdoors, and rests outdoors after feeding.

## Anopheles sacharovi

It is found in Italy, Greece, eastern Europe, Turkey, Syria, Jordan, Lebanon, Iran, Iraq and to central Russia; it is a malaria vector in Middle East countries. Larvae occur in fresh or brackish waters of coastal or inland marshes, pools and ponds, especially those with vegetation. They prefer sunlit habitats. The adult bites humans and animals indoors and outdoors, and usually rests in houses or animal shelters after feeding.

## Anopheles sergentii

It is found in Algeria, Tunisia, Egypt, Syria, Palestine, Saudi Arabia, Turkey, Afghanistan and Pakistan to north-west India. Larvae occur in rice fields, borrow pits, ditches, seepages, slow-flowing streams and sunlit or partially shaded habitats. The adult bites humans and animals indoors or outdoors, and rests in houses and caves after feeding.

## Anopheles stephensi

It is found in Egypt, Iraq, Iran, Saudi Arabia, Oman, Bahrain, Afghanistan, Pakistan, Sri Lanka, India, Myanmar, Thailand and China. It is an important vector over much of its range, especially in and around towns. It breeds in man-made habitats associated with towns, such as cisterns, wells, gutters, water-storage jars and containers, drains, fresh water or brackish waters, and even polluted waters, and in rural situations in grassy pools and alongside rivers. Adults bite humans indoors and outdoors and rest mainly indoors after feeding.

## Anopheles superpictus

It is found in the Mediterranean area, Iran, Iraq, Saudi Arabia, Palestine, Jordan, Turkey, Afghanistan and Pakistan. It prefers flowing waters such as torrents of shallow water over rocky streams, pools in rivers, muddy hill streams and where vegetation may be present. It prefers sunlight. The adult bites humans and animals indoors and outdoors, and after feeding rests mainly in houses and animal shelters, but also in caves.

## 3. MALARIA VECTORS OF THE INDIAN SUBCONTINENT AND PARTS OF SOUTH-EAST ASIA

## Anopheles culicifacies

It is found in Oman, Iran, Iraq, Bahrain, Afghanistan, Pakistan through India, Sri Lanka, Bangladesh, Myanmar, Thailand, Indonesia and southern China. It is probably the most important vector in much of Pakistan, India, Bangladesh and Sri Lanka. Larvae occur in a great variety of clean and polluted habitats, irrigation ditches, rice fields, swamp pools, wells, borrow pits, edges of streams, even occasionally brackish waters, and in sunlit or partially shaded habitats. The adult prefers domestic animals, but commonly bites humans indoors or outdoors, and rests mainly indoors after feeding.

## Anopheles dirus

There has been considerable confusion over the identities of this species and *A. balabacensis*, but the latter species has a more restricted distribution (see below). *A. dirus* is found in western India, Bangladesh, Thailand, southern China, Hainana Island, Vietnam, Laos, Myanmar, northern Malaysia, Sumatra and Java. Larvae colonize shaded pools and hoof prints in or at the edges of forests. Adults bite humans and domestic animals, mainly outdoors, and rest outdoors after feeding. It is basically a forest species.

## Anopheles flavirostris

It is found in the Philippines, Borneo and Java. Larvae occur in flowing waters, such as foothill streams, irrigation ditches, seepages and rice fields, preferring shaded to sunlit habitats. Adults bite mainly indoors, but sometimes outdoors, but rest mainly outdoors after feeding.

## Anopheles fluviatilis

It is found in Oman, Bahrain, Iran, Iraq, eastern Saudi Arabia, Pakistan, Afghanistan, India, Sri Lanka, Bangladesh, Myanmar, Thailand, Indonesia and Indochina. It is an important vector in Pakistan, India and Bangladesh. Larvae can occur in most flowing waters, such as hill streams, pools in riverbeds and irrigation ditches. They prefer sunlight. The adult bites humans and domestic animals indoors and outdoors, and rests both indoors and outdoors after feeding.

## Anopheles minimus

It is found in India, Sri Lanka, Myanmar, Malaysia, Thailand, Indochina, Taiwan, Sumatra, Java and the

Philippines to southern China. Larvae occur in flowing waters, such as foothill streams, springs, irrigation ditches, seepages, and also rice fields and borrow pits. They prefer shaded areas of sunlit habitats. Adults feed mainly on humans, but also domestic animals, mainly feeding and resting indoors.

## Anopheles stephensi (see Section 2)

## Anopheles sundaicus

It is found in India, Myanmar, Malaysia, Thailand, Indonesia, Java, Sumatra, Borneo, China and Indochina. Larvae occur in salt or brackish waters, lagoons, marshes, pools and seepages, especially with putrifying algae and aquatic weeds. It is mainly a coastal species, but is also found in fresh-water inland pools in Java and Sumatra. Larvae prefer sunlight. The adult bites humans and domestic animals indoors and outdoors, and rests mainly indoors after feeding.

## Anopheles superpictus (see Section 2)

## 4. MALARIA VECTORS OF SOUTH-EAST ASIA

## Anopheles aconitus

It is found in India, Sri Lanka, Malaysia, Indochina, Indonesia, Sumatra, Borneo and southern China. Larvae occur in rice fields, swamps, irrigation ditches, pools and streams with vegetation and prefer sunlit habitats. Adults feed indoors or outdoors on humans, but also commonly on animals; adults rest indoors or outdoors after feeding.

## Anopheles anthropophagus

This species occurs in Thailand, Malaysia, Borneo, Philippines, Korea and southern China to Japan. It is an important vector in the central plains and

eastern China. Larvae occur in cool, clean waters, including rice fields; some forms can occur in brackish water. Adults are mainly anthropophagic and endophilic, but will also bite cattle. Adults sometimes rest outdoors.

## Anopheles balabacensis

In the past, it was often confused with *A. dirus*. *A. balabacensis* is found in Sabah, Java, Borneo, Balbac Island and Palawan Island in the Philippines. Larvae are found in muddy and shaded forest pools, animal hoof prints and vehicle ruts. Adults bite humans and cattle, and rest outdoors. It is a forest species.

## Anopheles campestris

There has been considerable confusion over the identity of this species. It has sometimes been misidentified as *A. donaldi*, but more frequently as *A. barbirostris*. Many references in the literature refer to *A. barbirostris* as an important vector of both malaria and filariasis, but this species is predominantly zoophagic, although it bites humans in Timor and the Celebes, where it can be a malaria vector. Most references giving *A. barbirostris* as a vector refer in fact to *A. campestris*, a species found along the coasts and deltas of Malaysia and Thailand, and possibly in other mainland areas of South-east Asia, or to *A. donaldi*. Larvae of *A. campestris* are usually found in swamps or ponds having some vegetation. Partial shade is preferred. Larvae often accumulate in shaded corners of rice fields, and also ditches, earthern wells and sometimes in brackish waters. Adults bite humans and animals indoors and outdoors, with substantial numbers resting indoors after feeding.

## Anopheles culicifacies (see Section 3)

## Anopheles donaldi

In the past, has been confused with *A. campestris*. *A. donaldi* is found in Malaysia and Thailand

and possibly in Sumatra and Java. Larvae occur in shaded habitats such as tree-covered swamps, forest pools and rice fields. Adults bite livestock but also humans inside or outside houses, and rest mainly outdoors.

## Anopheles hyrcanus

This mosquito has been reported from Europe, the northern Mediterranean, North Africa, across central and northern Asia to Japan, but what was formerly considered a single species is now known to consist of a species group. Many records incriminating *A. hyrcanus* in the transmission of malaria refer to closely related species such as *A. anthropophagus*, *A. sinensis*. *A. hyrcanus* sensu stricto may be a vector in some areas.

## Anopheles letifer

It is found in Thailand, Malaysia, Philippines, Sumatra, Java and Borneo. This species is very similar to *A. umbrosus*, which has a similar distribution and has in the past been confused with it. *A. umbrosus*, however, is not, as formerly supposed, an important malaria vector because many sporozoites found in the salivary glands are of animal malarias. *A. letifer* bites humans more often than *A. umbrosus*, but also commonly feeds on animals; it seems to be a malaria vector in certain areas. Larvae are often found in stagnant waters, especially on coastal plains, such as pools, swamps and ponds. They prefer shade. Adults bite animals and humans mainly outdoors, and rest outdoors after feeding.

## Anopheles leucosphyrus

There has been confusion concerning the identity of three very similar species, namely, *A. leucosphyrus*, *A. balabacensis* and *A. dirus*. *A. leucosphyrus* occurs in Indonesia, Sumatra, Malaysia and Sarawak. Larvae commonly occur in clear seepage pools in forests. Adults bite humans inside or outside houses, but afterwards rest outdoors. It is a vector in Sumatra and Sarawak and possibly elsewhere.

## Anopheles maculatus

One of eight species in the *A. maculatus* complex, it is found in India, Malaysia, Indonesia, Indochina, Borneo, Philippines, Sumatra, Java and southern China. It occurs in or near hilly areas, in seepage waters, pools formed in streams, edges of ponds, ditches and rice fields, and prefers sunlight. Adults bite domestic animals and also humans indoors and outdoors, and rest mainly outdoors after feeding.

## Anopheles minimus (see Section 3)

## Anopheles nigerrimus

It is found in India, Sri Lanka, Myanmar, Thailand, Malaysia, Indochina, Borneo and China. Larvae like deep ponds, rice fields, irrigation ditches and swamps with much vegetation, and prefer sunlight. Adults bite humans and animals mainly outdoors, and rest mainly outdoors after feeding.

## Anopheles sinensis

In the past often confused with *A. anthropophagus*, *A. sinensis* occurs in the plains of China, where it is probably the only vector north of 34°N. Larvae are very common in rice fields, and also in marshes, ditches and grassy ponds. Adults bite cattle but also humans, feeding indoors or outdoors, but are sometimes found in houses.

## Anopheles subpictus

It is found in Iran, Pakistan, India, Sri Lanka, Myanmar, Malaysia, Thailand, Indochina, China, Papua New Guinea, Java and Sulawesi. It may be an important malaria vector in Sulawesi, Java and Indochina. Larvae occur in muddy pools near houses, gutters, borrow-pits and also in brackish waters. Adults mainly bite animals, but also humans indoors and outdoors, and rest indoors and outdoors after feeding.

*Anopheles sundaicus* (see Section 3)

# 5. MALARIA VECTORS OF MEXICO AND CENTRAL AMERICA

## *Anopheles albimanus*

It is found in Texas and Florida in the USA, through Central America to Colombia, Ecuador, Venezuela and the Antilles. Larvae occur in fresh or brackish waters such as pools, puddles, marshes, ponds and lagoons, especially those containing floating or grassy vegetation, and prefer sunlight. Adults feed on humans and domestic animals, indoors and outdoors; after feeding they rest mainly outdoors. It is a very important malaria vector in Mexico and Central America.

## *Anopheles albitarsis*

It is found in Central America to South America and Trinidad. Larvae nearly always occur in sunlit ponds, large pools and marshes with filamentous algae. Adults bite almost indiscriminately humans and domestic animals, outdoors and also indoors, and usually rest outdoors after feeding.

## *Anopheles aquasalis*

It is found in the Lesser Antilles, Trinidad, Tobago and other nearby islands, Central America to northern parts of Brazil. Larvae occur in tidal salt-water marshes, lagoons, salt-water regions of rivers and estuaries, rarely in fresh water. They occur in sunlit or shaded habitats. Adults bite humans and domestic animals, indoors and outdoors, and rest mainly outdoors.

## *Anopheles darlingi*

It is found in Mexico through Central America to Argentina and Chile. Larvae occur in fresh-water marshes, lagoons, rice fields, swamps, lakes and ponds, pools and edges of streams, especially with vegetation, and prefer shaded habitats. Adults feed mainly on humans indoors, and remain indoors after feeding.

## *Anopheles punctimacula*

It is found in Mexico through Central America to Peru, Brazil, Argentina and Trinidad. Larvae occur in small pools, swamps, grassy pools at edges of streams, and prefer shade. Adults bite humans and domestic animals, indoors and outdoors, and rest indoors or outdoors after feeding.

# 6. MALARIA VECTORS OF SOUTH AMERICA

## *Anopheles albimanus* (see Section 5)

## *Anopheles albitarsis* (see Section 5)

## *Anopheles aquasalis* (see Section 5)

## *Anopheles bellator*

It is found in Trinidad, Venezuela, Surinam, Guyana and Brazil. Larvae occur only in water collected in leaf axils of bromeliads, which are epiphytes of trees; they prefer partially shaded habitats. Adults bite humans during the daytime in shaded forests, as well as at night, and may enter houses to feed; they usually rest indoors after feeding. Although humans are the favoured host, domestic animals are also attacked.

## *Anopheles cruzii*

It is found in Costa Rica, Panama, Ecuador, Bolivia, Colombia, Peru, Brazil and Venezuela. Larvae occur in water collected in leaf axils of bromeliads, and partial shade is preferred. Adults bite humans indoors and outdoors, and after feeding rest indoors and outdoors. Its main importance is as a malaria vector in coastal areas of Brazil.

## *Anopheles darlingi* (see Section 5)

## *Anopheles nuneztovari*

It is found in Guyana, Venezuela, Colombia, Brazil and Bolivia. Larvae occur in muddy waters of pools, vehicle tracks, hoof prints and small ponds, especially in and around towns, and prefer sunlight. Adults mainly feed on animals, but also bite humans outdoors; they rest outdoors after feeding. It is an important vector in Colombia and Venezuela.

## Anopheles pseudopunctipennis

It is found in the Antilles, southern USA to Argentina. Larvae occur in pools, puddles, seepage waters and edges of streams, especially habitats with algae, and prefer sunlight. Adults feed almost indiscriminately on humans and domestic animals, indoors or outdoors, and rest outdoors after feeding.

## Anopheles punctimacula (see Section 5)

## 7. MALARIA VECTORS OF AUSTRALASIA

## Anopheles farauti

One of seven species in the A. farauti complex, it is found in Moluccas, Papua New Guinea, Solomon Islands, New Hebrides to northern Australia. Larvae usually occur in semi-permanent waters such as swamps, ponds and the edges of slow-flowing streams, but also in puddles, hoof prints, wells, water-storage pots and other man-made containers; water may be polluted, fresh or brackish, sunlit or shaded. Adults bite animals but also humans, indoors or outdoors; they rest mainly outside, but occasionally in houses.

## Anopheles koliensis

Found in Papua New Guinea and the Solomon Islands. Larvae found in marshy pools, irrigation

ditches and pools alongside forest streams. Adults bite humans and, more occasionally, animals; after feeding they rest indoors or outdoors.

## Anopheles punctulatus

One of a species complex of two species comprising A. koliensis and several sibling species of A. farauti. Found in Papua New Guinea, Solomon Islands and Moluccas. Larvae occur in swamps, muddy pools, hoof prints and edges of streams. Adults bite humans in preference to animals, either indoors or outdoors; they often rest indoors after feeding.

## NOTE

1. This tabulation of main larval habitats and feeding/resting behaviour of adults of some of the more important malaria vectors cannot indicate all the countries in which these occur. Moreover, their importance as vectors and their behaviour may differ in some areas of their distribution. As stressed by Service (2000), such notes are merely a guide. For greater detail of the behaviour and importance of Anopheles as malaria vectors in different countries, other reference works and books should he consulted.

## REFERENCE

Service MW. Medical entomology for students. Cambridge, Cambridge University Press, 2000.

# Index